SALEM HEALTH
GENETICS
& INHERITED CONDITIONS

Second Edition

SALEM HEALTH
GENETICS
& INHERITED CONDITIONS
Second Edition

Edited by Gary M. Flashner, M.D. and Deanna M. Neff, MPH

Volume 3

P–Z

First Edition edited by Jeffrey A. Knight, Ph.D.

SALEM PRESS
A Division of EBSCO Information Services, Inc.
Ipswich, Massachusetts
GREY HOUSE PUBLISHING

Publisher's Cataloging-In-Publication Data
(Prepared by The Donohue Group, Inc.)

Names: Flashner, Gary M., editor. | Neff, Deanna M., editor.

Title: Genetics & inherited conditions / editors, Gary M. Flashner, M.D., Deanna M. Neff, MPH.

Other Titles: Genetics and inherited conditions | Salem health | Salem health (Pasadena, Calif.)

Description: Second edition. | Ipswich, Massachusetts : Salem Press, a division of EBSCO Information Services, Inc. ; [Amenia, New York] : Grey House Publishing, [2017] | Includes bibliographical references and indexes. | Contents: Volume I. Aarskog syndrome - Friedreich ataxia -- Volume II. Galactokinase deficiency - Ovarian cancer -- Volume III. Palmoplantar keratoderma - Zellweger syndrome.

Identifiers: ISBN 9781682176030 (set) | ISBN 9781682178836 (v.1) | ISBN 9781682178843 (v.2) | ISBN 9781682178850 (v.3)

Subjects: LCSH: Genetic disorders--Encyclopedias. | Genetics--Encyclopedias.

Classification: LCC RB155.5 .G4616 2017 | DDC 616/.042--dc23

Contents

Complete List of Contents

Volume 1

Volume 2

Volume 3

SALEM HEALTH
GENETICS
& INHERITED CONDITIONS

Second Edition

P

Palmoplantar keratoderma

CATEGORY: Palmoplantar keratoderma (PPK) is a generic term for an heterogenous group of mostly hereditary disorders characterized by unusual thickening of the skin in soles of the feet and palms of the hands. Excessive or abnormal keratin production leads to hypertrophy of the stratum corneum (hyperkeratosis of the top layer of the skin). Their initial classification is based on whether they are inherited (congenital) or acquired. Hereditary variants result from several gene abnormalities that cause abnormal skin protein.

ALSO KNOWN AS: PPK; keratosis palmaris et plantaris; Palmoplantar keratosis; Hyperkeratosis of palms and soles; palmar plantar keratodermas.

DEFINITION

Palmoplantar keratoderma (PPK) is a generic term for an heterogenous group of mostly hereditary disorders characterized by unusual thickening of the skin in soles of the feet and palms of the hands. Excessive or abnormal keratin production leads to hypertrophy of the stratum corneum (hyperkeratosis of the top layer of the skin). Their initial classification is based on whether they are inherited (congenital) or acquired. Hereditary variants result from several gene abnormalities that cause abnormal skin protein.

RISK FACTORS

Hereditary predisposition is associated with the genetic PPK forms. Therefore, familial association is a common risk factor for patients. Mutations in up to sixteen different chromosomes have been identified as responsible for the inherited variants of PPK in an autosomal dominant or recessive manner. In certain populations, it is common to see a higher frequency of a particular inherited skin disorder, as seen with Naxos disease (the Greek island of Naxos), diffuse PPK (Norrbotten, Sweden), or Mal de Meleda (the island of Meleda, Yugoslavia).

ETIOLOGY AND GENETICS

Keratin is a tough fibrous structural protein and a component of the top layer of the skin, the epidermis. The keratinocyte is the epidermal cell that produces keratin. The normal keratinized skin provides waterproofing and works as a natural barrier to infection or harmful chemicals. Keratoderma is a disease of the skin marked by overgrowth of horny tissue or keratosis. In hyperkeratosis, there is an excess of keratin production in the skin.

Although PPK can manifest itself as an acquired condition, in the inherited form it is frequently present as the result of various genetic mutations. In the acquired type, the condition is not the result of genetic abnormalities and appears because of a shift in the patient's health or environmental factors. The most evident causes in the acquired variants are mechanical, vascular, endocrine, infective, or drug-induced.

The genetic PPK disorders are inherited from one or both parent(s) by their children. Generally, PPKs result from genetic abnormalities that affect the keratin protein expression, causing atypical thickening of the skin. Inheritance may occur either by an autosomal dominant or autosomal recessive pattern. In autosomal dominant keratodermas, each affected patient has at least one parent phenotypically affected and there is a transmission of the gene defect from generation to generation. There is a 50 percent chance that each offspring will be affected. For the autosomal recessive form, the affected patient has phenotypical unaffected parents and there is no transmission of the abnormal gene from generation to generation. People that carry the abnormal gene are referred to as carriers of the disease. Therefore, the carriers pass on the genetic defect to the next generation, but the children can only exhibit the disease if their other parent also is a carrier of the same abnormal gene and successfully passes it forward.

There is a 25 percent chance that each offspring will be affected by the autosomal recessive disorder. Recessive disorders are frequently found in families with increased consanguinity (descendent from a common ancestor).

More than eighty PPK disorders are indexed in the Online Mendelian Inheritance in Man (OMIM) catalog. These mutated genes code for structural skin proteins such as keratins or subcellular structures such as desmosomes. Additional mutations affect protein products related to keratinocyte cytoskeleton structure, cell-to-cell adhesion, connexins, and gap junctions. The physiologic role of other molecules related to PPK pathogenesis is not well understood. What is known is that all these affected protein structures interact in a highly regulated and integrated manner to keep epithelia and skin integrity. Keratin gene mutations are responsible for several types of hereditary PPK. Some of the main PPKs, with their corresponding protein product of its mutated gene in parenthesis, are Mal de Meleda (SLURP-1), Thost-Unna keratoderma (keratin-1), Vörner keratoderma (keratin-1 and 9), Vohwinkel mutilating keratoderma (Loricrin and Connexin-26), Papillon-Lefévre syndrome (Cathepsin C), Carrajo syndrome (Desmoplakin), Naxos disease (Plakoglobin), and Richner-Hanhart syndrome (tyrosine amino transferase).

When these PPK mutations alter the normal skin surface functions, the epidermal protective properties are compromised, giving the chance for bacterial and fungal infections, inflammatory skin reactions (eczema or psoriasis), or other severe conditions to arise that have an impact on quality of life or might worsen morbidity and mortality for the affected patient.

Only one pertinent PPK clinical study is listed and completed in ClinicalTrials.gov, and none are ongoing.

SYMPTOMS

In this cutaneous hereditary disorder, there is marked hyperkeratosis present over the palms and the soles of the patient. The three main clinical patterns of epidermal involvement are diffuse, focal, and punctate. In the diffuse form there is uniform hyperkeratosis of the palmoplantar surface. The focal pattern mainly affects pressure points or sites of constant friction. The punctate pattern consists of multiple, hyperkeratotic nodules or tiny bumps on the palms and soles. Generally, the abnormal thickening of the skin is seen only on the surface of the palms and soles (nontransgradient), but sometimes there is transmigration to close areas outside the palmoplantar surface (transgradient). The understanding of the pathogenesis is critical in narrowing down the target genes for each individual case. More apparent symptoms could be present such as knuckle pads, oral lesions, atrophy, blisters, deafness, mental retardation, starfish keratoses, nail changes, constricting bands, redness, malignancies, cardiomyopathies, or sclerodactyly. For some rare PPK types, organs in the body may be implicated so the keratoderma could be a marker of some internal abnormality.

SCREENING AND DIAGNOSIS

The rare and large group of hyperkeratotic disorders that inherited PPKs comprise are phenotypically characterized as extensively heterogeneous. Overcoming the diagnostic challenges posed by phenotypic and genotypic heterogeneity, several classification strategies have been designed using morphology, associated symptoms, distribution, and inheritance mode to improve screening between different genetic variants. Traditionally, diagnosis has been clinically based, but in recent years the molecular genetic classification is slowly being adopted and replacing the historical descriptive system. Clinical reference laboratories for genetic diagnostics are available, and information can be found through OMIM. Screening includes evaluation of the main genetic mutations that affect protein products associated to keratinocyte cytoskeleton structure, gap junctions, connexins, keratins, and subcellular structures such as desmosomes. Differential diagnosis might include blood tests, skin biopsy, histology, PCR, and mutation, microsatellite, and haplotype analysis. Knowledge of genetic mutations. associated with distinct clinical findings together with a systematic and comprehensive analysis makes the exact diagnosis possible by their molecular pathology. This integrative approach leads to the discovery of the real underlying genetic defect. A full personal and family history, regular medical examinations, and appropriate cancer screenings are crucial for early detection of any associated internal malignancies or cardiomyophathies for some of these patients or whether other skin findings are evident and/or other organs are affected. Dermatopathology plays in increasing role in the diagnosis.

TREATMENT AND THERAPY

Currently, there is no effective treatment for any PPK types. Common therapy alternatives mainly cause short-term improvements that are often aggravated by unacceptable adverse side effects. Treatment is tailored to the severity of the symptoms, the age of the patient, the affected areas, and the degree of hyperkeratosis. Generally, treatment will either focus on softening the thickened skin or making it less noticeable. Therapies may range from saltwater soaks and paring to emollients, topical keratolytics, topical or systemic retinoids, topical vitamin D ointment, potent topical steroids, careful footwear selection, or even reconstructive surgery in severe cases to excise the hyperkeratotoic skin, followed by grafting. When the PPK syndrome is also showcased as an associated feature with other diseases (such as deafness, corneal dystrophy, internal malignancy, cardiomyopathy, alopecia, and severe periodontitis), treatment and therapy are particularly adapted to the special needs of each case. Future studies on genotype/phenotype correlations in PPK and their treatment response are vital to improve the patient's quality of life. Palmoplantar keratoderma.

PREVENTION AND OUTCOMES

Since genetic factors play an important role in PPK inherited disorders and there is no effective way of prevention, genetic counseling should be provided. Disease management is difficult considering there is no effective treatment for any PPK variants. Early diagnosis is essential for disease management purposes, to mitigate some symptoms, and to define possible outcomes. The PPK inherited variant and the severity of the condition defines disease outcome. Outcome strategies for PPK with associated diseases, as with cardiomyopathies, internal malignancies, and systemic conditions, add another layer of variability, complexity, and challenge to disease management.

FURTHER READING

Bergman, Reuven. "Dermatopathology and Molecular Genetics." *Journal of the American Academy of Dermatology* 58, no. 3 (2008): 452-457.

Itin, Peter H., and Stephen Lautenschlager. "Palmoplantar Keratoderma and Associated Syndromes." *Seminars in Dermatology* 14, no. 2 (1995): 152-161.

Kimyai-Asadi, A., L. B. Kotcher, and M. H. Jih. "The Molecular Basis of Hereditary Palmoplantar Keratodermas." *Journal of the American Academy of Dermatology* 47, no. 3 (September, 2002): 327-343.

Lucker, G. P., P. C. Van de Kerkhof, and P. M. Steijlen. "The Hereditary Palmoplantar Keratoses: An Updated Review and Classification." *British Journal of Dermatology* 131, no. 1 (July, 1994): 1-14.

Torres, Gisela, et al. "'I Forgot to Shave My Hands': A Case of Spiny Keratoderma." *Journal of the American Academy of Dermatology* 58, no. 2 (2008): 344-348.

See also: Albinism; Chediak-Higashi syndrome; Epidermolytic hyperkeratosis; Hermansky-Pudlak syndrome; Ichthyosis; Melanoma.

Pancreatic cancer and genetics

CATEGORY: Diseases and syndromes
ALSO KNOWN AS: Cancer of the pancreas

DEFINITION

Pancreatic cancer is the growth of cancer cells in the pancreas. The pancreas is a long, flattened pear-shaped organ in the abdomen. It makes digestive enzymes and hormones, including insulin.

Cancer occurs when cells in the body divide with out of control order. If cells keep dividing uncontrollably, a mass of tissue forms. This is called a growth or tumor. The term "cancer" refers to malignant tumors. They can invade nearby tissue and spread to other parts of the body.

Pancreatic cancer is the fourth leading cause of cancer deaths, being responsible for 7% of all cancer-related deaths in both men and women. There are two main types:

1. Exocrine pancreatic cancer. Most of the cells of the pancreas are of the "exocrine" type. These cells make pancreatic enzymes that are released into the intestines to help with digestion of food.
2. Pancreatic endocrine tumors (also called neuroendocrine or islet cell tumors). These are

Pancreatic Cancer By Unknown photographer, via Wikimedia Commons

Cross section of a human liver, taken at autopsy examination, showing multiple large pale tumor deposits. The tumor is an adenocarcinoma derived from a primary lesion in the body of the pancreas. By Haymanj (Own work (photo by author)), via Wikimedia Commons

much less common (accounting for about 5% of all pancreatic cancers) and involve pancreatic cells that produce various hormones. There are many subtypes of these uncommon tumors (which may be benign or cancerous) categorized based on the type of hormone produced. Steve Jobs, former CEO of Apple, Inc was a victim of a pancreatic neuroendocrine cancer.

Risk Factors

Age is certainly a risk factor for developing pancreatic cancer. Almost all patients are older than age 45. Men and African-Americans are slightly more at risk than women and other races. Other risk factors include smoking and using smokeless tobacco, such as chewing tobacco; having diabetes; having chronic pancreatitis, cirrhosis of the liver, and workplace exposure to certain chemicals used in the dry cleaning and metal working industries. There may also be an increased risk in those with stomach ulcer problems.

Inherited gene mutations may cause as many as 10% of all pancreatic cancers. Sometimes these changes result in syndromes that include increased risks for developing pancreatic cancer as well as other cancers. A few examples of these syndromes are: hereditary pancreatitis, or familial nonpolyposis colon cancer syndrome; having a family or personal history of certain types of colon polyps or colon cancer; having a family history of pancreatic cancer, especially in Ashkenazi Jews with the *BRCA2* (breast cancer as sociated) gene. Others are described in the Etiology and Genetics section that follows.

ETIOLOGY AND GENETICS

While there is a substantial genetic component to the development of pancreatic cancer, the majority of new cases of the disease occur in families where there is no previous family history. Several genes, however, have been identified that are associated with an increased risk of pancreatic cancer. For ex ample, mutations in the *PRSS1* gene, found on the long arm of chromosome 7 at position 7q35, can cause hereditary pancreatitis, a condition that involves inflammation and swelling of the pancreas and severe abdominal pain. Affected individuals also have about a 40 percent risk of developing pancreatic cancer at some point in their adult years.

Most other cases of inherited pancreatic cancer result from mutations in any of several genes called tumor-suppressor genes, and these mutations can be inherited from either the male or female parent. Tumor-suppressor genes encode proteins that normally function in a variety of ways to limit or prevent cell growth and division. Mutations in these genes can lead to a loss in the ability to restrict tumor formation due to uncontrolled cell growth. When mutations occur in tumor-suppressor genes, it is not unusual to find that there is an in-creased risk for several different types of cancer to develop.

Peutz-Jeghers syndrome (PJS) is a rare condition in which affected individuals have multiple polyps in the digestive tract. People with PJS have about a 35 percent risk of developing pancreatic cancer, as well as an increased risk for skin, uterine, ovarian, breast, and lung cancers. Mutations in a single gene called *STK11* (at position 19p13.3) are responsible for this condition.

The two genes most commonly associated with an increased risk of breast and ovarian cancer are *BRCA1*, found on the long arm of chromosome 17 at position 17q21, and *BRCA2* (at position 13q12.3), yet mutations in these same two genes have also been linked to an increased risk of pancreatic cancer—about ten times greater than the average risk. These mutations are inherited in an autosomal dominant fashion, meaning that a single copy of the mutation is sufficient to cause the increased cancer risk. An affected individual has a 50 percent chance of transmitting the mutation to each of his or her children.

Individuals carrying a mutation that predisposes them to familial nonpolyposis colon cancer syndrome (Lynch syndrome) have been shown to have about an 8 to 10 percent risk of developing pancrea tic cancer, as well as a 20 to 50 percent risk of devel oping uterine cancer and a 10 percent increased risk for ovarian cancer. Four different genes have been identified in which such mutations might occur: *MLH1* (at position 3p21.3), *MSH2* (at position 2p22-p21), *MSH6* (at position 2p16), and *PMS2* (at position 7p22).

Finally, there is a condition known as familial atypical multiple mole melanoma and pancreatic cancer (FAMMM-PC), which is associated with mu tations in the *CDKN2A* gene (at position 9p21). Af fected individuals have a 15 to 17 percent risk of de veloping pancreatic cancer and as much as a 70 percent risk of developing melanoma skin cancer.

SYMPTOMS

Pancreatic cancer does not cause symptoms in its early stages. The cancer may grow for some time be fore it causes symptoms. When symptoms do appear, they may be very vague. In up to 80% of cases, the cancer has spread outside the pancreas by the time it is discovered.

Symptoms will vary depending on the location, size, and the type of tumor. More common exocrine cancers may have different symptoms compared to neuroendocrine cancers.

Symptoms of exocrine tumors may include nausea; loss of appetite; unexplained weight loss; pain in the upper abdomen, sometimes spreading to the back (a result of the cancer growing and spreading);

jaundice—yellowness of skin and whites of the eyes; dark urine (if the tumor blocks the common bile duct); tan stool or stool that floats to the top of the bowl; and weakness, dizziness, chills, muscle spasms, and diarrhea (especially if the cancer involves the is let cells that make insulin and other hormones).

Pancreatic neuroendocrine tumors release excess hormones into the bloodstream. Different types of tumors make different hormones, which can lead to different symptoms. A few of the many types are:

1. Gastrinomas. These tumors make gastrin, a hormone that tells the stomach to make more acid. This leads to stomach ulcers, which can cause pain, nausea, and loss of appetite. Severe ulcers can start bleeding. If the bleeding is mild, it can lead to anemia (too few red blood cells), which can cause symptoms like feeling tired and being short of breath. If the bleeding is more severe, it can cause stool to be black and tarry. Severe bleeding can itself be life-threatening. If the excess stomach acid reaches the intestines, it can also cause diarrhea and weight loss.

2. Glucagonomas. These tumors make glucagon, a hormone that increases glucose (sugar) levels in the blood. Excess glucagon can sometimes lead to the development of diabetes. This can cause symptoms such as feeling thirsty and hungry, and having to urinate often.

   People with these tumors can also have problems with diarrhea, weight loss, and malnutrition. The nutrition problems can lead to symptoms like irritation of the tongue and the corners of the mouth.

   The symptom that brings most people with glucagonomas to their doctor is a rash called *necrolytic migratory erythema*. This is a red rash with swelling and blisters that often travels from place to place on the skin.

3. Insulinomas. These tumors make insulin, which lowers blood glucose levels. Too much insulin leads to low blood sugar, which can cause symptoms like weakness, confusion, sweating, and rapid heartbeat. When blood sugar gets very low, it can lead to a person passing out or even going into a coma and having seizures.

All of these symptoms may also be caused by other, less serious and common health conditions. Anyone experiencing these symptoms should see a doctor.

SCREENING AND DIAGNOSIS

The doctor may ask about a patient's symptoms and medical history, and a physical exam may be done. The doctor may order blood and urine tests and may also check for hidden blood in bowel movements.

Tests may include an upper GI (gastrointestinal) series, a series of X rays of the upper digestive sys tem taken after drinking a barium solution; a com puted tomography (CT) scan, a type of X ray that uses a computer to make pictures of structures in side the abdomen; a magnetic resonance imaging (MRI) scan, a test that uses magnetic waves to make pictures of structures inside the abdomen; and ultrasonography, a test that uses sound waves to find tumors. Other tests may include an endoscopic ret rograde cholangiopancreatography (ERCP), a type of X ray that shows the pancreatic ductal system af ter dye has been sent through a tube down the throat and into the pancreas; percutaneous transhepatic chol angiography (PTC), a type of X ray test that shows blockages in the bile ducts of the liver; angiography, X rays of blood vessels taken af ter an injection of dye that makes the blood vessels show up on the X rays; a positron emission tomography (PET) scan which can help determine cancer activity in organs other than the pancreas: and a biopsy, the removal of a sample of pancreatic tissue to test for cancer cells.

If there is concern about the presence of a neu roendocrine tumor, a somatostatin receptor scintigraphy (SRS) scan may be recommended. If such a tumor is present, this scan can help with both diagnosis and treatment.

Blood tests that may be recommended can vary considerably depending on the type of tumor that is suspected.

TREATMENT AND THERAPY

Once cancer of the pancreas is found, staging is performed in order to plan appropriate treatments.

A staging system is a standard way for doctors to sum up how large a cancer is and how far it has spread. The system used most often is based on 3 key pieces of information:

- **T** describes the size of the main (primary) **tumor** and whether it has grown outside the pancreas and into nearby organs.
- **N** describes the spread to nearby (regional) lymph **nodes**, which are bean-sized collections of immune system cells to which cancers often spread first.

- **M** indicates whether the cancer has **metastasized** (spread) to other organs of the body. (The most common sites of pancreatic cancer spread are the liver, lungs, and the peritoneum, which is the lining that covers the organs in the abdomen.)

Treatments for pancreatic cancer depend on the stage of the cancer.

Treatments include surgery to remove the can cerous tumor and nearby tissue. Nearby lymph nodes may also need to be removed. Surgery may also be performed to relieve symptoms of pancreatic cancer. Surgeries include the Whipple procedure, which is the removal of the head of the pancreas, part of the small intestine, and some of the tissues around it; a total pancreatectomy, which is the removal of the whole pancreas, part of the small intestine, part of the stomach, the bile duct, the gall bladder, the spleen, and most of the lymph nodes in the area; and a distal pancreatectomy, which is the removal of the body and tail of the pancreas. After surgery, follow-up chemotherapy and radiation therapy may be helpful to prolong survival in some cases.

Radiation therapy (radiotherapy) uses radiation to kill cancer cells and shrink tumors. In external radiation therapy, radiation is directed at the tumor from a source outside the body; in internal radiation therapy, radioactive materials are placed into the body in or near the cancer cells.

Chemotherapy is the use of drugs to kill cancer cells. It may be given in many forms, including pill, injection, and via a catheter. The drugs enter the bloodstream and travel through the body, killing mostly cancer cells. Some healthy cells are also killed.

Biological therapy is the use of medications or substances made by the body in order to increase or restore the body's natural defenses against cancer. It is also called biologic response modifier (BRM) therapy.

Most times, pancreatic cancer is discovered at an advanced stage. Surgery may not be appropriate in these cases. If surgery cannot be done, then chemo therapy and radiation may be offered together to pro long sur vival.

PREVENTION AND OUTCOMES

There are no guidelines for preventing this dis ease; however, steps can be taken to decrease certain risks. Those steps include, but are not limited to, avoidance of all tobacco products; maintaining a healthy weight, limiting alcohol use, and avoiding exposure to workplace chemicals that are linked to pancreatic cancer. Individuals who think they are at risk for pan creatic cancer should talk to their doctors about ways to reduce their risk factors. Patients and doctors can work together to make an appropriate schedule for checkups.

Laurie LaRusso, M.S., ELS;
reviewed by Igor Puzanov, M.D.
"Etiology and Genetics" by Jeffrey A. Knight, Ph.D.;
updated by Gary M. Flashner, M.S., M.D.

FURTHER READING

Boffetta, P., et al. "Smokeless Tobacco and Cancer." *Lancet Oncology* 9, no. 7 (July, 2008): 667–675. Cameron, John L. *Pancreatic Cancer*. Hamilton, Ont.: B. C. Decker, 2001.

EBSCO Publishing. *Health Library: Pancreatic Cancer*. Ipswich, Mass.: Author, 2009. Available through http://www.ebscohost.com.

O'Reilly, Eileen, and Joanne Frankel Kelvin. *One Hundred Questions and Answers About Pancreatic Cancer*. 2d ed. Sudbur y, Mass.: Jones and Bartlett, 2010.

WEB SITES OF INTEREST

American Cancer Society
http://www.cancer.org

Canadian Cancer Society
http://www.cancer.ca

National Cancer Institute
https://www.cancer.org/cancer/pancreatic-cancer.html

Pancreatic Cancer Action Network
http://www.pancan.org
http://emedicine.medscape.com/article/280605-overview

See also: Cancer; Colon cancer; Hereditary diffuse gastric cancer; Hereditary leiomyomatosis and renal cell cancer; Hereditary mixed polyposis syndrome; Hereditary non-VHL clear cell renal cell carcinomas; Hereditary papillary renal cancer; Mutagenesis and cancer; Mutation and mutagenesis; Oncogenes; Ovarian cancer; Tumor-suppressor genes.

Parkinson disease and genetics

CATEGORY: Diseases and syndromes
ALSO KNOWN AS: Parkinson's disease; PD; paralysis agitans; shaking palsy

DEFINITION

Parkinson disease (PD) is one of the most progressive diseases of the nervous system and a movement disorder that causes muscle rigidity, tremor at rest, slowing down of movements (bradykinesia), difficulty moving, and gait instability. The disorder is caused by a loss of nerve cells in the brain, including loss in an area called the substantia nigra. This loss decreases the amount of dopamine in the brain. Low dopamine contributes to PD symptoms. More recent studies have shown that people with Parkinson disease also experience damage to the nerve endings that produce the neurotransmitter norepinephrine. This loss may explain some of the non-motor features seen in Parkinson disease, including fatigue and problems with blood pressure regulation.

RISK FACTORS

Individuals at increased risk for Parkinson dis ease include those who are age 60 or older, have family members with PD, and are nonsmokers. Men are somewhat more likely than women to develop PD. Other risk factors may include certain drugs and ongoing exposure to herbicides and pesticides Also, alterations in certain genes, including GBA and UCHL1, do not cause Parkinson disease but appear to modify the risk of developing the condition in some families.

ETIOLOGY AND GENETICS

The causes of Parkinson disease are complex and poorly understood, but it is clear that both genetic and environmental factors are involved. In about 85 percent of new cases, the disease appears in people with no family history of the disorder. In the re maining 15 percent of cases, mutations in any one of five different genes (*PARK2*, *PARK7*, *PINK1*, *LRRK2*, and *SNCA*) might be responsible.

The *PARK2* gene, found on chromosome 6 at po sition 6q25.2-q27, is a very large gene that specifies the protein called parkin. This protein is an impor tant component of a cellular system designed to rid the cell of damaged or excess proteins. Loss of par kin function because of a mutation in the gene

Parkinson's Disease. See a full animation of this medical topic By BruceBlaus (Own work), *via Wikimedia Commons*

could result in an accumulation of defective proteins in the nerve cells of the brain that can lead to cell death and the characteristic symptoms of Parkinson disease. The *PARK7* gene on chromosome 1 (at position 1p36.33-p36.12) encodes a protein called DJ-1, which has several functions, one of which is similar to parkin. The *PINK1* gene, also found at location 1p36, encodes the protein PTEN induced putative kinase 1. This protein is important for proper mitochondrial function, but it is unclear why the lack of this protein as a result of a mutation in the *PINK1* gene causes the death of nerve cells that lead to Parkinson disease.

Parkinson disease that results from mutations in any of these three genes is inherited in an autosomal recessive manner, which means that both copies of the gene must be deficient in order for the individual to be afflicted. Typically, an affected child is born to two unaffected parents, both of whom are carriers of the recessive mutant allele. The probable outcomes for children whose parents are both carriers are 75 percent unaffected and 25 percent affected.

The *LRRK2* gene (at position 12q12) specifies a protein called dardarin, which is a complex protein with at least three different enzyme activities. It is unclear why loss of this protein might contribute to the development Parkinson disease symptoms. Finally, the *SNCA* gene (at position 4q21) encodes the protein alpha synuclein, which is abundant in the presynaptic vesicles in brain neurons. Most mutations in this gene which cause Parkinson disease result in an excess production of alpha-synuclein, although it is unclear how this excess impairs proper nerve cell function.

Parkinson disease that results from mutations in either of these two genes is inherited in an auto somal

dominant fashion, meaning that a single copy of the mutation is sufficient to cause full expression of the disease. An affected individual has a 50 per cent chance of transmitting the mutation to each of his or her children.

SYMPTOMS

Symptoms of PD begin mildly, and they will worsen over time. Symptoms include a "pill-rolling" tremor in the hands. Tremors are present at rest, improve with movement, and are absent during sleep.

Other symptoms include stiffness and rigidity of muscles, usually beginning on one side of the body; difficulty and shuffling when walking; short steps; slowness of purposeful movements; trouble per forming usual tasks due to shaking in the hands; trouble speaking; a flat, monotonous voice; stut tering; a shaky, spidery handwriting; poor balance; difficulty rising from a sitting position; and "freezing." Anxiety; seborrhea (a skin problem that causes a red rash and white scales); a tendency to fall; stooped posture; an increasingly masklike face, with little variation in expression; trouble chewing and swallowing; depression; dementia; difficulty think ing; problems with memory; loss of or decreased sense of smell; and sleep problems, such as rapid eye movement (REM) behavior disorder, are also symptoms.

SCREENING AND DIAGNOSIS

The doctor may ask about a patient's symptoms and medical history and a physical exam may be done. There are no tests to definitively diagnose PD. A thorough medical history and physical exam can help to rule out other causes of a patient's symptoms.

Tests to rule out other conditions may include blood tests; urine tests; a computed tomography (CT) scan, a type of X ray that uses a computer to make pictures of structures inside the head; a magnetic resonance imaging (MRI) scan, a test that uses magnetic waves to make pictures of structures inside the head; and a positron emission tomography (PET) scan, a test that makes images that show forms of activity in the brain.

TREATMENT AND THERAPY

Currently, there is no cure for PD. There are also no proven treatments to slow or stop its progression.

The main goal of medical management of PD is to provide control of signs and symptoms for as long as possible while minimizing adverse effects. Studies demonstrate that a patient's quality of life

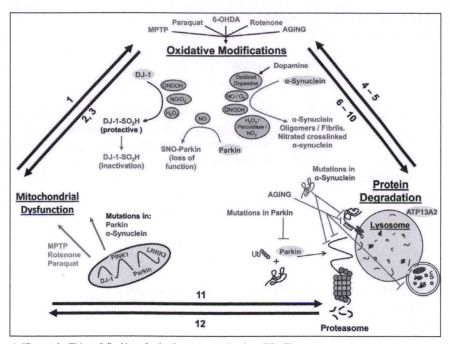

A *"Bermuda Triangle" of insults leads to neurondeath in PD. Known risk factors for the onset of Parkinson's disease (PD) include environmental (green), genetic (purple), and endogenous (blue) influences* By Malkus KA, Tsika E, Ischiropoulos H., *via Wikimedia Commons*

deteriorates quickly if treatment is not instituted at or shortly after diagnosis. In addition, it is now recognized that in PD, nonmotor symptoms may be as troublesome as, or more troublesome than, motor symptoms. Nonmotor symptoms can be categorized as autonomic, cognitive/psychiatric, and sensory and may include depression, dementia, hallucinations, rapid eye movement (REM) sleep behavior disorder (RMD), orthostatic hypotension, and constipation. Over time side effects may become troublesome, and the medications may lose their effectiveness.

The dopamine replacement medication levodopa/ carbidopa is still the "gold standard" for management of PD. Several other categories of medications may be helpful, and they include anticholinergics, dopamine agonists, non-selective monoamine oxidase (MAO)-B inhibitors, and inhibitors of catechol-O-methyl transferase, an enzyme involved in the degradation of neurotransmitters. In 2017, safinamide was the first new drug in 10 years to be approved as an adjunct in the treatment of PD. It is a selective monoamine oxidase (MAO) B inhibitor. Current research includes

the investigation of various forms of gene therapy in the treatment of PD.

Medicine may also be given to relieve the depression or hallucinations that may also occur with PD. These medications may include selective serotonin reuptake inhibitors (SSRIs) and antipsychotic cloza-pine. These drugs can worsen other symptoms. Patients who take them will need to be closely followed.

Different brain operations are available, and many more are being researched. Deep brain stimulation (DBS) involves implanting a device to stimulate certain parts of the brain. For several reasons (including the fact that no brain tissue is destroyed), it has become the surgical treatment of choice for PD. DBS can decrease tremor and rigidity. There are also destructive procedures known as neuroablative surgeries that do destroy sections of brain. These include thalamotomy and pallidotomy which improve tremor when medication does not work. These operations are not used as commonly as DBS. Research is being conducted about the possible use of nerve-cell transplants to increase the amount of dopamine made in the brain.

Physical therapy can improve muscle tone, strength, and balance; it will often include exercises and stretches. Patients with PD can also join a support group with other people who have the disorder. Participation in the support group will help patients learn how others are learning to live with the challenges of PD.

Prevention and Outcomes

There are no guidelines for preventing PD; however, there has been some evidence that caffeine may have a protective effect thus possibly slowly the nerve degeneration that yields the symptoms of the disease.

PD is both chronic, meaning it persists over a long period of time, and progressive, meaning its symptoms grow worse over time. Although some people become severely disabled, others experience only minor motor disruptions. It is currently not possible to predict which symptoms will affect an individual, and the intensity of the symptoms also varies from person to person. After the diagnosis is made, the long term survival can also vary greatly from person to person.

Rosalyn Carson-DeWitt, M.D.; reviewed by Rimas Lukas, M.D. "Etiology and Genetics" by Jeffrey A. Knight, Ph.D.; updated by Gary M. Flashner, M.S., M.D.

FURTHER READING

EBSCO Publishing. *DynaMed: Parkinson's Disease.* Ipswich, Mass.: Author, 2009. Available through http://www.ebscohost.com/dynamed.

_____. *Health Library: Parkinson Disease.* Ipswich, Mass.: Author, 2009. Available through http://www.ebscohost.com.

Goetz, Christopher G., ed. *Textbook of Clinical Neurology.* 3d ed. Philadelphia: Saunders Elsevier, 2007.

Rowland, Lewis P., ed. *Merritt's Neurology.* 11th ed. Philadelphia: Lippincott Williams & Wilkins, 2005.

Samii, A., J. G. Nutt, and B. R. Ransom. "Parkinson's Disease." *Lancet* 363, no. 9423 (May 29, 2004): 1783–1793.

Samuels, Martin A., and Steven K. Feske, eds. *Office Practice of Neurology.* 2d ed. Philadelphia: Chur chill Livingstone, 2003.

Siderowf, A., and M. Stern. "Update on Parkinson's Disease." *Annals of Internal Medicine* 138, no. 8 (April 15, 2003): 651–658.

Wider, C., and C. K. Wszolek. "Movement Disorders: Insights into Mechanisms and Hopes for Treatments. *Lancet Neurology* 8, no. 1 (Januar y, 2009): 8–10.

Liu R, Guo X, Park Y, Huang X, Sinha R, Freedman ND, et al. Caffeine Intake, Smoking, and Risk of Parkinson Disease in Men and Women. *Am J Epidemiol.* 2012 Apr 13

Pezzoli G, Cereda E. Exposure to pesticides or solvents and risk of Parkinson disease. *Neurology.* 2013 May 28. 80(22):2035–41.

Wirdefeldt K, Adami HO, Cole P, Trichopoulos D, Mandel J. Epidemiology and etiology of Parkinson's disease: a review of the evidence. *Eur J Epidemiol.* 2011 Jun. 26 Suppl 1:S1–58.

Hauser RA, Grosset DG. [(123) I]FP-CIT (DaTscan) SPECT Brain Imaging in Patients with Suspected Parkinsonian Syndromes. *J Neuroimaging.* 2011 Mar 16.

WEB SITES OF INTEREST

American Academy of Neurology
http://www.aan.com

Genetics Home Reference
http://ghr.nlm.nih.gov

Health Canada
http://www.hc-sc.gc.ca/index-eng.php

National Institute of Neurological Disorders and Stroke: NINDS Parkinson's Disease Information Page
http://www.ninds.nih.gov/disorders/parkinsons_disease/parkinsons_disease.htm

National Parkinson Foundation
http://www.parkinson.org/Page.aspx?pid=201

Parkinson Society Canada
http://www.parkinson.ca

Parkinson's Disease Foundation, Inc.
http://www.pdf.org

U.S. Food and Drug Administration: "FDA Announces Voluntary Withdrawal of Pergolide Products"
http://www.fda.gov/NewsEvents/Newsroom/ PressAnnouncements/2007/ucm108877.htm

http://emedicine.medscape.com/article/1831191-overview

http://www.medscape.com/viewarticle/877524

https://www.fda.gov/newsevents/newsroom/pressannouncements/ucm547852.htm

https://www.ncbi.nlm.nih.gov/pubmed/20182024

See also: Adrenoleukodystrophy; Alexander disease; Alzheimer's disease; Amyotrophic lateral sclerosis; Arnold-Chiari syndrome; Ataxia telangiectasia; Canavan disease; Cerebrotendinous xanthomatosis; Charcot-Marie-Tooth syndrome; Chediak-Higashi syndrome; Dandy-Walker syndrome; Deafness; Epilepsy; Essential tremor; Friedreich ataxia; Huntington's disease; Jansky-Bielschowsky disease; Joubert syndrome; Kennedy disease; Krabbé disease; Leigh syndrome; Leukodystrophy; Limb girdle muscular dystrophy; Maple syrup urine disease; Metachromatic leukodystrophy; Myoclonic epilepsy associ ated with ragged red fibers (MERRF); Narcolepsy; Nemaline myopathy; Neural tube defects; Neurofibromatosis; Prion diseases: Kuru and Creutzfeldt Jakob syndrome; Spinal muscular atrophy; Vanishing white matter disease.

Paroxysmal nocturnal hemoglobinuria

CATEGORY: Diseases and syndromes
ALSO KNOWN AS: PNH

DEFINITION

Paroxysmal nocturnal hemoglobinuria (PNH) is a rare noninherited polyclonal genetic disorder caused by somatic mutations of the hematopoietic stem cells, which normally give rise to the trilineage cell lines including white blood cells, red blood cells, and platelets. The abnormal stem cells in PNH give rise to cells that are deficient in an anchor protein that normally bind certain proteins to cell membranes.

Paroxysmal nocturnal hemoglobinuria (PNH) is a hematological disorder characterized by complement-mediated hemolytic anemia, thrombophilia, and bone marrow failure. By E. Uthman, MD (http://www.flickr.com/photos/euthman/2989437967), via Wikimedia Commons

Resultant complications can lead to hemolysis, aplastic anemia, venous thrombosis, and acute leukemia.

RISK FACTORS

PNH is a rare disorder, with a general prevalence of about 0.5 to 1.5 in 1 million, as reported by the National Organization for Rare Disorders (NORD) in 2014. It frequently affects those who are middle-aged and affects both sexes at all age ranges. It is usually diagnosed in those with an existing diagnosis of myelodysplastic syndrome or aplastic anemia, the latter of which is a risk factor for the development of PNH.

A micrograph of red blood cells, (erythrocytes) taken from [1], specifically [2]. The images are due to the NIH, a US government agency. The photos are attributed to Drs. Noguchi, Rodgers, and Schechter of NIDDK.

ETIOLOGY AND GENETICS

PNH is an acquired disorder due to somatic mutations of the phosphatidylinositol glycan class A (*PIGA*) gene *pig-*A gene on the X chromosome of hematopoietic stem cells. This defect leads to an absent or defective protein product that normally is involved in the synthesis of the glycosyl-phosphatidylinositol (GPI) anchor protein that is required for binding of cell membrane surface proteins. The majority of *PIGA* defects are due to frame-shift mutations that end with an early stop codon, leading to a lack of the protein product. Substitution mutations are also possible that may lead to protein products that are less effective in the synthesis of the GPI anchor. NORD stated in 2014 that PNH patients are believed have more than one type of mutation, leading to a polyclonal population of stem cells admixed with a population of normal stem cells. Most of these mutations are unique to each patient.

Because this defect occurs in hematopoietic stem cells, all cell lines are affected, including red blood cells, white blood cells, and platelets. The critical cell membrane surface proteins that are lacking on red blood cells include the decay-accelerating factor (also known as CD55), membrane inhibitor

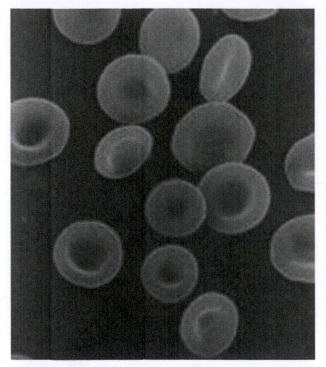

A micrograph of red blood cells, (erythrocytes) taken from, specifically. The images are due to the NIH, a US government agency. The photos are attributed to Drs. Noguchi, Rodgers, and Schechter of NIDDK. public domain via wikimedia commons

to the preferential selection of defective cells characteristic of PNH.

SYMPTOMS

One of the defining manifestations of PNH is dark urine in the morning, which is due to the leakage of hemoglobin from breakdown of red blood cells. Other symptoms vary depending on the degree of disease progression. Yellowing of the skin (jaundice) can occur with prolonged red blood cell breakdown; bleeding can occur with an abnormally low platelet count; risks for infections can occur with low white blood cell count; and headache, abdominal pain, and skin findings can occur due to vessel thrombosis.

SCREENING AND DIAGNOSIS

The principal diagnostic test of PNH is flow cytometry, which is able to detect the CD55 and CD59 glycoproteins on the surface of red blood cells. The absence or the reduced expression of both such glycoproteins, along with clinical and laboratory features, is diagnostic of PNH. Another more specific method is using fluorescently labeled inactive bacterial toxin aerolysin, which normally initiates hemolysis by binding to GPI anchors on RBCs. The lack of such binding suggests an absence of GPI and is also diagnostic of PNH.

TREATMENT AND THERAPY

Therapy for PNH includes addressing clinical issues related to anemia, leukopenia, thrombocytopenia, and thrombosis. Blood or platelet transfusions are indicated in clinically indicated anemia or thrombocytopenia. Other therapies such as folic acid, glucocorticoids, and eculizumab (an agent that inhibits terminal complement pathway activation) have been used. Treatment of thrombosis includes thrombolysis to break up blood clots in life-threatening thrombosis or with anticoagulation agents such as heparin or warfarin for preventive measures. Hematopoietic stem cell transplants and medical agents such as cyclosporine or antithymocyte globulin have been used to address the issue of aplastic anemia. Stem cell transplantation is the only known cure. Gene therapy is theoretically possible since the *PIGA* gene was cloned in 1993 and may one day be a reality.

of reactive lysis (also known as CD59), homologous restriction factor (HRF), and C8 binding protein. These surface proteins normally interact and slow down the complement process, notably through proteins C3b and C4b. Their absence therefore leads to the unhampered destruction of the red cell membrane by the complement system, leading to intravascular hemolysis.

Though the *PIGA* gene defect appears to be a necessary component for the development of PNH, it is not clear if this is sufficient, since *PIGA* mutations have been found in small numbers in many, if not most, normal individuals. The abnormal population increases in aplastic anemia and becomes overwhelmingly large in PNH. The Luzzatto-Young hypothesis on the development of PNH notes that the processes that lead to aplastic anemia tend to suppress the proliferation of normal cells and not defective cells, therefore leading

Prevention and Outcomes

Although PNH is a chronic disorder, many patients are able to live for extended periods of time, and spontaneous recovery is possible. A 2008 study published in *Blood* found the median survival after the onset of disease to be twenty-two years, with longer lifespans for those diagnosed after 1986. The majority of deaths and morbidity are related to complications from venous thrombosis.

Further Reading

Gross, Matthew B., and Cassandra L. Kniffin. "#300818 Paroxysmal Nocturnal Hemoglobinuria 1; PNH1." *OMIM.org.* Johns Hopkins U, 21 Apr. 2014. Web. 5 Aug. 2014.

Kaushansky, Kenneth, et al. *Williams Hematology.* 8th ed. McGraw-Hill, 2010. Print.

Omime, M. *Paroxysmal Nocturnal Hemoglobinuria and Related Disorders.* New York: Springer, 2003. Print.

"Paroxysmal Nocturnal Hemoglobinuria (PNH)." *Aplastic Anemia & MDS International Foundation.* Aplastic Anemia and MDS International Foundation, 18 Dec. 2013. Web. 5 Aug. 2014.

"Paroxysmal Nocturnal Hemoglobinuria (PNH)." *Medline Plus.* US Natl. Lib. of Medicine, 24 Feb. 2014. Web. 5 Aug. 2014.

"Paroxysmal Nocturnal Hemoglobinuria (PNH)." *RareDiseases.org.* Natl. Organization for Rare Diseases, 28 Jan. 2014. Web. 5 Aug. 2014.

Peffault de Latour, Régis, et al. "Paroxysmal Nocturnal Hemoglobinuria: Natural History of Disease Subcategories." *Blood* 112.8 (2008): 3099–3106. PDF file.

Young, Neal S., and Joel Moss, eds. *PNH and the GPI-Linked Proteins.* New York: Academic, 2000. Print.

See also: ABO blood types; Chronic myeloid leukemia; Fanconi anemia; Hemophilia; Hereditary spherocytosis; Infantile agranulocytosis; Myelodysplastic syndromes; Rh incompatibility and isoimmunization; Sickle-cell disease.

Parthenogenesis

Category: Genetic engineering and biotechnology
Significance: Parthenogenesis is unisexual reproduction through the development of unfertilized eggs, which produces offspring that are genetically alike and allows rapid expansion of a population of well-adapted individuals into a rich environment. This clonal reproduction strategy is used by a number of species for rapid reproduction under favorable conditions, and it appears to offer a selective advantage to creatures living in disturbed habitats.

Key terms

adaptive advantage increased fertility in offspring as a result of passing on favorable genetic information

diploid: having two sets of homologous chromosomes

fertilization: the fusion of two cells (egg and sperm) in sexual reproduction

haploid: having one set of chromosomes

meiosis: nuclear division that reduces the chromosome number from diploid to haploid in the production of the sperm and the egg

zygote: the product of fertilization in sexually reproducing organisms

The Nature of Parthenogenesis

Parthenogenesis is derived from two Greek words that mean "virgin" (*parthenos*) and "origin" (*genesis*) and describes a form of reproduction in which females lay diploid eggs (containing two sets of chromosomes) that develop into offspring without fertilization—there is no fusion of a sperm nucleus with the ovum nucleus to produce the new diploid individual. This is a form of clonal reproduction because all of the offspring are genetically identical

A baby Komodo dragon born by parthenogenesis, photographed at Chester Zoo Neil at en.wikipedia, via Wikimedia Commons

to the mother and to each other. The mechanisms of parthenogenesis do not show any single pattern and have evolved independently in different groups of organisms. In some organisms, such as rotifers and aphids, parthenogenesis alternates with normal sexual reproduction. When there is a rich food source, such as new rose bushes emerging in the early spring, aphids reproduce by parthenogenesis; late in the summer, however, as the food source is decreasing, sexually reproducing females appear.

The same pattern has been observed in rotifers, in which a decrease in the quality of the food supply leads to the appearance of females that produce haploid eggs by normal meiosis that require fertilization for development. The strategy appears to involve the clonal production of large numbers of genetically identical individuals that are well suited to the environment when the conditions are favorable and the production of a variety of different types, by the recombination that occurs during normal meiosis and the mixing of alleles from two individuals in sexual reproduction, when the conditions are less favorable. In social insects, such as bees, wasps, and ants, parthenogenesis is a major factor in sex determination, although it may not be the only factor. In these insects, eggs that develop by parthenogenesis remain haploid and develop into males, while fertilized eggs develop into diploid, sexually reproducing females.

In algae and some forms of plants, parthenogenesis also allows rapid reproduction when conditions are favorable. In citrus plants seed development by parthenogenesis maintains the favorable characteristics of each plant. For this reason, most commercial citrus plants are propagated by asexual means, such as grafting. Parthenogenesis has also been induced in organisms that do not show the process in natural populations. In sea urchins, for example, development can be induced by mechanical stimulation of the egg or by changes in the chemistry of the medium. Even some vertebrate eggs have shown signs of early development when artificially stimulated, but haploid vertebrate cells lack all of the information required for normal development, so such "zygotes" cease development very early.

PARTHENOGENESIS IN VERTEBRATES

Parthenogenesis has been observed in certain populations of vertebrates such as fish, frogs, and lizards. In these parthenogenetic populations, all organisms

All of the aphids are females; they reproduce by parthenogenesis (clones of the mother) and they bear live young (nymphs). By aroid from San Luis Obispo, CA, USA (Milkweed aphid, Aphis nerii), via Wikimedia Commons

are female, so reproduction of the clone is restricted to parthenogenesis. Parthenogenetic fish often occur in populations along with sexually reproducing individuals. The parthenogenetic forms produce diploid eggs that develop without fertilization; in rare cases, however, fertilization of a parthenogenetic egg gives rise to a triploid individual that has three sets of chromosomes rather than the normal two sets (two from the diploid egg and one from the sperm). In some groups, penetration of a sperm is necessary to activate development of the zygote, but the sperm nucleus is not incorporated into the zygote.

Evidence indicates that in each of these vertebrate situations, the parthenogenetic populations have resulted from a hybridization between two different species. The parthenogenetic forms always occur in regions where the two parental species overlap in their distribution, often an area that is not the most favorable habitat for either species. The hybrid origin has been confirmed by the demonstration that the animals have two different forms of an enzyme that have been derived from the two different species in the region. Genetic identity has also been confirmed using skin graft studies. In unrelated organisms, skin grafts are quickly rejected because of genetic incompatibilities; clonal animals, on the other hand, readily accept grafts from related donors. Parthenogenetic fish from the same clone accept grafts that confirm their genetic identity, but rejection of grafts by other parthenogenetic forms from different populations shows that they are different clones and must have a different origin. This makes it possible to better understand the structure of the populations and helps in the study of the origins of parthenogenesis within those populations. Comparisons using nuclear and mitochondrial DNA also allow the determination of species origin and the maternal species of the parthenogenetic form since the mitochondria are almost exclusively transmitted through the vertebrate egg. Within the hybrid, a mechanism has originated that allows the egg to develop without fertilization, although, as already noted, penetration by a sperm may be required to activate development in some of the species. The advantage of parthenogenesis appears to be the production of individuals that are genetically identical. Since the parthenogenetic form may, at least in vertebrates, be a hybrid, it is heterozygous at most of its genetic loci. This provides greater variation that may provide the animal with a greater range of responses to the environment. Maintaining this heterozygous genotype may give the animals an advantage in environments where the parental species are not able to reproduce successfully and may be a major reason for the persistence of this form of reproduction. Many vertebrate parthenogenetic populations are found in disturbed habitats, so their unique genetic composition may allow for adaptation to these unusual conditions.

MECHANISMS OF DEVELOPMENT

The mechanisms of diploid egg development are as diverse as the organisms in which this form of reproduction is found. In normal meiosis, the like chromosomes of each pair separate at the first division and the copies of each chromosome separate at the second division (producing four haploid cells). During the meiotic process in the egg, three small cells (the polar bodies), each with one set of chromosomes, are produced, and one set of chromosomes remains as the egg nucleus. In parthenogenetic organisms, some modification of this process occurs that results in an egg nucleus with two sets of chromosomes—the diploid state. In some forms, the first meiotic division does not occur, so two chromosome sets remain in the egg following the second division. In other forms, one of the polar bodies fuses back into the cell so that

there are two sets of chromosomes in the final egg. In another variation, there is a replication of chromosomes after the first division, but no second division takes place in the egg, so the chromosome number is again diploid. In all of these mechanisms, the genetic content of the egg is derived from the mother's genetic content, and there is no contribution to the genetic content from male material.

The situation may be even more complex, however, because some hybrid individuals may retain the chromosomal identity of one species by a selective loss of the chromosomes of the other species during meiosis. The eggs may carry the chromosomes of one species but the mitochondria of the other species. The haploid eggs must be fertilized, so these individuals are not parthenogenetic, but their presence in the population shows how complex reproductive strategies can be and how important it is to study the entire population in order to understand its dynamics fully: A single population may contain individuals of the two sexual species, true parthenogenetic individuals, and triploid individuals resulting from fertilization of a diploid egg.

FURTHER READING

Beatty, Richard Alan. *Parthenogenesis and Polyploidy in Mammalian Development.* Cambridge: Cambridge UP, 1957. Print.

Booth, Warren, et al. "New Insights on Facultative Parthenogenesis in Pythons." *Biological Journal of the Linnean Society* 112.3 (2014): 461–68.

Print. Cocco, J. et al. "Sex Produces as Numerous and Long-Lived Offspring as Parthenogenesis in a New Parthenogenetic Insect." *Canadian Journal of Zoology* 91.3 (2013): 187–90.

Print. Elzinga, Jelmer A., Jukka Jokela, and Lisa N. S. Shama. "Large Variation in Mitochondrial DNA of Sexual and Parthenogenetic Dahlica Triquetrella (Lepidoptera: Psychidae) Shows Multiple Origins of Parthenogenesis." *BMC Evolutionary Biology* 13.1 (2013): 1–9. Print.

Kaufman, Matthew H. *Early Mammalian Development: Parthenogenetic Studies.* New York: Cambridge UP, 1983. Print. Lim, Hwa A. *Multiplicity Yours: Cloning, Stem Cell Research, and Regenerative Medicine.* Hackensack: World Scientific, 2006. Print.

Schon, Isa, Koen Martens, and Peter van Dijk, eds. *Lost Sex: The Evolutionary Biology of Parthenogenesis.* New York: Springer, 2009. Print.

See also: Totipotency.

Patau syndrome

CATEGORY: Diseases and syndromes
ALSO KNOWN AS: Trisomy 13; Patau's syndrome; D trisomy syndrome; Bartholin-Patau syndrome

DEFINITION

Patau syndrome is a severe systemic disorder that affects many essential body systems and functions. Typically, each cell in the body will have an extra copy of chromosome 13, thus yielding a total of 47 chromosomes per cell instead of the usual 46.

RISK FACTORS

The only consistently reported risk factor is advanced maternal age, since the extra copy of chromosome 13 most commonly arises from an error in meiosis during egg cell maturation. Sex does not appear to be a significant risk factor, with the incidence in female fetuses being 52 percent as compared to 48 percent in males, as reported in a 2012 *Pediatrics*study by K. E. Nelson, K. R. Hexem, and C. Feudtner.

ETIOLOGY AND GENETICS

The presence of an extra chromosome 13 in the cells of a developing fetus results from a type of error called nondisjunction. Nondisjunction which can occur during gamete (sperm or egg) production in either parent. Either the failure of homologous chromosomes to separate from each other during the first meiotic division or the failure of sister chromatids to

Risk for Trisomy 13 (Patau syndrome) in relation to maternal age (X axis) and gestation (Hbd, marked by color). By Filip em (Own work), via Wikimedia Commons

A 37 2/7 week gestational age male infant with Patau syndrome demonstrating alobar holoprosencephaly with cyclopia. Facial features included sloping forehead with a proboscis superior to a single central palpebral fissure. By Chan A et al, via Wikimedia Commons

separate from each other during the second meiotic division will result in mature sperm cells or egg cells that have either one extra or one missing chromosome. Since each chromosome contains thousands of genes, it is not surprising that individuals with extra or missing chromosomes in all cells would have a severe imbalance of genetic information and suffer from multiple developmental anomalies. In fact, only three autosomal trisomies (conditions in which each cell has three copies of a nonsex chromosome) are generally known to be consistent with full-term delivery, and Patau syndrome is the least common and most severe of these. The most common and least severe is Down syndrome (trisomy 21). Edwards syndrome (trisomy 18), like Patau syndrome, results in affected newborns with multiple structural and developmental problems, and survival beyond the first year is rare.

Very occasionally, a case of trisomy 13 occurs in which the extra copy of chromosome 13 does not appear as a separate chromosome but rather is physically attached onto the end of another chromosome; such cases are known as translocation Patau syndrome. While the clinical features of the affected newborn do not differ from the usual form of the syndrome, it is particularly important to identify this variety of Patau, since it may be transmitted with high frequency by a normal-appearing parent who carries the translocation chromosome.

One additional variant that is infrequently encountered is known as mosaic trisomy 13. The bodies of mosaic individuals are composed of two distinctly different cell lines, in which only some of the cells have the extra chromosome 13, while the remainder have a normal chromosome complement. The severity of the clinical presentation in these cases depends on the type and number of cells that carry the extra chromosome, but in almost all cases a less severe form of the syndrome is manifested.

SYMPTOMS

The most consistent symptoms present at birth include microcephaly (small head), cleft lip and/or palate, and polydactyly (extra fingers or toes). Ears are often low-set and malformed, and the nose can be oddly shaped or occasionally altogether absent. Most affected individuals are presumed to be hearing impaired, and many are blind as well. Other neurological problems are common, including profound intellectual disability and failure of the brain to divide into its proper hemispheres during gestation. About 80 percent of affected newborns are reported to have moderate to severe heart defects, as reported by the National Organization for Rare Diseases.

SCREENING AND DIAGNOSIS

According to the University of Chicago, Patau syndrome occurs in about 1 out of 5,000 live births, and diagnosis is most often immediately apparent, although there is some overlap of symptoms with Edwards syndrome. Genetic studies should be performed to confirm the diagnosis. Ultrasound examinations and imaging studies should be done to check for more extensive developmental problems. They include brain, heart, and kidney defects as well as an extra spleen, rotated intestines, and defects of the liver and pancreas. Males may have undescended testes, while females frequently have a divided uterus.

TREATMENT AND THERAPY

Because of the heterogeneous nature of each clinical presentation, treatment is usually specifically directed to the particular physical problems with which each affected child is born. As reported by the University of Chicago, about 44 percent of affected newborns die within the first month and more than 70 percent die within a year. Most die from serious heart defects or severe neurological problems. Historically, medical treatment has focused primarily on patient comfort and noninvasive symptom treatment rather than on prolonging life. Surgery may be performed to repair heart defects or cleft lip and palate. In those cases where survival extends beyond one or two years, additional surgeries and physical therapy are often undertaken to allow the affected child to reach his or her full developmental potential. Nelson, Hexem, and Feudtner's study indicates that children born with Patau syndrome are surviving for increasingly longer periods and that neonatal interventions may improve survival rates.

PREVENTION AND OUTCOMES

Except for the rare translocation form of Patau syndrome, there is no effective means of prevention. Genetic counseling should always be available for parents of an affected child, and amniocentesis is an option for older at-risk mothers. According to the University of Chicago, only up to 30 percent of affected newborns survive the first year of life and survival into the teenage years is exceedingly rare.

Jeffrey A. Knight, Ph.D.

FURTHER READING

Cummings, Michael R. *Human Heredity: Principles and Issues*. 10th ed. Belmont: Brooks/Cole, 2014. Print.

De la Rocha, Kelly. "Chromosomal Abnormalities: Trisomy 13 and 18." *Health Library*. EBSCO, 28 May 2014. Web. 5 Aug. 2014.

Lewis, Ricki. *Human Genetics*. 10th ed. New York: McGraw, 2011. Print.

Nelson, Katherine E., Kari R. Hexem, and Chris Feudtner. "Inpatient Hospital Care of Children with Trisomy 13 and Trisomy 18 in the United States." *Pediatrics* 129.5 (2012): 1–8. PDF file.

Nussbaum, Robert L., Roderick R. McInnes, and Huntington F. Willard. *Thompson and Thompson Genetics in Medicine*. 7th ed. New York: Saunders, 2007. Print. "Trisomy 18 (Edwards), Trisomy 13 (Patau)." *Pediatrics Clerkship, University of Chicago*. U of Chicago, 2013. Web. 13 Aug. 2014.

See also: Apert syndrome; Brachydactyly; Carpenter syndrome; Cleft lip and palate; Congenital defects; Cornelia de Lange syndrome; Cri du chat syndrome; Crouzon syndrome; Down syndrome; Edwards syndrome; Ellis-van Creveld syndrome; Holt-Oram syndrome; Ivemark syndrome; Meacham syndrome; Opitz-Frias syndrome; Polydactyly; Robert syndrome; Rubinstein-Taybi syndrome.

Patents on life-forms

CATEGORY: Bioethics; Human genetics and social issues

SIGNIFICANCE: In 1980, the US Supreme Court upheld the right to patent a live, genetically altered organism. The decision was opposed by many scientists and theologians who believed that such organisms would pose a threat to the future of humanity. Although "legally" settled, the debate has continued, opponents arguing that patenting life-forms and DNA sequences imposes too great a cost and greatly inconveniences genetic research.

KEY TERM

patent: a grant made by the government that gives the creator or inventor the sole right to make, use, or sell that invention for a specific period of time, usually twenty years in the United States

PATENT ON LIFE-FORM UPHELD

On June 16, 1980, the U.S. Supreme Court voted 5 to 4 that living organisms could be patented under federal law. The case involved Ananda M. Chakrabarty, a scientist who, while working for General Electric General Electric in 1972, had created a new form of bacteria, *Pseudomona originosa* which could break down crude oil, and, therefore, could be used to clean up oil spills. Chakrabarty filed for a patent, but an examiner for the Patent Office rejected the application on the ground that living things are not patentable subject matter under existing patent law. Commissioner of Patents

Old Patent Office Building in Washington, D.C public domain via wikimedia commons

and Trademarks Sidney A. Diamond supported this view. Federal patent law provided that a patent could be issued only to a person who invented or discovered any new and useful "manufacture" or "composition of matter." The U.S. Court of Customs and Patent Appeals reversed that decision in 1979, concluding that the fact that microorganisms are alive has no legal significance. It held that a live, human-made bacterium is a patentable item since the microorganism was manufactured by crossbreeding four existing strains of bacteria and had never existed in nature.

Writing for the majority, Supreme Court Chief Justice Warren E. Burger upheld the patent appeals court judgment, making a distinction between the new bacterium and "laws of nature, physical phenomena and abstract ideas," which are not patentable. In the Court majority's view, Chakrabarty had invented a form of life that did not exist in the natural world, so it could not be considered part of nature. Instead, it was a product of human "ingenuity and research" that deserved patent protection. Items not patentable include new minerals that are discovered in the earth or a new species of plant found in a distant forest. These things occur naturally and are not created by humans. Burger also stressed that physicist Albert Einstein could not have patented his formula $E = mc^2$, since it is a law of nature, nor could Sir Isaac Newton have received a patent for the law of gravity. Discoveries such as these are part of the natural world and cannot be owned by a single individual.

Chakrabarty, on the other hand, had not found an unknown, natural species, nor had he discovered a law of nature. His new bacterium had a distinctive name and was developed in the laboratory for a specific purpose. None of the characteristics of the new organism could be found in nature. His discovery, Burger reemphasized, was patentable because he had created it.

OPPOSITION TO THE RULING

The court majority refused to consider arguments made in friend-of-the-court briefs filed by opponents of genetic engineering. The briefs were presented by groups representing scientists, including several Nobel Prize winners, and religious organizations. One brief suggested that genetic research posed a dangerous and serious threat to the future of humanity and should, therefore, be prohibited. Possible dangers included the spread of pollution and disease by newly created bacteria, none of which would have any natural enemies. Other threats involved the possible loss of genetic diversity patents on life-forms if, for instance, only the "best" form of laboratory-created plant seeds were grown. Research into human genetics could lead to newly designed gene material that could be used to build a "master race," thereby devaluing other human lives. Chief Justice Burger concluded, however, that humans could be trusted not to create such horrible things. Quoting William Shakespeare's *Hamlet*, the chief justice asserted that it is sometimes better "to bear those ills we have than to fly to others that we know not of." People can try to guess what genetic manipulation could lead to, but it would also be a good idea to expect good things from science rather than "a gruesome parade of horribles." Besides, he then said, it did not matter whether a patent was granted in this case; in either case, scientific research would continue into the nature of genes.

The People's Business Commission, a nonprofit educational foundation, had argued that granting General Electric and Chakrabarty a patent would give corporations the right "to own the processes of life in the centuries to come" through genetic manipulation. Chief Justice Burger wrote that the Court was "without competence to entertain these arguments." They did not have enough information available to determine whether to ignore such fears "as fantasies generated by fear of the unknown" or accept them. Such a determination was not the responsibility of the Court, however. Questions of the morality of genetic research and manipulation were better left to Congress and the political process. How to proceed in these matters could only be resolved "after the kind of investigation, examination, and study that legislative bodies can provide and courts cannot."

Supreme Court Justice William J. Brennan, presented a brief dissenting opinion. He noted that Congress had twice, in 1930 and 1970, permitted new types of plants to be patented. However, those laws made no mention of bacteria. Thus, Brennan argued, Congress had indicated that only plants could receive patents and that the legislators had thus clearly indicated that other life-forms were excluded from the patent process. The Court majority rejected this view, arguing that Congress had not specifically excluded other life-forms.

THE U.S. PATENT AND TRADEMARK OFFICE (USPTO)

Those opposed to patents on DNA sequences have a wide variety of contentions, ranging from the concern

Patent Office 2 By Tony Hisgett from Birmingham, UK (Patent Office 2 Uploaded by tm), via Wikimedia Commons

that sole privileges will impede research to the notion that genes represent the very basis of life and thus no one should have exclusive rights to them.

In 2001, the USPTO thoughtfully considered whether genetic discoveries were patentable by evaluating opposition comments from thirty-five individuals and seventeen organizations. Their decisions were published in the *Federal Register*. To address the contention that a gene is not a new invention because it exists in nature, the USPTO emphasized that only DNA in an unnatural form, excised and purified from its chromosome or synthesized in a laboratory, is patentable. To tackle the notion that no one person or company should own a human gene sequence because it inherently belongs to all humans, the USPTO asserted that progress is promoted and secrecy reduced when a patent gives an inventor purely the legal right to exclude others from making, using, selling, or importing the gene for twenty years, not ownership. To avoid reckless patenting of any gene sequence found, the USPTO stipulated that the utility of a gene or expressed sequence tag (EST), not just its sequence, must be known when filing for sole rights. Examples of a gene's utility include being involved in the cell regulation, coding for a useful protein, or flagging a disease.

The USPTO established these four criteria when considering a patent grant on a gene, gene fragment, single nucleotide polymorphism (SNP), gene test, protein, or stem cell: novelty, usefulness, nonobviousness, and enablement, whereby the life-form could be reproduced by someone skilled in the biochemistry field. Patentees must deposit a sample of the unique life-form in one of twenty-six worldwide culture depositories.

SHARING KNOWLEDGE, LICENSING, AND COMMERCIALIZING LIFE-FORMS

Measures have been taken by key institutions to even the genomics playing field for all researchers. The Human Genome Project publically lists the genome for free on the Internet. In April, 1999, the UK Wellcome Trust vowed unrestricted access to the 1.5 million SNPs they identified and patented in order to prevent others from gaining exclusive rights to them first.

As one of the United States' primary financial supporters of scientific research, the National Institutes of Health (NIH) weighed in on the patenting debate in 2004 by developing its "Best Practices for the Licensing of Genomic Inventions." These guidelines leave room for researchers to protect their work with patents, especially when there is potential to commercialize their product through the private sector for society's health benefit, but the NIH also strongly encourages investigators to propagate information by granting nonexclusive licenses to other universities receiving NIH funding.

In 1980, Congress passed the Bahy-Dole Act, which permits universities to commercialize via private industry their federally funded discoveries. This prompted colleges to establish a campus Technology Transfer Office and implement a material transfer agreement (MTA). Material transfer agreement (MTA) Academic researchers now need to obtain an MTA before they disclose information to other investigators, adding another potential hurdle to the flow of knowledge. A 2005 survey of ninety-three agricultural biology departments found that MTAs have taken the lead over patents as the hindrance of conveying scientific information. This study and others have found that patents are not aggressively enforced and not truly encumbering academic research. Since the human genome was sequenced in 2003, the genomics industry has increased in prominence, to the point that many have questioned the ethical nature of genes patents. In 2013, in a unanimous decision, the Supreme Court ruled that genes could not be patented (though those produced synthetically could). The case in question involved a lawsuit by the American Civil Liberties Union and the Public Patent Foundation against molecular diagnostics company Myriad Genetics, which owned the patents to several genes, including BRCA1 and BRCA2, linked to breast and ovarian cancers. The decision was seen as an landmark in the protection of individual rights and in the development of personalized and inclusive medical care.

FURTHER READINGY

Barfield, Claude, and John E. Calfee. *Biotechnology and the Patent System: Balancing Innovation and Property Rights.* Washington, DC: AEI Press, 2007. Print. Baran, George R., Mohammad F. Kiani, and Solomon Praveen Samuel. *Healthcare and Biomedical Technology in the Twenty-First Century: An Introduction for Non-Science Majors.* New York: Springer, 2014. Digital file.

Chapman, Audrey R., ed. *Perspectives on Genetic Patenting: Religion, Science, and Industry in Dialogue.* Washington, DC: American Assn. for the Advancement of Science, 1999. Print.

Diamond, Commissioner of Patents and Trademarks v. Chakrabarty. 447 U.S. 303. Supreme Court of the US. 1980. Print. Doll, John. "Talking Gene Patents." *Scientific American* Aug. 2001. Print. Ghosh, Shubha. *Identity, Invention, and the Culture of Personalized Medicine Patenting.* New York: Cambridge UP, 2013. Print.

Hanson, Mark J. "Religious Voices in Biotechnology: The Case of Gene Patenting." *Hastings Center Law Report* Nov.-Dec. 1997. Print.

Hope, Janet. *Biobazaar, the Open Source Revolution and Biotechnology.* Cambridge: Harvard UP, 2008. Print.

Resnick, David B. *Owning the Genome: A Moral Analysis of DNA Patenting.* Albany: State U of New York P, 2004. Print.

Specter, Michael. *Can We Patent Life? New Yorker.* Condé Nast, 1 Apr. 2013. Web. 6 Aug. 2014.

"Supreme Court Issues Compromise Ruling on Landmark BRCA Gene Patenting Case." *New York Daily News.* NYDailyNews.com, 14 June 2013. Web. 6 Aug. 2014.

US Patent and Trademark Office. *Federal Register* 66.4 (2001): 1092–99. Print.

Vogel, Fredrich, and Reinhard Grunwald, eds. *Patenting of Human Genes and Living Organisms.* New York: Springer, 1994. Print.

See also: Genetic engineering: Historical development; Genetic engineering: Industrial applications; Genetic engineering: Social and ethical issues; Human genetics; Human Genome Project; Hybridization and introgression; Model organism: Mus musculus; Transgenic organisms.

Berlin Museum of Natural History, "Developments – 60 Years Discovery of the Structure of DNA", parental testing By Hwaja Götz (Museum für Naturkunde Berlin), via Wikimedia Commons

Paternity tests

CATEGORY: Human genetics and social issues

SIGNIFICANCE: Establishing paternity can be important for establishing legal responsibility for child support, health insurance, veterans' and social security benefits, and legal access to medical records. It may also affect a child's future as it relates to inherited diseases.

KEY TERMS

forensic genetics: the use of genetic tests and principles to resolve legal questions

human leukocyte antigens (HLA) antigens produced by a cluster of genes that play a critical role in the outcome of transplants; because they are made up of a large number of genes, they are used in individual identification and the matching of parents and offspring

paternity exclusion: the indication, through genetic testing, that a particular man is not the biological father of a particular child

GENETIC PRINCIPLES OF PATERNITY TESTING

The basic genetic principles utilized in paternity testing have remained the same from the first applications of ABO blood groups paternity testing to applications of DNA fingerprinting. Available tests may positively exclude a man from being a child's biological father. Evidence supporting paternity, however, cannot be considered conclusive. Ultimately, a court must decide whether a man is determined to be the legal father based on all lines of evidence.

The genetic principles can be illustrated with a very simple example that uses ABO blood types. The four blood groups (A, B, AB, and O) are controlled by three pairs of genes. In the example, however, only three of the blood groups will be used to demonstrate the range of matings with the possible children for each of them (see the table headed "Blood Types, Genes, and Possible Offspring").

Example 1: A man is not excluded.

Mother: A

Child: A

Putative Father: AB

It can be seen that the mothers in matings 1 and 4 satisfy the condition of the mother being A and possibly having a child being A. Mating 4 satisfies the condition of a father being AB, the mother A, and a possible child being A. Results indicate that the putative father could be the father. He is not excluded.

Example 2: A man is excluded.

Mother: A

Child: A

Putative Father: B

Again, it is seen that the mothers in matings 1, 4, and 7 satisfy the condition of the mother being A and possibly having a child being A. Mating 7 satisfies the condition of a father being B and the mother A, but mating 7 cannot produce a child being A. The putative father cannot be the father, and he is excluded.

DNA FINGERPRINTING

After the initial use of ABO blood groups in paternity testing, it became apparent that there were many cases in which the ABO phenotypes did not permit exclusion. Other blood group systems have also been used, including the MN and Rh groups. As more blood groups are utilized, the probability of exclusion (or nonexclusion) increases. Paternity tests have not been restricted to blood groups alone; tissue types and serum enzymes have also been used.

The most powerful tool developed has been DNA testing. DNA fingerprinting was developed in England by Sir Alec Jeffreys. DNA is extracted from white blood cells and broken down into fragments by bacterial enzymes (restriction endonucleases).

Paternity test - a single genetic profile based on STR analysis By Armaron (Own work), via Wikimedia Commons

The fragments are separated by size, and specific fragments are identified. Each individual has a different DNA profile, but the profiles of parents and children have similarities in greater proportion than those between unrelated people. Also, frequencies of different fragments tend to vary among ethnic groups. It is possible not only to exclude someone who is not the biological father but also to determine actual paternity with a probability approaching 100 percent. The personal, social, and economic implications involved in paternity testing have far-reaching consequences. Blood-group analysis is cheaper but less consistent than DNA testing. Paternity can often be excluded but rarely proven with the same degree of accuracy that DNA testing provides. Human leukocyte antigen (HLA) testing can also be used but suffers from many of the same problems as blood-group analysis. The development of DNA testing after 1984 revolutionized the field of paternity testing. DNA fingerprinting has made decisions on paternity assignments virtually 100 percent accurate. The same technique has also been applied in cases of individual identification, and results have helped to release people who have been falsely imprisoned as well as convict other people with the analysis of trace evidence.

FURTHER READING

Anderlik, Mary R., and Mark A. Rothstein. "DNA-Based Identity Testing and the Future of the Family: A Research Agenda." *American Journal of Law and Medicine* 28.2-3 (2002): 215. Print.

Cohen, Warren. "Kid Looks Like the Mailman? Genetic Labs Boom as the Nation Wonders Who's Daddy." *US News and World Report* 122.3 (1997): 62. Print. Goodman, Christi. *Paternity, Marriage, and DNA.* Denver: Natl. Conf. of State Legis., 2001. Print.

Goodwin, William, Adrian Linacre, and Sibte Hadi. *An Introduction to Forensic Genetics.* 2nd ed. Oxford: Wiley-Blackwell, 2011. Print.

Lasarow, Avi. *Who Is Really Who? The Comprehensive Guide to DNA Paternity Testing.* London: Blake, 2006. Print.

Rothstein, Mark A., et al., eds. *Genetic Ties and the Family: The Impact of Paternity Testing on Parents and Children.* Baltimore: Johns Hopkins UP, 2005. Print.

Shewale, Jaiprakash G., and Ray H. Liu. *Forensic DNA Analysis: Current Practices and Emerging Technologies.* Boca Raton: CRC Press, 2014. Print.

Sonenstein, Freya L., Pamela A. Holcomb, and Kristin S. Seefeldt. *Promising Approaches to Improving Paternity Establishment Rates at the Local Level.* Washington, DC: Urban Inst., 1993. Print.

Weir, Bruce S. *Human Identification: The Use of DNA Markers.* New York: Kluwer, 1995. Print.

See also: DNA fingerprinting; Forensic genetics; Repetitive DNA

Pattern baldness

CATEGORY: Diseases and syndromes
ALSO KNOWN AS: Male pattern baldness; MPB; androgenetic alopecia

DEFINITION

Pattern baldness, or androgenetic alopecia, refers to the most common form of scalp hair loss. Male pattern baldness follows a typical progression that begins with mild frontal hairline recession, developing to more noticeable frontal hair loss and vertex loss. Female hair loss does not typically follow this same pattern and may have a different underlying etiology.

RISK FACTORS

The three main risk factors for pattern baldness are male gender, age, and family history. Early-onset baldness is almost entirely dependent on genetic predisposition. By middle age, more than half of the male population will have some degree of pattern baldness. By age eighty, more than 80 percent of men will have pattern baldness. The incidence is much lower in females.

ETIOLOGY AND GENETICS

Anecdotally, pattern baldness is often described as being autosomal dominant or X-linked in inheritance. In reality, opulation studies and genetic research suggest that male pattern baldness is a complex, multifactorial condition. A combination of both genetic predisposition and environmental factors leads to an individual's risk for baldness.

The environmental factors involved in baldness development are poorly defined and appear to be significantly less influential than genetic factors. Preliminary studies of multiple different environmental exposures and influences have yet to find a significant association to male-pattern baldness.

While genetic predisposition to baldness appears to be the strongest risk factor, researchers are still identifying the genes involved. Pattern baldness is androgen-dependent, and therefore, early investigations into the genetics of baldness relied on the candidate gene approach, focusing on genes involved in the sex steroid pathway. The 5 alpha-reductase, aromatase,

Bald head Smobserver at en.wikipedia, from Wikimedia Commons

and androgen receptor genes have all been investigated, with only the androgen receptor (*AR*) gene *AR* gene showing a clear association with pattern baldness.

The androgen receptor gene is approximately 90 kilobases (kb) long and is located on the X chromosome. Mutations in this gene have been associated with other genetic conditions, but research has not found a specific mutation or functional alteration in men with pattern baldness. Different polymorphisms in the *AR* gene have been investigated but not confirmed. Current research is focusing on the regulatory regions of the gene, splicing variants, or other epigenetic factors in an attempt to identify specific genetic changes involved in baldness predisposition. *AR* has been postulated to be the primary genetic factor in the development of early-onset pattern baldness, possibly accounting for up to 40 percent of the total genetic risk.

While other genes in the sex-steroid pathway have not shown a significant association to pattern baldness in previous studies, new technologies and considerations warrant further investigation into these candidate genes. Male-pattern baldness has been associated with coronary heart disease, disorders of insulin resistance, and prostate cancer. Investigation of genes involved in these conditions may lead to further identification of predisposition genes.

Genome-wide association studies (GWAS) have yielded new susceptibility variants for pattern baldness. A locus on chromosome 20p11 has shown significant association with male-pattern baldness, and was identified by this method. This locus appears to have a strong influence on the development of

Male pattern baldness By Originally uploaded by Lkinkade (Transferred by XenonX3) (Originally uploaded on en.wikipedia), via Wikimedia Commons

early-onset hair loss, and does not show an association to the androgen pathway. Additionally, another locus at chromosome 3q26 has been identified and is being investigated. In discovering more about these loci, additional information about the molecular basis for hair loss will be gained. Ultimately, this may lead to improved treatments, and advance the molecular understanding of the complex diseases that have been associated with pattern baldness.

SYMPTOMS

The degree of male-pattern baldness is defined by the Hamilton-Norwood baldness scale, which contains seven distinct categories of hair loss. As baldness progresses, the hair in the affected region becomes shorter, finer, and less pigmented. Ultimately, the hair follicle is incapable of producing a noticeable hair, rendering the area bald.

SCREENING AND DIAGNOSIS

The diagnosis of male-pattern baldness is made by clinical assessment of scalp hair loss. As female scalp hair loss does not typically follow the same pattern as males, the diagnosis cannot be made by the degrees defined by the Hamilton-Norwood baldness scale. Genetic testing for a predisposition to baldness is being developed.

TREATMENT AND THERAPY

Current treatments for hair loss mainly involve medications that were originally intended for other uses but found to have hair growth as a side effect. The best-known treatment, minoxidil, was originally prescribed for hypertension. Its mechanism for stimulation of hair growth is unknown, but as with other similar medications, it is not curative. Other medications that inhibit the actions of 5 alpha-reductase have also been effective and are the basis of future studies.

Ideally, a more complete understanding of an individual's personal predisposition to hair loss, and the molecular pathways involved, will allow for a more targeted approach to treatment.

PREVENTION AND OUTCOMES

There are no known preventive measures for male-pattern baldness.

FURTHER READING

Chin, Evelyn Y. "Androgenetic Alopecia (Male Pattern Hair Loss) in the United States: What Treatments Should Primary Care Providers Recommend?" *Journal of the American Association of Nurse Practitioners* 25.8 (2013): 395–401. *Academic Search Alumni Edition*. Web. 7 Aug. 2014.

Ellis, Justine A., and Stephen B. Harrap. "The Genetics of Androgenetic Alopecia." *Clinical Dermatology* 19 (2001): 149–54. Print

Ellis, Justine A., and Rodney D. Sinclair. "Male Pattern Baldness: Current Treatments, Future Prospects." *Drug Discovery Today* 13 (2008): 791–97. Print.

Haupt, Angela. "What Causes Hair Loss? Nine Myths about Baldness." *US News and World Report—Health*. US News and World Report, 22 Feb. 2011. Web. 7 Aug. 2014.

Hillmer, Axel M., et al. "Genetic Variation in the Human Androgen Receptor Gene Is the Major Determinant of Common Early-Onset Androgenetic Alopecia." *American Journal of Human Genetics* 77 (2005): 140–48. Print.

Judd, Sandra J. *Men's Health Concerns Sourcebook*. 4th ed. Detroit: Omnigraphics, 2013. Digital file.

Yamada, Tomohide, et al. "Male Pattern Baldness and Its Association with Coronary Heart Disease: A Meta-Analysis." *BMJ Open* 3.4 (2013): *MEDLINE Complete*. Web. 7 Aug. 2014.

See also: Albinism; Chediak-Higashi syndrome; Epidermolytic hyperkeratosis; Hermansky-Pudlak syndrome; Ichthyosis; Melanoma; Palmoplantar keratoderma.

Pearson syndrome

CATEGORY: Diseases and syndromes
ALSO KNOWN AS: Pearson's syndrome; Pearson's disease; Pearson's marrow-pancreas syndrome

DEFINITION

Pearson syndrome—named for Howard Pearson, a pediatric hematologist oncologist—is a rare, generally fatal disorder of infancy that affects the hematopoietic system (the bone marrow functions that produce red blood cells, white blood cells, and platelets) and exocrine pancreas, with vari able kidney, liver, and endocrine failure. Pearson syndrome is commonly caused by mitochondrial DNA (mtDNA) deletions or duplications, with high levels of heteroplasmy (proportion of mutant mitochondrial genomes) in the affected tissues.

Risk Factors

There are no specific risk factors for mtDNA de letions, which usually arise de novo, either in the oocyte or early in embryogenesis. There is no race or sex specific association for Pearson syndrome. Siblings of affected individuals are rarely affected. Males do not transmit mitochondrial disease, while affected females occasionally transmit mtDNA dele tions.

Etiology and Genetics

Mitochondria are the cell's energy-producing organelles. They contain hundreds to thousands of copies of mtDNA, a small double-stranded circular genome that encodes thirteen subunits of respira tory chain enzymes and part of the protein synthetic machinery necessary to translate these mitochondrial transcripts, two ribosomal RNA genes, and twenty-two transfer RNA genes. Pearson syndrome is caused by deletions or, less commonly, duplica tions/rearrangements of mtDNA. Depending on their size, mtDNA deletions can disrupt protein coding sequences or decrease their expression by removing rRNA and tRNA genes. The proportion of deleted mitochondrial genomes varies between tis sues and can change over time. When heteroplasmy levels reach a critical threshold, oxidative metabo lism is impaired and cells experience an energy defi cit. Abnormal iron metabolism also occurs in Pearson syndrome, which may contribute to cellular damage.

An important feature of different diseases involving mtDNA mutations is that, depending on the level of heteroplasmy and/ or tissue-specific factors, a single mutation can cause different multisystemic disorders. MtDNA de letions are associated with three overlapping syn dromes, with a general correspondence between the level of heteroplasmy and the affected tissue. Pearson syndrome primarily involves bone marrow and exocrine pancreas, but rare survivors may accu mulate mtDNA deletions as the mitochondrial ge nome rep licates in nerve and muscle, leading to Kearns-Sayre syndrome or progressive external oph thalmoplegia (paralysis of extraocular eye muscle).

Most mitochondrial diseases show maternal in heritance because mtDNA is transmitted exclusively in oocytes. However, mitochondrial DNA deletion syndromes (like Pearson syndrome) usually occur sporadically. In rare inherited cases, mtDNA deletions are transmitted maternally, but the mother is usually affected with a later onset syndrome that involves other tissues, such as Kearns-Sayre syndrome.

Symptoms

An affected newborn may be pale from birth, and birth weight may be low with poor subsequent weight gain. An infant may have had previous illnesses or hospitalizations that may have included episodes of anorexia, vomiting, fever, and lethargy in association with electrolytic abnormalities, lactic acidosis, and hepatic dysfunction.

Development may be abnormal with the presence of neuromuscular abnormalities such as tremor, abnormal tone, and lethargy.

Neutrophils public domain via wikimedia commons

Pancreas and related structures model. Showing the (on the ante rios side) duodenum, duct of Wirsung and the spleen By Süleyman Habib 04:02, 19 April 2007 (UTC) (Own work), via Wikim

The major organ problems in those with Pearson syndrome are bone marrow failure resulting in pancytopenia (reduced number of red and white blood cells and platelets) and exocrine pancreas dysfunction (problems with digestive enzymes, leading to chronic diarrhea and malabsorption). Typically sideroblastic anemia occurs despite the presence of sufficient iron (sideroblasts are nucleated erythrocytes with cytoplasmic iron granules because they cannot incorporate iron into hemoglobin). Often the patient is transfusion-dependent. Defective oxidative phosphorylation leads to lactic acidemia, which can be persistent or intermittent. The liver and kidneys are variably affected.

Symptoms begin during infancy and early childhood. Parents notice paleness due to anemia, chronic diarrhea and fatty stools, and failure to thrive. Death is usually caused from sepsis, hepatic failure, or metabolic crisis.

SCREENING AND DIAGNOSIS

A background history may be helpful in raising suspicion about the presence of this rare disease. It is important to note a history of medication exposure that may have included contact with drugs that may have damaged the bone marrow. Family history of unexplained pancytopenia, failure to thrive, acidosis, pancreatic insufficiency, neuromuscular dysfunction, or early death are important to document.

In Pearson syndrome, mtDNA deletions are usually more common in blood than in muscle. However, a bone marrow biopsy is the most reliable mechanism for diagnosis, because less-involved tissues may have lower levels of heteroplasmy that can reduce the chance of detection. Although the junction-fragment created by an mtDNA deletion can be detected by poly-merase chain reaction (PCR), deletions occur in normal individuals as part of the aging process, and PCR tests can thus give false positive results; Southern blot analysis is preferred. Molecular genetic analysis may be recommended and is usually performed on blood isolated before transfusions to avoid false negative results caused by dilution of the patient's abnormal blood with transfused donor blood.

The following lab tests may also be recommended: Complete blood count; tests of pancreatic function; Urinalysis; Serum Lactic Acid; Liver enzymes; and endocrinologic studies as some have deficiencies of thyroid, parathyroid, and/or growth hormone.

TREATMENT AND THERAPY

There is no specific therapy, but individual symptoms have corresponding treatments: infection (antibiotics), metabolic acidosis (bicarbonate supplements or dichloracetic acid, DCA, which can be neurotoxic), pancytopenia (transfusions, with erythropoietin to possibly decrease their frequency), neutropenia (granulocyte colony-stimulating factor), and malabsorption (pancreatic enzyme replacement and vitamins). Supplementation with fat-soluble vitamins (ADEK) may also be needed. Other endocrine imbalances are treated with the appropriate hormones. One study suggests that high carbohydrate diets should be avoided, as those diets may stress the liver. Transplantation is not effective due to the multisystemic nature of the disease.

PREVENTION AND OUTCOMES

Pearson syndrome is usually sporadic. Prenatal screening for females with mtDNA deletions is problematic because of unknown levels of heteroplasmy in untested fetal tissues. Pearson syndrome is usually fatal in childhood (before age 4 years), but survivors may develop Kearns-Sayre syndrome and should be monitored for abnormalities in cardiac and muscle function.

Toni R. Prezant, Ph.D.; updated by
Gary M. Flashner, M.S., M.D.

FURTHER READING

Bernes, S. M., et al. "Identical Mitochondrial DNA Deletion in Mother with Progressive External Ophthalmoplegia and Son with Pearson Marrow Pancreas Syndrome." *Journal of Pediatrics* 123 (1993): 598–602. Demonstration of identical mtDNA deletion with different clinical outcomes.

Rotig, A., et al. "Pearson's Marrow-Pancreas Syndrome: A Multisystem Mitochondrial Disorder in Infancy." *The Journal of Clinical Investigation* 86 (1990): 1601–1608. A technical investigation that identifies the pathogenic mechanism in five infants with Pearson syndrome.

Van den Ouweland, J. M. W., et al. "Characterization of a Novel Mitochondrial DNA Deletion in a Patient with a Variant of the Pearson Marrow Pancreas Syndrome." *European Journal of Human Genetics* 8 (2000): 195–203. A patient with multisystemic disease that resembles Pearson syndrome, but without pancreas involvement, has a similar genetic cause.

Williams TB, Daniels M, Puthenveetil G, Chang R, Wang RY, Abdenur JE. Pearson syndrome: unique endocrine manifestations including neonatal diabetes and adrenal insufficiency. *Mol Genet Metab.* 2012 May. 106(1):104–7.

Crippa BL, Leon E, Calhoun A, Lowichik A, Pasquali M, Longo N. Biochemical abnormalities in Pearson syndrome. *Am J Med Genet A.* 2015 Mar. 167A (3):621–8.

Baertling F, Meissner T, Troeger A, Pillekamp F, Mayatepek E, Laws HJ, et al. Granulocyte colony stimulating factor for treatment of neutropenia-associated infection in Pearson syndrome. *Klin Padiatr.* 2014 May. 226(3):190–1.

WEB SITES OF INTEREST

eMedicine Pediatrics: Pearson Syndrome (Charles Quinn)
http://emedicine.medscape.com/article/957186-print

GeneReviews: Mitochondrial DNA Deletion Syndromes
http://www.ncbi.nlm.nih.gov/bookshelf/br.fcgi?book=gene&part=kss

Online Mendelian Inheritance in Man: Pearson Marrow Pancreas Syndrome
http://www.ncbi.nlm.nih.gov/entrez/dispomim.cgi?id=557000

https://rarediseases.info.nih.gov/diseases/7343/pearson-syndrome

http://emedicine.medscape.com/article/957186-overview

See also: Adrenomyelopathy; Androgen insensitivity syndrome; Autoimmune polyglandular syndrome; Congenital hypothyroidism; Diabetes insipidus; Graves' disease; Obesity; Pancreatic cancer; Pancreatitis; Steroid hormones.

Pedigree analysis

CATEGORY: Population genetics; Techniques and methodologies

SIGNIFICANCE: Charts called pedigrees are used to represent the members of a family and to indicate which individuals have particular inherited traits. A pedigree is built of shapes connected by lines to indicate relationships. Pedigrees are used by genetic counselors to help families determine the risk of genetic disease and by research scientists to study how particular traits are inherited.

KEY TERMS

alleles: alternate forms of a gene locus, some of which may cause disease

autosomal trait: a trait that typically appears just as frequently in either sex because an autosomal chromosome, rather than a sex chromosome, carries the gene

dominant allele: an allele that is expressed even when only one copy (instead of two) is present *hemizygous*: male humans are considered to be hemizygous for X-linked traits, because they have only one copy of X-linked genes

heterozygous carriers: individuals who have one copy of a particular recessive allele that is expressed only when present in two copies

homozygote: an organism that has identical alleles at the same locus

recessive allele: an allele that is expressed only when there are two copies present

X-linked trait: a trait caused by a gene carried on the X chromosome, which has different patterns of inheritance in females and males because females have two X chromosomes while males have only one

OVERVIEW AND DEFINITION

Pedigree analysis involves the construction of family trees that can be used to trace inheritance of a trait over several generations. It is a graphical representation of the appearance of a particular trait or disease in related individuals, along with the nature of the relationships.

Standardized symbols are used in pedigree charts. Male individuals are designated by squares, and female individuals by circles. The symbols representing individuals affected by a trait are shaded, while those for unaffected individuals are not. Heterozygous carriers are indicated by shading of half of the symbol, and carriers of X-linked recessive traits have a dot in the middle of the symbol. Matings are indicated by horizontal lines linking the mated individuals. Offspring of the mated individuals are linked to their parents by a vertical line intersecting with the horizontal mating line.

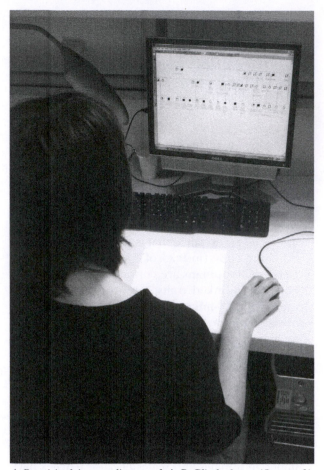

A Geneticist doing a pedigree analysis By Plindenbaum (Own work), via Wikimedia Commons

The classic way to determine the mode of inheritance of a trait in animals is to conduct experimental matings of large numbers of individuals. Such experimental matings between humans are neither ethical nor feasible, so it is necessary to infer the mode of inheritance of traits in humans through the use of pedigrees. Large families with good historical records are the easiest to analyze. Once a pedigree is established, it can be used to determine the likely mode of inheritance of a particular trait and, if the mode of inheritance can be determined with certainty, to determine the risk of the trait appearing in offspring.

TYPICAL PEDIGREES

There are four common modes of inheritance that can be detected using pedigree analysis: autosomal dominant, autosomal recessive, X-linked dominant, and X-linked recessive. Autosomal traits are governed by genes found on one of the autosomes (chromosomes 1–22), while the genes that cause X-linked traits are found on the X chromosome. Males and females are equally likely to be affected by autosomal traits, whereas X-linked traits are never passed on from father to son but can be passed from father to daughter, and all affected males in a family received the mutant allele from their mothers.

The pattern of autosomal dominant inheritance is perhaps the easiest type of Mendelian inheritance to recognize in a pedigree. A trait that appears in successive generations and is found only among offspring when at least one of the parents is affected is normally due to a dominant allele.

If neither parent has the characteristic phenotype displayed by the child, the trait is recessive. For recessive traits, on average, the recurrence risk to the unborn sibling of an affected individual is one in four. The majority of X-linked traits are recessive. The hallmark of X-linked recessive inheritance is that males are much more likely to be affected than females, because males are hemizygous—that is, they possess only one X chromosome, while females have two X chromosomes. Therefore, a recessive trait on the X chromosome will be expressed in all males who possess that X chromosome, while females with one affected X chromosome will be asymptomatic carriers unless their other X chromosome also carries the recessive trait.

X-linked dominant traits are rare but distinctive. If a male is affected and a female is unaffected, all of the pair's daughters will be affected, and none of their sons will be. If the female is affected and the male is not, their risk of having an affected child is one in two, regardless of the sex of the child. In the general population, females are more likely to be affected than males, but males are usually more severely affected, and the trait may be lethal in males.

USEFULNESS

Pedigrees are important both for helping families identify the risk of transmitting an inherited disease and as starting points for researchers in identifying the genes responsible for inherited diseases. Mendelian ratios do not apply in individual human families because of the small size. Pooling of families is possible.

However, even using large, carefully constructed records, pedigrees can be difficult to construct and interpret for several reasons. Tracing family relationships can be complicated by adoption, children born out of wedlock, and assisted reproductive technologies that result in children who may not be genetically related to their parents. Additionally, people are sometimes hesitant to supply information because they are embarrassed by genetic conditions.

Many traits do not follow clear-cut Mendelian ratios. There are numerous extensions and exceptions to Mendel's laws that can confound efforts to develop a useful pedigree. In diseases with variable expressivity, some of the symptoms of the disease are always expressed but may range from very mild to severe. In autosomal dominant diseases with incomplete penetrance, some individuals who possess the dominant allele may not express the disease phenotype at all. Some traits have a high recurrent mutation rate. An example is achondroplasia, in which 85 percent of cases are due to new mutations in offspring whose parents both have normal phenotypes. Traits due to multifactorial inheritance have variable expression as a result of the involved genes' interactions with the environment. Early-acting lethal alleles can lead to embryonic death and a resulting dearth of expected affected individuals. Pleiotropy, which refers to a situation in which a single gene controls several functions and therefore has several effects, can result in different symptoms in different affected individuals. Finally, one trait can have a different basis of inheritance in different families. For example, mutations in any one of more than four hundred different genes can result in hereditary deafness.

MODERN APPLICATIONS

Genetic counseling is one of the key areas in which pedigrees are employed. A genetic counseling session usually begins with the counselor taking a family history and sketching a pedigree with paper and pencil, followed by use of a computer program to create an accurate pedigree. The Human Genome Project has greatly increased the number of genetic disorders that can be detected by heterozygote and prenatal screening. A large part of the genetic counselor's job is to determine which, if any, specific genetic tests are appropriate for whom.

Although genetic tests for many disorders are now available, the genes involved in many others have yet to be identified. Therefore, most human gene mapping utilizes molecular DNA markers, which reflect variation at noncoding regions of the DNA near the affected gene, rather than biochemical, morphological, or behavioral traits. A DNA marker is a piece of DNA of known size, representing a specific locus, that comes in identifiable variations. These allelic variations segregate according to Mendel's laws, which means it is possible to follow their transmission as one would any gene's transmission. If a particular allelic variant of the DNA marker is found in individuals with a particular phenotype, the DNA marker can be used to develop a pedigree. The DNA from all available family members is examined, and the pedigree is constructed using the presence of the DNA marker rather than phenotypic categories. This method is particularly useful for late-onset diseases such as Huntington's disease, as affected individuals may not know they carry the deleterious allele until they are in their forties or fifties, well past reproductive years. Although using DNA markers is a powerful method, crossover in the chromosome between the marker and the gene can cause an individual to be normal but still have the marker that suggests presence of the mutant allele. Thus, for all genetic tests there is a small percentage of false positive and false negative results, which must be factored into the advice given during genetic counseling.

FURTHER READING

Bennett, Robin L. *The Practical Guide to the Genetic Family History.* 2nd ed. Hoboken: Wiley, 2010. Print.

Bennett, Robin L., et al. "Recommendations for Standardized Human Pedigree Nomenclature." *American Journal of Human Genetics* 56.3 (1995): 745–52. *PubMed Central.* Web. 21 Jan. 2016.

Cummings, Anna C., et al. "Evaluating Power and Type 1 Error in Large Pedigree Analyses of Binary Traits." *PLOS ONE* 8.5 (2013): n. pag. *Academic Search Complete.* Web. 21 Jan. 2016.

Cummings, Michael R. *Human Heredity: Principles and Issues.* 10th ed. Belmont: Brooks, 2014. Print.

Powell, Joseph E., et al. "Congruence of Additive and Non-Additive Effects on Gene Expression Estimated from Pedigree and SNP Data." *PLOS Genetics* 9.5 (2013): n. pag. *Academic Search Complete.* Web. 21 Jan. 2016.

Thompson, James N., Jr., et al. *Primer of Genetic Analysis: A Problems Approach.* 3rd ed. New York: Cambridge UP, 2007. Print.

Wolff, G., T. F. Wienker, and H. Sander. "On the Genetics of Mandibular Prognathism: Analysis of Large European Noble Families." *Journal of Medical Genetics* 30.2 (1993): 112–16. *MEDLINE Complete.* Web. 21 Jan. 2016.

Pelizaeus-Merzbacher disease

CATEGORY: Diseases and syndromes

ALSO KNOWN AS: Pelizaeus Merzbacher brain sclerosis; sudanophilic leukodystrophy; Cockayne-Pelizaeus-Merzbacher disease; PMD

Overview of Nervous System By OpenStax College, via Wikimedia Commons

DEFINITION

Pelizaeus-Merzbacher disease (PMD) is an X-linked neurological disorder caused by mutation or duplication of the proteolipid protein gene (*PLP1*) and characterized by dysmyelination, resulting in permanent hypomyelination or lack of the myelin sheath, the fatty covering of nerve cells.

RISK FACTORS

PMD occurs in 1 out of every 200,000 to 500,000 male newborns in the United States. It is an X-linked disorder, predominantly affecting males who inherit it from their mothers, who are carriers. The condition rarely affects females. For females who carry the *PLP1* gene, there is a 50 percent risk of passing it on with every pregnancy—sons have a 50 percent chance of inheriting the gene and having PMD, while daughters are at a 50 percent risk of being carriers. Genetic counseling and in utero testing are advised for those with a family history.

ETIOLOGY AND GENETICS

PMD is one of the leukodystrophies, a group of inherited and progressive metabolic diseases affecting myelination of the nervous system and the development of white matter in the brain. Each disorder has a separate gene abnormality that affects a different enzyme (protein). In PMD, the defect is in the *PLP1* gene, caused by a point mutation (substitution of a single AT or GC base), which results in misfolding of the proteolipid protein 1 and DM20 protein, or a duplication of the entire gene, causing overexpression of the protein. These mutant proteins are toxic to the oligodendrocyte cells that make myelin.

Myelin constitutes the myelin sheath, which is a fatty covering surrounding axons in the central and peripheral nervous systems and acts as an electrical insulator, allowing impulses to be transmitted quickly along the nerve cells. Without myelin, impulses leak out and nerves cannot function normally. Normal myelination is a step-by-step, ordered process that begins at about five months gestation and continues until a child is two to three years old. In PMD, myelin simply never develops, resulting in permanent hypomyelination and axonal degeneration, primarily in the subcortical region of the cerebrum, cerebellum, and/or brain stem. This prevents impulses from being transmitted from neuron to neuron and causes a range of neurological and motor dysfunctions. It is now known that duplication of the *PLP1* gene accounts for 50 to 75 percent of PMD cases.

The gene encoding the PLP protein is located on the long arm of the X chromosome at band Xq22 and is about 17 kilobases in size, consisting of seven exons and six introns. Two transcript variants encoding distinct isoforms (Isoform 1 and Isoform DM-20) have been identified. The normal PLP protein is a four-transmembrane domain structure that correlates well with one exon of the gene, except at the C terminal end, and binds strongly to other copies of itself.

Many mutations in the *PLP1* gene have been reported. Molecular analysis of the gene revealed a variety of mutations, deletions, and duplications, including two mutations in the 5 untranslated region, missense mutations in exon 2, and an A-to-T transition in exon 4 leading to an Asp-to-Val substitution at residue 202. Exonic mutations tend to be more severe than simple point mutations. Forms of the disorder include the classical X-linked PMD, a severe acute infantile (connatal) PMD, and an autosomal dominant late-onset PMD.

White matter By OpenStax College, via Wikimedia Commons

SYMPTOMS

Symptoms of PMD are typically progressive and can appear in the first year of life. In the case of connatal PMD, symptoms can begin in infancy. The first symptom in infants is usually involuntary oscillatory movements of the eyes (nystagmus) and may be concomitant with labored and noisy breathing (stridor) and lack of muscle tone/floppiness (hypotonia). Involuntary muscle spasms (spasticity) and associated muscle and joint stiffness develop. With time, other symptoms become evident, such as impaired ability to coordinate movement (ataxia), developmental delays, loss of motor function and head/trunk control, and deterioration of intellectual abilities.

SCREENING AND DIAGNOSIS

DNA-based testing can be used to diagnose PMD in symptomatic patients, as well as in utero, and to determine carrier status in family members. Identification of pathologic mutations and copies of the *PLP1* gene is the definitive test, using sequence analysis and quantitative polymerase chain reaction (PCR) or fluorescence in situ hybridization (FISH) methods, respectively. Pathological signs of dysmyelination can be examined using magnetic resonance imaging (MRI), once a child is one to two years old when white matter pathways in the brain are maturing and hypomyelination can be detected.

TREATMENT AND THERAPY

PMD cannot be cured and there is no effective treatment. Currently, treatment is symptomatic and supportive, but medications are available to alleviate stiffness or spasticity and to control seizures. Cell-based therapies are being investigated, including transplantation of a functioning neuregulin gene into unmyelinated nerve cells, which may reprogram cells to produce myelin and the use of human adult-derived glial progenitor cells as vectors.

PREVENTION AND OUTCOMES

There are no means of preventing PMD, but genetic counseling and testing isavailable for couples who have the *PLP1* gene mutation. The prognosis for patients with PMD varies by the severity of mutation and form of PMD, with survival as short as early childhood and as long as into the sixties.

FURTHER READING

Hannigan, Steve, and National Information Centre for Metabolic Diseases. *Inherited Metabolic Diseases: A Guide to 100 Conditions.* Abingdon: Radcliffe, 2007. Print.

Martenson, Russell. *Myelin—Biology and Chemistry.* New York: CRC, 1992. Print. Mori, Tatsuo, et al. "Age-Related Changes in a Patient with Pelizaeus-Merzbacher Disease Determined by Repeated 1H-Magnetic Resonance Spectroscopy." *Journal of Child Neurology* 29.2 (2014): 283–88. Print.

"Pelizaeus-Merzbacher Disease." *Genetics Home Reference.* National Library of Medicine, 4 Aug 2014. Web. 8 Aug. 2014. "*PLP1.*" *GeneticsHome Reference.* National Library of Medicine, 4 Aug. 2014. Web. 8 Aug. 2014.

Sims, Katherine B. *Handbook ofPediatric Neurology.* Philadelphia: Lippincott, 2014 Print.=Southwood, Cherie M., et al. "Potential for Cell-Mediated Immune Responses in Mouse Models of Pelizaeus-Merzbacher Disease." *Brain Sciences* 3.4 (2013): 1417–44. Print.

Swaiman, Kenneth F., Stephen Ashwal, Donna M. Ferriero, and Nina F. Schor. *Swaiman's Pediatric Neurology: Principles and Practice.* 5th ed. Edinburgh: Elsevier, 2012. Print.

Vinken, Pierre, G. W. Bruyn, Christopher Goetz, et al. *Neurodystrophies and Neurolipidoses.* Amsterdam: Elsevier Science, 1992. Print.

See also: Adrenoleukodystrophy; Alzheimer's disease; Alzheimer's disease; Amyotrophic lateral sclerosis; Arnold-Chiari syndrome; Ataxia telangiectasia; Canavan disease; Cerebrotendinous xanthomatosis; Charcot-Marie-Tooth syndrome; Chediak-Higashi syndrome; Dandy-Walker syndrome; Deafness; Epilepsy;

Essential tremor; Friedreich ataxia; Huntington's disease; Jansky-Bielschowsky disease; Joubert syndrome; Kennedy disease; Krabbé disease; Leigh syndrome; Leukodystrophy; Limb girdle muscular dystrophy; Maple syrup urine disease; Metachromatic leukodystrophy; Myoclonic epilepsy associated with ragged red fibers (MERRF); Narcolepsy; Nemaline myopathy; Neural tube defects; Neurofibromatosis; Parkinson disease; Prion diseases: Kuru and Creutzfeldt-Jakob syndrome; Spinal muscular atrophy; Vanishing white matter disease.

Pendred syndrome

CATEGORY: Diseases and syndromes

ALSO KNOWN AS: Autosomal recessive sensorineural hearing impairment and goiter; deafness with goiter; goiter-deafness syndrome; Pendred's syndrome

DEFINITION

Pendred syndrome (PS), first described by English physician Vaughan Pendred in 1896, is a genetic condition caused by mutations in the *SLC26A4* gene. PS is one of the most common forms of syndromic hearing loss, accounting for about 10 percent of all cases of hereditary hearing loss. PS is associated with developmental abnormalities of the innerear and is characterized by enlarged vestibular aqueducts (EVA) and severe to profound sensorineural

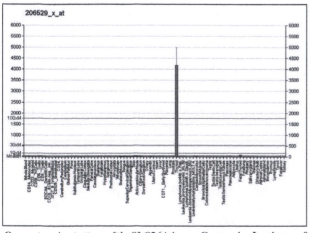

Gene expression pattern of the SLC26A4 gene. Genomics Institute of the Novartis Research Foundation, via Wikimedia Commons

hearing loss that is evident at birth. Individuals with PS may also have cochlea malformations (Mondini dysplasia) and goiter (enlarged thyroid gland), which typically forms between late childhood and early adulthood.

RISK FACTORS

There are no reported factors associated with an increased risk for having achild with PS; it is diagnosed in both males and females and in all ethnicities. The exact prevalence for PS is unknown.

ETIOLOGY AND GENETICS 50 PERCENT

PS is associated with mutations in the *SLC26A4* gene located on the long arm of chromosome 7 (7q21-34) and is inherited in an autosomal recessivemanner, in which a condition has to be inherited by both parents. A person who has one working gene and one nonworking gene is referred to as a carrier. A carrier is unaffected by the condition. However, when two carriers of the same nonworking gene have children, they have a 25 percent chance of both passing on the nonworking gene and thus, of having a child affected with the condition. This is also a 75 percent chance with each pregnancy that the child will not have PS. If one parent has PS, the chance of having an affected child depends upon the carrier status of the other parent. If both parents have PS, every child born will also have PS. *SLC26A4*, a member of the solute carrier 26 gene family, codes for the protein pendrin. Pendrin is involved in the transport of chloride, iodide, and bicarbonate ions into and out of cells, which is important for the normal function of the inner ear and thyroid. Ion transport is disrupted when *SLC26A4* mutations alter the function or structure of pendrin. Currently more than sixty mutations have been reported. Mutations in *SLC26A4* are also associated with nonsyndromic enlarged vestibular aqueduct (DFNB4). DFNB4 is similar to PS, but thyroid abnormalities are not associated with it.

Genetic testing is available for individuals suspected of having PS However only 50 percent of individuals from families where multiple people are affected have a mutation identified. Families with only one individual affected have approximately a 20 percent chance of gene detection. Therefore PS is likely a genetically heterogeneous condition (caused by more than one gene).

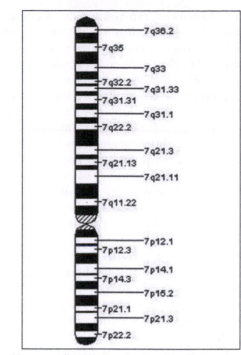

7q36.2
7q35
7q33
7q32.2
7q31.33
7q31.31
7q31.1
7q22.2
7q21.3
7q21.13
7q21.11
7q11.22
7p12.1
7p12.3
7p14.1
7p14.3
7p15.2
7p21.1
7p21.3
7p22.2

Human Chromosom 7 public domain via wikimedia commons

SYMPTOMS

PS is characterized by bilateral, severe to profound sensorineural hearing loss. Although mild-to-moderate and progressive hearing loss has been reported, hearing loss is usually nonprogressive and congenital. Individuals with PS have inner ear abnormalities of the temporal bones. In fact, more than 60 percent of individuals have bilateral enlarged vestibular aqueducts (EVA). Approximately 75 percent of individuals have evidence of goiter on clinical examination. In approximately 40 percent the goiter develops in late childhood or early puberty and for 60 percent in early adult life. There is significant interfamilial and intrafamilial variability.

SCREENING AND DIAGNOSIS

A clinical diagnosis is given to individuals with sensorineural hearing loss, bilateral enlarged vestibular aqueducts, and either a goiter or an abnormal perchlorate discharge test (a test to determine if the thyroid is working properly). Molecular genetic testing is available clinically to confirm the diagnosis if PS is suspected, to clarify risks for family members, and for prenatal diagnosis. Population screening for PS is not available.

TREATMENT AND THERAPY

There is no cure for PS. However, benefits are gained from early detection and treatment with hearing aids or cochlear implants and speech and language therapy. EVA may cause increased intracranial pressure that can cause a decline in hearing; therefore activities such as weightlifting, contact sports, and scuba diving should be avoided, and head protection for activities such as bicycling should be encouraged. The abnormal thyroid function should be treated in the standard manner. For optimal care, patients should see a variety of specialists, including a clinical geneticist, genetic counselors, otolaryngologists, audiologists, speech-language pathologists, and an endocrinologist.

PREVENTION AND OUTCOMES

Genetic counseling should be made available for individuals with personal or family histories. Prenatal or preimplantation genetic diagnosis is available if the cause is known. Most individuals with PS have normal intelligence and life expectancies.

FURTHER READING

Kochhar, A., M. S. Hildebrand, and R. J. H. Smith. "Clinical Aspects of Hereditary Hearing Loss." *Genetics in Medicine* 9 (2007): 393–409. Print.

Kontorinis, Georgios, et al. "Cochlear Implantation in Pendred Syndrome." *Cochlear Implants International. An Interdisciplinary Journal* 12.3 (2011): 157–63. *EBSCO Academic Search Complete.* Web. 11 Aug. 2014.

Landa, Priya, et al. "Lack of Significant Association between Mutations of *KCNJ10* or *FOXI1* and *SLC26A4* Mutations in Pendred Syndrome/ Enlarged Vestibular Aqueducts." *BMC Medical Genetics* 14.1 (2013): 1–7. *EBSCO Academi-c Search Complete.* Web. 11 Aug. 2014.

Ladsous, Miriam, et al. "Analysis of the Thyroid Phenotype in 42 Patients with Pendred Syndrome and Nonsyndromic Enlargement of the Vestibular Aqueduct." *Thyroid* 24.4 (2014): 639–48. *EBSCO Academic Search Complete.* Web. 11 Aug. 2014.

Maciaszczyk, K., and A. Lewinski. Phenotypes of SLC26A4 Gene Mutations: "Pendred Syndrome and Hypoacusis with Enlarged Vestibular Aqueduct." *Neuroendocrinology Letters* 29.1 (2008): 29–36. Print "Pendred Syndrome." *Genetics Home Reference.* National Library of Medicine, 4 Aug. 2014. Web. 11 Aug. 2014.

"*SLC26A4.*" *Genetics Home Reference.* National Library of Medicine, 4 Aug. 2014. Web. 11 Aug. 2014.

See also: Adrenoleukodystrophy; Alexander disease; Alzheimer's disease; Amyotrophic lateral sclerosis; Arnold-Chiari syndrome; Ataxia telangiectasia; Canavan disease; Cerebrotendinous xanthomatosis; Charcot-Marie-Tooth syndrome; Chediak-Higashi syndrome; Dandy-Walker syndrome; Deafness; Epilepsy; Essential tremor; Friedreich ataxia; Huntington's disease; Jansky-Bielschowsky disease; Joubert syndrome; Kennedy disease; Krabbé disease; Leigh syndrome; Leukodystrophy; Limb girdle muscular dystrophy; Maple syrup urine disease; Metachromatic leukodystrophy; Myoclonic epilepsy associated with ragged red fibers (MERRF); Narcolepsy; Nemaline myopathy; Neural tube defects; Neurofibromatosis; Parkinson disease; Pelizaeus-Merzbacher disease; Prion diseases: Kuru and Creutzfeldt-Jakob syndrome; Spinal muscular atrophy; Vanishing white matter disease.

Penetrance

CATEGORY: Population genetics

SIGNIFICANCE: Penetrance is a measure of how frequently a specific genotype results in the same, predictable phenotype. Such variable expression of the same genotype is the result of different genetic backgrounds and the effects of variations in the environment. Geneticists desire 100 percent penetrance for desirable genes that offer disease resistance but reduced penetrance and low expressivity for others that may contribute to human diseases.

GENE EXPRESSION AND ENVIRONMENT

Gene expression results in a chemical product (protein) with a specific function. The genotype (genetic makeup, or gene) and environmental conditions determine the phenotype of an individual.

PENETRANCE AND EXPRESSIVITY

Gene expression is dependent upon environmental factors and may be modified, enhanced, silenced, and/or timed by the regulatory mechanisms of the cell in response to internal and external forces. A range of phenotypes can result from a genotype in response to different environments; the phenomenon is called "norms of reaction" or "phenotypic plasticity." Phenotypic plasticity represent the expression of phenotypic variability in individuals of a single genotype.

The question of which is more important in the formation of an organism, nature (genotype) or nurture (environment). Nature vs. nurture has been debated for centuries. The answer is that it depends. The genotype defines phenotypic potential. The environment works on the plasticity of expression to produce different phenotypes from similar genotypes.

Penetrance is the proportion of individuals with a specific genotype who display a defined phenotype. Some individuals may not express a gene if modifiers, epistatic genes, or suppressors are also present in the genome. Penetrance is the likelihood, or probability, that a condition or disease phenotype will, in fact, appear when a given genotype is present. If every person carrying a gene for a dominantly inherited disorder has the mutant phenotype, then the gene is said to have 100 percent penetrance. If only 30 percent of those carrying the mutant allele exhibit the mutant phenotype, the penetrance is 30 percent. Sometimes an individual with a certain genotype fails to express the expected phenotype, and then the allele is said to be nonpenetrant in the individual. If the phenotype is expressed to any degree, the genotype is penetrant.

Given a particular phenotypic trait and a genotype, penetrance can be expressed as the probability of the phenotype given the genotype. For example, penetrance can be the probability of round seeds, a phenotype, given the genotype G; it can also be the probability of wrinkled seeds, another phenotype, given the genotype G. One could label the specific phenotype of interest as P_{ii} (Pi might refer to either the round or wrinkled seeds) and the specific genotype among many possibilities as G_j. The penetrance would then be the probability of P_{ii} given G_j. These penetrances can all be expressed using the mathematical notation of conditional probabilities as follows:

Case 1: $\Pr(\text{round}|G)$
Case 2: $\Pr(\text{wrinkled}|G)$
Case 3: $\Pr(P_{ii}|Gj)$

A 100 percent penetrance means that all individuals who possess a particular genotype express the phenotype (common in all homozygous lethal genes). Tay-Sachs disease shows complete, or 100 percent,

It is transmitted by an autosomal dominant gene with complete penetrance and variable expressivity, affecting males and females equally. By Herbert L. Fred, MD, Hendrik A. van Dijk (http://cnx.org/content/m15026/latest/), via Wikimedia Commons

These mice developed bilateral retinoblastoma with 100% penetrance and a short latency See page for author, via Wikimedia Commons

penetrance, as all homozygotes for this allele develop the disease and die.

An allele, *Fu*, in mice causes fusion in the tail in heterozygotes, *Fufu*, and extremely fused and abnormal tails in the homozygotes, *FuFu*. From testcross matings of *Fufu* × *fufu*, 87 fused-tailed mice and 129 nonfused-tailed mice resulted. Genetic analyses of the 129 nonfused-tailed mice revealed that 22 were genotypically *Fufu*. The number of fused-tailed mice was 87 and the number of mice with the *Fufu* genotype but nonfused tails was 22. The total number of fused-tailed mice expected was (87 + 22) = 109. Therefore, penetrance was calculated at 87/109 = 0.798

EXPRESSIVITY

Whereas penetrance describes the frequency with which a genotype is expressed as a specified phenotype, expressivity describes the range of variation in the phenotype when expression is observed. Expressivity is variation in allelic expression when the allele is penetrant. Not all traits are expressed 100 percent of the time even though the allele is present. Expressivity is the range of variation in a phenotype; it refers to the degree of expression of a given trait or combination of traits that is associated with a gene. Affected individuals may have severe or mild symptoms; they may have symptoms that show up in one organ or combination of organs in one individual but not in the same locations in other individuals.

Phenotype may be altered by heterogeneity of other genes that affect the expression of a particular locus in question, or by environmental influence. Variable expressivity is a common feature of a variety of cancers. The lower the penetrance, the fewer individuals will be affected. In humans, the dominant allele *P* produces polydactyly—extra toes and/or fingers. Matings between two normal appearing parents sometimes produce offspring with polydactyly. The parent with the *Pp* genotype exhibits reduced penetrance for the *P* allele.

Manjit S. Kang, Ph.D.

FURTHER READING

Fairbanks, Daniel J., and W. Ralph Anderson. *Genetics: The Continuity of Life.* New York: Brooks, 1999. Print.

Finegold, David N. "Inheritance of Single-Gene Disorders." *Merck Manual Home Health Handbook.* Merck, Aug. 2013. Web. 6 Aug. 2014.

Kang, Manjit S. "Using Genotype-by-Environment Interaction for Crop Cultivar Development." *Advances in Agronomy* 62 (1997): 199–252. Print.

Kang, Manjit S., and Hugh G. Gauch, Jr. *Genotype-by-Environment Interaction.* Boca Raton: CRC, 1996. Print.

Snustad, D. Peter, and Michael J. Simmons. "Gene Action: From Genotype to Phenotype." *Principles of Genetics.* 6th ed. Hoboken: Wiley, 2011. Print.

Strachan, Tom, and Andrew P. Read. "Complications to the Basic Mendelian Pedigree Patterns." *Human Molecular Genetics.* 4th ed. New York: Garland, 2010. Print.

See also: Hereditary diseases; Pedigree analysis.

Periodic paralysis syndrome

CATEGORY: Diseases and syndromes
ALSO KNOWN AS: Hypokalemic periodic paralysis; Hyperkalemic periodic paralysis; Andersen-Tawil syndrome; paraneoplastic periodic paralysis

DEFINITION

Familial periodic paralyses is a group of rare inherited conditions that cause occasional episodes of severe muscle weakness. These disorders are inherited and are usually associated with alterations in levels of blood potassium. The two most common types of periodic paralysis are hypokalemic and hyperkalemic. They sometimes include a type of muscle spasm called myotonia which is an inability to relax voluntary muscle after vigorous effort.

RISK FACTORS

Risk factors include a family history of periodic paralysis as well as identified genetic defects associated with the condition. In patients with hyperthyroid disease, periodic paralysis is a rare complication and can be life threatening. This specific type of periodic paralysis is most often found in young Asian males.

ETIOLOGY AND GENETICS

"Familial periodic paralyses" is a general term that refers to any of several rare genetic diseases, all of which are inherited as autosomal dominant disorders. This means that a single copy of the defective gene is sufficient to cause the disease, al though not all family members who carry the gene are affected to the same extent. An affected individual has a 50 percent chance of transmitting the mutation to each of his or her children. Many cases of periodic paralysis syndrome, however, re sult from a spontaneous new mutation, so in these instances affected individuals will have unaffected parents.

Mutations in at least four different genes are known to cause this syndrome. All these genes en code ion channel proteins, which form bridges across cell membranes to facilitate the movement of electrically charged ions, such as potassium, sodium, and calcium. Mutations can result in non functional or partially functioning ion channels that allow ions to leak in or out of muscle cells and result in the symptoms associated with the syndrome.

In hypokalemic periodic paralysis, potassium leaks into muscle cells from the blood. This condition is usually caused by two mutations of *CACNA1S* gene, R528H and R1239H. 25.3). Most cases of hyperkalemic PP are due to two mutations in *SCN4A*, *T704M*, and *M1592V.*, in which potassium leaks out of muscle cells.

A fourth gene, *KCNJ2* (at position 17q23.1-q24.2), is associated with Andersen-Tawil syndrome, a con dition that sometimes involves changes in heart rhythms and other developmental abnormalities in addition to the characteristic periodic muscle weakness. It en codes an ion channel protein that is particularly prevalent in cardiac muscle, as well as skeletal muscle.

The physiologic basis of the flaccid weakness in this disorder is the inexcitability of the muscle membrane (ie, sarcolemma). Alteration of serum potassium level is **not** the principal defect in primary PP. In fact, the altered potassium metabolism is a **result** of the PP. In primary and thyrotoxic PP, flaccid paralysis may occur with relatively small changes in the serum potassium level, whereas in secondary PP, serum potassium levels are markedly abnormal.

HypoKalemic Periodic Paralysis By Miansari66 (Own work), via Wikimedia Commons

SYMPTOMS

While muscle strength returns to normal between attacks, repeated bouts may lead to chronic muscle weakness later in life. An individual remains alert and aware during attacks, and there is no accompanying loss of sensation.

Episodic bouts of severe weakness in the arms and legs are the most prominent symptom of periodic paralysis. Typically, these bouts occur during sleep, especially after strenuous activity. Cold, stress, and alcohol may also produce attacks. Other symptoms are specific to the type of periodic paralysis.

In the hypokalemic type, potassium levels are low during attacks. Weakness may range from slight transient weakness of an isolated muscle group to severe generalized weakness. Severe attacks begin in the morning, often with strenuous exercise or a high carbohydrate meal on the preceding day. Sometimes, the time between premonitory symptoms to full-blown attack is in order of minutes. Attacks may also be provoked by stress, including infections, menstruation, lack of sleep, and certain medications (eg, beta-agonists, insulin, corticosteroids). Patients wake up with severe symmetrical weakness, often with truncal involvement. Mild attacks are frequent and involve only a particular group of muscles, and may be unilateral, partial, or affecting only one limb. This may affect predominantly legs; sometimes, extensor muscles are affected more than flexors. Duration varies from a few hours to several days but seldom exceeds 72 hours. The attacks are intermittent and infrequent in the beginning but may increase in frequency until attacks occur almost daily.

Attacks usually begin in adolescence, but they can occur before age ten. The frequency starts diminishing by age 30 years, and they rarely occur after age 50.

Thyrotoxic periodic paralysis is the most common secondary hypokalemic periodic paralysis. It is most common in adults aged 20–40 years. Hyperinsulinemia, a carbohydrate load, and exercise are important in precipitating paralytic attacks. Weakness is proximal and, if severe, may involve respiratory or bulbar muscles. Attacks last hours to days.

In the hyperkalemic type, potassium levels are high or normal during attacks. Patients usually describe a sense of heaviness or stiffness in the muscles. Weakness starts in the thighs and calves, which then spreads to arms and neck. Proximal weakness predominates; distal muscles may become involved after vigorous exercise. In children, a myotonic lid lag (lagging of upper eyelid on downward gaze) may be the earliest symptom. Complete paralysis is rare and some residual mobility remains. Respiratory muscle involvement is rare. Sphincter muscles of the bowel and bladder are not involved. Weakness occurs during rest after a period of strenuous exercise or during fasting. It also may be provoked by potassium, cold, ethanol, or stress. It may be relieved by mild prolonged exercise or carbohydrate intake. Some families have no myotonia.

Attacks are usually shorter (lasting one to two hours), more frequent, and less severe than in the hypokalemic form; breathing and swallowing difficulties are extremely rare. Between attacks, patients often experience muscle spasms or difficulty relaxing their muscles, a condition known as myotonia; but some families never experience this. If it is present, it is less severe compared to the hypokalemic form of the disease

Andersen-Tawil syndrome is characterized by variable expression of the triad of dysmorphic features, periodic paralysis, and abnormal heart rhythms, the latter not found in other forms of the disease. Patients may have short stature, wide-set eyes, low-set ears, a small jaw, fifth finger clinodactyly (a bending or curvature of the finger in the plane of the palm), and scoliosis. Episodic weakness lasting a few hours to several days may arise spontaneously but usually follows physical activity. The periodic paralysis is not associated with myotonia. A prolonged QT interval and ventricular arrhythmias are the most common cardiac manifestations; but other heart rhythm abnormalities may be present. Some patients may have no symptoms. Others may

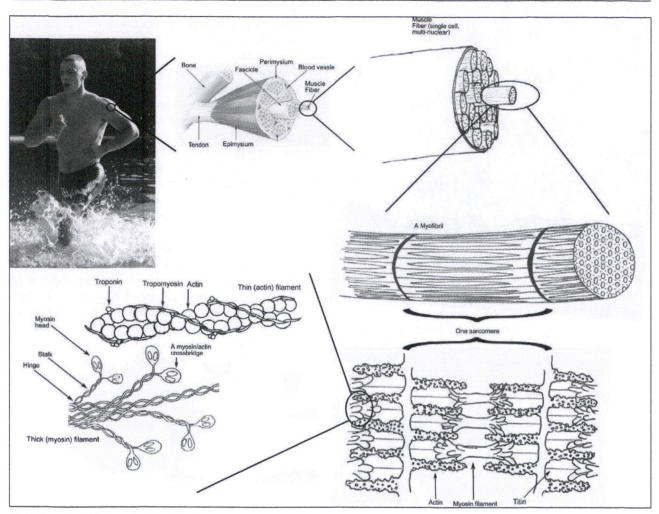

Skeletal muscle public domain via wikimedia commons

experience palpitations, syncopal episodes, and cardiac arrest. Sudden cardiac death is less frequent in these patients when compared with other types of long QT syndromes.

Previously, it has been suggested that individuals with some types of periodic paralysis are at risk for a condition known as malignant hyperthermia, a rare, often fatal, condition which can occur during the use of general anesthesia. Anyone with a family history of peri odic paralysis and/or past episode of malignant hyperthermia needs to notify the anesthesiologist of this history prior to any surgery requiring general anesthesia.

SCREENING AND DIAGNOSIS

Because this primarily is an inherited condition, the most important aspect of diagnosis is obtaining a family histor y. In addition to asking about symptoms and a patient's medical history, a physical exam may also be done.

Several blood tests may be helpful in making the diagnosis, and ideally, the blood can be drawn during an actual attack to look for either high or low levels of potassium. The doctor may also recommend provoking an attack and then doing the blood tests while the attack is in progress. If this is done, it is often done under careful monitoring by an experienced neurologist and/or cardiologist in an intensive care setting. Genetic testing is also available to look for one or more of the mutations associated with the disorder.

Other tests that might be considered include an electrocardiogram (ECG), a test that records the heart's activity by measuring electrical currents through the heart muscle; and electromyography

(EMG) to test the functioning of nerves and muscles; a specialized muscle cooling test, a needle electrode exam, and specific types of exercise testing. If the diagnosis is in question, the doctor may recommend doing a muscle biopsy.

TREATMENT AND THERAPY

Treatment is often necessary for acute attacks of hypokalemic periodic paralysis but not needed as often for hyperkalemic periodic paralysis unless potassium levels become dangerously high. Prophylactic treatment is necessary when the attacks are frequent.

Dichlorphenamide, a carbonic anhydrase inhibitor, was approved by the FDA in August 2015 for the management of primary hyperkalemic periodic paralysis, primary hypokalemic periodic paralysis, and related variants. In the past, acetazolamide has been used; but it was never an officially approved treatment for periodic paralysis.

Individuals can adopt a few behaviors to reduce the frequency and severity of attacks. For individuals with hypokalemic period paralysis, these lifestyle changes include eating a low-carbohydrate, low-sodium diet and avoiding strenuous exercise. Individuals with the hyperkalemic type can eat a low-potassium diet; stay warm; and avoid fasting, alcohol, and heavy exercise.

For patients with the hypokalemic type, potassium in pill or liquid form may stop an attack. Intravenous potassium is reserved for those with potassium levels low enough to cause abnormal heart rhythms and/or weakness/paralysis of airway muscles. Avoiding certain commonly prescribed medications (such as diuretics that cause loss of potassium) may help reduce the onset of attacks. At the same time, medications that lead to the retention of potassium may be helpful. If these patients also have thyroid conditions, those conditions are usually managed as well.

Medications for patients with hyperkalemic periodic paralysis include thiazide diuretics, or water pills, which cause loss of potassium in the urine. Glucose, glucose plus insulin, or calcium carbonate may be effective treatments for the rapid lowering of very high potassium levels.

In patients with Anderson-Tawill syndrome, Dichlorphenamide or acetazolamide is used as well as potassium supplements to reverse low potassium levels. If abnormal heart rhythms exist, medications used to control those rhythms are the same ones used when those rhythms are found in patients who do not have Anderson-Tawill.

PREVENTION AND OUTCOMES

Familial periodic paralysis cannot be prevented. Because it can be inherited, genetic counseling may be advised for couples at risk of passing on the disorder.

For the hypokalemic type, patients may reduce attacks by avoiding corticosteroids and high sugar intake and following a diet low in carbohydrates and sodium and rich in potassium. For the hyperkalemic type, patients may reduce attacks by avoiding high-potassium foods, fasting, and drugs known to increase potassium levels. Patients may also decrease attacks by engaging in regular, mild exercise.

If diligent prevention measures are implemented and acute attacks are well managed, most patients will be able to participate in work and most activities and experience a normal life expectancy. In severe cases left completely untreated, potential complications may lead to progressive loss of muscle function or early death.

Jill Buchanan;

reviewed by J. Thomas Megerian, M.D., Ph.D., F.A.A.P. "Etiology and Genetics" by Jeffrey A. Knight, Ph.D.; updated by Gary M. Flashner, M.S., M.D.

FURTHER READING

Chaudhry MA, Wayangankar S. Thyrotoxic Periodic Paralysis: A Concise Review of the Literature. *Curr Rheumatol Rev.* 2016. 12 (3):190–194.

EBSCO Publishing. *DynaMed: Hyperkalemic Period Paralysis.* Ipswich, Mass.: Author, 2009. Available through http://www.ebscohost.com/dynamed.

Health Library: Periodic Paralysis Syndrome. Ipswich, Mass.: Author, 2009. Available through http://www.ebscohost.com.

Jurkat-Ratt, K., and F. Lehmann-Horn. "Paroxysmal Muscle Weakness: The Periodic Paralyses." *Journal of Neurology* 253, no. 11 (November, 2006):1391–1398.

Levitt, J., P. Cochran, and J. Jankowiak. "Patient Page: Attacks of Immobility Caused by Diet or Exercise? The Mystery of Periodic Paralyses." *Neurology* 63, no. 9 (November 9, 2004): E17–18.

Matthews E, Portaro S, Ke Q, et al. Acetazolamide efficacy in hypokalemic periodic paralysis and the predictive role of genotype. *Neurology.* 2011 Nov 29. 77(22):1960–4.

Miller, T. M., et al. "Correlating Phenotype and Genotype in the Periodic Paralyses." *Neurology* 63, no. 9 (November 9, 2004): 1647–1655.

Neki NS. Hyperthyroid hypokalemic periodic paralysis. *Pakistan Journal of Medical Sciences.* 2016;32(4):1051–1052. doi:10.12669/pjms.324.11006.

Ropper, Allan H., and Martin A. Samuels. *Adams and Victor's Principles of Neurology.* 9th ed. New York: McGraw-Hill Medical, 2009.

WEB SITES OF INTEREST

Genetics Home Reference http://ghr.nlm.nih.govHealth Canada
http://www.hc-sc.gc.ca/index-eng.php

Muscular Dystrophy Association
http://www.mdausa.org

Muscular Dystrophy Canada
http://www.mdac.ca
National Institute of Neurological Disorders and Stroke: NINDS Familial Periodic Paralyses Information Page
https://www.ninds.nih.gov/Disorders/All-Disorders/Familial-Periodic-Paralyses-Information-Page

National Organization for Rare Disorders
http://www.rarediseases.org

Periodic Paralysis Resource Center, Periodic Paralysis Association
http://www.periodicparalysis.org

http://emedicine.medscape.com/article/1171678-overview

http://www.medscape.com/viewarticle/862364

See also: Adrenoleukodystrophy; Alexander disease; Alzheimer's disease; Amyotrophic lateral sclerosis; Arnold-Chiari syndrome; Ataxia telangiectasia; Canavan disease; Cerebrotendinous xanthomatosis; Charcot-Marie-Tooth syndrome; Chediak-Higashi syndrome; Dandy-Walker syndrome; Deafness; Epilepsy; Essential tremor; Friedreich ataxia; Huntington's disease; Jansky-Bielschowsky disease; Joubert syndrome; Kennedy disease; Krabbé disease; Leigh syndrome; Leukodystrophy; Limb girdle muscular dystrophy; Maple syrup urine disease; Metachromatic leukodystrophy; Myoclonic epilepsy associated with ragged red fibers (MERRF); Narcolepsy; Nemaline myopathy; Neural tube defects; Neurofibromatosis; Parkinson disease; Pelizaeus-Merz bacher disease; Pendred syndrome; Prion diseases: Kuru and Creutzfeldt-Jakob syndrome; Spinal muscular atrophy; Vanishing white matter disease.

Pfeiffer Syndrome

CATEGORY: Diseases and syndromes
ALSO KNOWN AS: ACS5; Pfeiffer type acrocephalosyndactyly; Acrocephalosyndactyly, type 5; Acrocephalosyndactyly type 5

DEFINITION
Pfeiffer syndrome is an inherited genetic disorder that affects the development of the bones in the skull, hands, and feet. It is caused by mutations in the *FGFR1* or *FGFR2* genes and is inherited in an autosomal dominant manner. Pfeiffer syndrome is divided into three subtypes (type I, type II and type III) based on the presence and severity of specific features. The incidence of the disorder is about 1 in every 100,000 births. Management typically includes various surgical interventions.

RISK FACTORS
The main risk factor for developing Pfeiffer syndrome is having a family member who has the disorder diagnosed with the aid of genetic testing. In addition, advanced paternal age is associated with an increased risk for new mutations that can lead to Pfeiffer syndrome.

The risk of passing the abnormal gene from an affected parent to offspring is 50 percent for each pregnancy. The risk is the same for males and females.

ETIOLOGY AND GENETICS
Pfeiffer syndrome is an autosomal dominant disorder caused by a single recurring mutation (Pro252Arg) of the *FGFR1* gene and several mutations involving the *FGFR2* gene. About 5 percent of type I cases are attributed to mutations in the *FGFR1* gene. The remainder of type I cases and all type II and type III cases are attributed to mutations in the FGFR2 gene.

Signs and Symptoms

The presence and severity of features of Pfeiffer syndrome may differ depending on the type of Pfeiffer syndrome a person has. Type I is considered mild compared to types II and III.

In Pfeiffer syndrome type I, infants have craniosynostosis that causes the head to appear vertically elongated. Distinctive facial features may include a high, full forehead; underdeveloped mid-facial regions (midface hypoplasia); widely spaced eyes (ocular hypertelorism); an underdeveloped upper jaw (hypoplastic maxilla) with a prominent lower jaw and dental abnormalities. People with type I usually have normal intelligence and a good prognosis with a normal life span.

In Pfeiffer syndrome type II, people typically have more severe craniosynostosis, more severe hand and foot abnormalities, and additional malformations of the limbs. Infants with type II have a form of craniosynostosis that causes the skull to have a "tri-lobed" appearance (called a "cloverleaf skull" deformity). This is often associated with hydrocephalus, which causes increased pressure on the brain. Distinctive facial features may include an abnormally high, broad forehead; severe protrusion of the eyes (ocular proptosis); midface hypoplasia; a "beak-shaped" nose; and low-set ears. Infants may also have lack of mobility of the elbow joints and/or various abnormalities in some of the internal organs. Infants with type II often have intellectual disabilities and neurological problems due to severe brain involvement. The physical abnormalities associated with type II can lead to life-threatening complications without appropriate treatment.

Pfeiffer syndrome type III is very similar to type II, but people with type III do not have the cloverleaf skull deformity. The features associated with type III may include a shortened base of the skull; the abnormal presence of teeth at birth (natal teeth); ocular proptosis; and/or various abnormalities of internal organs. As in type II, people with type III often have intellectual disabilities and severe neurological problems.

Screening and Diagnosis

The clinical features of Pfeiffer syndrome generally lead to further investigation that helps to determine if the patient has Pfeiffer syndrome or different disorder.

In most cases, genetic testing will help confirm the diagnosis, particularly when the clinical diagnosis is questionable. At the same time, the sensitivity of this testing is lower for Pfeiffer syndrome than for some other types of craniosynostoses.

An algorithm to increase efficiency and cost-effectiveness of molecular testing in craniosynostosis disorders involves initial performance of targeted analysis for recurrent pathogenic variants followed by selective gene sequencing. When working to confirm or rule out Pfeiffer syndrome, it is recommended to do sequence analysis of exons 8 and 10 (in which approximately 80 percent of FGFR2 pathogenic variants are located). If normal, it is then recommended to do sequence analysis of FGFR2 exons 3, 5, 11, 14, 15, 16, and 17 (in which an additional 10 percent of pathogenic variants are located) and targeted analysis for the *FGFR3* pathogenic variant p.Pro250Arg. Although the *FGFR3* gene has not specifically been associated with Pfeiffer syndrome, one of the specific mutations found in *FGFR1* and *FGFR2* has been identified in the *FGFR3* gene. This has been associated with a much more variable clinical presentation that includes mental retardation unrelated to appropriate management of craniosynostosis. There may also be a need to carry out *FGFR1* testing for Pfeiffer syndrome if a pathogenic variant in *FGFR2* is not identified and/or the patient has a milder phenotype.

Pre-natal screening is available for high-risk pregnancies. If the pathogenic allele of an affected family member has been identified, prenatal diagnosis for pregnancies at 50 percent risk may be available from a clinical laboratory that offers either testing for the gene of interest or custom prenatal testing. In a pregnancy not previously identified to be at risk for craniosynostosis in which an abnormal skull shape is detected on a prenatal ultrasound examination, prenatal testing is more difficult. Although testing for pathogenic variants in *FGFR1*, *FGFR2*, or *FGFR3* is possible, the yield is likely to be low. Furthermore, identification of a pathogenic variant in one of these genes would not clarify the prognosis, which is determined by clinical findings. For example, the prognosis for cloverleaf skull is generally poor regardless of the molecular defect or nature of hand and foot findings.

In order to evaluate the extent of the disease, further diagnostics are often recommended once a diagnosis of Pfeiffer's syndrome is confirmed. They may include:

- Assessment for hydrocephalus by brain CT or MRI with close observation in those with pathogenic variants known to cause a more severe phenotype
- Assessment for upper-airway obstruction or a condition called "tracheal sleeve" (in *FGFR2*-related Pfeiffer syndrome)
- Assessment for exposure keratopathy (damage to the cornea that occurs primarily from prolonged exposure of the ocular surface to the outside environment)
- Spinal x-rays to evaluate for vertebral anomalies
- Imaging of the gastrointestinal system to evaluate for the presence of intestinal malrotation or esophageal atresia

TREATMENT AND THERAPY

Children with Pfeiffer syndrome or any of the *FGFR*-related craniosynostosis syndromes benefit from the multidisciplinary team approach practiced in most craniofacial clinics affiliated with major pediatric medical centers. The specialists usually include plastic surgeons, neurosurgeons, ENT specialists, and dentists as well as audiologists, speech pathologists, developmental pediatricians, social workers, medical geneticists, and genetic counselors. The team can usually identify and address physical and developmental problems as well as psychosocial and other issues.

Early treatment of craniofacial anomalies may reduce the risk for secondary complications such as hydrocephalus and cognitive impairment; ophthalmologic lubrication can prevent exposure keratopathy in those with severe proptosis. Individuals with syndromic craniosynostosis usually require a series of staged surgical procedures; the number and type are tailored to the individual's needs. Three-dimensional skull CT can be used for morphologic mapping to help plan surgical treatment. Some individuals with syndromic craniosynostosis require a dozen or more surgeries over a lifetime. Seldom is the correction perfect, but significant cosmetic improvement is often possible.

PREVENTION AND OUTCOMES

Although there is no means for preventing Pfeiffer syndrome, per se, genetic counseling is often recommended for parents who currently have a child with this disorder and are thinking of having more children. Because inheritance is autosomal dominant, there is a 50 percent chance of passing on the pathogenic variant to future offspring. In addition, in a circumstance where a couple includes an older male, counseling may be given regarding the increased risk of Pfeiffer syndrome as well as other conditions associated with advanced paternal age.

Because Type I disease is fairly mild, the outcome for these patients is good and a normal lifespan may be anticipated. Because the defects are much more severe for those with Type II and Type III disease, the prognosis is more guarded and very dependent on timely surgical interventions. Even when these patients receive all appropriate care, it is reasonable to anticipate intellectual disabilities and neurological problems due to severe brain involvement.

Gary M Flashner MS MD

FURTHER READING

Cohen MM Jr. "Pfeiffer syndrome update, clinical subtypes, and guidelines for differential diagnosis." *Am J Med Genet.* 1993;45:300–7.

Cornejo-Roldan LR, Roessler E, Muenke M. "Analysis of the mutational spectrum of the *FGFR2* gene in Pfeiffer syndrome." *Hum Genet.* 1999;104:425–31.

Glaser RL, Jiang W, Boyadjiev SA, Tran AK, Zachary AA, Van Maldergem L, Johnson D, Walsh S, Oldridge M, Wall SA, Wilkie AO, Jabs EW. "Paternal origin of *FGFR2* mutations in sporadic cases of Crouzon syndrome and Pfeiffer syndrome." *Am J Hum Genet.* 2000;66:768–77.

Muenke M, Schell U, Robin NH, et al. "Variable clinical spectrum in Pfeiffer syndrome: correlation between phenotype and genotype." *Proc Green Genet Ctr.* 1995;15:126.

Robin NH, Scott JA, Arnold JE, Goldstein JA, Shilling BB, Marion RW, Cohen MM Jr. "Favorable prognosis for children with Pfeiffer syndrome types II and III: implications for classification." *Am J Med Genet.* 1998;75:240–4

WEB SITES OF INTEREST

https://rarediseases.info.nih.gov/diseases/7380/pfeiffer-syndrome

https://ghr.nlm.nih.gov/condition/pfeiffer-syndrome

https://www.ncbi.nlm.nih.gov/books/NBK1455/

https://www.ncbi.nlm.nih.gov/pmc/articles/PMC1051023/

See also: Apert Syndrome, Crouzon syndrome, Muenke syndrome, Jackson-Weiss syndrome, Beare-Stevenson syndrome, Saethre-Chotzen Syndrome, Carpenter Syndrome

Phenylketonuria (PKU)

CATEGORY: Diseases and syndromes

DEFINITION

Phenylketonuria is a relatively common genetic disease affecting about one in every ten thousand newborn babies. Phenylketonuria, or PKU, was dis covered in 1934 by Asbjørn Følling in Nor way. Følling discovered that the urine of retarded children turned green when ferric chloride, a chemical used to detect ketones in the urine of diabetics, was added. The urine of diabetics normally turns purple or burgundy with the addition of ferric chloride. Følling conducted further investigations and discov ered that the substance responsible for turning urine green upon addition of ferric chloride was phenylpyruvic acid. Følling discovered that the ori gin of phenylpyruvic acid was the amino acid phe nylalanine.

RISK FACTORS

Both of a child's parents must pass along the mu tated *PAH* gene in order for the child to develop this condition. Children who have only one parent with this gene are not at risk. PKU primarily affects white people of Northern European ancestry and is much less common in African Americans.

ETIOLOGY AND GENETICS

PKU can be caused by a mutation in the *PAH* gene. This gene encodes the information for the liver enzyme phenylalanine hydroxylase (PAH), which catalyzes the conversion of phenylalanine to tyro-sine. In people with normal metabolisms, phe nylalanine, an essential amino acid, must be con sumed in the diet. Phenylalanine is either incorpo rated into the body's proteins or converted by the enzyme phenylalanine hydroxylase into tyrosine, an other amino acid. Tyrosine is either incorporated into protein or converted into other important bio logical molecules, such as dopamine, epinephrine, norepinephrine, and melanin. Alternatively, tyro sine can be completely metabolized and eliminated from the body.

People with PKU cannot metabolize phenylala nine into tyrosine at normal rates. The disease caus ing mutant PKU gene is autosomal recessive. Thus, in order for a person to have PKU, he or she must inherit two copies of the mutant gene. Approximately one in every fifty people in the United States is a heterozygous carrier for the disease. About one in every ten thousand newborn babies has the disease.

The PKU gene was isolated in 1992, and soon after ward it was discovered that there is no one type of PKU mutation. Instead, the disease can be caused by a variety of defects affecting the PKU gene. Many of these defects are "point" mutations resulting in single base-pair changes in the DNA which lead to amino acid substitutions in the *PAH* gene. Other de fects include base-pair changes leading to splicing defects in *PAH* messenger RNA (mRNA), deletions resulting in one or more miss ing amino acids in PAH, and insertions resulting in mRNA reading frame shifts. More than four hun dred mutations have been found in the PKU gene. The variety of different defects in the PKU gene leads to variability in the activity of PAH and the severity of the disease.

Normally, blood phenylalanine concentrations are between 2 and 6 milligrams per deciliter (mg/dl), but in PKU phenylalanine accumulates to 20 mg/dl or more. Phenylalanine is normally con verted to tyrosine, and tyrosine is a critical com ponent of biochemical pathways leading to the production of melanin, dopamine, norepineph rine,and epinephrine. The disruption of these pathways leads to a deficiency of these important compounds, which probably contributes to the development of symptoms characteristic of the disease.

The high levels of phenylalanine may also inter fere with the transport of other important amino ac ids into the brain. Since several amino acids use the same transport system as phenylalanine, phenylala nine is preferentially transported at the expense of the others. This may also contribute to the develop ment of symptoms characteristic of

PKU. Additionally, since phenylalanine cannot be metabolized normally, it is metabolized into abnormal compounds such as phenylpyruvic acid, which further contributes to the development of PKU symptoms.

SYMPTOMS

Signs and symptoms of untreated disease can vary from mild to severe. Common characteristics of untreated patients with PKU are mental retardation, light-colored skin and hair, seizures, delayed development, hyperactivity, schizophrenia, tremors, and eczema. PKU also has major metabolic effects.

SCREENING AND DIAGNOSIS

Robert Guthrie developed a screening test for phenylketonuria in the early 1960s. In this test, bacteria are grown on an agar medium that contains an inhibitor of growth that can be overcome by exogenously added phenylalanine. If a small piece of filter paper containing blood is placed on the agar medium with the bacteria, the phenylalanine in the blood leaches out of the filter paper and stimulates growth of the bacteria. The extent of the growth around the filter paper is directly proportional to the amount of phenylalanine in the blood. Guthrie published his procedure in 1961. In 1963 Massachusetts became the first state to legislate mandatory PKU screening of all newborns. It is now mandatory in all fifty states and currently only requires a small sample of blood obtained from the baby's heel at age 24–48 hours. The blood sample is analyzed by tandem mass spectrometry as opposed to using the Guthrie bacterial inhibition assay.

If the screening test is abnormal, then additional testing may be recommended to measure plasma phenylalanine and tyrosine and tests to rule out other conditions. DNA testing is available but is generally not needed.

Prenatal diagnosis is available but rarely used since the disorder is so treatable. Prenatal diagnosis can be accomplished by DNA mutation analysis following chorionic villous sampling or amniocentesis.

TREATMENT AND THERAPY

The treatment of choice for PKU is dietary or nutritional intervention. PKU babies placed on very low phenylalanine diets show normal cognitive development. The PKU diet eliminates high-protein foods, which are replaced with low-phenylalanine foods and supplemented with a nutritional formula that may contain tyrosine, vitamins, minerals, and other micronutrients.

It is recommended that dietary intervention begin as soon as possible after birth and continue for life. It is especially important that pregnant PKU women adhere closely to the diet, or their babies will be mentally retarded. Studies have shown that if children or adults are taken off the diet, some PKU symptoms may develop.

The U.S. Food and Drug Administration (FDA) in December, 2007, approved the drug sapropterin dihydrochloride (Kuvan) for treatment of some people with PKU, to be used in combination with a PKU diet. Since Kuvan has been introduced, it has been found to be safe and effective, and in some cases, permits relaxation in some of the dietary restrictions required for effective management.

In most cases, patients are treated in specialty metabolic disease clinics that include a nutritionist and a psychologist.

PREVENTION AND OUTCOMES

If PKU is not detected and treatment is not begun within the first few weeks of life, the child will develop various neurological symptoms, including retardation. If the disease is detected shortly after birth and dietary treatment is instituted, symptoms characteristic of the disease usually will not develop.

Women with PKU can prevent birth defects by maintaining a low-phenylalanine diet before they become pregnant. Individuals with PKU, or those who have a close relative or child with the condition, may benefit from genetic counseling before deciding to have a child.

Those who optimally manage the disease have a very good chance of a normal lifespan and no restrictions in activity.

Charles L. Vigue, Ph.D.; updated by Rebecca Kuzins;
updated by Gary M. Flashner, M.S., M.D.

FURTHER READING

Kaufman, Seymour. *Overcoming a Bad Gene: The Story of the Discovery and Successful Treatment of Phenylketonuria, a Genetic Disease That Causes*

Mental Retar dation. Bloomington, Ind.: Author-House, 2004. Kaufman, who was chief of the laboratory of neurochemistry at the National Institutes of Health, recounts the history of PKU's discovery and the subsequent research to learn more about the disease. He also provides a thorough explana tion of the disease's symptoms, treatment, diagnosis, and how it can cause mental retardation.

Koch, Jean Holt. *Robert Guthrie, the PKU Stor y: A Crusade Against Mental Retardation.* Pasadena, Calif.: Hope, 1997. A longtime friend profiles the scien tific work and personal life work of Robert Guthrie. *National PKU News.* This newsletter, published in Se attle, Washington, three times a year, provides in formation about PKU.

Parker, James N. *The Official Parent's Sourcebook on Phenylketonuria.* San Diego: Icon Health, 2002. rare disease database that enables users to retrieve information about phenylketonura, as well as a list of other names for the disease and a list of related organizations. See also: Biochemical mutations; Genetic screen ing; Genetic testing; Hereditary diseases; Inborn errors of metabolism. This resource, created for parents with PKU children, tells parents how and where to look for in formation about PKU.

Surendran, Sankar, et al. "Neurochemical Changes and Therapeutical Targets in Phenylketonuria (PKU)." In *Neurochemistry of Metabolic Diseases: Lysosomal Storage Diseases, Phenylketonuria, and Canavan Disease,* 2007, edited by Surendran. Kerala, India: Transworld Research Network, 2007. Focuses on PKU and other health condi tions in which a single gene defect hampers nor mal metabolic activity, resulting in pathophysio logical abnormalities.

Hood A, Antenor-Dorsey JA, Rutlin J, Hershey T, Shimony JS, McKinstry RC, et al. "Prolonged exposure to high and variable phenylalanine levels over the lifetime predicts brain white matter integrity in children with phenylketonuria." *Mol Genet Metab.* 2015 Jan. 114 Vockley J, Andersson HC, Antshel KM, Braverman NE, Burton BK, Frazier DM, et al. "Phenylalanine hydroxylase deficiency: diagnosis and management guideline." *Genet Med.* 2014 Feb. 16 (2):188–200.

Bilder DA, Kobori JA, Cohen-Pfeffer JL, Johnson EM, Jurecki ER, Grant ML. "Neuropsychiatric comorbidities in adults with phenylketonuria: A retrospective cohort study." *Mol Genet Metab.* 2017 Mar 6 Bell SM, Wendt DJ, Zhang Y, Taylor TW, Long S, Tsuruda L, et al. "Formulation and PEGylation optimization of the therapeutic PEGylated phenylalanine ammonia lyase for the treatment of phenylketonuria." *PLoS One.* 2017. 12 (3):e0173269.

WEB SITES OF INTEREST

Genetic and Rare Diseases Information Center, Phenylketonuria
https://rarediseases.info.nih.gov/diseases/7383/phenylketonuria
Links to online resources that explain the disease and provide management guidelines and information about newborn screening.

Genetics Home Reference
http://ghr.nlm.nih.gov/condition=phenylketonuria
Describes the disease and explains how it results from a mutation in the PAH gene. Links to other on line resources.

Medline Plus
http://www.nlm.nih.gov/medlineplus/phenylketonuria.html
Contains a brief description of PKU and numer ous links to additional information.

National Organization for Rare Disorders
http://www.rarediseases.org
This site contains an index of rare diseases and a rare disease database that enables users to retrieve information about phenylketonura, as well as a list of other names for the disease and a list of related organizations.
https://www.dovepress.com/update-on-the-treat-ment-of-phenylketonuria-long-term-safety-and-ef-fica-peer-reviewed-article-RRED

See also: Biochemical mutations; Genetic screen ing; Genetic testing; Hereditary diseases; Inborn errors of metabolism.

Pierre Robin Syndrome

CATEGORY: Diseases and syndromes

ALSO KNOWN AS: Pierre Robin sequence; Glossoptosis, micrognathia, and cleft palate; Pierre Robin Anomalad; Pierre Robin Complex; Pierre Robin Deformity; Pierre Robin Malformation Sequence; Pierre Robin Triad

DEFINITION

Pierre Robin sequence is a condition present at birth, in which the infant has a smaller than normal lower jaw (micrognathia), a tongue that is placed further back than normal (glossoptosis), and an opening in the roof of the mouth (cleft palate). This combination of features can lead to difficulty breathing and problems with eating early in life. Pierre Robin sequence may occur alone (isolated) or as a feature in multiple defect disorders (described as syndromic). In about 20 to 40 percent of cases, the condition occurs alone. The exact causes of Pierre Robin syndrome are unknown. Changes (mutations) in DNA near the *SOX9* gene are the most common genetic cause of isolated cases of Pierre Robin sequence. Treatment is focused on the specific needs of each patient, but may include surgery to help improve breathing and feeding functions and to help prevent choking. The disorder is present in about 1 out of every 8500 births and equally affects males and females.

RISK FACTORS

The main known risk factor is having a family member who has isolated Pierre Robin and found to be secondary to autosomal recessive or, less often, X-linked inheritance.

ETIOLOGY AND GENETICS

At present, the exact cause of Pierre Robin sequence is unknown. Pierre Robin sequence is a condition with multiple causes. At about 7–10 weeks into a pregnancy, the lower jaw grows rapidly, allowing the tongue to descend from between the two halves of the palate. If, for some reason, the lower jaw does not grow properly, the tongue can prevent the palate from closing, resulting in a cleft palate. The small or displaced lower jaw also causes the tongue to be positioned at the back of the mouth causing breathing difficulties when the child is born. This "sequence of events" is the reason why the condition has been classified as a sequence.

Possible mechanisms for the sequence include genetic causes; low volume of amniotic fluid (oligohydramnios), which may limit chin growth; weakness of the facial muscles (myotonia); or connective tissue disease.

The genetic causes for some of the isolated cases (Pierre Robin sequence without any associated malformations) may include mutations or deletions of parts of the DNA neighboring the *SOX9* gene (located in chromosome 17 (17q24)). These may be inherited in an autosomal recessive fashion. The *SOX9* gene provides instructions for making a protein (protein SOX9) that plays an important role in the formation of many different tissues and organs during embryonic development. The SOX9 protein regulates the activity of other genes, especially those involved in the development of the skeleton, including the jaw.

An X-linked variant has also been reported involving cardiac malformations and clubfeet.

In about one-third of cases, Pierre Robin occurs as part of a syndrome with multiple malformations. Pierre Robin sequence has been reported as occurring in association with Stickler syndrome (20 percent–25 percent of these cases), campomelic dysplasia, trisomy 11q syndrome, deletion 4q syndrome, CHARGE association, velocardiofacial syndrome, and Treacher-Collins syndrome.

SIGNS AND SYMPTOMS

The defects associated with Pierre Robin syndrome are present at birth. They generally include a smaller than normal lower jaw (micrognathia), a tongue that is placed further back than normal (glossoptosis), and an opening in the roof of the mouth (cleft palate). But there may be significant variability as regards the presence of other defects. This partly depends on whether the disease was generated by a defect in the *SOX9* gene, or by the rare X-linked variety or if the three defects are part of a more complex syndrome.

The downward placement of the tongue, coupled with an unusually small jaw, may obstruct normal breathing and cause respiratory distress, feeding problems, and failure to thrive. Sleep disorders, including obstructive sleep apnea, a condition in which breathing temporarily stops, may occur.

Cardiovascular and lung conditions, such as benign heart murmurs, high blood pressure in the arteries of the lungs (pulmonary hypertension), and narrowing of the opening between the lung artery and the right ventricle of the heart (pulmonary stenosis) may also be present. A large variety of musculoskeletal abnormalities may be seen that may affect the arms, legs, feet, and vertebral column. These are fairly common and occur in about 70–80 percent of cases.

Inflammation of the middle ear (otitis media) occurs in about 80 percent of patients, and hearing loss occurs in about 60 percent. These problems are certainly associated with a variety of different anatomic defects that may be present. A variety of eye defects are noted in about 10 percent to 30 percent of patients.

Softening of the tissue that makes up the voice box (laryngomalacia) occurs in about 10–15 percent of patients. A failure of the ability to temporarily close the communication between the nasal cavity and the mouth (velopharyngeal insufficiency) may also be present. If present, both of these problems contribute to speech defects in these patients.

SCREENING AND DIAGNOSIS
Although it is possible to detect the defects of Pierre Robin syndrome with ultrasound while the fetus is still in the womb, pre-delivery ultrasound examinations are not generally carried out specifically to make this diagnosis except possibly in cases where expectant parents already have a child with isolated Pierre Robin syndrome.

The diagnosis is first suspected when an infant is born with the combination of jaw, tongue and palate abnormalities described above. X-rays and a full genetic analysis can help to rule out other conditions. Because of the common sleep, breathing and feeding problems that occur in these infants, sleep studies are often performed as well as direct visualization of the entire nose and throat (using a procedure called "nasopharyngoscopy") and a detailed evaluation by a feeding specialist.

TREATMENT AND THERAPY
Infants with Pierre Robin syndrome are usually treated by a knowledgeable and experienced multidisciplinary team capable of providing a comprehensive assessment, a realistic plan of treatment, and appropriate follow-up. This often includes engaging the family in the early stages of the evaluation, the ongoing medical investigations, the issues regarding the child's care, and future planning.

Immediately after birth, critical care services are needed in a neonatal intensive care unit mainly because of the potential for life-threatening compromise to the airway. For those with particularly severe airway problems, one of several surgical procedures may be recommended in order to decrease the chances of the infant experiencing a complete airway obstruction. More frequently than not, this will involve a procedure to help move the tongue into a more normal position or will involve surgical placement of a tracheostomy. In some cases, feeding can be successfully done by mouth; but in more severe cases, a temporary feeding tube may be necessary.

At some point, there is a need to repair the cleft palate. This usually is done between ages 10 and 18 months; however, it may be delayed if the infant has had more severe airway problems. Addressing problems associated with a small jaw or one that is displaced backwards of a normal position is handled on a case-by-case basis. In some cases, specialized surgical repair may be recommended, and in other cases, it may not.

Genetic counseling is often offered to parents who already have a child with Pierre Robin syndrome and are considering having more children. In discussing autosomal recessive inheritance, they are generally advised that recessive genetic disorders occur when an individual inherits the same abnormal gene for the same trait from each parent. If an individual receives one normal gene and one gene for the disease, he or she will be a carrier of the disease, but usually will not show symptoms. The risk of two carrier parents both passing the defective gene and having an affected child is 25 percent with each pregnancy. The risk of having a child who is a carrier like the parents is 50 percent with each pregnancy. The chance of having a child who receives normal genes from both parents and is genetically normal for that particular trait is 25 percent. The risk is the same for males and females.

PREVENTION AND OUTCOMES
Over a relatively short period of time, most of these infants will experience "catch-up" growth of the jaw (usually in the first three months) thus decreasing

the initial critical issues connected with compromised breathing and feeding. Feeding and speech assessments continue to be needed, and breathing capacity must be monitored. Eventually, the cleft palate must be closed, and long-term orthodontic care is often required.

If management of the clinical manifestations is successful during the first year of life, the prognosis is favorable. The tongue displacement together with the feeding and respiratory problems usually resolve during the first two years of life and growth of the mandible leads to correction of the jaw deformity within three to six years. The cleft palate can be corrected by surgical intervention before the age of nine months. The neurological prognosis for these patients is also good. However, the persistent risk of ear infections, hearing loss and speech difficulties necessitate follow-up by an ear, nose, and throat specialist and speech therapist.

FURTHER READING

Bütow KW, Hoogendijk CF, Zwahlen RA. "Pierre Robin sequence: Appearances and 25 years of experience with an innovative treatment protocol." *J Pediatr Surg.* 2009 Nov. 44(11):2112–8.

Costa MA, Tu MM, Murage KP, Tholpady SS, Engle WA, Flores RL. "Robin sequence: mortality, causes of death, and clinical outcomes." *Plast Reconstr Surg.* 2014 Oct. 134 (4):738–45.

Evans AK, Rahbar R, Rogers GF, et al. "Robin sequence: a retrospective review of 115 patients." *Int J Pediatr Otorhinolaryngol.* 2006 Jun. 70(6):973–80.

Rathe M, Rayyan M, Schoenaers J, Dormaar JT, Breuls M, Verdonck A, et al. "Pierre Robin sequence: Management of respiratory and feeding complications during the first year of life in a tertiary referral centre." *Int J Pediatr Otorhinolaryngol.* 2015 Aug. 79 (8):1206–12.

WEB SITES OF INTEREST

https://rarediseases.info.nih.gov/diseases/4347/ pierre-robin-syndrome

https://ghr.nlm.nih.gov/condition/ isolated-pierre-robin-sequence

https://rarediseases.org/rare-diseases/ pierre-robin-sequence/
https://ghr.nlm.nih.gov/gene/SOX9#conditions
http://emedicine.medscape.com/ article/844143-overview

http://emedicine.medscape.com/ article/995706-overview
http://www.orpha.net/consor/cgi-bin/OC_Exp. php?Lng=GB&Expert=718

See also: Stickler syndrome, Campomelic dysplasia, Trisomy 11q syndrome, Deletion 4q syndrome, CHARGE association, Velocardiofacial syndrome, and Treacher-Collins syndrome

Gary M Flashner MS MD

Plasmids

CATEGORY: Molecular genetics

SIGNIFICANCE: Plasmids are DNA molecules that exist separately from the chromosome. Plasmids exist in a commensal relationship with their host and may provide the host with new abilities. They are used in genetic research as vehicles for carrying genes. In the wild, they promote the exchange of genes and contribute to the problem of antibiotic resistance.

KEY TERMS

commensalism: a relationship in which two organisms rely on each other for survival

gene: a region of DNA containing instructions for the manufacture of a protein

transposon: a piece of DNA that can copy itself from one location to another

PLASMID STRUCTURE

The structure of plasmids is usually circular, although linear forms do exist. Their size ranges from a few thousand base pairs to hundreds of thousands of base pairs. They are found primarily in bacteria but have also been found in fungi, plants, and even humans.

In its commensal relationship with its host, the plasmid can be thought of as a molecular parasite whose primary function is to maintain itself within its host and to spread itself as widely as possible to other hosts. The majority of genes that are present on a plasmid will be dedicated to this function. Researchers have discovered that despite the great diversity of plasmids, most of them have similar genes, dedicated to this function. This relative simplicity of plasmids makes them ideal models of gene function, as well as useful tools for molecular biology.

Genes of interest can be placed on a plasmid, which can easily be moved in and out of cells. Using plasmids isolated from the wild, molecular biologists have designed many varieties of artificial plasmids, which have greatly facilitated research in molecular biology.

PLASMID REPLICATION

To survive and propagate, a plasmid must be able to copy itself, or replicate. The genes that direct this process are known as the replication genes. These genes do not carry out all the functions of replication, but instead coopt the host's replication machinery to replicate the plasmid. Replication allows the plasmid to propagate by creating copies of itself that can be passed to each daughter cell when the host divides. In this manner, the plasmid propagates along with the host.

A second function of the replication genes is to control the copy number of the plasmid. The number of copies of a plasmid that exist inside a host can vary considerably. Plasmids can exist at a very low copy number (one or two copies per cell) or at a higher copy number, with dozens of copies per cell. Adjusting the copy number is an important consideration for a plasmid. Plasmid replication is an expensive process that consumes energy and resources of the host cell. A plasmid with a high copy number can place a significant energy drain on its host cell. In environments where the nutrient supply is low, a plasmid-bearing cell may not be able to compete successfully with other, non-plasmid-containing cells. Wild plasmids often exist at a low copy number, or create a high copy number for only a brief period of time.

PLASMID PARTITIONING

Because the presence of a plasmid is expensive in terms of energy, a cell harboring a plasmid will grow more slowly than a similar cell with no plasmid. This can cause a problem for a plasmid if it fails to partition properly during its host's division. If the plasmid does not partition properly, then one of the host's daughter cells will not contain a plasmid. Since this cell does not have to spend energy replicating a plasmid, it will gain an ability to grow faster, as will all of its offspring. In such a situation, the population of non-plasmid-containing cells could outgrow the population of plasmid-containing cells and use up all the nutrients in the environment. To avoid this problem, plasmids have evolved strategies to prevent improper partitioning. One strategy is for the plasmid to contain partitioning genes. Partitioning genes encode proteins that actively partition plasmids into each daughter cell during the host cell's division. Active partitioning greatly reduces the errors in partitioning that might occur if partitioning were left to chance.

A second strategy that plasmids use to prevent partitioning errors is the plasmid addition system. In this strategy, genes on the plasmid direct the production of both a toxin and an antidote. The antidote protein is very unstable and degrades quickly, but the toxin is quite stable. As long as the plasmid is present, the cytoplasm of the cell will be full of toxin and antidote. Should a daughter cell fail to receive a plasmid during division, the residual antidote and toxin present in the cytoplasm from the mother cell will begin to degrade, since there is no longer a plasmid present to direct the synthesis of either toxin or antidote. Since the antidote is very unstable, it will degrade first, leaving only toxin, which will kill the cell.

PLASMID TRANSFER BETWEEN CELLS

Propagation of plasmids can occur through the spread of plasmids from parent cells to their offspring (referred to as vertical transfer), but propagation can also occur between two different cells (referred to as horizontal transfer). Many plasmids are able to transfer themselves from one host to another through the process of conjugation. Conjugal plasmids contain a collection of genes that direct the host cell that contains them to attach to other cells and transfer a copy of the plasmid. In this manner, the plasmid can spread itself to other hosts and is not limited to spreading itself only to the descendants of the original host cell.

One of the first plasmids to be identified was discovered because of its ability to conjugate. This plasmid, known as the F plasmid, or F factor, is a plasmid found in the bacterium *Escherichia coli*. Cells harboring the F plasmid are designated F+ cells and can transfer their plasmid to other *E. coli* cells that do not contain the F plasmid (called F- cells).

Conjugal plasmids can be very specific and transfer only between closely related members of the same species (such as the F plasmid), or they can be very promiscuous and allow transfer between unrelated species. An extreme example of cross-species transfer is the Ti plasmid of the bacterial species *Agrobacterium tumefaciens*. The Ti plasmid is capable of transferring part of itself from *A. tumefaciens* into the cells of dicotyledonous plants. Plant cells that receive parts of the Ti plasmid are induced to grow and form a tumorlike structure, called a gall, that provides a hospitable environment for *A. tumefaciens*.

HOST BENEFITS FROM PLASMIDS

In most commensal relationships, there is an exchange of benefits between the two partners. The same is true for plasmids and their hosts. In many cases, plasmids provide their host cells with a collection of genes that enhance the ability of the host cell to survive. Enhancements include the ability to metabolize a wider range of materials for food and the ability to survive in hostile environments. One particular hostile environment in which plasmids can provide the ability to survive is the human body. A number of pathogenic microorganisms gain their ability to inhabit the human body, and thus cause disease, from genes contained on plasmids. An example of this is *Bacillus anthracis*, the agent that causes anthrax. Many of the genes that allow this organism to cause disease are contained on one of two plasmids, called pXO1 and pXO2. *Yersinia pestis*, the causative agent of bubonic plague, also gains its disease-causing ability from plasmids.

R FACTORS

Another example of plasmids conferring on their hosts the ability to survive in a hostile environment is antibiotic resistance. Plasmids known as R factors contain genes that make their bacterial hosts resistant to antibiotics. These R factors are usually conjugal plasmids, so they can move easily from cell to cell. Because the antibiotic resistance genes they carry are usually parts of transposons, they can readily copy themselves from one piece of DNA to another. Two different R factors that happened to be together in one cell could exchange copies of each other's antibiotic resistance genes. A number of R factors exist that contain multiple antibiotic resistance genes. Such plasmids can result in the formation of "multidrug resistant" (MDR) strains of pathogenic bacteria, which are difficult to treat. There is much evidence to suggest that the widespread use of antibiotics has contributed to the development of MDR pathogens, which are emerging as an important health concern.

ROLE OF PLASMIDS IN EVOLUTION

Through conjugation, plasmids can transfer genetic information from one species of bacterial cell to another. During its stay in a particular host, a plasmid may acquire some of the chromosomal genes of the host, which it then carries to a new host by conjugation. These genes can then be transferred from the plasmid to the chromosome of the new host. If the new host and the old host are different species, this gene transfer can result in the introduction of new genes, and thus new traits, into a cell. Bacteria, being asexual, produce daughter cells that are genetically identical to their parent. The existence of conjugal plasmids, which allow for the transfer of genes between bacterial species, may represent an important mechanism by which bacteria generate diversity and create new species.

GENETIC ENGINEERING OF PLASMIDS

The identification of restriction endonuclease sites within plasmids allowed scientists to manipulate the organization and makeup of these molecules. Researchers were now able to insert genes of interest into these restriction sites within the plasmids and have the recombined plasmid vector taken up by bacteria through the process of transformation. Transcription of the inserted gene by the host bacterium is dependent on an upstream promoter that is active in that bacterial strain. The use of genetic engineering and the creation of artificial plasmid vectors have revolutionized basic research and have led to the creation of modern industrial microbiology. Because bacteria containing the vector are able to express proteins encoded by the inserted gene(s) at a high level, mass quantities of desired proteins can be produced on an industrial scale. Vectors have been used to express medically important proteins such as insulin, human growth hormone, and human factor IX, a blood-clotting factor. Vectors have also been used to express proteins within eukaryotic cells. Additional DNA elements are necessary for the optimal production of proteins in these cells. Viral or mammalian promoters recognized by host RNA polymerases, as well as enhancer sequences, allow proteins to be expressed from the vector. Poly-adenylation sequences are added downstream of the inserted gene for proper messenger RNA (mRNA) expression.

The ability to express proteins within mammalian cells has enabled the development of DNA vaccines in which antigenic proteins are expressed from plasmids. These plasmids are taken up by cells following introduction into the animal or human subject by injection or alternate means of inoculation. Expression of these proteins in the cell then allows for an immunological response by the vaccine.

Expression of cytokine or other immunomodulatory molecules from the same plasmid has been explored as a means of enhancing the immune response to the coexpressed antigenic protein using DNA vaccines. Plasmid DNA itself can sometimes have immunostimulatory effects due to the presence of CpG dinucleotides. Clinical trials using DNA vaccines targeting cancer have demonstrated the immunogenicity of these vaccines in humans. Veterinary applications of DNA vaccines have been approved for use. Plasmids have also been used as delivery vehicles for the expression of double-stranded RNAs (dsRNAs) in order to suppress specific mRNAs by RNA interference (RNAi). Because of the abbreviated length (about 21 nucleotides) and need for a distinction termination point of these dsRNAs, RNA polymerase III promoters and the accompanying termination signals have often been included on the plasmids to express these transcripts within cells. Delivery of the RNAi expression plasmids to the desired location within the body remains a challenge for the development of this technology.

Douglas H. Brown, Ph.D.;
updated by Daniel E. McCallus, Ph.D.

Further Reading

Bower, D. M., and K. L. J. Prather. "Engineering of Bacterial Strains and Vectors for the Production of Plasmid DNA." *Applied Microbiology and Biotechnology* 82, no. 5 (2009): 805-813. Discusses innovations in both plasmid vectors and the bacterial strains that produce them in current biotechnology practice.

Levy, Stuart B. "The Challenge of Antibiotic Resistance." *Scientific American* 278 (1998): 46-53. A discussion on the growing problem of antibiotic resistance. Written by one of the experts in the field.

Summers, David K. *The Biology of Plasmids*. Malden, Mass.: Blackwell, 1996. A comprehensive book on plasmid biology written for college undergraduates.

Thomas, Christopher M. "Paradigms of Plasmid Organization." *Molecular Microbiology* 37, no. 3 (2000): 485-491. A review that clearly discusses the evolution and organization of plasmid genes.

Van Gaal, E. V. B., W. E. Hennink, D. J. A. Crommelin, and E. Mastrobattista. "Plasmid Engineering for Controlled and Sustained Gene Expression for Nonviral Gene Therapy." *Pharmaceutical Research* 23, no. 6 (2006): 1053-1074. Indepth review describing

the factors and genetic regions necessary for optimal expression of proteins from plasmid vectors.

Web Sites of Interest
Plasmid Sequencing
http://www.sanger.ac.uk/Projects/Plasmids

Plasmid.org
http://www.plasmid.org

Plasmids: History of a Concept
http://histmicro.yale.edu/mainfram.htm

See also: Anthrax; Antisense RNA; Archaea; Bacterial genetics and cell structure; Bacterial resistance and super bacteria; Biopesticides; Biopharmaceuticals; Blotting: Southern, Northern, and Western; Cloning; Cloning vectors; DNA sequencing technology; Emerging and remerging infectious diseases; Extrachromosomal inheritance; Gene regulation: Bacteria; Genetic engineering; Genetic engineering: Agricultural applications; Genetic engineering: Historical development; Genetic engineering: Industrial applications; Genome size; Genomics; High-yield crops; Human growth hormone; Immunogenetics; Model organism: *Chlamydomonas reinhardtii*; Model organism: *Escherichia coli*; Model organism: *Saccharomyces cerevisiae*; Model organism: *Xenopus laevis*; Noncoding RNA molecules; Polymerase chain reaction; Proteomics; Shotgun cloning; Transgenic organisms; Transposable elements.

PMS genes

Category: Molecular genetics
Significance: *PMS* genes function in DNA mismatch repair, where they help correct errors that arise during replication. If these errors go uncorrected, mutations will accumulate in the genome, eventually leading to cancer. Deficiency in the *PMS2* gene can cause hereditary nonpolyposis colon cancer as well as Turcot syndrome.

Genetics

There are two genes in the *PMS* family, *PMS1* and *PMS2*. *PMS* stands for postmeiotic segregation, the name given to the yeast homologue due to its role in regulating recombination during meiosis. In humans, *PMS1* is located on chromosome 2q31-33, and *PMS2* is located on 7p22.

MMR AND CANCER

The main cellular role for the *PMS* genes is in mismatch repair. When cells divide, the DNA is replicated by enzymes called polymerases that use the existing strand as a copy for the new strand. The polymerases occasionally make an error, creating a mismatch between the template strand and the newly replicated strand. MMR functions to correct these errors before they become mutations. The *PMS* genes are part of the MutL heterodimer. *PMS2* is in MutLalpha, where it binds *MLH1*. *PMS1* also binds MLH1, as part of MutLbeta. The MutL heterodimer gets recruited to mismatched bases in the DNA by the MutS heterodimer, typically MutSalpha, which is composed of *MSH2* and *MSH6*. Once bound to DNA, MutS and MutL recruit downstream factors that excise the newly replicated strand in the area of the mismatch and fill it in with the correct base. If MMR is compromised, then the mismatched bases will go uncorrected and become mutations in the next round of replication. An increased rate of mutation accumulation can eventually lead to cancer.

If a mismatch repair gene is defective, it causes hereditary nonpolyposis colon cancer, or Lynch syndrome. The majority of HNPCC cases are caused by mutations in either *MLH1* or *MSH2*; less than 5 percent of HNPCC cases are due to inherited mutations in *PMS2* and no HNPCC-causing mutations have been definitively attributed to *PMS1*. However, *PMS2* has a number of pseudogenes that have made detecting mutations in *PMS2* difficult. HNPCC is an autosomal dominant disorder; only one copy of *PMS2* must be mutated to cause the disease. Eventually, the remaining copy of *PMS2* is lost in a subset of cells. These cells have a high mutation rate, increasing the likelihood of activating genes that promote cancer as well as altering genes that prevent it.

In addition to its role in repairing replication errors, *PMS2* also responds to damage caused by methylating agents. Methylating agents damage DNA by creating lesions that cannot be repaired by normal cellular repair mechanisms. The cells then signal apoptosis in order to prevent the damaged cells from continuing to proliferate. *PMS2* is necessary for cells to signal apoptosis in response to methylation. Cells deficient in *PMS2* will continue to grow in the presence of methylating agents.

TURCOT SYNDROME

Turcot syndrome also known as mismatch repair cancer syndrome, is caused by mutation in both alleles of a mismatch repair gene, including *PMS2*. It differs from HNPCC in that it causes early-onset malignancies of the central nervous system as well as colorectal tumors. In addition, patients often present with light brown spots on the skin, termed café-au-lait spots. Due to having mutations in both copies of *PMS2*, the severity of Turcot syndrome is increased compared to HNPCC, with cancers presenting much earlier.

IMPACT

The *PMS* genes are an essential component of mismatch repair, which is necessary to maintain genomic stability in the cell. Mutation in one copy of *PMS2* can lead to HNPCC, while mutation in both copies can cause Turcot syndrome. Furthermore, *PMS2* was the first MMR gene to be identified as causing Turcot syndrome. It was later shown that the other MMR genes could cause Turcot syndrome as well. *PMS2* also responds to DNA damage caused by methylating agents, signaling cell death. Such methylating agents are often used in chemotherapeutic settings; for example, 6-mercaptopurine, which is used to treat childhood leukemias. Functioning MMR is necessary for these drugs to be effective. It has been demonstrated that tumors can become resistant to these drugs by mutating MMR.

Jennifer Johnson

FURTHER READING

Alberts, Bruce, et al. *Molecular Biology of the Cell.* New York: Garland, 2002. Print.

Hodgson, S. V., et al. *A Practical Guide to Human Cancer Genetics.* London: Springer, 2013. *eBook Collection (EBSCOhost).* Web. 7 Aug. 2014.

Kufe, Donald W., et al., eds. *Cancer Medicine.* Hamilton: BC Decker, 2003. Print.

Nussbaum, Robert L., Roderick McInnes, and Huntington F. Willard. *Genetics in Medicine.* 7th ed. New York: Saunders, 2007. Print.

Tomsic, J, et al. "Recurrent and Founder Mutations in the PMS2 Gene." *Clinical Genetics* 83.3 (2013): 238–43. *Academic Search Elite.* Web. 7 Aug. 2014.

Vogelsang, Matjaž. *DNA Alterations in Lynch Syndrome: Advances in Molecular Diagnosis and Genetic Counseling.* New York: Springer, 2013. Digital file.

See also: *BRAF* gene; *BRCA1* and *BRCA2* genes; *MLH1* gene; *RB1* gene; *RhoGD12* gene; *SCLC1* gene.

Polycystic kidney disease

CATEGORY: Diseases and syndromes
ALSO KNOWN AS: PKD; autosomal dominant poly cystic kidney disease; AKPKD; adult polycystic disease; polycystic kidney disease type 2

DEFINITION

The word polycystic means many cysts. Polycystic kidney disease (PKD) is a group of inherited disorders that causes many cysts to form in the kidneys.

Cysts, which are sacs filled with fluid, grow in both kidneys causing them to become enlarged. The number of cysts can range from a few to a great number. The size of the cysts can vary from extremely small to cysts larger than the kidney itself.

PKD can be painful and interfere with the nor mal functioning of the kidney, resulting in infection, kidney stones, high blood pressure, and, eventually, kidney failure. PKD is a potentially serious condition that requires care from team of clinicians.

RISK FACTORS

The primary risk factor for PKD is having a parent with the disease. In autosomal dominant disease, fifty percent of children born to a parent with the PKD gene develop the disease. In about 10 percent of cases, the gene for the disease was not inherited, but mutated. PKD affects men and women equally.

Risk factors for progression to end-stage kidney disease include:

- *PKD1* genotype
- Large kidneys
- Several episodes of gross hematuria
- Severe and frequent kidney infections
- Hypertension
- Multiple pregnancies
- Black racial background
- Male sex

ETIOLOGY AND GENETICS

The majority of cases of adult-onset polycystic kidney disease result from a genetic disorder, but some cases are known in which the disease has been acquired, usually after years of dialysis for kidney failure of unrelated origin. The most common genetic forms result from autosomal dominant mutations in either the genes, *PKD1*, or *PKD2* genes; but there is also an association with the *GANAB* gene. About 85 percent of these cases result from mutations in *PKD1*, found on the short arm of chromosome 16 at position 16p13.3. This gene encodes a large protein called polycystin-1, which normally spans the membrane of kidney cells and receives chemical signals from outside the cell that help the cell respond properly under varying environmental conditions. The protein interacts with polycystin-2 (the product of the *PKD2* gene, found on chromosome 4 at position 4q21-q23) to trigger a cascade of cellular reactions. A missing or altered polycystin-1 protein disrupts this signaling, and cells in the renal tissue may grow and divide abnormally, resulting in the cyst development that is characertistic of the disease. Mutations in *PKD2*, which account for the remaining 15 percent of adult cases, result in abnor mal polycystin-2 proteins that lead to similar physio logical malfunctions. Mutations in either gene are inherited in an autosomal dominant fashion, mean ing that a single copy of the mutation is sufficient to cause full expression of the disease. An affected in dividual has a 50 percent chance of transmitting the mutation to each of his or her children. About 10 percent of cases of polycystic kidney disease, how ever, result from a spontaneous new mutation, so in these instances affected individuals will have unaf fected parents.

A rare severe form of polycystic kidney disease that usually is diagnosed at birth or in early infancy results from mutations in the *PKHD1* gene (at posi tion 6p12.2). The protein encoded by this gene is fibrocystin, a membrane-spanning protein with func tions similar to polycystin-1. This often lethal form of the disease is inherited in an autosomal recessive manner, which means that both copies of the *PKHD1* gene must be deficient in order for the individual to be afflicted. Typically, an affected child is born to two unaffected parents, both of whom are carriers of the recessive mutant allele. The probable out comes for children whose parents are both carriers are 75 percent unaffected and 25 percent affected.

SYMPTOMS

During the early stages of PKD, there are often no symptoms. Some people are never diagnosed be cause there are no symptoms or their symptoms are mild. Most symptoms begin to appear in middle age.

Frequently, the first symptom is pain in the back or flank area. Other signs of PKD include high blood pressure, blood in the urine, urinary tract infection, and kidney stones. Cysts may also form in other organs, particularly the liver. These patients also have a higher risk of developing abnormalities in heart valves as well as both thoracic aortic and cerebral aneurysms, a condition involving weakness and bulging of blood vessels that could eventually become life-threatening. Additional, less common symptoms may include nail abnormalities, painful menstruation, joint pain, fatigue, breathlessness, weakness, and malaise.

Individuals who experience any of these symptoms should not assume it is due to PKD. These symptoms may be caused by other, more common health conditions. Individuals who experience any one of the symptoms should see their physicians.

SCREENING AND DIAGNOSIS

The doctor may ask about a patient's symptoms and medical history and may perform a physical exam. Signs of the disease may include, high blood pressure, enlarged or tender kidneys, enlarged liver, and protein and/or blood in the urine. Much less commonly, there may be signs of kidney failure such as pale, dry skin as well as leg and abdominal swelling.

An abdominal ultrasound is usually the test of first choice to detect the presence of cysts on the kidneys. If cysts are not detected by ultra sound and the diagnosis is still in question, an abdominal computed tomography (CT) scan or a magnetic resonance imaging (MRI) scan may be recommended. Genetic testing is also available.

Between 10 and 40 percent of patients with PKD also have an aneur ysm (a weakness in the wall of a blood vessel) in the brain. If a patient is diagnosed with PKD and there is a family history of a brain aneurysm, magnetic resonance angiography may be recommended.

TREATMENT AND THERAPY

Most treatments for PKD treat the disease symp toms or prevent complications. Treatment often includes antihypertensive medications to control high blood pressure. Medications may also be needed to maintain appropriate electrolyte levels in the face of failing kidney function.

Pain medications may be used cautiously, since some of them can cause further damage to the kid neys. In the event of a urinary tract or cyst infection, aggressive treatment with antibiotics is required to avoid further damage to the kidneys. Adequate hydration is often recommended especially in those who develop blood in the urine.

Tolvaptan is a drug that has been approved in Canada, Europe, and Japan for treatment of autosomal dominant PKD, but not in the United States where it is still being studied in clinical trials. It is indicated to slow the progression of cyst development and renal insufficiency in these patients when, at the initiation of treatment, there is Stage 1-3 chronic kidney disease with evidence of rapid progression.

Cysts may be drained through surgery to relieve pain, blockage, infection, or bleeding. Cyst drainage

Cat scan of person with polycystic kidney disease. PKD is a progressive, genetic disorder of the kidneys. By Sb2207 (Own work), via Wikimedia Commons

Gross pathology of polycystic kidneys. See page for author, via Wikimedia Commons

may also temporarily lower blood pressure. Some times one or both kidneys may need to be removed if pain is severe and cannot be controlled any other way. In there is severe involvement of the liver, partial removal of the liver or liver transplantation may be recommended.

A low-protein diet may reduce stress on the kidney. Avoiding salt can help maintain normal blood pressure, and drinking lots of water can help reduce the risk of kidney stones.

More than half of PKD patients develop end-stage kidney disease and require dialysis. Dialysis is used to re move wastes from the blood, since the kidneys can not. At this stage, dialysis will be a lifelong requirement. In many cases, an eventual kidney transplant needs to be considered.

Recent research has led to the development of several drugs that may slow the progression of cyst formation and enlargement in patients with autosomal dominant PKD. An example is octreotide, an analogue of somatostatin. This may one day be available to help slow the progression to end-stage kidney disease in these patients.

Prevention and Outcomes

PKD is an inherited disease and is not pre ventable. Even with optimal treatment, up to 50% of patients with autosomal dominant disease will require a kidney transplant by age 60. Individuals who have a family history of PKD may want to talk to their doctors about genetic testing.

Patricia Griffin Kellicker, B.S.N.;
reviewed by Adrienne Carmack, M.D.
"Etiology and Genetics" by Jeffrey A. Knight, Ph.D.;
updated by Gary M. Flashner, M.S., M.D.

Further Reading

Chang, M. Y., and A. C. Ong. "Autosomal Dominant Polycystic Kidney Disease: Recent Advances in Pathogenesis and Treatment." *Nephron: Physiology* 108, no. 1 (2008): 1-7.

EBSCO Publishing. *DynaMed: Autosomal Dominant Polycystic Kidney Disease.* Ipswich, Mass.: Author, 2009. Available through http://www.ebscohost.com/dynamed.

_____. *Health Library: Polycystic Kidney Disease.* Ipswich, Mass.: Author, 2009. Available through http://www.ebscohost.com.

McPhee, Stephen J., and Maxine A. Papadakis., eds. *Current Medical Diagnosis and Treatment 2009.* 48th ed. New York: McGraw-Hill Medical, 2008.

Irazabal MV, Huston J 3rd, Kubly V, Rossetti S, Sundsbak JL, Hogan MC, et al. "Extended follow-up of unruptured intracranial aneurysms detected by presymptomatic screening in patients with autosomal dominant polycystic kidney disease." *Clin J Am Soc Nephrol.* 2011 Jun. 6(6):1274-85

Pirson Y. "Extrarenal Manifestations of Autosomal Dominant Polycystic Kidney Disease." *Adv Chronic Kidney Dis.* 2010 Mar. 17(2):173-180.

Porath B, Gainullin VG, Cornec-Le Gall E, Dillinger EK, Heyer CM, Hopp K, et al. "Mutations in GANAB, Encoding the Glucosidase IIα Subunit, Cause Autosomal-Dominant Polycystic Kidney and Liver Disease." *Am J Hum Genet.* 2016 Jun 2. 98 (6):1193-207

Akoh JA. "Current management of autosomal dominant polycystic kidney disease." *World J Nephrol.* 2015 Sep 6. 4 (4):468-79

Cornec-Le Gall E, Audrézet MP, Chen JM, Hourmant M, Morin MP, Perrichot R, et al. "Type of PKD1 mutation influences renal outcome in ADPKD." *J Am Soc Nephrol.* 2013 May. 24 (6):1006-13.

Higashihara E, Nutahara K, Okegawa T, Tanbo M, Mori H, Miyazaki I, Nitatori T, Kobayashi K. "Safety study of somatostatin analogue octreotide for autosomal dominant polycystic kidney disease in Japan." *Clin Exp Nephrol.* 2015 Aug;19(4):746-52. doi: 10.1007/s10157-014-1047-1. Epub 2014 Oct 29.

Web Sites of Interest

American Academy of Family Physicians: Polycystic Kidney Disease http://familydoctor.org/online/famdocen/home/common/kidney/142.html

American Urological Association: Renal Dysplasia and Cystic Disease
http://www.urologyhealth.org/auafhome.asp

Genetics Home Reference
http://ghr.nlm.nih.gov
HealthLink B. C. (British Columbia)
http://www.healthlinkbc.ca/kbaltindex.asp

The Kidney Foundation of Canada
http://www.kidney.ab.ca

https://rarediseases.info.nih.gov/diseases/7419/polycystic-kidney-disease

http://emedicine.medscape.com/article/244907-overview

https://ghr.nlm.nih.gov/gene/GANAB#conditions

https://www.ncbi.nlm.nih.gov/gene/23193

MedLine Plus: Polycystic Kidney Disease
http://www.nlm.nih.gov/medlineplus/ency/article/000502.htm

PKD Foundation
http://www.pkdcure.org

See also: Alport syndrome; Bartter syndrome; Hereditary leiomyomatosis and renal cell cancer; Hereditary non-VHL clear cell renal cell carcinomas; Hereditary papillary renal cancer.

Polydactyly

CATEGORY: Diseases and syndromes
ALSO KNOWN AS: Polydactylia; polydactylism; hyper dactyly; extra digits; supernumerary digits

DEFINITION

Polydactyly is a relatively common congenital deformity that occurs due to errors during fetal development and results in the presence of one or more extra digits on the hand and/or foot. It occurs as follows: preaxial duplication—thumb side of hand/ hallux (big toe) side of foot; central duplication— middle digit area of hand/foot; postaxial duplica tion—little digit side of hand/foot.

Extra digits are usually smaller in size and abnor mal in appearance. However, they range from barely noticeable and consisting solely of soft tissue to fully developed and possibly functional.

RISK FACTORS

Polydactyly can occur spontaneously (familial polydactyly) or in conjunction with a number of genetic disorders. The following are examples of genetic disorders that often include polydactyly: Asphyxiating thoracic dystrophy (Jeune syndrome) is a bone growth disorder. Car penter syndrome is an acrocephalopolysyndactyly (ACPS) disorder that affects bone growth. Ellis-van Creveld syndrome (chondroectodermal dysplasia) is a bone growth disorder involving growth hormone derficiency; the highest incidence rate of this syndrome occurs in Old Order Amish from Lancas ter County, Pennsylvania. Laurence-Moon-Biedl syn drome is a mitochondrial myopathic disorder char acterized by mental retardation and possibly short stature. Genetics and Inherited Conditions Polydactyly • 985 Rubinstein-Taybi syndrome is a rare disorder characterized by mental retardation and short stat ure. Smith-Lemli-Opitz syndrome is a disorder char acterized by microcephaly (small head circumfer ence), hypotonia (weak muscle tonus), and possible organ malformations; the highest incidence of this syndrome occurs in Caucasians of Central European ancestry. Trisomy 13 (Patau syndrome) is a usually fatal disorder characterized by multiple structural and developmental abnormalities.

Familial polydactyly may occur independent of any other symptoms or disease. The highest incidence of sixth digit inheritance occurs in African Americans. In those rare instances where polydactylism causality cannot be definitively attributed to genetic abnormality, it is hypothesized that a womb abnormality or exposure to toxins may be contribut ing factors.

Other factors associated with postaxial hand polydactyly include twinning, low maternal education, parental consanguinity, occurrence in first-degree relatives, and maternal bleeding in the first trimester. Despite the associations, there is no clear cause-and-effect.

ETIOLOGY AND GENETICS

Although it can occur independent of genetic factors, polydactyly is most commonly a heritable, autosomal dominant trait involving a single gene that is capable of causing several variations in ex pression. Therefore, inheritance is not gender linked and does not require that both parents have the trait. It most likely occurs as the result of duplication of a single embryologic bud. Polydactyly is most often autosomal recessive when it occurs as a part of the manifestation of a syndrome such as those listed under "Risk Factors".

Despite being a common malformation, the true incidence of polydactyly is not fully known. The incidence rate for all cases of polydactyly of the hand is estimated to be approximately 1 per 1,000 births in Caucasian populations and upwards of 10 times this in

Polydactyly Rhand By en:User:Drgnu23, subsequently altered by en:user:Grendelkhan, en:user: Raul654, and en:user:Solipsist (Original work by author), via Wikimedi

Polydactyly By Sreeakhileee (Own work), via Wikimedia Commons

African-American populations. It is the most common hand anomaly and occurs most frequently as preaxial (thumb) polydactyly in those of Asian ancestry who have the trait and as postaxial (little finger) polydactyly in those of African ancestry who have the trait. It occurs in a male-to-female ratio of 2.5 to 1 and is most often unilateral. Incidence rate for polydactyly of the foot is ap proximately 1 to 2 per 1,000 births. In approximately 50 percent of all cases, it occurs bilaterally although not necessarily symmetrically. In approx imately 33 percent of all cases, it occurs in conjunc tion with polydactyly of the hand. Incidence of fused extra digits indicates the con comitant occurrence of polydactyly and syndactyly (fusion of digits) and is termed polysyndactyly.

SYMPTOMS
The only symptom of polydactyly is the presence of one or more extra digits. The presence of other symptoms may indicate the possibility of a concomi tant genetic disorder.

SCREENING AND DIAGNOSIS
Fetal finger buds can be seen using transvaginal ultrasound as early as 9 weeks and reliably by 13 weeks of pregnancy. Once polydactyly is established, a thorough ultrasound evaluation, especially of the heart, nervous system, limbs, and kidneys, to identify an associated syndrome might be recommended. Follow-up ultrasound between 17 and 34 weeks with biometric profile may be recommended to establish the diagnosis of isolated polydactyly.

After birth, x-rays of the affected limb may be recommended to show whether the rudimentary digit contains skeletal elements. The degree of deviation of the digit and the size of the articulating metacarpal or metatarsal also may be helpful for surgical planning.

Additional screening may include a comprehensive medical history and performing chromosome studies to rule out a syndrome that includes polydactyly. Other tests may enzyme tests, metabolic studies, and genetic testing.

TREATMENT AND THERAPY
A child with distal extremity anomalies frequently experiences emotional stress. By age 3 years, the child has become aware of the anomaly. By age 7 years, the child has begun to experience the close scrutiny of peers at school. For these reasons, along with others, surgical correction is often recommended early in life.

Surgical management depends greatly on the complexity and location of the deformity as well as the degree of bone, ligament, and tendon involvement. In order to reduce the risk of anesthesia yet allow for the maximum potential for remodeling, surgical excision usually occurs when a baby is between about 9 and 12 months of age. For the most part, traditional suture ligation for post-axial polydactyly has been abandoned due to the increased risk for developing painful neuromas.

PREVENTION AND OUTCOMES

There is no known means for preventing spontaneous polydactyly. Possible prevention of polydactyly that occurs in conjunction with genetic disorders would require genetic screening and counseling of prospective parents. The prognosis for isolated polydactyly is extremely favorable with surgical excision. Most patients have good-to-excellent results after surgery. Careful surgery helps to ensure better cosmetic and functional outcomes.

Cynthia L. De Vine;
updated by Gary M. Flashner, M.S., M.D.

FURTHER READING

Barnhill, Raymond L., and A. Neil Crowson. *Textbook of Dermatopathology.* 2d ed. New York: McGraw Hill, 2004. A comprehensive, illustrated reference written for professionals and scholars yet comprehensible for nonprofessionals; includes photomicrographs.

McGlamry, Dalton, et al. *McGlamr y's Comprehensive Textbook of Foot and Ankle Surger y.* 3d ed. Philadelphia: Lippincott, Williams & Wilkins, 2001. A standard, core pediatric textbook written for physicians, researchers, and students.

Tickle, C. "Embryology." In *The Growing Hand: Diagnosis and Management of the Upper Extremity in Children,* edited by A. Gupta, S. P. J. Kay, and L. R. Scheker. London: Mosby, 2000.

Wattanarat O, Kantaputra PN. "Preaxial polydactyly associated with a MSX1 mutation and report of two novel mutations." *Am J Med Genet A.* 2015 Oct 13. Klaassen Z, Shoja MM, Tubbs RS, Loukas M. "Supernumerary and absent limbs and digits of the lower limb: a review of the literature." *Clin Anat.* 2011 Jul. 24(5):570-5 Dijkman R, Selles R, van Rosmalen J, Hülsemann W, Mann M, Habenicht R, et al. "A clinically weighted approach to outcome assessment in radial polydactyly." *J Hand Surg Eur* Vol. 2015 Aug 28.

WEB SITES OF INTEREST

Children's Craniofacial Association
http://www.ccakids.com/syn.asp#Carpenter_Syndrome

Children's Hospital Boston
http://www.childrenshospital.org/az/Site1073/mainpageS1073P0.html

Genetics Home Reference; US National Library of Medicine
http://ghr.nlm.nih.gov/

March of Dimes Pregnancy & Newborn Health Education Center
http://www.marchofdimes.com/pnhec/4439_4136.asp

MedlinePlus Medical Encyclopedia; U.S. National Library of Medicine and the National Institutes of Health
http://www.nlm.nih.gov/medlineplus/ency/article/003176.htm

Penn State Milton Hershey Medical Center College of Medicine
http://www.hmc.psu.edu/healthinfo/pq/poly.htmUniversity of Mar yland Medical Center
http://www.umm.edu/news/

Wheeless' Textbook of Orthopaedics; Duke University Medical Center's Division of Orthopaedic Surgery
http://www.wheelessonline.com/ortho/polydactyly_of_foot
http://www.wheelessonline.com/ortho/polydactyly_of_the_handhttp://www.mdedge.com/amjorthopedics/article/99409/hand-wrist/polydactyly-hand
http://emedicine.medscape.com/article/1113584-overview

See also: Apert syndrome; Brachydactyly; Carpenter syndrome; Cleft lip and palate; Congenital defects; Cornelia de Lange syndrome; Cri du chat syndrome; Crouzon syndrome; Down syndrome; Edwards syndrome; Ellis-van Creveld syndrome; Holt-Oram syndrome; Ivemark syndrome; Meacham syndrome; Opitz-Frias syndrome; Patau syndrome; Robert syndrome; Rubinstein-Taybi syndrome.

Polygenic inheritance

CATEGORY: Classical transmission genetics
SIGNIFICANCE: Polygenically inherited traits—characterized by the amount of some attribute that they possess but not by their presence or absence—are central to plant and animal breeding, medicine, and evolutionary biology. Most of the economically important traits in plants and animals—for example, yield and meat production—are polygenic

in nature. Quantitative genetic principles are applied to improve such traits.

Discovery of Polygenic Inheritance

Soon after the rediscovery of Gregor Mendel's laws of heredity in 1900, Herman Nilsson-Ehle, a Swedish geneticist, showed in 1909 how multiple genes with small effects could collectively affect a continuously varying character. He crossed dark, red-grained wheat with white-grained wheat and found the progeny with an intermediate shade of red. Upon crossing the progeny among themselves, he obtained grain colors ranging from dark red to white. He could classify the grains into five groups in a symmetric ratio of 1:4:6:4:1, with the extreme phenotypes being one-sixteenth dark red and one-sixteenth white. This suggested two-gene segregation. For a two-gene ($n = 2$) model, the number and frequency of phenotypic classes ($2n + 1 = 5$) can be determined by expanding the binomial $(a + b)4$, where a represents the number of favorable alleles and b represents the number of nonfavorable alleles.

Subsequently, Nilsson-Ehle crossed a different variety of red-grained wheat with white-grained wheat. He found that one-sixty-fourth of the plants produced dark red kernels and one-sixty-fourth produced white kernels. There were a total of seven phenotypic (color) classes instead of five. The segregation ratio corresponded to three genes: $(a + b)^6 = 1a^6 + 6a^5b^1 + 15a^4b^2 + 20a^3b^3 + 15a^2b^4 + 6a^1b^5 + 1b^6$. Here, a^6 means that one of sixty-four individuals possessed six favorable alleles, $20a^3b^3$ means that twenty of sixty-four individuals had three favorable and three nonfavorable alleles, and b^6 means that one individual had six nonfavorable alleles. An assumption was that each of the alleles had an equal, additive effect. These experiments led to what is known as the multiple-factor hypothesis, or polygenic inheritance (Kenneth Mather coined the terms "polygenes" and "polygenic traits"). Around 1920, Ronald Aylmer Fisher, Sewall Green Wright, and John Burdon Sanderson Haldane developed methods of quantitative analysis of genetic effects.

Polygenic traits are characterized by the amount of some attribute that they possess but not by presence or absence, as is the case with qualitative traits that are controlled by one or two major genes. Environmental factors generally have little or no effect on the expression of a gene or genes controlling a qualitative trait, whereas quantitative traits are highly influenced by the environment and genotype is poorly represented by phenotype. Genes controlling polygenic traits are sometimes called minor genes.

Examples and Characteristics of Polygenic Traits

Quantitative genetics encompasses analyses of traits that exhibit continuous variation caused by polygenes and their interactions among themselves and with environmental factors. Such traits include height, weight, and some genetic defects.

Diabetes and cancer are considered to be threshold traits because all individuals can be classified as affected or unaffected (qualitative). They are also continuous traits because severity varies from nearly undetectable to extremely severe (quantitative). Because it is virtually impossible to determine the exact genotype for such traits, it is difficult to control defects with a polygenic mode of inheritance.

skin color varation is an example of polygenic inheritance By Henry M. Trotter at en.wikipedia, from Wikimedia Commons *cleft palate is an example of polygenic inheritance By CDC.MooreSvn at en.wikipedia, from Wikimedia Commons*

DETECTION OF GENES CONTROLLING POLYGENIC TRAITS

The detection of genes controlling polygenic traits is challenging and complex for the following reasons.

(1) The expression of genes controlling such traits is modified by fluctuations in environmental and/or management factors.

(2) A quantitative trait is usually a composite of many other traits, each influenced by many genes with variable effects.

(3) Effects of allele substitution are small because many genes control the trait.

(4) Expression of an individual gene may be modified by the expression of other genes and environment.

Polygenic traits are best analyzed with statistical methods, the simplest of which are estimation of arithmetic mean, standard error, variance, and standard deviation. Two populations can have the same mean, but their distribution may be different. Thus, one needs information on variances for describing the two populations more fully. From variances, effects of genes can be ascertained in the aggregate rather than as individual genes.

The issues in quantitative genetics are not only how many and which genes control a trait but also how much of what is observed (phenotype) is attributable to genes (heritability) and how much to the environment. The concept of heritability in the broad sense is useful for quantitative traits, but heritability itself does not give any clues to the total number of genes involved. If heritability is close to 1.0, the variance for a trait is attributable entirely to genetics, and when it is close to zero, the population's phenotype is due entirely to the variation in the underlying environment. Environmental effects mask or modify genetic effects.

Distribution or frequency of different classes in segregating populations—for example, F2—may provide an idea about the number of genes, particularly if the gene number is small (say, three to four). Formulas have been devised to estimate the number of genes conditioning a trait, but these estimates are not highly reliable. Genes controlling quantitative traits can be estimated via use of chromosomal translocations or other cytogenetic procedures. The advent of molecular markers, such as restriction fragment length polymorphisms, RFLP analysis has made it easier and more reliable to pinpoint the location of genes on chromosomes of a species of interest. With much work in a well-characterized organism, these polygenes can be mapped to chromosomes as quantitative trait loci.

Manjit S. Kang, Ph.D.

FURTHER READING

Jurmain, Robert, et al. "Heredity and Evolution." *Introduction to Physical Anthropology.* 13th ed. Florence: Wadsworth, 2011. Print.

Kang, Manjit S. *Quantitative Genetics, Genomics, and Plant Breeding.* Wallingford: CABI, 2002. Print.

Khoury, M. J., A. C. J. W. Janssens, and D. F. Ransohoff. "How Can Polygenic Inheritance Be Used in Population Screening for Common Diseases?" *Genetics in Medicine* 15.6 (2013): 437–43. *Global Health.* Web. 7 Aug. 2014.

Krimsky, Sheldon, and Jeremy Gruber. *Genetic Explanations: Sense and Nonsense.* Cambridge: Harvard UP, 2013. Print.

Lynch, Michael, and Bruce Walsh. *Genetics and Analysis of Quantitative Traits.* Sunderland: Sinauer, 1998. Print.

Young, Ian D. "Polygenic Inheritance and Complex Diseases." *Medical Genetics.* New York: Oxford UP, 2005. Print.

See also: Congenital defects; Genetic engineering; Hereditary diseases; Neural tube defects; Pedigree analysis; Plasmids; Quantitative inheritance.

Polymerase chain reaction

CATEGORY: Genetic engineering and biotechnology; Molecular genetics; Techniques and methodologies

SIGNIFICANCE: Polymerase chain reaction (PCR) is the in vitro (in the test tube) amplification of specific nucleic acid sequences. In a few hours, a single piece of DNA can be copied one billion times. Because this technique is simple, rapid, and very sensitive, it is used in a very wide range of applications, including forensics, disease diagnosis, molecular genetics, and nucleic acid sequencing.

KEY TERMS

DNA polymerase: an enzyme that copies or replicatesDNA; it uses a single-stranded DNA as a templat for synthesis of a complementary new strand and requires an RNA primer or a small section of double-stranded DNA to initiate synthesis

molecular cloning: the process of splicing a piece of DNA into a plasmid, virus, or phage vector to obtain many identical copies of that DNA

THE DEVELOPMENT OF THE POLYMERASE CHAIN REACTION

The polymerase chain reaction (PCR) was developed by Kary B. Mullis in the mid-1980's. The technique revolutionized molecular genetics and the study of genes. One of the difficulties in studying genes is that a specific gene can be one of approximately twenty-one thousand genes in a complex genome. To obtain the number of copies of a specific gene needed for accurate analysis required the time-consuming techniques of molecular cloning and detection of specific DNA sequences. The polymerase chain reaction changed the science of molecular genetics by allowing huge numbers of copies of a specific DNA sequence to be produced without the use of molecular cloning. The tremendous significance of this discovery was recognized by the awarding of the 1993 Nobel Prize in Chemistry to Mullis for the invention of the PCR method. (The 1993 prize was also awarded to Michael Smith, for work on oligonucleotide-based, site-directed mutagenesis and its development for protein studies.)

HOW POLYMERASE CHAIN REACTION WORKS

PCR begins with the creation of a single-stranded DNA template to be copied. This is done by heating double-stranded DNA to temperatures near boiling (about 94 to 99 degrees Celsius, or about 210 degrees Fahrenheit). This is followed by the annealing (binding of a complementary sequence) of pairs of oligonucleotides (short nucleic acid molecules about ten to twenty nucleotides long) called primers. Because DNA polymerase requires a doublestranded region to prime (initiate) DNA synthesis, the starting point for DNA synthesis is specified by the location at which the primer anneals to the template. The primers are chosen to flank the DNA to be amplified. This annealing is done at a lower temperature (about 30-65 degrees Celsius, or about 86- 149 degrees Fahrenheit). The final step is the synthesis by DNA polymerase of a new strand of DNA complem entary to the template starting from the primers. This step is carried out at temperatures about 65-75 degrees Celsius (149-167 degrees Fahrenheit). These three steps are repeated many times (for many cycles) to amplify the template DNA. The time for each of the three steps is typically one to two minutes. If, in each cycle, one copy is made of each of the strands of the template, the number of DNA molecules produced doubles each cycle. Because of this doubling, more than one million copies of the template DNA are made at the end of twenty cycles.

The PCR reaction is made more efficient by the use of heat-stable DNA polymerases, isolated from bacteria that live at very high temperatures in hot springs or deep-sea vents, and by the use of a programmable water bath (called a thermal cycler) to change the temperatures of samples quickly to each of the temperatures needed in each of the steps of a cycle.

IMPACT AND APPLICATIONS

PCR is extremely rapid. One billion copies of a specific DNA can be made in a few hours. It is also extremely sensitive. It is possible to copy a single DNA molecule. Great care must be taken to avoid contamination, however, for even trace contaminants can readily be amplified by this method.

PCR is a useful tool for many different applications. It is used in basic research to obtain DNA for sequencing and other analyses. PCR is used in disease diagnosis, in prenatal diagnosis, and to match donor and recipient tissues for organ transplants. Because a specific sequence can be amplified greatly, much less clinical material is needed to make a diagnosis. The assay is also rapid, so results are available sooner. PCR is used to detect pathogens, such as the causative agents for Lyme disease or for acquired immunodeficiency syndrome (AIDS), that are difficult to culture. PCR can even be used to amplify DNA from ancient sources such as mummies, bones, and other museum specimens PCR is an important tool in forensic investigations Target DNA from trace amounts of biological material such as semen, blood, and hair roots can be amplified. There are probes for regions of human DNA that show hypervariability in the population and therefore make good markers to identify the source of the DNA. PCR can therefore be used to evaluate evidence at the scene of a crime, help identify missing people, and resolve paternity cases.

Susan J. Karcher, Ph.D.

FURTHER READING

Budowle, Bruce, et al. *DNA Typing Protocols: Molecular Biology and Forensic Analysis.* Natick, Mass.:Eaton, 2000. Discussion includes DNA extraction and PCR-based analyses. Illustrations, bibliography, index.

Chen, Bing-Yuan, and Harry W. Janes, eds. *PCR Cloning Protocols.* Rev. 2d ed. Totowa, N.J.: Humana Press, 2002. Presents helpful introductory chapters with each section and guidelines for PCR cloning. Illustrations, bibliographies, index.

Dorak, M. Tevfik, ed. *Real-Time PCR.* New York: Taylor and Francis, 2006. Focuses on the practical aspects of PCR techniques, emphasizing how these methods can be used in the laboratory.

Guyer, Ruth L., and Daniel E. Koshland, Jr. "The Molecule of the Year." *Science* 246, no. 4937 (December 22, 1989): 1543-1546. Reviews the "major scientific development of the year," the polymerase chain reaction, noting that the technique, although introduced earlier, "truly burgeoned" in 1989.

Innis, Michael A., David H. Gelfand, and John J. Sninsky, eds. *PCR Applications: Protocols for Functional Genomics.* San Diego: Academic Press, 1999. Discusses gene discovery, genomics, and DNA array technology. Includes entries on nomenclature, expression, sequence analysis, structure and function, electrophysiology, and information retrieval. Illustrations, bibliography, index.

Kochanowski, Bernd, and Udo Reischl, eds. *Quantitative PCR Protocols.* Totowa, N.J.: Humana Press, 1999. Outlines protocols and includes methodological and process notes. Illustrations, bibliography, index.

Lloyd, Ricardo V., ed. *Morphology Methods: Cell and Molecular Biology Techniques.* Totowa, N.J.: Humana Press, 2001. Includes an overview of PCR. Illustrations, bibliography, index.

Logan, Julie, Kirstin Edwards, and Nick Saunders, eds. *Real-Time PCR: Current Technology and Applications.* Norfolk, England: Caister Academic Press, 2009. Discusses PCR technologies and tools, as well as applications for PCR in gene expression, mutation detection, diagnosis of fungal infections, and determination of food authenticity.

McPherson, M. J., and S. G. Møller. *PCR.* 2d ed. New York: Taylor and Francis, 2006. Provides introductory information about PCR theory, background, and protocols. Illustrations, bibliography, index.

Mullis, Kary B. "The Unusual Origin of the Polymerase Chain Reaction." *Scientific American* 262, no. 4 (April, 1990): 56. Nobel laureate Mullis describes the initial development of the technique for the general audience.

Watson, James D., et al. *Recombinant DNA—Genes and Genomes: A Short Course.* 3d ed. New York: W. H. Freeman, 2007. Summarizes polymerase chain reaction and its applications. Full-color illustrations, diagrams, bibliography, index.

WEB SITES OF INTEREST

Dolan DNA Learning Center, Biology Animation Library
http://www.dnalc.org/resources/animations/pcr.html
Viewers can watch an animated demonstration of PCR.

Library, University of California, Berkeley, PCR Project
http://sunsite3.berkeley.edu/PCR
An introductory overview to PCR prepared by professors and librarians at the university, including Paul Rainbow, an anthropology professor who wrote the book *Making PCR: A Story of Biotechnology* (1996). Provides access to several papers discussing the fundamentals of PCR, applications of PCR basics, and technical variations in basic PCR methods.

University of Utah, Genetic Science Learning Center, PCR Virtual Lab
http://learn.genetics.utah.edu/content/labs/pcr
The virtual lab provides a demonstration of PCR.

See also: Ancient DNA; Anthrax; Bioinformatics; Blotting: Southern, Northern, and Western; Central dogma of molecular biology; Cloning vectors; DNA fingerprinting; DNA sequencing technology; Forensic genetics; Genetic engineering: Historical development; Human Genome Project; In vitro fertilization and embryo transfer; Mitochondrial diseases;

Molecular genetics; Paternity tests; Repetitive DNA; Reverse transcription polymerase chain reaction (RT-PCR); RFLP analysis; RNA isolation.

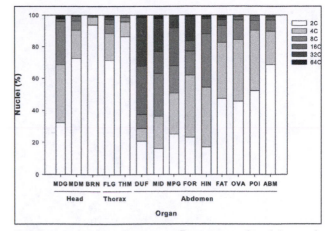

Distribution of ploidy among organs. Percentage of nuclei at each of the ploidy levels observed (2C–64C) within each organ analyzed. Organs are presented by body segment in descending order of cycle value. By Scholes D, Suarez A, Smith A, Johnston S, Paige K (2014), via Wikimedia Commons

Polyploidy

CATEGORY: Population genetics

SIGNIFICANCE: Olyploids have three or more complete sets of chromosomes in their nuclei instead of the two sets found in diploids. Polyploids are especially common in plants, with some examples also existing in animals, and have a prominent role in the evolution of species. Some tissues of diploid organisms are polyploid, while the remaining cells in the organism are diploid.

THE FORMATION OF POLYPLOIDY

Most animals are diploid, meaning that they have two homologous sets of chromosomes in their cells; and their gametes (eggs and sperm) are haploid, that is, having one set of chromosomes. Plants, a variety of single-celled eukaryotes, and some insects have individual or parts of an individual's life cycle when they are haploid. In any case, when there are more than two sets of homologous chromosomes, the cell or organism is considered polyploid. A triploid organism has three sets of homologous chromosomes, a tetraploid has four sets, a dodecaploid has twelve sets, and there are organisms known to have many more than a dozen sets of homologous chromosomes.

How polyploids are formed in nature is still debated. Regardless of what theory is accepted, the first step certainly involves a failure during cell division, in either meiosis or mitosis. For example, if cytokinesis (division of the cytoplasm) fails at the conclusion of meiosis II, the daughter cells will be diploid. If, by chance, a diploid sperm fertilizes a diploid egg, the resulting zygote will be tetraploid. Although polyploidy might occur this way, biologists have proposed an alternative model involving a triploid intermediate stage.

The triploid intermediate model has been applied primarily to plants, in which polyploidy is better studied. Hybrids between two species are often sterile, but occasionally a diploid gamete from one of the species joins with a normal haploid gamete from the other species, which produces a triploid hybrid. Triploids are also sterile, for the most part, but do produce a small number of gametes, many of which are diploid. This makes the probability that two diploid gametes will join, to form a tetraploid, much higher. This hypothesis is supported by the discovery of triploid hybrid plants that do produce a small number of viable gametes. This type of polyploid, formed as a result of hybridization between two species, is called an allopolyploid. Allopolyploids are typically fertile and represent a new species.

Polyploidy can also occur within a single species, without hybridization, in which case it is called an autopolyploid. Autopolyploids can form in the same way as allopolyploids, but they can also occur as the result of a failure in cell division in a bud. If a cell in the meristematic region (a rapidly dividing group of cells at the tip of a bud) completes mitosis but not cytokinesis, it will be a tetraploid cell. All daughter cells from this cell will also be tetraploid, so that any flowers borne on this branch will produce diploid gametes. If the plant is self-compatible, it can then produce tetraploid offspring from these flowers. Autopolyploids are often a little larger and more robust than the diploids that produce them, but they are often so similar they cannot be easily distinguished. An autopolyploid, when formed, represents a new species but is not generally recognized as such unless it looks different enough physically from diploids.

Polyploidy occurs in goldfish. By Azaz.sayyad (Own work), via Wikimedia Commons

THE GENETICS OF POLYPLOIDS

A polyploid has more copies of each gene than a diploid. For example, a tetraploid has four alleles at each locus, which means tetraploids can contain much more individual variability than diploids. This has led some evolutionists to suggest that polyploids should have higher fitness than the diploids from which they came. With more variation, the individual would be preadapted to a much wider range of conditions. Because there are so many extra copies of genes, a certain amount of gene silencing (loss of genes through mutation or other processes) occurs, with no apparent detriment to the plant.

The pairing behavior of chromosomes in polyploids is also unique. In a diploid, during meiosis, homologous chromosomes associate in pairs. In an autotetraploid there are four homologous chromosomes of each type which associate together in groups of four. In an allotetraploid, the chromosomes from the two species from which they are derived are commonly not completely homologous and do not associate together. Consequently, the pairs of homologous chromosomes from one parent species associate together in pairs, as do the chromosomes from the other parent species. For this reason, sometimes allopolyploids are referred to as amphidiploids, because their pairing behavior looks the same as it does in a diploid. This is also why an allopolyploid is fertile (because meiosis occurs normally), but a hybrid between two diploids commonly is not, because the chromosomes from the two species are unable to pair properly.

POLYPLOID PLANTS AND ANIMALS

In the plant kingdom, it is estimated by some that 95 percent of pteridophytes (plants, including ferns, that reproduce by spores) and perhaps as many as 80 percent of angiosperms (flowering plants that form seeds inside an ovary) are polyploid, although there is high variability in its occurrence among families of angiosperms. In contrast, polyploidy is uncommon in gymnosperms (plants that have naked seeds that are not within specialized structures). Extensive polyploidy is observed in chrysanthemums, in which chromosome numbers range from 18 to 198. The basic chromosome number (haploid or gamete number of chromosomes) is 9. Polyploids from triploids (with 27 chromosomes) to 22-ploids (198 chromosomes) are observed. The stonecrop *Sedum suaveolens*, which has the highest chromosome number of any angiosperm, is believed to be about 80-ploid (720 chromosomes). Many important agricultural crops, including wheat, corn, sugarcane, potatoes, coffee, apples, and cotton, are polyploid.

Polyploid animals are less common than polyploid plants but are found among some groups, including crustaceans, earthworms, flatworms, and insects such as weevils, sawflies, and moths. Polyploidy has also been observed in some vertebrates, including tree frogs, lizards, salamanders, and fish. It has been suggested that the genetic redundancy observed in vertebrates may be caused by ancestral polyploidy.

POLYPLOIDY IN TISSUES

Most plants and animals contain particular tissues that are polyploid or polytene, while the rest of the organism is diploid. Polyploidy is observed in multinucleate cells and in cells that have undergone endomitosis, in which the chromosomes condense but the cell does not undergo nuclear or cellular division. For example, in vertebrates, liver cells are binucleate and therefore tetraploid. In addition, in humans, megakaryocytes can have polyploidy levels of up to sixty-four. A megakaryocyte is a giant bone-marrow cell with a large, irregularly lobed nucleus that is the precursor to blood platelets. A megakaryocyte does not circulate, but forms platelets by budding. A single megakaryocyte can produce three thousand to four thousand platelets. A platelet is an enucleated, disk-shaped cell in the blood that has a role in blood coagulation. In polytene cells, the replicated copies of the chromosomal DNA remain associated to produce giant chromosomes that have a continuously visible banding pattern. The trophoblast cells of the mammalian placenta are polytene.

IMPORTANCE OF POLYPLOIDS TO HUMANS

Most human polyploids die as embryos or fetuses. In a few rare cases, a polyploid infant is born that lives for a few days. In fact, polyploidy is not tolerated in most animal systems. Plants, on the other hand, show none of these problems with polyploidy. Some crop plants are much more productive because they are polyploid. For example, wheat (*Triticum aestivum*) is an allohexaploid and contains chromosome sets that are derived from three different ancient types. Compared to the species from which it evolved, *T. aestivum* is far more productive and produces larger grains of wheat. *Triticum aestivum* was not developed by humans but appears to have arisen by a series of chance events in the past, humans simply recognizing the better qualities of *T. aestivum*. Another fortuitous example involves three species of mustard that have given rise to black mustard, turnips, cabbage, broccoli, and several other related crops, all of which are allotetraploids.

Polyploids may be induced by the use of drugs such as colchicine, which halts cell division. Because of the advantages of the natural polyploids used in agriculture, many geneticists have experimented with artificially producing polyploids to improve crop yields. One prime example of this approach is *Triticale*, which represents an allopolyploid produced by hybridizing wheat and rye. Producing artificial polyploids often produces a new variety that has unexpected negative characteristics, so that only a few such polyploids have been successful. Nevertheless, research on polyploidy continues.

Susan J. Karcher, Ph.D.;
updated by Bryan Ness, Ph.D.

FURTHER READING

Adams, Keith L., et al. "Genes Duplicated by Polyploidy Show Unequal Contributions to the Transcriptome and Organ-Specific Reciprocal Silencing." *Proceedings of the National Academy of Sciences* 100 (2003): 4649–4654. Print.

Gregory, T. Ryan, ed. *The Evolution of the Genome.* N.p.: Academic, 2011. Digital file.

Hunter, Kimberley L., et al. "Investigating Polyploidy: Using Marigold Stomates and Fingernail Polish." *American Biology Teacher* 64.5 (2002): 364. Print.

Leitch, Illia J., and Michael D. Bennett. "Polyploidy in Angiosperms." *Trends in Plant Science* 2.12 (1997): 470–476. Print.

Lewis, Ricki. *Human Genetics: Concepts and Applications.* 11th ed. [S.I.]: McGraw, 2014. Print.

Linder, H. Peter, and Nigel P. Barker. "Does Polyploidy Facilitate Long-Distance Dispersal?" *Annals of Botany* 113.7 (2014): 1175–1183. Digital file.

Madlung, A. "Polyploidy and Its Effect on Evolutionary Success: Old Questions Revisited with New Tools." *Heredity* 110.2 (2013): 99–104. *MEDLINE with Full Text.* Web. 7 Aug. 2014.

Miller, Orlando J., and Eeva Therman. *Human Chromosomes.* 4th ed. New York: Springer, 2001. Print.

Soltis, Pamela S., and Douglas E. Soltis. *Polyploidy and Genome Evolution.* Berlin; New York: Springer, 2012. Digital file.

Sumner, Adrian T. *Chromosomes: Organization and Function.* Hoboken: Wiley, 2008. Digital file.

See also: Cell division; Cytokinesis; Gene families; Genome size; Hereditary diseases; High-yield crops; Nondisjunction and aneuploidy.

Pompe disease

CATEGORY: Diseases and syndromes
ALSO KNOWN AS: Lysosomal storage disease; acid maltase deficiency disease; glycogen storage disease type II

DEFINITION

Pompe disease is a metabolic disorder caused by mutations in the acid alpha-glucosidase (*GAA*) gene. GAA, an enzyme responsible for breaking down glycogen in the cells, is either absent (resulting in the rapidly progressive infantile form of Pompe disease) or deficient (resulting in the late-onset juvenile or adult form). As a result, glycogen builds up in the lysosomes of cells and tissues, primarily in cardiac and skeletal muscles, affecting their function and causing progressive weakness and organ failure.

RISK FACTORS

This is an autosomal recessive disorder; therefore, each parent must carry a defective *GAA* gene, both of which are inherited by the affected child. The National Institute of Neurological Disorders and

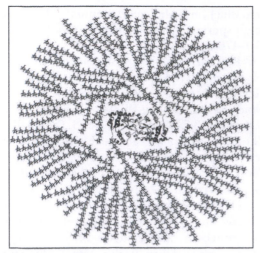

Muscle biopsy showing large vacuoles in a case of pompes disease (acid maltase deficiency, HE stain, frozen section). By Jensflorian (Own work), via Wikimedia Commons

glycogen By Mikael Häggström, via Wikimedia Commons By Mikael Häggström, via Wikimedia Commons

Stroke (NINDS) reports (2013) that the incidence is estimated at 1 in 40,000 people worldwide. About one-third of patients have the infantile-onset form. Both sexes are equally affected, although the incidence does vary by geography and ethnic group.

ETIOLOGY AND GENETICS

The *GAA* gene, located on the long arm of chromosome 17, is the only gene associated with Pompe disease. More than three hundred mutations have been identified throughout the gene. Some defects are more common than others. For example, more than half of Caucasians with late-onset Pompe disease share a common splice-site mutation. According to the Emory University School of Medicine in 2010, some infantile-onset mutations are observed more frequently in certain geographic regions (such as southern China and Taiwan) or ethnic populations (such as African Americans).

In general, the type and combination of mutations inherited determine the residual level of GAA activity and thus the severity of the disease. If both chromosomes are fully compromised, GAA activity is nonexistent. Combinations of one severely mutated allele and one mildly affected allele usually preserve some GAA activity, meaning a slower disease progression, although the age of onset can vary. Researchers are cautious about correlating genotype with clinical features, however, because both infantile and late-onset forms have been observed in the same family.

Several factors explain how glycogen buildup in the lysosomes likely disrupts muscle function. As the lysosomes become bloated, they can displace myofibrils in neighboring cells, disrupting the muscle's ability to contract and transmit force. In late-onset Pompe disease, swollen lysosomes can rupture or release other enzymes into surrounding tissues, damaging muscles. Disuse and oxidative stress may also play a role in muscle wasting.

SYMPTOMS

Manifestations of Pompe disease vary depending on age of onset and level of residual GAA activity. In the classic infantile-onset form, symptoms are observed shortly after birth and include an enlarged heart, poor muscle tone (inability to hold the head up, roll over), feeding problems (difficulty swallowing, enlarged tongue), and respiratory distress (frequent lung infections). In the nonclassic infantile form, cardiac involvement is moderate and muscle weakness is delayed. In late-onset Pompe disease, symptoms can appear from two to seventy years. Muscle weakness and pain, primarily in the legs and trunk (difficulty climbing stairs or playing sports, frequent falls) and respiratory distress (shortness of breath, sleep apnea) are typical. In all cases, early diagnosis is critical for disease management.

SCREENING AND DIAGNOSIS

Pompe disease shares many symptoms with other muscle disorders, complicating diagnosis. Initial clinical studies include chest radiography and electrocardiograms, as well as muscle tests, electromyography, and nerve conduction tests in adults. The diagnosis is confirmed through tests of GAA activity (blood tests, skin fibroblasts cultures, and/or muscle biopsy in adults) or through DNA analysis. DNA analysis is also useful for identifying familial mutations and carriers and for newborn screening.

TREATMENT AND THERAPY

Historically, patients with Pompe disease were given supportive care only. However, enzyme replacement therapy (ERT) using recombinant human GAA has become a promising treatment, especially in infants younger than six months who do not yet require ventilatory assistance. As reported by the National Center for Biotechnology Information (2012), clinical trials of ERT in late-onset Pompe disease are ongoing and also show promise. Other treatment is multidisciplinary and aimed at preventing secondary complications such as infections, treating symptoms, and maintaining function as long as possible. These treatments include frequent cardiac evaluations, use of bronchodilators, steroids, and mechanical ventilation, and special diets and tube feeding. Physical, occupational, and speech therapies and immunizations are also advised.

PREVENTION AND OUTCOMES

Before ERT, patients with infantile-onset Pompe disease typically died of cardiac and/or respiratory complications by one year of age. ERT has enhanced ventilator-free survival for many young patients; reduced heart size and improvements in cardiac and skeletal muscle function have also been seen. In late-onset Pompe disease, juvenile patients are usually more severely affected than adults and rarely survive past the second or third decade of life due to respiratory failure. They often require mechanical ventilation and wheelchairs. Older patients may also experience steadily progressive debilitation and premature mortality. However, improved screening techniques that enhance early diagnosis have become available. NINDS (2013) reports that not only ERT, but new drugs show promise for treatment.

Judy Majewski

FURTHER READING

Acton, Q. Ashton, ed. *Pompe's Disease: New Insights for the Healthcare Professional.* Atlanta: ScholarlyEditions, 2012. Print.

Akman, Hasan O., Anders Oldfors, and Salvatore DiMauro. "Glycogen Storage Diseases of Muscle." *Neuromuscular Diseases of Infancy, Childhood, and Adolescence: A Clinician's Approach.* 2nd ed. Ed. Basil T. Darras, et al. Boston: Academic, 2015. 735–60. Print.

Anand, Geeta. *The Cure: How a Father Raised $100 Million—And Bucked the Medical Establishment in a Quest to Save His Children.* New York: Harper, 2006. Print.

Hirschhorn, R., and A. J. Reuser. "Glycogen Storage Disease Type II: Acid Alpha-glucosidase (Acid Maltase) Deficiency." *The Metabolic and Molecular Bases of Inherited Disease.* Ed. Charles Scriver, et al. 8th ed. New York: McGraw, 2001. Print.

Hoffman, Georg F., et al. *Inherited Metabolic Diseases.* New York: Springer, 2010. Print.

Houser, Christine N. *Pediatric Genetics and Inborn Errors of Metabolism: A Practically Painless Review.* New York: Springer, 2014. Print.

Kishnani, Priya S., et al. "Pompe Disease Diagnosis and Management Guidelines." *Genetics in Medicine* 8.5 (2006): 267–88. Print.

Lim, Jeong-a, et al. "Pompe Disease: Shared and Unshared Features of Lysosomal Storage Disorders." *Rare Diseases* 3.1 (2015): n. pag. PDF file.

"Pompe Disease." *Genetics Home Reference.* Natl. Lib. of Medicine, 4 Aug. 2014. Web. 6 Aug. 2014.

WEBSITES OF INTEREST

Acid Maltase Deficiency Association (AMDA)
http://www.amda-pompe.org/

Association for Glycogen Storage Disease
http://www.agsdus.org/

Pompe Disease
http://ghr.nlm.nih.gov/condition=pompedisease

Pompe Registry
http://www.lsdregistry.net/pomperegistry/

See also: Andersen's disease; Forbes disease; Galactokinase deficiency; Galactosemia; Gaucher disease; Glucose galactose malabsorption; Glucose-6-phosphate dehydrogenase deficiency; Glycogen storage diseases; Hereditary diseases; Hers disease; Inborn errors of metabolism; McArdle's disease; Tarui's disease.

Population genetics

CATEGORY: Population genetics

SIGNIFICANCE: Population genetics is the study of how genes behave in populations. It is concerned with both theoretical and experimental investigations of changes in genetic variation caused by various forces; therefore, the field has close ties to evolutionary biology. Population genetics models can be used to explore the evolutionary histories of species, make predictions about future evolution, and predict the behavior of genetic diseases in human populations.

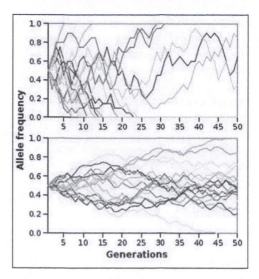

allele frequency Esurnir at the English language Wikipedia, from Wikimedia Commons

KEY TERMS

allele: one of the different forms of a particular gene (locus)

fitness: a measure of the ability of a genotype or individual to survive and reproduce compared to other genotypes or individuals

gene pool : all of the alleles in all the gametes of all the individuals in a population

genetic drift: random changes in genetic variation caused by sampling error in small populations

genotype: the pair of alleles carried by an individual for a specific gene locus

Hardy-Weinberg law: a mathematical model that predicts, under particular conditions, that allele frequencies will remain constant over time, with genotypes in specific predictable proportions

modern synthesis: the merging of the Darwinian mechanisms for evolution with Mendelian genetics to form the modern fields of population genetics and evolutionary biology

neutral theory of evolution: Motoo Kimura's theory that nucleotide substitutions in the DNA often have no effect on fitness, and thus changes in allele frequencies in populations are caused primarily by genetic drift

THE HARDY-WEINBERG LAW

The branch of genetics called population genetics is based on the application of nineteenth century Austrian botanist Gregor Mendel's principles of inheritance to genes in a population. (Although, for some species, "population" can be difficult to define, the term generally refers to a geographic group of interbreeding individuals of the same species.) Mendel's principles can be used to predict the expected proportions of offspring in a cross between two individuals of known genotypes, where the genotype describes the genetic content of an individual for one or more genes. An individual carries two copies of all chromosomes (except perhaps for the sex chromosomes, as in human males) and therefore has two copies of each gene. These two copies may be identical or somewhat different. Different forms of the same gene are called alleles. A genotype in which both alleles are the same is called a homozygote, while one in which the two alleles are different is a heterozygote. Although a single individual can carry no more than two alleles for a particular gene, there may be many alleles of a gene present in a population.

It would be essentially impossible to track the inheritance patterns of every single mating pair in a population, in essence tracking all the alleles in the gene pool. However, by making some simplifying assumptions about a population, it is possible to predict what will happen to the gene pool over time. Working independently in 1908, the British mathematician Godfrey Hardy and the German physiologist Wilhelm Weinberg were the first to formulate a simple mathematical model describing the behavior of a gene (locus) with two alleles in a population. In this model, the numbers of each allele and of each genotype are not represented as actual numbers but as proportions (known as allele frequencies and genotype frequencies, respectively) so that the model can be applied to any population regardless of its size. By assuming Mendelian inheritance of alleles, Hardy and Weinberg showed that allele frequencies in a population do not change over time and that genotype frequencies will change to specific proportions, determined by the allele frequencies, within one generation and remain at those proportions in future generations. This result is known as the Hardy-Weinberg law, and the stable genotype proportions predicted by the law are known as Hardy-Weinberg equilibrium. It was shown in subsequent work by others that the Hardy-Weinberg law remains true in more complex models with more than two alleles and more than one locus.

In order for the Hardy-Weinberg law to work, certain assumptions about a population must be true:

(1) The gene pool must be infinite in size.
(2) Mating among individuals (or the fusion of gametes) must be completely random.
(3) There must be no new mutations.
(4) There must be no gene flow (that is, no alleles should enter or leave the population.
(5) There should be no natural selection.

Since real populations cannot meet these conditions, it may seem that the Hardy-Weinberg model is too unrealistic to be useful, but, in fact, it can be useful. First, the conditions of a natural population may be very close to Hardy-Weinberg assumptions, so the Hardy-Weinberg law may be approximately true for at least some populations. Second, if genotypes in a population are not in Hardy-Weinberg equilibrium, it is an indication that one or more of these assumptions is not met. The Hardy-Weinberg law has been broadly expanded, using sophisticated mathematical modeling, and with adequate data can be used to determine why a population's allele and genotype frequencies are out of Hardy-Weinberg equilibrium.

GENETIC VARIATION AND MATHEMATICAL MODELING
Sampling and genetic analyses of real populations of many different types of organisms reveal that there is usually a substantial amount of genetic variation, meaning that for a fairly large proportion of genes (loci) that are analyzed, there are multiple alleles, and therefore multiple genotypes, within populations. For example, in the common fruit fly _Drosophila melanogaster_ (an organism that has been well studied genetically since the very early 1900s), between one-third and two-thirds of the genes that have been examined by protein electrophoresis have been found to be variable. Genetic variation can be measured as allele frequencies (allelic variation) or genotype frequencies (genotypic variation). A major task of population geneticists has been to describe such variation, to try to explain why it exists, and to predict its behavior over time.

The Hardy-Weinberg law predicts that if genetic variation exists in a population,

Linkage tree for 9 population clusters showing genetic distances (F_{ST})
(Cavalli-Sforza _et al._, 1994:80)

F_{ST} distance matrix for the 9 clusters shown above
(x10,000 with standard errors obtained by bootstrap analysis)

	AFR	NEC	EUC	NEA	ANE	AME	SEA	PAI	NGA
African	0.0								
Non-European Caucasian	1340.0 ± 301	0.0							
European Caucasian	1655.6 ± 416	154.7 ± 29	0.0						
Northeast Asian	1979.1 ± 452	640.4 ± 134	938.2 ± 217	0.0					
Arctic Northeast Asian	2008.5 ± 387	708.2 ± 160	746.7 ± 210	459.7 ± 98	0.0				
Amerindian	2261.4 ± 434	955.5 ± 204	1038.2 ± 276	746.5 ± 183	577.4 ± 89	0.0			
Southeast Asian	2206.3 ± 529	939.6 ± 262	1240.4 ± 339	630.5 ± 299	1039.4 ± 326	1341.7 ± 418	0.0		
Pacific Islander	2505.4 ± 648	953.7 ± 230	1344.7 ± 354	723.8 ± 262	1181.2 ± 331	1740.7 ± 544	436.7 ± 87	0.0	
New Guinean and Australian	2472.0 ± 536	1179.1 ± 189	1345.7 ± 231	734.4 ± 118	1012.5 ± 257	1457.9 ± 283	1237.9 ± 277	808.7 ± 264	0.0

Linkage tree By Varoon Arya (Own work), via Wikimedia Commons

it will remain constant over time, with genotypes in specific proportions. However, the law cannot begin to explain natural variation, since genotypes are not always found in Hardy-Weinberg proportions, and studies that involve sampling populations over time often show that genetic variation can be changing. The historical approach to explaining these observations has been to formulate more complex mathematical models based on the simple Hardy-Weinberg model that violate one or more of the implicit Hardy-Weinberg conditions.

Beginning in the 1920s and 1930s, a group of population geneticists, working independently, began exploring the effects of violating Hardy-Weinberg assumptions on genetic variation in populations. In what has become known as the "modern synthesis," Ronald A. Fisher, J. B. S. Haldane and Sewall Wright merged Charles Darwin's theory of natural selection with Mendel's theory of genetic inheritance to create a field of population genetics that allows for genetic change. They applied mathematics to the problem of variation in populations and were eventually able to incorporate what happens when each, or combinations, of the Hardy-Weinberg assumptions are violated.

ASSORTATIVE MATING AND INBREEDING

One of the implicit conditions of the Hardy-Weinberg model is that genotypes form mating pairs at random. In most cases mates are not selected based on genotype. Unless the gene in question has some direct effect on mate choice, mating with respect to that gene is random. However, there are conditions in natural populations in which mating is not random. For example, if a gene controls fur color and mates are chosen by appropriate fur color, then the genotype of an individual with respect to that gene will determine mating success. For this gene, then, mating is not random but rather "assortative." Positive assortative mating means that individuals tend to choose mates with genotypes like their own, while negative assortative mating means that individuals tend to choose genotypes different than their own.

Variation in a population for a gene subject to assortative mating is altered from Hardy-Weinberg expectations. Although allele frequencies do not change, genotype frequencies are altered. With positive assortative mating, the result is higher proportions of homozygotes and fewer heterozygotes, while the opposite is true when assortative mating

is negative. Sometimes random mating in a population is not possible because of the geographic organization of the population or general mating habits. Truly random mating would mean that any individual can mate with any other, but this is nearly impossible because of gender differences and practical limitations. In natural populations, it is often the case that mates are somewhat related, even closely related, because the population is organized into extended family groups whose members do not (or cannot, as in plants) disperse to mate with members of other groups. Mating between relatives is called inbreeding. Because related individuals tend to have similar genotypes for many genes, the effects of inbreeding are much like those of positive assortative mating for many genes. The proportions of homozygotes for many genes tend to increase. Again, this situation has no effect on allelic variation, only genotypic variation. Clearly, the presence of nonrandom mating patterns cannot by itself explain the majority of patterns of genetic variation in natural populations but can contribute to the action of other forces, such as natural selection.

MIGRATION AND MUTATION

In the theoretical Hardy-Weinberg population, there are no sources of new genetic variation. In real populations, alleles may enter or leave the population, a process called migration or "gene flow" (a more accurate term, since migration in this context means not only movement between populations but also successful reproduction to introduce alleles in the new population). Also, new alleles may be introduced by mutation, the change in the DNA sequence of an existing allele to create a new one, as a result of errors during DNA replication or the inexact repair of DNA damage from environmental influences such as radiation or mutagenic chemicals. Both of these processes can change both genotype frequencies and allele frequencies in a population. If the tendency to migrate is associated with particular genotypes, a long period of continued migration tends to push genotype and allele frequencies toward higher proportions of one type (in general, more homozygotes) so that the overall effect is to reduce genetic variation. However, in the short term, migration may enhance genetic variation by allowing new alleles and genotypes to enter. The importance of migration depends on the particular population. Some populations may be relatively isolated from others so that migration is a relatively weak force affecting genetic variation, or there may be frequent migration among geographic populations. There are many factors involved, not the least of which is the ability of members of the particular species to move over some distance.

Mutation, because it introduces new alleles into a population, acts to increase genetic variation. Before the modern synthesis, one school of thought was that mutation might be the driving force of evolution, since genetic change over time coming about from continual introduction of new forms of genes seemed possible. In fact, it is possible to develop simple mathematical models of mutation that show resulting patterns of genetic variation that resemble those found in nature. However, to account for the rates of evolution that are commonly observed, very high rates of mutation are required. In general, mutation tends to be quite rare, making the hypothesis of evolution by mutation alone unsatisfactory.

The action of mutation in conjunction with other forces, such as selection, may account for the low-frequency persistence of clearly harmful alleles in populations. For example, one might expect that alleles that can result in genetic diseases (such as cystic fibrosis) would be quickly eliminated from human populations by natural selection. However, low rates of mutation can continually introduce these alleles into populations. In this "mutation-selection balance," mutation tends to introduce alleles while selection tends to eliminate them, with a net result of continuing low frequencies in the population.

GENETIC DRIFT

Real populations are not, of course, infinite in size, though some are large enough that this Hardy-Weinberg condition is a useful approximation. However, many natural populations are small, and any population with less than about one thousand individuals will vary randomly in the pattern of genetic variation from generation to generation. These random changes in allele and genotype frequencies are called genetic drift. The situation is analogous to coin tossing. With a fair coin, the expectation is that half of the tosses will result in heads and half in tails. On average, this will be true, but in practice a small sample will not show the expectation. For example, if a coin is tossed ten times, it is unlikely that the result will be exactly five heads and five tails. On the other hand, with a thousand tosses, the results will

be closer to half and half. This higher deviation from the expected result in small samples is called a sampling error. In a small population, there is an expectation of the pattern of genetic variation based on the Hardy-Weinberg law, but sampling error during the union of sex cells to form offspring genotypes will result in random deviations from that expectation. The effect is that allele frequencies increase or decrease randomly, with corresponding changes in genotype frequencies. The smaller the population, the greater the sampling error and the more pronounced genetic drift will be.

Genetic drift has an effect on genetic variation that is similar to that of other factors. Over the long term, allele frequencies will drift until all alleles have been eliminated but one, eliminating variation. (For the moment, ignore the action of other forces that increase variation.) Over a period of dozens of generations, however, drift can allow variation to be maintained, especially in larger populations in which drift is minimal.

In the early days of population genetics, the possibility of genetic drift was recognized but often considered to be a minor consideration, with natural selection as a dominant force. Fisher in particular dismissed the importance of genetic drift, engaging over a number of years in a published debate with Wright, who always felt that drift would be important in small populations. Beginning in the 1960's with the acquisition of data on DNA-level population variation, the role of drift in natural populations became more recognized. It appears to be an especially strong force in cases in which a small number of individuals leave the population and migrate to a new area where they establish a new population. Large changes can occur, especially if the number of migrants is only ten or twenty. This type of situation is now referred to as a founder effect.

NATURAL SELECTION

Natural selection in a simple model of a gene with two alleles in a population can be easily represented by assuming that genotypes differ in their ability to survive and produce offspring. This ability is called fitness. In applying natural selection to a theoretical population, each genotype is assigned a fitness value between zero and one. Typically, the genotype in a population that is best able to survive and can, on average, produce more offspring than other genotypes is assigned a fitness value of one, and genotypes with lower fitness are assigned fitnesses with fractional values relative to the high-fitness genotype.

The study of this simple model of natural selection has revealed that it can alter genetic variation in different ways, depending on which genotype has the highest fitness. In the simple one-gene, two-allele model, there are three possible genotypes: two homozygotes and one heterozygote. If one homozygote has the highest fitness, it will be favored, and the genetic composition of the population will gradually shift toward more of that genotype (and its corresponding allele). This is called directional selection. If both homozygotes have higher fitness than the heterozygote (disruptive selection), one or the other will be favored, depending on the starting conditions. Both of these situations will decrease genetic variation in the population, because eventually one allele will prevail. Although each of these types of selection (particularly directional) may be found for genes in natural populations, they cannot explain why genetic variation is present, and is perhaps increasing, in nature.

Heterozygote advantage, in which the heterozygote has higher fitness than either homozygote, is the other possible situation in this model. In this case, because the heterozygote carries both alleles, both are expected to be favored together and therefore maintained. This is the only condition in this simple model in which genetic variation may be maintained or increased over time. Although this seems like a plausible explanation for the observed levels of natural variation, studies in which fitness values are measured almost never show heterozygote advantage in genes from natural populations. As a general explanation for the presence of genetic variation, this simple model of selection is unsatisfactory.

Studies of more complex theoretical models of selection (for example, those with many genes and different forms of selection) have revealed conditions that allow patterns of variation very similar to those observed in natural populations, and in some cases it seems clear that natural selection is a major factor determining patterns of genetic change. However, in many cases, selection does not seem to be the most important factor or even a factor at all.

EXPERIMENTAL POPULATION GENETICS AND THE NEUTRAL THEORY

Population genetics has always been a field in which the understanding of theory is ahead of empirical observation and experimental testing, but these have not been neglected. Although Fisher, Haldane, and Wright were mainly theorists, there were other architects of the modern synthesis who concentrated on testing theoretical predictions in natural populations. Beginning in the 1940s, for example, Theodosius Dobzhansky showed in natural and experimental populations of *Drosophila* species that frequency changes and geographic patterns of variation in chromosome variants are consistent with the effects of natural selection.

Natural selection was the dominant hypothesis for genetic changes in natural populations for the first several decades of the modern synthesis. In the 1960s, new techniques of molecular biology allowed population geneticists to examine molecular variation, first in proteins and later, with the use of restriction enzymes in the 1970s and DNA sequencing in the 1980s and 1990s, in DNA sequences. These types of studies only confirmed that there is a large amount of genetic variation in natural populations, much more than can be attributed to only natural selection. As a result, Motoo Kimura proposed the "neutral theory of evolution," the idea that most DNA sequence differences do not have fitness differences and that population changes in DNA sequences are governed mainly by genetic drift, with selection playing a minor role. This view, although still debated by some, was mostly accepted by the 1990s, although it was recognized that evolution of proteins and physical traits may be governed by selection to a greater extent.

IMPACT AND APPLICATIONS

The field of population genetics is a fundamental part of the current field of evolutionary biology. One possible definition of evolution would be "genetic change in a population over time," and population geneticists try to describe patterns of genetic variation, document changes in variation, determine their theoretical causes, and predict future patterns. These types of research have been valuable in studying the evolutionary histories of organisms for which there are living representatives, including humans.

In addition to the scientific value of understanding evolutionary history better, there are more immediate applications of such work. In conservation biology, data about genetic variation in a population can help to assess its ability to survive in the future. Data on genetic similarities between populations can aid in decisions about whether they can be considered as the same species or are unique enough to merit preservation.

Population genetics has had an influence on medicine, particularly in understanding why "disease genes," while clearly harmful, persist in human populations. The field has also affected the planning of vaccination protocols to maximize their effectiveness against parasites, since a vaccine-resistant strain is a result of a rare allele in the parasite population. In the 1990s it began to be recognized that effective treatments for medical conditions would need to take into account genetic variation in human populations, since different individuals might respond differently to the same treatment.

Stephen T. Kilpatrick, Ph.D.;
updated by Bryan Ness, Ph.D.

FURTHER READING

Christiansen, Freddy B. *Population Genetics of Multiple Loci*. New York: Wiley, 2000. Print.

Dobzhansky, Theodosius. *Genetics and the Origin of Species*. 3rd ed. New York: Columbia UP, 1951. Print.

Gillespie, John H. *Population Genetics: A Concise Guide*. 2nd ed. Baltimore: Johns Hopkins UP, 2004. Print.

Hamilton, Matthew B. *Population Genetics*. Hoboken: Wiley, 2009. Print.

Hartl, Daniel L. *A Primer of Population Genetics*. Rev. 3rd ed. Sunderland: Sinauer, 2000. Print.

Hedrick, Philip W. *Genetics of Populations*. 4th ed. Boston: Jones, 2011. Print.

Landweber, Laura F., and Andrew P. Dobson, eds. *Genetics and the Extinction of Species: DNA and the Conservation of Biodiversity*. Princeton: Princeton UP, 1999. Print.

Lewontin, Richard C. *The Genetic Basis of Evolutionary Change*. New York: Columbia UP, 1974. Print.

Masel J. "Genetic Drift." *Current Biology* 21.20 (2011): R837–38. Print.

Papiha, Surinder S., Ranjan Deka, and Ranajit Chakraborty, eds. *Genomic Diversity: Applications in Human Population Genetics*. New York: Kluwer, 1999. Print.

Peng, Bo, Christopher I. Amos, and Marek Kimmel. *Forward-Time Population Genetics Simulations: Methods, Implementation, and Applications*. Hoboken: Wiley, 2012. Digital file.

Provine, William B. *The Origins of Theoretical Population Genetics*. 2nd ed. Chicago: U of Chicago P, 2001. Print.

Relethford, John. *Human Population Genetics*. Hoboken: Wiley, 2012. Print.

Slatkin, Montgomery, and Michel Veuille, eds. *Modern Developments in Theoretical Population Genetics: The Legacy of Gustave Malécot*. New York: Oxford UP, 2002. Print.

Templeton, Alan R. *Population Genetics and Microevolutionary Theory*. Hoboken: Wiley, 2006. Print.

Derived from: "Population genetics." *Genetics & Inherited Conditions*. Salem Press. 2010.

See also: Artificial selection; Behavior; Consanguinityand genetic disease; Emerging and reemerging infectious diseases; Evolutionary biology; Genetic load; Genetics: Historical development; Hardy- Weinberg law; Heredity and environment; Hybridization and introgression; Inbreeding and assortative mating; Lateral gene transfer; Natural selection; Polyploidy; Punctuated equilibrium; Quantitative inheritance; Sociobiology; Speciation.

Porphyria

CATEGORY: Diseases and syndromes

DEFINITION

The term "porphyria" refers to a group of blood disorders. They do differ in some ways, but all share the same problem: defects of enzymes needed at various steps of hemesynthesis that result in distinct clinical syndromes known as porphyrias. Heme is a critical part of the hemoglobin molecule, and the hemoglobin molecule is a critical part of red blood cells and the transport of oxygen all over the body.

These syndromes can be clinically classified into those predominantly involving the skin, those involving the liver/nervous system, and a combination involving all three buildup of porphyrins in the body. Porphyrins help to make heme, a part of the red blood cell. However, a buildup of the porphyrins in the body causes damage. It most often affects the nervous system and skin.

Some porphyria disorders include acute intermit tent porphyria, porphyria cutanea tarda, and er ythropoietic protoporphyria. Another disorder, congenital erythropoietic protoporphyria, is present from birth. Some types of porphyria start in early

Acute photosensitivity reaction in EPP. By see above, via Wikimedia Commons

Chronic skin lesions of EPP: The skin of an adult face that is thickening with a waxy or leathery appearance, also with areas of hyperkeratosis

childhood, some at puberty, and others during adulthood. Attacks may be separated by long periods of time. The attacks can be triggered by drugs, infections, alcohol consumption, and dieting.

RISK FACTORS

The most common risk factor for porphyria is having a family member with this disease. Caucasians are at greater risk than blacks or Asians, and females also have an increased risk (related to their menstrual cycles). Most onsets happen between the ages of twenty and forty.

ETIOLOGY AND GENETICS

Porphyrias can be inherited or (rarely) acquired. With the exception of congenital erythropoietic porphyria (CEP), which is autosomal recessive, and X-linked protoporphyria, which is X-linked, all other inherited porphyrias are autosomal dominant disorders. Mutations in at least eight different genes are known to be responsible. The protein products of these genes are all enzymes necessary for the biosynthesis of heme, so a mutation which results in a missing or altered form of any of the enzymes could severely limit the amount of heme produced in various body tissues.

The *CPOX* gene (found on chromosome 3 at position 3q12) specifies an enzyme known as coproporphyrinogen oxidase; *HMBS* (at position 11q23.3) encodes the enzyme hydroxymethylbilane synthase; *PPOX* (at position 1q22) specifies protoporphyrinogen oxidase; and UROD (at position 1p34) encodes uroporphyrinogen decarboxylase. Mutations in any of these four genes can result in an autosomal dominant form of porphyria, meaning that a single

copy of the mutation is sufficient to cause full expression of the disease. An affected individual has a 50 per cent chance of transmitting the mutation to each of his or her children. Many cases of autosomal dominant porphyria, however, result from a spontaneous new mutation, so in these instances affected individuals will have unaffected parents.

The *ALAD* gene (at position 9q34) specifies the enzyme delta-aminolevulinate dehydratase, and the *UROS* gene (at position 10q25.2-q26.3) encodes uroporphyrinogen III synthase. Mutations in either of these two genes cause autosomal recessive forms of porphyria, which means that both copies of the gene must be deficient in order for the individual to be afflicted. Typically, an affected child is born to two unaffected parents, both of whom are carriers of the recessive mutant allele. The probable outcomes for children whose parents are both carriers are 75 percent unaffected and 25 percent affected.

The *FECH* gene (at position 18q21.3), which encodes the enzyme ferrochelatase, is unique in that it is associated with both autosomal dominant and autosomal recessive porphyria, depending on the specific molecular nature of the mutation. Finally, the *ALAS2* gene (at position Xp11.21), which specifies the enzyme aminolevulinate,delta-,synthase 2, is associated with an extremely rare X-linked dominant form of porphyria. A single copy of the mutation is sufficient for disease expression, but while an affected woman will transmit the mutation to one-half of her children, regardless of sex, an affected father will transmit the disease to all of his daughters and none of his sons.

Although there are various forms of inherited porphyrias, the most common form seen in clinical practice (porphyria cutanea tarda) is acquired in 80% of patients who have this disorder. Acquired porphyria has previously occurred in large populations exposed to polyhalogenated aromatic hydrocarbons that are toxic to the liver. There are other items toxic to the liver that are associated with the development of porphyria cutanea tarda including, but not limited to, ethanol intake, estrogen therapies, and hepatitis and human immunodeficiency viral infections. All of these conditions effect iron metabolism and accumulation of iron contributes to the development of the disease. Hepatic tumors producing excess porphyrins are rare causes of porphyria cutanea tarda–like disorders.

SYMPTOMS

Symptoms may vary depending on the type of porphyria. The most common presenting symptom is abdominal pain. Muscle weakness and focal neurologic deficits such as tetraparesis (weakness of all four limbs) may be the presenting feature, especially in women of child-bearing age. Limb pain is common. Anxiety problems and even evidence of psychosis may be seen. Many will have high blood pressure during an acute attack. Seizures may occur; but are less frequent that previously described.

Urine from some types of the disorder may be reddish in color due to the presence of excess porphyrins. The urine may darken after standing in the light.

Attacks can last from days to weeks and symptoms of future attacks resemble the initial episode.

In those with porphyria cutanea tarda (PCT) symptoms may include sun sensitivity, and sun-exposed skin may be fragile. Minor injury may damage the skin. Additional symptoms may include blisters on the face, hands, arms, feet, and legs; skin that heals slowly; skin susceptible to infection; skin that thickens and scars; skin color changes; excess hair growth; and reddish urine in infancy or childhood.

SCREENING AND DIAGNOSIS

The doctor may ask about symptoms and may obtain a medical and family history. A physical exam may also be done. The symptoms can be veryvague. As a result, the diagnosis is often delayed.

Tests differ for the various types of porphyria and may include blood, urine, and/or stool tests. These tests check for excess porphyrin or a specific enzyme deficiency. In some cases, specific genetic testing is available and may be recommended.

MRI scanning of the brain and liver may be helpful because of fairly characteristic abnormalities that reverse once appropriate treatment has been given.

The utility of prenatal testing is questionable as many heterozygous carriers live healthy lives. The prenatal testing might not be recommended unless pregnancy termination is being considered.

TREATMENT AND THERAPY

For all types of porphyria, treatment includes withdrawal of known triggers and drugs that can precipitate an attack. Porphyria that affects the skin requires special attention to protect the skin from injury and/or infection.

Specific treatment depends on the type of porphyria. Patients with acute intermittent porphyria may need to be hospitalized during an attack. In the hospital, they may be given hemin by vein (intravenous); glucose by vein; and drugs to control symptoms, such as pain, nausea, anxiety, and insomnia. Electrolytes may need to be given to reverse low levels of sodium and magnesium. Magnesium may also be used to control seizures as many more common anti-seizure medications cannot be used. Blood pressure medication may be needed to control high blood pressure during an acute attack. Breathing support may become necessary if muscle weakness affects the diaphragm.

Porphyria cutanea tarda treatment may include blood removal weekly to monthly; low doses of antimalarial drugs, such as chloroquine (Aralen Phosphate) or hydroxychloroquine (Plaquenil); and radiological imaging to monitor for increased risk of liver cancer.

Erythropoietic protoporphyria treatment may include oral beta-carotene; maintaining normal iron levels with food or supplements; medication to aid excretion of porphyrins in the stool, such as activated charcoal, cholestyramine, blood transfusions, and hemin by vein; and splenectomy, the removal of the spleen.

Treatment for congenital erythropoietic protoporphyria may include oral beta-carotene; oral charcoal, to aid excretion of porphyrins in the stool; blood transfusions; splenectomy, the removal of the spleen; and bone marrow transplantation.

PREVENTION AND OUTCOMES

Genetic testing may identify individuals at risk for porphyria. An individual who has a family member with the diagnosis of porphyria may be eligible for testing. An individual whose family member has had a test that showed DNA changes can also be tested for these changes.

A genetic counselor can review family history. The counselor can help find the risks for this disorder in an individual and in his or her offspring. The counselor may also discuss appropriate testing.

Genetic mutations cannot be corrected. However, attacks can be anticipated, prevented, or controlled. Steps to avoid porphyria attacks and complications include protecting skin from injury or infection and avoiding drugs and other triggers such as alcohol consumption, smoking. If a patient needs to undergo surgery, filters may be used to protect the skin from exposure to surgical lighting.

Triggers for acute intermittent porphyria include drugs, such as barbiturates; sulfa drugs; seizure drugs; and steroid hormones, such as estrogen and progesterone. Other triggers include hormonal changes related to the menstrual cycle, weight-loss diets or fasting, infections, alcohol, stress, surger y, and cigarette smoke.

Triggers for porphyria cutanea tarda include al cohol, estrogens, hydrocarbons, and certain pesti cides or chemicals. Sunlight and weight-loss diets or fasting can trigger erythropoietic protoporphyria. Sunlight can trigger congenital erythropoietic pro toporphyria.

Long-term complications in patients with acute intermittent porphyria include chronic hypertension, chronic kidney insufficiency, chronic pain syndrome, and liver cancer. Patients with variegate porphyria have also shown increased incidences of liver cancer. As a result, ongoing surveillance of the liver may be recommended.

Erythropoietic porphyria is a persistent, severely painful, socially disabling disease with a marked impact on quality of life.

Debra Wood, R.N.; reviewed by Igor Puzanov, M.D.
"Etiology and Genetics" by Jeffrey A. Knight, Ph.D.;
updated by Gary M. Flashner, M.S., M.D.

FURTHER READING

Beers, Mark H., ed. *The Merck Manual of Medical In formation.* 2d home ed., new and rev. Whitehouse Station, N.J.: Merck Research Laboratories, 2003. Conn, H. F., and R. E. Rakel. *Conn's Current Therapy.* 53d ed. Philadelphia: W.B. Saunders, 2001. EBSCO Publishing. *Health Library: Porphyria.* Ipswich, Mass.: Author, 2009. Available through http://www.ebscohost.com.

Fauci, Anthony S., et al., eds. *Harrison's Principles of Internal Medicine.* 17th ed. New York: McGraw-Hill Medical, 2008.

Goldman, Lee, and Dennis Ausiello, eds. *Cecil Medicine.* 23d ed. Philadelphia: Saunders Elsevier, 2008.

Kuo HC, Huang CC, Chu CC, Lee MJ, Chuang WL, Wu CL, et al. "Neurological complications of acute intermittent porphyria." *Eur Neurol.* 2011. 66(5):247-52.

Singal AK, Anderson KE. "Variegate Porphyria." Pagon RA et al. *Gene Reviews.* Feb. Seattle: University of Washington; 2013.

Van Meter JR, Tierney KR, Pittelkow MR. "Iron, genes, and viruses: the porphyria cutanea tarda triple threat." *Cutis.* 2011 Aug. 88(2):73-6.

Gucev Z, Slavevska N, Tasic V, Laban N, Pop-Jordanova N, Danilovski D, et al. "Congenital erythropoietic porphyria with two mutations of the uroporphyrinogen III synthase gene" (Cys73Arg, Thr228Met). *Indian J Hum Genet.* 2011 May. 17(2):104-7

Seager MJ, Whatley SD, Anstey AV, Millard TP. "X-linked dominant protoporphyria: a new porphyria." *Clin Exp Dermatol.* 2014 Jan. 39(1):35-7.

WEB SITES OF INTEREST

American Liver Foundation
http://www.liverfoundation.org

The American Porphyria Foundation
http://porphyriafoundation.com

Canadian Liver Foundation
http://www.liver.ca/Home.aspx

Canadian Organization for Rare Disorders
http://www.cord.ca

Genetics Home Reference
http://ghr.nlm.nih.gov

MedLine Plus: Porphyria
http://www.nlm.nih.gov/medlineplus/porphyria.
  html

National Institute of Diabetes and Digestive and Kidney Diseases
http://www2.niddk.nih.gov

National Organization for Rare Disorders
https://rarediseases.org/
  rare-diseases/x-linked-protoporphyria/
https://rarediseases.info.nih.gov/diseases/10353/
  porphyria

See also: ABO blood types; Chronic myeloid leuke mia; Fanconi anemia; Hemophilia; Hereditary sphe rocytosis; Infantile agranulocytosis; Myelodysplastic syndromes; Paroxysmal nocturnal hemoglobinuria; Rh incompatibility and isoimmunization; Sickle-cell disease.

Prader-Willi and Angelman syndromes

CATEGORY: Diseases and syndromes

DEFINITION

Prader-Willi syndrome (PWS) is a genetic condition that affects many parts of the body. Angelman syndrome (AS) is a genetic disorder that primarily affects the nervous system. Both are caused by errors at the same site in the long arm of chromosome 15, but the clinical outcomes of these errors are markedly different. In each condition, the chromo somes containing the errors come from different parents. These syndromes offer a striking ex ample of the genetic concept known as parental imprinting.

RISK FACTORS

In most cases, the defects and deletions in pater nal genes that are the cause of PWS occur randomly and are not inherited. However, in rare instances a genetic mutation inherited from the father may cause this disorder.

Similarly, it is not known what causes the genetic defect that results in most cases of AS. The majority of people with AS do not have a family history of the

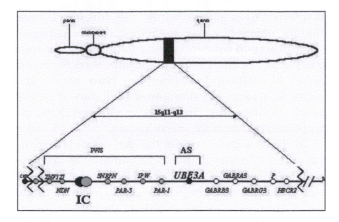

Circles in gray indicate genes implicated in Prader-Willi syndrome (PWS). By Ramujana at en.wikibooks [Public domain], from Wikimedia Commons

disease. However, in rare cases, AS may be inherited from the mother. In view of the above, there are no clear known risk factors that lead to an increased risk of developing either of these disorders

ETIOLOGY AND GENETICS

The primary cause of both syndromes appears to be a small deletion on the long arm of chromosome 15 (del 15q11-q13). The deleted area is estimated to be about 4 million base pairs (bp), small by molecu lar standards but large enough to contain several genes. This area of chromosome 15 is known to con tain several genes that are activated or inactivated depending on the chromosome's parent of origin (that is, a gene may be turned on in the chromo some inherited from the mother but turned off in the chromosome inherited from the father). This parent-specific activation

Prader-Willi syndrome By Schüle B et al [CC-BY-2.0 (http://creativecommons.org/licenses/by/2.0)], via Wikimedia Commons

is referred to as genetic imprinting. It is now known that the deletions caus ing AS appear in the chromosome inherited from the mother, while those causing PWS occur in the chromosome inherited from the father. Since the genes of only one chromosome are active at a time, any disruption (deletion or inactivation) in the active chromosome will lead to the effects seen in one of these syndromes.

In 1997 a gene within the AS deletion region called UBE3A was found to be mutated in approximately 5 percent of AS individuals. These mutations can be as small as a single base pair. This gene codes for a protein/enzyme called a ubiquitin protein ligase, and loss of function or absence of the UBE3A gene is believed to be the causative problem in AS. UBE3A is an enzymatic component of a complex protein degradation system termed the ubiquitin proteasome pathway. This pathway is located in the cytoplasm of all cells. The pathway involves a small protein molecule (ubiquitin) that can be attached to proteins, thereby causing them to be degraded. In the normal brain, UBE3A inherited from the father is almost completely inactive, so the maternal copy performs most of the ubiquitin-producing function. Inheritance of a UBE3A mutation from the mother causes AS; inheritance of the mutation from the father has no apparent effect on the child. In some families, AS caused by a UBE3A mutation can occur in more than one family member.

Another cause of AS (3 percent of cases) is pater nal uniparental disomy (UPD). In this case a child inherits both copies of chromosome 15 from the fa ther, with no copy inherited from the mother. Even though there is no deletion or mutation, the child is still missing the active UBE3A gene because the paternally derived chromosomes only have brain inactivated UBE3A genes.

A fourth class of AS individuals (3-5 percent) have chromosome 15 copies inherited from both parents, but the copy inherited from the mother functions in the same way as a paternally inherited one would. This is referred to as an "imprinting de fect." Some individuals may have a very small dele tion of a region known as the imprinting center (IC), which regulates the activity of UBE3A from a distant location. The mechanism for this is not yet known.

While there are several genetic mechanisms for AS, all of them lead to the typical clinical features found in AS individuals, although minor differences in incidence of features may occur between each group.

The primary genes involved in PWS are SNRPN, a gene that encodes the small ribonucleotide poly peptide SmN that is found in the fetal and adult brain, and ZFN127, a gene that encodes a zinc finger protein of unknown function. SNRPN is involved in messenger RNA (mRNA) processing, an intermediate step between DNA transcription and protein formation. A mouse model of PWS has been developed with a large deletion that includes the SNRPN region and the PWS imprinting center and shows a phenotype similar to that of infants with PWS.

It is probable that the hypothalamic problems (such as overeating) associated with PWS might re sult from a loss of SNRPN. The production of this protein is found mainly in the hypothalamic regions of the brain and in the olfactory cortex. Thus, dis ruption of hypothalamic functions such as satiety are a likely result of this defect. Prader-Willi syndrome is the most common genetic cause of obesity. In addition to its role in satiety, the hypothalamus regulates growth, sexual development, metabolism, body temperature, pigmentation, and mood—all functions that are affected in those with PWS.

PWS may also be caused by uniparental disomy, as seen in AS. However, in PWS both copies of chro mosome 15 are derived from the mother instead of from the father.

As mentioned above, the imprinting center may be involved in at least some cases of both syndromes. This chromosome 15 IC is about 100 kilobase pairs (kb) long and includes exon 1 of the SNRPN gene. Mutations in this area appear to pre vent the paternal-to-maternal imprinting switch in the AS families and prevents the maternal-to-paternal switch in PWS families. Therefore, it is possible that the IC is needed to regulate alternate RNA splicing in the SNRPN gene transcripts.

Few examples of known parental imprinting oc cur in the human, so AS and PWS provide rare op portunities for geneticists and biologists to study this important phenomenon. Examples of nonhu man parental imprinting are well known, but the ge netic and biochemical mechanisms have not been established. Detailing the IC for chromosome 15 will be key to understanding how imprinting occurs and how the effects of AS and PWS are manifested.

The suggestion has been made that PWS (and therefore disruption of the IC) may also, at least in some cases, have an environmental trigger. A high association of PWS with fathers employed in hydro carbon-related occupations (such as factory workers, lumbermen, machinists, chemists, and mechanics) at the time of conception has been reported by one investigative team. This is an area that needs further exploration.

Symptoms

Angelman syndrome was first described in 1965 by Dr. Harry Angelman, who described three chil dren with a stiff, jerky gait, absent speech, excessive laughter, and seizures. Newer reports include severe mental retardation and a characteristic face that is small with a large mouth and prominent chin. Other features of this condition include developmental delay, intellectual disability, severe speech impairment, problems with movement and balance (ataxia), epilepsy, and a small head size. Individuals with Angelman syndrome typically have a happy, excitable demeanor with frequent smiling, laughter, and hand-flapping movements. These characteristics give rise to the alternate name for the syndrome, that being "happy puppet syndrome." The syndrome is fairly rare, with an incidence estimated to be between one in fifteen thousand to one in thirty thousand. It is usually not recognized at birth or in infancy, since the developmental problems are nonspecific during this period.

Prader-Willi syndrome, by comparison, is charac terized by mental retardation, hypotonia (decreased muscle tone), skin picking, short stature, cr yt orchidism (undescended testes), hypogonadism, and in later infancy or early childhood, hyperphagia (overeating leading to severe obesity). Delayed motor and language development are common, as is intellectual and cognitive impairment (the average IQ is about 70), and distinctive behavioral characteristics such as temper tantrums, stubbornness, and obsessive-compulsive tendencies. The syndrome was first described by Doctors Andrea Prader, Alexis Labhart, and Hein rich Willi in 1956. Like Angelman syndrome, PWS has a fairly low incidence, estimated at one in fifteen thousand. Neither condition is race-specific, and neither is considered to be a familial disease.

Screening and Diagnosis

The usual chromosome studies carried out dur ing prenatal diagnosis are interpreted as normal in fetuses with AS and PWS syndromes, since the small abnormalities on chromosome 15 are not detected by this type of study. Likewise, fetal ultrasound of fers no help in detecting physical abnormalities re lated to AS or PWS, since the affected fetus is well formed. Amniotic fluid volume and alpha-feto protein levels also appear normal.

Specific forms of genetic testing are needed in order to confirm the diagnosis when these disorders are suspected. Fluorescence in situ hybridization (FISH) is an extremely sensitive assay for determining the presence of deletions on chromosomes. It uses a fluorescence-tagged segment of DNA that binds to the DNA region being studied. Specialized chromosome 15 FISH studies are needed to determine the presence of either syndrome resulting from chromosomal deletions. Testing for parent-specific methylation imprints at the 15q11-q13 locus detects more than 95 percent of cases. For cases caused by uniparental disomy, polymerase chain reaction (PCR) testing can be used.

Treatment and Therapy

Treatment for both PWS and AS focuses on man aging the medical and development problems that are caused by these conditions. Most people with PWS will require specialized care throughout their lives. Many infants who have this disorder need a high-calorie formula to help them gain weight early on. Older children will need to maintain a reduced calorie diet in order to control their weight and en sure proper nutrition.

Some children with PWS receive human growth hormones to increase growth and reduce body fat. Over time, it has been found that lower doses may be just as effective and carry lower long-term risks. This treatment is carried out in consultation with an endocrinologist—a specialist who treats hormonal disorders—to determine if it is the right approach. Recent evidence has also shown that low-dose intranasal oxytocin therapy may reduce appetite drive in patients with PWS, as well as improve socialization, anxiety, and repetitive behaviors. The endocrinologist may also recommend that a child receive hormone re placement therapy (testosterone for males or estro gen and progesterone for females) to replenish low levels of sex hormones.

Children with PWS may also receive physical, speech, occupational, and developmental therapies in order to improve movement and language skills, learn to perform everyday tasks, behave ap propriately, and acquire social and interpersonal skills.

In addition, a psychologist or psychiatrist may be needed to address a child's psychological prob lems, including mood or obsessive-compulsive disor ders.

Along with all of the above, those with PWS are usually monitored for scoliosis, cryptorchidism, and complications of obesity as all of these, if severe enough, may need surgical correction. As regards complications of obesity, monitoring include evalu ation of obstruction sleep apnea which might lead to removal of tonsils and adenoids. Note that past expe rience has shown that gastric bypass surgery has not been effective for long-term weight control.

Treatment for AS may include antiseizure medi cation to control the seizures caused by the disor der. Physical therapy can help children walk and improve other mobility problems; behavioral therapy can teach children to overcome their hyperactivity and short attention spans. Because people with AS usually have limited verbal language skills, commu nication therapy can help them develop nonverbal language skills through sign language and picture communication.

PREVENTION AND OUTCOMES

There is no cure for PWS or AS. For those with PWS, complications due to obesity (eg, slipped capital fem oral epiphyses, sleep apnea, cor pulmonale, type 2 diabetes mellitus and early atherosclerosis adding to risk for heart attack and stroke) and behavioral problems are major contributors to morbidity and mortality. In one study of of 152 patients with PWS, choking episodes were reported as the cause of death in 7.9%.,

Most of those with AS will have severe develop mental delays, speech limitations, and motor difficul ties. However, they can have normal life spans and not show developmental regression as they age. Early diagnosis and tailored interventions and therapies can help improve quality of life.

Kerry L. Cheesman, Ph.D.;
updated by Rebecca Kuzins and Gary M. Flashner,
M.S., M.D.

FURTHER READING

Butler, Merlin G., Phillip D. K. Lee, and Barbara Y. Whitman, eds. *Management of Prader-Willi Syn drome*. 3d ed. New York: Springer, 2006. Collec tion of articles describing the diagnosis, genetics, medical physiology, and treatment of PWS. The majority of the articles examine how to manage the lives of PWS patients, including discussions of associated speech and language disorders, the education of children and adolescents, vocational training, and behavior management.

Cassidy, S. B., and S. Schwartz. "Prader-Willi and Angelman Syndromes: Disorders of Genomic Im printing." *Medicine* (Baltimore) 77, no. 2 (March, 1998): 140-151. A review of these syndromes writ ten for health care professionals.

Dan, Bernard. *Angelman Syndrome*. London: Mac Keith Press, 2008. Reviews the genetic issues, re search, and treatment of Angelman syndrome, as well as specific clinical problems associated with the syndrome, such as motor impairment, behav ior, learning difficulties, communication, sleep, and epilepsy.

Eiholzer, Urs. *Prader-Willi Syndrome: Coping with the Disease, Living with Those Involved*. New York: Karger, 2005. Designed for family members and others who have contact with PWS-afflicted chil dren, this book provides information about the genetic cause of PWS, the results of research about the syndrome, and treatment options.

Hall, J. G. "Genomic Imprinting: Nature and Clini cal Relevance." *Annual Review of Medicine* 48, no. 1 (1997): 35-44. A well-documented review that in cludes discussion of both AS and PWS as examples of human genomic imprinting.

Lai, L. W., R. P. Erickson, and S. B. Cassidy. "Clin ical Correlates of Chromosome Fifteen Dele tions and Maternal Disomy in Prader-Willi Syn drome." *American Journal of Diseases of Children* 147, no. 11 (November, 1993): 1217-1223. Dis cusses the signs and symptoms of PWS, includ ing those that are needed to make a clinical diagnosis in children.

Lalalande, M. "Parental Imprinting and Human Dis ease." *Annual Review of Genetics* 30, no. 1 (1996): 173-195. A well-written, well-documented review of imprinting and how it relates to both AS and PWS. Good reading for undergraduate students.

Mann, M. R., and M. S. Bartolomei. "Towards a Mo lecular Understanding of Prader-Willi and Angel man Syndromes." *Human Molecular Genetics* 8, no. 10 (1999): 1867-1873. Details the molecular mech anisms, rather than the clinical correlates, of AS and PWS; fairly technical but readable by students of biology.

Nicholls, R. D. "Genomic Imprinting and Unipa rental Disomy in Angelman and Prader-Willi

Syndromes: A Review." *American Journal of Medical Genetics* 46, no. 1 (April 1, 1993): 16-25. Not as far-reaching as Lalalande, but a well-written re-

Canadian Agency for Drugs and Technologies in Health. *Human Growth Hormone Treatment for Prader-Willi Syndrome in Adolescent and Adult Patients: Clinical Evidence, Safety, and Guidelines.* Ottawa, ON: 2015 Nov 06.

Gito M, Ihara H, Ogata H, et al. "Gender Differences in the Behavioral Symptom Severity of Prader-Willi Syndrome." *Behav Neurol.* 2015. 2015:294127.

Bakker NE, Siemensma EP, van Rijn M, Festen DA, Hokken-Koelega AC. "Beneficial Effect of Growth Hormone Treatment on Health-Related Quality of Life in Children with Prader-Willi Syndrome: A Randomized Controlled Trial and Longitudinal Study." *Horm Res Paediatr.* 2015. 84 (4):231-9.

Miller JL, Tamura R, Butler MG, et al. "Oxytocin treatment in children with Prader-Willi syndrome: A double-blind, placebo-controlled, crossover study." *Am J Med Genet A.* 2017 May. 173 (5):1243-50.

Miller JL, Lynn CH, Driscoll DC, et al. "Nutritional phases in Prader-Willi syndrome." *Am J Med Genet A.* 2011 May. 155(5):1040-9.

Whittington, Joyce, and Tony Holland. "Prader-Willi Syndrome: Development and Manifestations." New York: Cambridge University Press, 2004. The authors participated in a major PWS study at Cambridge University and the study's findings are the basis for this book, which describes how to manage the medical, nutritional, psychological, educational, social, and therapeutic needs of patients with PWS.

WEB SITES OF INTEREST

Angelman Syndrome Foundation

http://www.angelman.org

This support group's Web site features an online booklet entitled "The Facts About Angelman Syndrome" and an alphabetical list of topics of importance to patients and their families.

Genetics Home Reference

http://ghr.nlm.nih.gov and https://ghr.nlm.nih.gov/gene/SNRPN and https://ghr.nlm.nih.gov/condition/angelman-syndrome

Users can search the "Genetic Disorders A to Z" section of the site to find individual pages about the Prader-Willi and Angelman syndromes. The pages describe the genetic changes and inheritance pat

terns related to both conditions and provide links to additional information.

National Organization for Rare Disorders

http://www.rarediseases.org

This site contains an index of rare diseases and a rare disease database that enables users to retrieve information about the Prader-Willi and Angelman syndromes, as well as a list of related organizations.

https://rarediseases.info.nih.gov/diseases/5575/prader-willi-syndrome

https://rarediseases.info.nih.gov/diseases/5810/angelman-syndrome

http://emedicine.medscape.com/article/947954-overview

https://www.angelman.org/conferences-symposia/2016-scientific-symposium/

http://www.mayoclinic.org/diseases-conditions/angelman-syndrome/diagnosis-treatment/diagnosis/dxc-20307412

Prader-Willi Syndrome Association

http://www.pwsausa.org Offers background information on the syndrome, a research/medical section, and links to other re sources.

See also: Amniocentesis; Chorionic villus sampling; Chromosome structure; Congenital defects; Down syndrome; Fragile X syndrome; Hereditary diseases; Human growth hormone; Huntington's disease; In telligence; Polymerase chain reaction; Prenatal di agnosis.

Prenatal diagnosis

CATEGORY: Human genetics and social issues

SIGNIFICANCE: Tests ranging from ultrasound and maternal blood tests to testing fetal cells from the amniotic fluid or placenta are performed to detect genetic disorders that the fetus may have. Although tests may show the absence of specific genetic defects, the detection of a genetic defect can produce an ethical dilemma for the parents and their physician.

KEY TERMS

amniotic fluid: the liquid that surrounds the developing fetus *neural tube*: the embryonic structure that becomes the brain and spinal cord

placenta: an organ composed of both fetal and maternal tissue through which the fetus is nourished

trisomy: the presence of three copies (instead of two) of a particular chromosome in a cell

PRENATAL TESTING

Prenatal testing is administered to a large number of women, and the tests are becoming more informative. Some of the tests are only mildly invasive to the mother, but others involve obtaining fetal cells. Some are becoming routine for all pregnant women; others are offered only when an expectant mother meets a certain set of criteria. Some physicians will not offer the testing (especially the more invasive procedures). Others will order testing, believing that test results will give the parents time to prepare themselves for a baby with special needs. The test results are also used to determine whether additional medical teams should be present at the delivery to deal with a newborn who is not normal and healthy. Most often, prenatal testing

Antero-posterior radiographic view, showing missing ribs, absent lumbosacral vertebrae, hypoplastic pelvis and "frog-like" position of the lower extremities. By see above, via Wikimedia Commons

is offered if the mother is age thirty-five or older, if a particular disorder is present in relatives on one or both sides of the family, or if the parents have already had a child with a genetic disorder.

MATERNAL BLOOD TESTS AND ULTRASOUND

Screening maternal blood for the presence of alpha fetoprotein (AFP) is offered to pregnant women who are about eighteen weeks into a pregnancy. Although AFP is produced by the fetal liver, some will cross the placenta into the mother's blood. Elevated levels of AFP can indicate an open neural tube defect (such as spina bifida), although it can also indicate twins. Unusual AFP findings are usually followed up by ultrasound examination of the fetus.

Other tests of maternal blood measure the amounts of two substances that are produced by the fetal part of the placenta: hCG and UE3. Lower-than-average levels of AFP and UE3, combined with a higher-than-average amount of human chorionic gonadotropin (hCG), increases the risk that the woman is carrying a fetus with Down syndrome (trisomy 21). For example, a nineteen-year-old woman has a baseline risk of conceiving a fetus with Down syndrome of 1 in 1,193. When blood-test results show low AFP and UE3 along with high hCG, the probability of Down syndrome rises to 1 in 145.

During an ultrasound examination, sound waves are bounced off the fetus from an emitter placed on the surface of the mother's abdomen or in her vagina. They are used to make a picture of the fetus on a television monitor. Measurements on the monitor can often be used to determine the overall size, the head size, and the sex of the fetus, and whether all the arms and legs are formed and of the proper length. Successive ultrasound tests will indicate if the fetus is growing normally. Certain ultrasound findings, such as shortened long bones, may indicate an increased probability for a baby with Down syndrome. Because Down syndrome is a highly variable condition, normal ultrasound findings do not guarantee that the child will be born without Down syndrome. Only a chromosome analysis can determine this for certain.

AMNIOCENTESIS, KARYOTYPING, AND FISH

Amniocentesis is the process of collecting fetal cells from the amniotic fluid. Fetal cells collected by amniocentesis can be grown in culture; then the fluid around the cells is collected and analyzed for enzymes produced by the cells. If an enzyme is missing (as in the case of Tay-Sachs disease), the fetus may be diagnosed with the

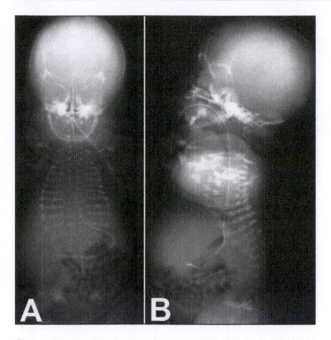

Postmortem anteroposterior (A) and lateral (B) whole-body radiographs of the baby. By see below, via Wikimedia Commons

disorder before birth. Because disorders such as Tay-Sachs disease are untreatable and fatal, a woman who has had one Tay-Sachs child may not wish to give birth to another. Early diagnosis of a second Tay-Sachs fetus may prompt the mother to terminate the pregnancy.

Chromosomes in the cells obtained by amniocentesis may be stained to produce a karyotype. In a normal karyotype, the chromosomes will be present in pairs. If the fetus has Down syndrome (trisomy 21), there will be three copies of chromosome 21. Other types of chromosome abnormalities that also appear in karyotypes are changes within a single chromosome. If a chromosome has lost a piece, it is said to contain a deletion. Large deletions will be obvious when a karyotype is analyzed because the chromosome will appear smaller than normal. Sometimes the deletion is so small that it is not visible on a karyotype.

If chromosome analysis is needed early in pregnancy before the volume of amniotic fluid is large enough to permit amniocentesis, the mother and doctor may opt for chorionic villus sampling (CVS). The embryo produces fingerlike projections (villi) into the uterine lining. Because these projections are produced by the embryo, their cells will have the same chromosome number as the rest of the embryonic cells. After growing in culture, the cells may

be karyotyped in the same way as those obtained by amniocentesis. Both amniocentesis and CVS carry risks of infection and miscarriage. Normally these procedures are not offered unless the risk of having an affected child is found to be greater than the risk of complications from the procedures.

If the doctor is convinced that the fetus has a tiny chromosomal defect that is not visible on a karyotype, it will then be necessary to probe (or "FISH") the fetal chromosomes; the initials "FISH" stand for fluorescence in situ hybridization. A chromosome probe is a piece of DNA that is complementary to DNA within a gene. Complementary pieces of DNA will stick together (hybridize) when they come in contact. The probe also has an attached molecule that will glow when viewed under fluorescent light. A probe for a particular gene will stick to the part of the chromosome where the gene is located and make a glowing spot. If the gene is not present because it has been lost, no spot will appear. Probes have been developed for many individual genes that cause developmental abnormalities when they are deleted from the chromosomes.

Cells obtained by amniocentesis can be probed in less time than it takes to grow and prepare them for karyotyping. Probes have been developed for the centromeres of the chromosomes that are frequently present in extra copies, such as 13, 18, 21, X, and Y. Y chromosomes that have been probed appear as red spots, X chromosomes as green spots, and number 18 chromosomes as aqua spots. A second set of probes attached to other cells from the same fetus will cause number 13 chromosomes to appear as green spots and number 21 chromosomes to appear as red spots. Cells from a girl with trisomy 21 would have two green spots and two aqua spots, but no red spot when the first set of probes is used. Some other cells from the same girl will show two red spots, but three green ones, when the second set of probes is used.

Tests for many more genetic defects using advanced molecular genetics tests have been developed. DNA can be isolated from fetal cells, obtained by one of the methods already described, which is then probed for single gene defects. Hundreds of potential genetic defects can be detected in this way, although only a few such tests are generally available. Another barrier to their use is their high cost. Costs will likely drop in the future as the tests are perfected and are used more widely. These same tests may be performed on the parents to determine whether they are carriers of certain genetic diseases.

IMPACT AND APPLICATIONS

Until the development of prenatal techniques, pregnant women had to wait until delivery day to find out the sex of their child and whether or not the baby had any genetic or congenital abnormalities. Now much more information is available to both the woman and her doctor months before the baby is due. Even though tests are not available for all possible birth defects, normal blood tests, karyotypes, or FISH can be very comforting. On the other hand, abnormal test results give the parents definite information about birth defects, as opposed to the possibilities inherent in a statement of risk. The parents must decide whether to continue the pregnancy. If they do, they must then prepare to care for a child with special needs. When properly administered, the test results are explained by a genetic counselor who is also equipped to help the parents deal with the strong emotions that such news can produce.

Nancy N. Shontz, Ph.D.;
updated by Bryan Ness, Ph.D.

FURTHER READING

Bianchi, Diana W., Timothy M. Crombleholme, Mary E. D'Alton, and Fergal D. Malone. *Fetology: Diagnosis and Management of the Fetal Patient.* 2nd ed. New York: McGraw-Hill, 2010. Print.

Coady, Anne Marie, and Sarah Bower, eds. *Twining's Textbook of Fetal Abnormalities.* 3rd ed. Edinburgh: Churchill Livingstone, 2014. Print.

De Crespigny, Lachlan, and Frank Chervenak. *Prenatal Tests: The Facts.* New York: Oxford UP, 2006. Print.

Evans, Mark I., et al., eds. *Prenatal Diagnosis.* New York: McGraw-Hill Medical, 2006. Print.

Heyman, Bob, and Mette Henriksen. *Risk, Age, and Pregnancy: A Case Study of Prenatal Genetic Screening and Testing.* New York: Palgrave, 2001. Print.

McConkey, Edwin H. *Human Genetics: The Molecular Revolution.* Boston: Jones and Bartlett, 1993. Print.

Milunsky, Aubrey, and Jeff M. Milunsky. *Genetic Disorders and the Fetus: Diagnosis, Prevention, and Treatment.* 7th ed. Hoboken: Wiley, 2015. Print.

New, Maria I., ed. *Diagnosis and Treatment of the Unborn Child.* Reddick: Idelson-Gnocchi, 1999. Print.

Petrikovsky, Boris M., ed. *Fetal Disorders: Diagnosis and Management.* New York: Wiley-Liss, 1999. Print.

Pilu, Gianluigi, and Kypros H. Nicolaides. *Diagnosis of Fetal Abnormalities: The Eighteen-Twenty-three-Week Scan.* New York: Parthenon Group, 1999. Print.

Rodeck, Charles H., and Martin J. Whittle, eds. *Fetal Medicine: Basic Science and Clinical Practice.* New York: Churchill Livingstone, 1999. Print

Weaver, David D., and Ira K. Brandt. *Catalog of Prenatally Diagnosed Conditions.* 3rd ed. Baltimore: Johns Hopkins UP, 1999. Print.

See also: Albinism; Amniocentesis; Androgen insensitivity syndrome; Burkitt's lymphoma; Chorionic villus sampling; Color blindness; Congenital defects; Consanguinity and genetic disease; Cystic fibrosis; Down syndrome; Dwarfism; Fragile X syndrome; Gender identity; Genetic counseling; Genetic screening; Genetic testing; Genetic testing: Ethical and economic issues; Heart disease; Hemophilia; Hereditary diseases; Hermaphrodites; Human genetics; Human Genome Project; Huntington's disease; In vitro fertilization and embryo transfer; Inborn errors of metabolism; Klinefelter syndrome; Metafemales; Monohybrid inheritance; Neural tube defects; Pedigree analysis; Phenylketonuria (PKU); Polymerase chain reaction; Prader-Willi and Angelman syndromes; Pseudohermaphrodites; RFLP analysis; Sickle-cell disease; Tay-Sachs disease; Thalidomide and other teratogens; Turner syndrome; XYY syndrome.

Prion diseases: Kuru and Creutzfeldt-Jakob syndrome

CATEGORY: Diseases and syndromes

SIGNIFICANCE: Kuru and Creutzfeldt-Jakob syndrome are rare, fatal diseases of the brain and spinal cord. Nerve cell death is caused by the accumulation of a protein called a prion, which appears to be a new infectious agent that interferes with gene expression in nerve cells. Understanding these diseases has far-reaching implications for the study of other degenerative mental disorders.

KEY TERMS

dementia: mental deterioration ranging from forgetfulness and disorientation to complete unresponsiveness

prion: short for "proteinaceous infectious particle," an element consisting mainly of protein and generally lacking nucleic acid (DNA and RNA), which is often the causative agent behind various spongiform encephalopathies

CAUSES, SYMPTOMS, AND TREATMENT

Kuru and Creutzfeldt-Jakob syndrome, degenerative diseases of the human central nervous system, are among a group of diseases that also affect cattle (mad cow disease)and sheep (scrapie). They have been classified in several ways, including "slow-virus" infections (because of the extremely long incubation period between contact and illness) and "spongiform encephalopathies" (because of the large holes seen in the brain after death). However, a virus that may cause such a disease has never been found, and the body does not respond to the disease as an infection. The only clue to the cause is the accumulation of a transmissible, toxic protein known as a prion; therefore, these disorders are now known simply as "prion diseases." Cdc cjd2 Histopathologic changes in frontal cerebral cortex of the patient who died of variant Creutzfeldt-Jakob disease i Variant Creutzfeldt-Jakob disease (vCJD), H&E Magnified 100X, and stained with H&E (hematoxylin and eosin) staining technique, this light photomicrograph of brain tissue reveals the presence of prominent spongiotic changes in the cortex, and loss of neurons in a case of variant Creutzfeldt-Jakob dise

Creutzfeldt-Jakob syndrome is rare: Approximately 250 people die from it yearly in the United States. It usually begins in middle age with symptoms that include rapidly progressing dementia, jerking spastic movements, and visual problems. Within one year after the symptoms begin, the patient is comatose and paralyzed, and powerful seizures affect the

entire body. Death occurs shortly thereafter. The initial symptom of the illness (rapid mental deterioration) is similar to other disorders; therefore, diagnosis is difficult. No typical infectious agent (bacteria or viruses) can be found in the blood or in the fluid that surrounds the brain and spinal cord. X rays and other scans are normal. There is no inflammation, fever, or antibody production. Brain wave studies are, however, abnormal, and at autopsy, the brain is found to have large holes and massive protein deposits in it.

Kuru is found among the Fore tribe of Papua New Guinea. Until the early 1960's, more than one thousand Fore died of kuru each year. Anthropologists recording their customs described their practice of eating the brains of their dead relatives in order to gain the knowledge they contained. Clearly, some infectious agent was being transmitted during this ritual. Such cannibalism has since stopped, and kuru has declined markedly. Kuru, like Creutzfeldt-Jakob syndrome, exhibits the same spongiform changes and protein deposits in the brain after death. Similarly, early symptoms include intellectual deterioration, spastic movements, and visual problems. Within a year, the patient becomes unresponsive and dies.

Magnified 100X, and stained with H&E (hematoxylin and eosin) staining technique, this light photomicrograph of brain tissue reveals the presence of prominent spongiotic changes in the cortex, and loss of neurons in a case of variant Creutzfeldt-Jakob dise. By Content Providers(s): CDC/ Teresa Hammett Photo Credit: Sherif Zaki; MD; PhD; Wun-Ju Shieh; MD; PhD; MPH (Public Health Image Library (PHIL) ID#: 10131), via Wikimedia Commons

Histopathologic changes in frontal cerebral cortex of the patient who died of variant Creutzfeldt-Jakob disease i. See page for author, via Wikimedia Commons

The outbreak of "mad cow" disease in the mid-1990's in Great Britain led to widespread fear. Thousands of cattle were killed to prevent human consumption of contaminated beef. The cows were infected by supplemental feedings tainted by infected sheep meat. Animal-to-human transmission of these diseases appears to occur, and research has shown that human-to-animal infection is possible as well.

Both kuru and Creutzfeldt-Jakob syndrome, as well as the animal forms, have no known treatment or cure. Because of the long incubation period, decades may pass before symptoms appear, but once they do, the central nervous system is rapidly destroyed, and death comes quickly. It is likely that many more people die of these disorders than is known because they are so rarely diagnosed.

PROPERTIES OF PRIONS

Most of the research on prion diseases has focused on scrapie in sheep. It became clear that the infectious particle had novel properties: It was not a virus as had been suspected, nor did the body react to it as an invader. It was discovered that this transmissible agent was an abnormal version of a common protein, which defied medical understanding. This protein is normally secreted by nerve cells and is found on their outer membranes. Its gene is on chromosome 20 in humans. The transmissible, infectious fragment of the prion somehow disrupts the nerve cell, causing it to produce the abnormal fragment instead of the normal protein. This product accumulates to toxic levels in the tissue and fluid of the brain and spinal cord over many years, finally destroying the central nervous system.

Prion infection appears to occur from exposure to infected tissues or fluids. Transmission has occurred accidentally through nerve tissue transplants and neurosurgical instruments. Prions are not affected by standard sterilization techniques; prevention requires careful handling of infected materials and extended autoclaving of surgical instruments (for at least one hour) or thorough rinsing in chlorine bleach. The agent is not spread by casual contact or air, and isolating the patient is not necessary.

Other human degenerative nervous system diseases whose causes remain unclear also show accumulations of proteins to toxic levels. Alzheimer's disease is the best-studied example, and it is possible that a process similar to that in prion diseases is at work. The discovery of prions has far-reaching implications for genetic and cellular research. Scientists have already learned a startling fact: Substances as inert as proteins and far smaller than viruses can act as agents of infection.

Connie Rizzo, M.D., Ph.D.

FURTHER READING

Aguzzi, Adriano, and Charles Weismann. "Prion Research: The Next Frontiers." *Nature* 389, no. 6653 (October 23, 1997): 796. An overview of the history of research into prions and prion diseases.

Baker, Harry F., ed. *Molecular Pathology of the Prions.* Totowa, N.J.: Humana Press, 2001. Overview of research on prion diseases. Illustrated, bibliography, index.

Goldman, Lee, and Dennis Ausiello, eds. *Cecil Textbook of Medicine.* 23rd ed. Philadelphia: Saunders Elsevier, 2008. A classic medical reference text that covers prion diseases. Bibliography, index.

Groschup, Martin H., and Hans A. Kretzschmar, eds. *Prion Diseases: Diagnosis and Pathogenesis.* New York: Springer, 2000. Comprehensive collection of research articles on the pathogenesis of prion diseases in humans and other animals, pharmacology, epidemiology, and diagnosis. Illustrations (some color), bibliography.

Harris, David A., ed. *Prions: Molecular and Cellular Biology.* Portland, Oreg.: Horizon Scientific Press, 1999. Focuses on the cellular, biochemical, and genetic aspects of prion diseases. Illustrations, bibliography, index.

Klitzman, Robert. *The Trembling Mountain: A Personal Account of Kuru, Cannibals, and Mad Cow Disease.* New York: Plenum Trade, 1998. Autobiographical account of a study of kuru disease in Papua New Guinea. Illustrations, index.

Max, D. T. *The Family That Couldn't Sleep: A Medical Mystery.* New York: Random House, 2006. Traces the understanding of prion diseases beginning in 1765, when members of a Venetian family began to die of a mysterious inability to sleep.

Prusiner, Stanley B. "The Prion Diseases." *Scientific American* 272, no. 1 (January, 1995): 48. Discusses how meat consumption by humans can lead to prion diseases.

_____, ed. *Prion Biology and Diseases.* 2d ed. Cold Spring Harbor, N.Y.: Cold Spring Harbor Laboratory Press, 2004. Prusiner, who won the 1997 Nobel Prize in Medicine for his discovery of prions, and contributors provide an overview of research. Illustrations (some color), bibliography, index.

Rabenau, Holger F., Jindrich Cinatl, and Hans Wilhelm Doerr, eds. *Prions: A Challenge for Science, Medicine, and Public Health System.* 2d ed, rev. and extended. New York: Karger, 2004. Focuses on the etiological, clinical, and diagnostic aspects of prion diseases, as well as epidemiology, disease management, and how prions might be inactivated. Illustrations, bibliography, index.

Ratzan, Scott C., ed. *The Mad Cow Crisis: Health and the Public Good.* New York: New York University Press, 1998. A look at the disease from scientific, historical, political, health, preventive, and management perspectives. Illustrations, bibliography, index.

Yam, Philip. *The Pathological Protein: Mad Cow, Chronic Wasting, and Other Deadly Prion Diseases.* New York: Copernicus, 2003. Chronicles medical and scientific efforts to discover and understand prions and to devise treatments for the diseases they create.

See also: Alzheimer's disease; Huntington's disease.

Progressive external ophthalmoplegia

CATEGORY: Diseases and syndromes
ALSO KNOWN AS: PEO

DEFINITION
Progressive external ophthalmoplegia (PEO) is a mitochondrial myopathy disorder that is characterized by painless, slowly progressive paralysis of certain eye muscles. PEO is typically caused by a mitochondrial DNA (mtDNA) deletion in the skeletal muscle during oogenesis or embryogenesis.

RISK FACTORS
Males and females are affected equally by this mutation. Onset of symptoms tends to begin in young adulthood. Although the mutation occurs almost always as a sporadic point mutation, it can be inherited as a point mutation of maternal mitochondrial tRNA or as autosomal dominant and autosomal recessive deletions of mtDNA, with the autosomal recessive inheritance usually being more severe. However, the

A headshot daguerreotype of an unidentified male presenting with ptosis of the eyelid in 1852. By William Bell, via Wikimedia Commons

mother of a child with PEO is usually unaffected. The risk to siblings is extremely low as no+ cases of maternal transmission to more than one child have been reported. The offspring of males with an mtDNA mutation are not at risk.

ETIOLOGY AND GENETICS
Mitochondrial diseases affect the mitochondria, which are found in almost all cells and are responsible

Congenital Ptosis. By Andrewya (Own work), via Wikimedia Commons for providing the energy that cells need to survive. Since most cells rely on mitochondria for energy, a mitochondrial disease can affect many different types of cells. When a mitochondrial disease causes prominent muscular complications, it is called a mitochondrial myopathy. PEO is a mitochondrial myopathy that is characterized by slowly progressive paralysis of the six muscles that control the movement of the human eye (extraocular muscles).

PEO involves multiple mtDNA deletions in the skeletal muscles. Several types of deletions of varying lengths have been identified in PEO. Most mitochondrial DNA deletions associated with PEO typically range in size from two to ten kilobases. The same person may have variable proportions of deleted mtDNA in different tissues throughout their body which can ultimately determine how significantly the tissue is clinically affected. However, no correlation exists between the size or location of the mtDNA deletion and phenotype.

Mitochondrial DNA deletions are almost always caused by a point mutation. Specifically in PEO, deletions of mtDNA have been identified by mutations in the *MT-TL1* mitochondrial gene as well as in *SLC25A4*, *POLG*, and *C10orf2*, which are nuclear genes involved with mtDNA maintenance. When PEO is caused by *MT-TL1* mutations, it is always transmitted by maternal inheritance; various mtDNA point mutations have been found in people with maternally inherited PEO. When PEO is the result of mutations in nuclear genes, the inheritance pattern is usually autosomal dominant. Some mutations in the *POLG* nuclear gene cause PEO inherited via an autosomal recessive pattern, while somatic mutations in this gene are not inherited but happen during a person's lifetime (GHR 2014).

Symptoms

Severity and phenotypic variability of symptoms vary greatly with PEO. This often makes an early diagnosis more difficult. The most consistent symptoms usually begin to manifest in late adolescence or young adulthood. Symptoms typically progress slowly. The defect in ocular motility is usually bilateral and symmetric so most patients do not complain of double vision. Primary symptoms include reduced superior visual field, corneal dryness and ulceration due to poor blinking reflexes, droopy eyelids, loss of Bell's reflex (eyes roll upward when lids are closed), muscle weakness and wasting, exercise intolerance, muscle cramps, and low energy.

Screening and Diagnosis

Diagnosis of PEO relies upon the presence of characteristic physical findings as well as through laboratory and imaging studies. When PEO is suspected, a complete ophthalmologic exam including a dilated retinal exam, a cranial nerve test, and a forced duction test should be performed. Thin, symmetrical extraocular muscles are often found during magnetic resonance imaging (MRI), computed tomography (CT), and ultrasound studies. Laboratory testing is often used to differentiate between PEO and other conditions with similar physical symptoms (such as myasthenia gravis). Serum creatine kinase is usually measured since this may be elevated in mitochondrial disease. In addition, deletions in mtDNA in PEO patients can be detected in muscle tissue by Southern blot analysis of samples taken from a muscle biopsy. Genetic tests can be performed to screen for known mutations/deletions.

Treatment and Therapy

There is no cure for PEO, but treatments do exist for the alleviation of some of the associated symptoms. Mechanical devices such as placement of eyelid slings have helped to decrease severe drooping. Surgical procedures can also be performed to lift a drooping eyelid. However, since poor blink responses are often associated with PEO, the cornea of the eye can become dry or scratched following surgical intervention. The use of artificial tears and/or eye patching at night can often help to alleviate this problem. Recently, dietary supplements such as coenzyme Q10 and L-carnitine, which are involved in increasing ATP production in the cells, have shown modest results in some people. Physical and occupational therapy as well as treatments aimed at preventing/treating symptoms of depression which are often present in people suffering from a chronic disease are also frequently incorporated into the overall treatment strategy for PEO.

Prevention and Outcomes

There is no effective means of prevention of PEO. Genetic counseling enables people to make more informed medical and personal decisions and should always be encouraged and available to patients and their families especially regarding options for at-risk mothers. PEO is not a fatal disease; however, associated disabilities may affect mortality.

Kimberly Lynch

Further Reading

Bau, Viktoria, and Stephan Zierz. "Update on Chronic Progressive External Ophthalmoplegia." *Strabismus* 13.3 (2005): 133–142. Print.

Cohen, Bruce H., Patick F. Chinnery, and William C. Copeland. "*POLG*-Related Disorders." *GeneReviews*. Ed. Roberta A. Pagon et al. Seattle: U of Washington, Seattle, 1993–2014. *NCBI Bookshelf*. Natl. Center for Biotechnology Information, 11 Oct. 2012. Web. 19 Aug. 2014.

DiMaura, Salvatore, and Michio Hirano. "Mitochondrial DNA Deletion Syndromes." *GeneReviews*. Ed. Roberta A. Pagon et al. Seattle: U of Washington, Seattle, 1993–2014. *NCBI Bookshelf*. Natl. Center for Biotechnology Information, 3 May 2011. Web. 19 Aug. 2014.

Genetics Home Reference. "Progressive External Ophthalmoplegia." *Genetics Home Reference*. US NLM, 18 Aug. 2014. Web. 19 Aug. 2014.

Lewin, Benjamin. *Genes X*. 10th ed. Sudbury: Jones, 2011. Print.

Riordan-Eva, Paul, et al. *Vaughan & Asbury's General Ophthalmology*. 18th ed. New York: McGraw, 2011. Print.

See also: Aniridia; Best disease; Choroideremia; Color blindness; Congenital muscular dystrophy; Corneal dystrophies; Duchenne muscular dystrophy; Glaucoma; Gyrate atrophy of the choroid and retina; Kennedy disease; Limb girdle muscular dystrophy; McArdle's disease; Macular degeneration; Myotonic dystrophy; Nemaline myopathy; Norrie syndrome; Retinitis pigmentosa; Retinoblastoma.

Prostate cancer and genetics

Category: Diseases and syndromes
Also known as: Prostatic carcinoma, Acinar adenocarcinoma, Ductal adenocarcinoma, Transitional cell (or urothelial) cancer, Squamous cell cance of the prostate, Small cell prostate cancer

Definition

Prostate cancer is a disease in which cancer cells grow in the prostate gland. The prostate is a walnut sized gland in men. The prostate makes a fluid that is part of semen.

Cancer occurs when cells in the body (in this, case prostate cells) divide without control or order. Normally, cells divide in a regulated manner. If cells keep dividing uncontrollably when new cells are not needed, a mass of tissue forms, called a growth or tumor. The term "cancer" refers to malignant tumors, which can invade nearby tissue and spread to other parts of the body. A benign tumor does not invade or spread.

The sooner prostate cancer is treated, the better the outcome. Men should contact their doctors right away if they think they have this condition.

Risk Factors

Although no factors have shown clear cause-and-effect, there are factors that are associated with a higher risk of prostate cancer. One of the most prominent is age – the older the person, the higher the risk of prostate cancer. In addition, some of these factors are more associated with non-aggressive tumors and others with aggressive tumors. For example, smoking and low intake of vegetables in diet seem to be associated with aggressive prostate cancer but not slow-growing tumors. Other risk factors for aggressive prostate cancer include: tall height; lack of exercise and a sedentary lifestyle; high calcium intake; African-American race; family history and Agent Orange exposure. There are also a number of genes that appear associated with an increased risk of developing the disease (see "Etiology and Genetics").

Etiology and Genetics

Prostate cancer is a complex condition that may involve both genetic and environmental determinants. About 75 percent of cases are sporadic, with no known underlying genetic basis. An additional 15 to 20 percent of cases are termed "familial" because they run in families, and these probably result from a combination of shared genes and shared life styles. Only 5 to 10 percent of cases are termed "hereditary," yet mutations in a dozen or more genes have been identified that may increase an individual's susceptibility to prostate cancer. Mutations in susceptibility genes for hereditary prostate cancer probably account for about half of the cases of disease in patients aged 50 years or younger. In these cases, the vast majority show an autosomal dominant pattern of transmission, meaning that a single copy of the mutation is sufficient to cause the increased susceptibility. An affected individual has a

Prostate Cancer. By Otis Brawley (Photographer), via Wikimedia Commons

50 percent chance of transmitting the mutation to each of his or her children. Other cases of hereditary prostate cancer, however, result from a spontaneous new mutation, so in these instances affected individuals will have an unaffected father.

A number of genes have been identified as being associated with in creased susceptibility to the small number of men who develop hereditary prostate cancer. Examples include HPC1 (found on chromosome 1 at position 1q25), HPC2 (located on chromosome 17 at position 17p11), HPCX (at position 11p11.22 and X-linked), HSPG2 at the CAPB locus (at position 1p36.1-p35), PCA3 (at position 9q21-q22), and TMPRSS2 (at position 21q22.3). Additionally, muta tions in the BRCA1 and BRCA2 genes, most com monly associated with hereditary breast and ovarian cancer, also confer an increased risk for prostate cancer. One study suggests that men with BRCA1 mutations have a slightly increased risk, while men with BRCA2 mutations may have as much as a 20 percent risk of developing prostate cancer.

SYMPTOMS

Men who have any of these symptoms should not assume it is due to prostate cancer. These symptoms may also be caused by other, less serious health con ditions, such as benign prostatic hyperplasia (BPH) or an infection. Symptoms may include a need to urinate fre quently, especially at night; difficulty starting urina tion or holding back urine; an inability to urinate; a weak or interrupted urine flow; and painful or burning urination. Additional symptoms include difficulty having an erection, painful ejaculation, blood in urine or semen, and frequent pain or stiff ness in the lower back, hips, or upper thighs.

SCREENING AND DIAGNOSIS

Because prostate cancers are so common, much research has been done to try to identify effective screening methods that will not only identify disease very early but will also improve overall outcomes such as reduction in prostate cancer morbidity, including urinary obstruction and painful metastases, and mortality. There continue to be concerns that the benefits of screening are outweighed by the potential harms to quality of life, including the substantial risks for overdiagnosis, diagnostic procedure complications (such as from obtaining biopsies) and treatment complications. This subject is a very dynamic one and continues to be the subject of a great deal of ongoing research. There is currently no single test or combination of tests that has been found effective for meeting these goals.

When there is a concern about a patient having prostate cancer, the doctor may ask about symptoms and medical history and may perform a physical exam. An exam might include a digital rectal exam, in which the doctor will insert a gloved finger into the rectum in order to ex amine the prostate; however, this exam is no longer recommended as part of prostate cancer screening. Urine tests may be done to check for blood or infection; and blood tests to measure prostate specific antigen (PSA) and prostatic acid phosphatase (PAP) may be recommended.

Other available tests to learn more about the cause of a patient's symptoms include blood tests a such as PSA velocity, Free PSA, ProPSA, Kallikrein assays, and an assay for prostate cancer antigen 3 gene (PCA3). Available imaging studies include transrectal ultrasonography, a test that uses sound waves and a probe inserted into the rectum to find tumors; intravenous pyelogram, a series of X rays of the organs of the urinary tract; cystoscopy, in which the doctor looks into the urethra and bladder through a thin, lighted tube; and biopsy, the removal of a sample of prostate tissue to test for cancer cells.

TREATMENT AND THERAPY

Once prostate cancer is found, tests are done to find out if the cancer has spread and, if so, to what extent. Treatment depends on how far the cancer has spread. Patients most often work with a urologist, who can discuss the benefits and risks of each treatment option and provide guidance as to the best treatment plan.

Cut section of the prostate showing carcinomatous growth. By Netha Hussain (Own work), via Wikimedia Commons

Standard options include watchful waiting. There is no treatment with watchful waiting. The doctor will do tests to see if the cancer is growing. Watchful waiting is used for early-stage prostate cancer that seems to be growing slowly, for older prostate cancer patients, and those with serious medical problems that may make the treatment risks outweigh the possible benefits.

For those who are candidates for surgery, there are various surgical approaches and techniques. Surgery involves removing the cancerous tumor, nearby tissues, and possibly the nearby lymph nodes. Surgery always carries the potential for risks and complications, and these are discussed by the patient and operating surgeon before making a final decision to undergo an operation.

Types of surgery include pelvic lymphadenectomy, the removal of lymph nodes in the pelvis to determine if they contain cancer. If they do, removal of the prostate and other treatment may be recommended. Radical retropubic prostatectomy is the removal of the entire prostate and nearby lymph nodes through an incision in the abdomen. Radical perineal prostatectomy is the removal of the entire prostate through an incision between the scrotum and the anus; nearby lymph nodes are sometimes removed through a separate incision in the abdomen.

Transurethral resection of the prostate (TURP) is the removal of part of the prostate with an instrument inserted through the urethra. TURP is not a cancer surgery, but it can be used to remove a blockage in the urethra in patients who have prostate can-

cer. Prostate cancer surgery can cause impotence, and it can also cause urine leakage from the bladder or stool from the rectum. Nerve-sparing surgery may reduce these risks. However, this surgery may not treat very large tumors or tumors that are very close to nerves. Robotic surgery and laparoscopic surgery are other options. These minimally invasive techniques may reduce side effects, blood loss, and recovery time. Radiation therapy involves the use of radiation to kill cancer cells and shrink tumors. Radiation may be external beam radiation therapy (EBRT), in which radiation is directed at the tumor from a source outside the body, or internal radiation therapy, in which radioactive materials are placed into the body near the cancer cells. Advances in EBRT have led to special types of this form of treatment. Conformal radiation therapy uses three dimensional radiation beams that are conformed into the shape of the diseased prostate. This treatment spares nearby tissue the damaging effects of radiation. Intensity-modulated radiation therapy (IMRT) uses radiation beams of different intensities to deliver higher doses of radiation therapy to the tumor and lower doses to nearby tissues at the same time.

Internal radiation therapy is often used for treating earlier-stage cancers. Radiation therapy for prostate cancer may cause impotence and urinary problems. When comparing impotence problems between those who have undergone radiation and those who have undergone surgery, there does not seem to be much long-term difference between the two. Men who have had radiation may see a general decrease in function over time (up to several years after radiation). In contrast, after surgery most men have problems right away and then have a chance to recover in the first 2 years following surgery. About 4 years after either treatment, the percentage of men reporting erectile dysfunction is about the same. Treatments exist that can often help recover these functions whether there has been past surgery or radiation. Incontinence also occurs less frequently following radiation therapy than it does following prostatectomy. However, there is a slightly increased risk of radiation cystitis (an irritation of the bladder) that can lead to blood in the urinary and burning during urination.

Hormone therapy is used for patients whose prostate cancer has spread beyond the prostate or has recurred after treatment. The goal of hormone therapy is to lower levels of male hormones called androgens. The main androgen is testosterone. Lowering androgen levels can cause prostate cancers to shrink or grow more slowly, but it does not cure cancer.

Methods of hormone therapy include orchiectomy, a surgical procedure to remove one or both of the testicles, which are the main source of male hormones. Orchiectomy decreases hormone production, which can shrink or slow the growth of most prostate cancers.

Hormone therapy also includes medications. Luteinizing hormone-releasing hormone (LHRH) agonists are injections that can decrease the amount of testosterone made by the testicles. Antiandrogens, such as flutamide or bicalutamide, are medications that can block the action of androgens. These medications may be used in combination with orchiectomy or LHRH agonists, a combination called total androgen blockade. Second line forms of hormone therapy include the use of the drugsketoconazole or aminoglutethimide, that prevent the adrenal glands from making androgens; and estrogens, drugs that prevent the production of testosterone in the testicles. Estrogens are rarely used today because of the risk of serious side effects. Hormone therapy for prostate cancer may cause hot flashes, impaired sexual function, loss of sexual desire, and weakened bones.

A newer medication called Degarelix is now available. Degarelix is a peptide mimetic that acts as a GnRH receptor antagonist. It binds GnRH receptors in the pituitary gland and blocks LH and FSH release from the pituitary. LH normally binds LH receptors on Leydig cells in the testes and activates testosterone production. In more advanced cases where the cancer has spread to other parts of the body, and androgen suppression drugs are not working, chemotherapy drugs may be recommended to kill the cancer cells. These may be given in many forms, including pill, injection, and via a catheter. The drugs enter the bloodstream and travel through the body, killing mostly cancer cells, but also some healthy cells. Several of these drugs are available including Docetaxel (Taxotere), Cabazitaxel (Jevtana), Mitoxantrone (Novantrone), and Estramustine (Emcyt).

Treatment of the cancer is often accompanied by treatment of known side effects of the medications used. One of these effects is the loss of bone density in areas such as the thigh, hip, and low back thus making the patient more apt to experience broken bones. As a result, patients are frequently advised to take supplemental vitamin D, calcium, and medications that can help slow the loss of bone during hormone therapy. One example of a drug used to maintain bone health is denosumab.

PREVENTION AND OUTCOMES
There is no way to actually prevent prostate cancer; however, risk factors can certainly be reduced with guidance and education. Men who have no symptoms and are over age 50 may consider a conversation with a physician about steps that can be taken to modify risk factors as well as monitoring for prostate cancer if there are significant risk factors for developing the disease. Any screening recommended will likely be the result of shared decision-making between the patient and the physician.

The prognosis for slow, non-aggressive tumors is very good, and the affected person may live a normal lifespan. For those with more aggressive tumors, the prognosis and outcomes will vary greatly depending upon the stage of the tumor, age of the patient, tolerance for recommended treatments, surgical complications, etc.

Krisha McCoy, M.S.; reviewed by Igor Puzanov, M.D.
"Etiology and Genetics" by Jeffrey A. Knight, Ph.D.;
updated by Gary M. Flashner, M.S., M.D.

FURTHER READING
American Cancer Society. "Quick Facts Prostate Cancer: What You Need to Know—Now." Atlanta: Author, 2007.

Berthold, D. R., et al. "Docetaxel Plus Prednisone or Mitoxantrone for Advanced Prostate Cancer: Updated Survival of the TAX 327 Study." *Journal of Clinical Oncology* 26, no. 2 (January 10, 2008): 242-245.

Burnett, Arthur. *The Johns Hopkins Patients' Guide to Prostate Cancer.* Sudbury, Mass.: Jones and Bartlett, 2010.

EBSCO Publishing. *Health Library: Prostate Cancer.* Ipswich, Mass.: Author, 2009. Available through http://www.ebscohost.com.

Klein, Eric A. *The Cleveland Clinic Guide to Prostate Cancer.* New York: Kaplan, 2009.

Tannock, I. F., et al. "Docetaxel Plus Prednisone or Mitoxantrone Plus Prednisone for Advanced Prostate Cancer." *New England Journal of Medicine* 351, no. 15 (October 7, 2004): 1502-1512. Bell KJ, Del Mar C, Wright G, et al. *Prevalence* of incidental prostate cancer: A systematic review of autopsy studies. *Int J Cancer* 2015; 137:1749. Pinsky PF, Prorok PC, Yu K, et al. "Extended mortality results for prostate cancer screening in the PLCO trial with median follow-up of 15 years." *Cancer* 2017; 123:592.

Andriole GL, Bostwick D, Brawley OW, et al. "The effect of dutasteride on the usefulness of prostate specific antigen for the diagnosis of high grade and clinically relevant prostate cancer in men with a previous negative biopsy: results from the REDUCE study." *J Urol* 2011; 185:126.

Vickers AJ, Till C, Tangen CM, et al. "An empirical evaluation of guidelines on prostate-specific antigen velocity in prostate cancer detection." *J Natl Cancer Inst* 2011; 103:462. Filella X, Giménez N. "Evaluation of [-2] proPSA and Prostate Health Index (phi) for the detection of prostate cancer: a systematic review and meta-analysis." *Clin Chem Lab Med* 2013; 51:729. Yang Z, Yu L, Wang Z. "PCA3 and TMPRSS2-ERG gene fusions as diagnostic biomarkers for prostate cancer." *Chinese Journal of Cancer Research.* 2016;28(1):65-71. doi:10.3978/j.issn.1000-9604.2016.01.05.

Web Sites of Interest

American Cancer Society
https://www.cancer.org/cancer/prostate-cancer/

American Urological Association
http://www.auanet.org

Hormone Refractory Prostate Cancer
http://www.hrpca.org/index.htm

National Cancer Institute
http://www.cancer.gov\

Prostate Cancer Canada
http://www.prostatecancer.ca/english/home
https://www.uptodate.com/contents/screening-for-prostate-cancerhttps://www.cancer.org/cancer/prostate-cancer/treating/radiation-therapy.htmlhttps://www.pcf.org/c/prostate-cancer-risk-factors/https://ghr.nlm.nih.gov/condition/prostate-cancer#genes http://www.medscape.com/viewarticle/837934

Prostate Cancer Canada Network
http://www.cpcn.org
Zero: The Project to End Prostate Cancer http://www.zerocancer.org/index.html https://www.cancer.org/treatment/treatments-and-side-effects/physical-side-effects/fertility-and-sexual-side-effects/sexuality-for-men-with-cancer/erections-and-treatment.html

See also: BRAF gene; BRCA1 and BRCA2 genes; Breast cancer; Burkitt's lymphoma; Chemical mutagens; Chromosome mutation; Chronic myeloid leukemia; Colon cancer; Cowden syndrome; DPC4 gene testing; Familial adenomatous polyposis; Gene therapy; Harvey ras oncogene; Hereditary diffuse gastric cancer; Hereditary diseases; Hereditary leiomyomatosis and renal cell cancer; Hereditary mixed polyposis syndrome; Hereditary non-VHL clear cell renal cell carcinomas; Hereditary papillary renal cancer; Homeotic genes; HRAS gene testing; Hybridomas and monoclonal antibodies; Li Fraumeni syndrome; Lynch syndrome; Mutagenesis and cancer; Multiple endocrine neoplasias; Mutation and mutagenesis; Nondisjunction and an euploidy; Oncogenes; Ovarian cancer; Pancreatic cancer; Tumor-suppressor genes; Wilms' tumor aniridia-genitourinary anomalies-mental retardation (WAGR) syndrome.

Protein structure

Category: Molecular genetics

Significance: Proteins have three-dimensional structures that determine their functions, and slight changes in overall structure may significantly alter their activity. Correlation of protein structure and function can provide insights into cellular metabolism and its many interconnected processes. Because most diseases result from improper protein function, advances in this field could lead to effective molecular-based disease treatments.

Key terms

amino acid : the basic subunit of a protein; there are twenty commonly occurring amino acids, any of which may join together by chemical bonds to form a complex protein molecule

enzymes: proteins that are able to increase the rate of chemical reactions in cells without being altered in the process

hydrogen bond: a weak bond that helps stabilize the folding of a protein

polypeptide : a chain of amino acids joined by chemical bonds

R group: a functional group that is part of an amino acid that gives each amino acid its unique properties

PROTEIN STRUCTURE AND FUNCTION

Proteins consist of strings of individual subunits called amino acids that are chemically bonded together with peptide bonds. Once amino acids are bonded, the resulting molecule is called a polypeptide. The properties and arrangement of the amino acids in the polypeptide cause it to fold into a specific shape or conformation that is required for proper protein function. Proteins have been called the "workhorses" of the cell because they perform most of the activities encoded in the genes of the cell. Proteins function by binding to other molecules, frequently to other proteins. The precise three-dimensional shape of a protein determines the specific molecules it will be able to bind to, and for many proteins binding is specific to just one other specific type of molecule.

In 1973, Christian B. Anfinsen performed experiments that showed that the three-dimensional structure of a protein is determined by the sequence of its amino acids. He used a protein called ribonuclease (RNase), an enzyme that degrades RNA in the cell. The ability of ribonuclease to degrade RNA is dependent upon its ability to fold into its proper three-dimensional shape. Anfinsen showed that if the enzyme was completely unfolded by heat and chemical treatment (at which time it would not function), it formed a linear chain of amino acids. Although there were 105 possible conformations that the enzyme could take upon refolding, it would refold into the single correct functional conformation upon removal of heat and chemicals. This established that the amino acid sequences of proteins, which are specified by the genes of the cell, carry all of the information necessary for proteins to fold into their proper three-dimensional shapes.

To understand protein conformation better, it is helpful to analyze the underlying levels of structure that determine the final three-dimensional shape. The primary structure of a polypeptide is the simplest level of structure and is, by definition, its amino acid sequence. Because the primary structure of polypeptides ultimately determines all succeeding levels of structure, knowing the primary structure should theoretically allow scientists to predict the final three-dimensional structure. Building on a detailed knowledge of the structure of many proteins, scientists have developed computer programs that are able to predict three-dimensional shape with some degree of accuracy.

PRIMARY PROTEIN STRUCTURE

There are twenty naturally occurring amino acids that are commonly found in proteins, and each of these has a common structure consisting of a nitrogen-containing amino group (—NH2), a carboxyl group (—COOH), a hydrogen atom (H), and a unique functional group referred to as an R group, all bonded to a central carbon atom (known as the alpha carbon, or Cα) as shown in the following figure:

The uniqueness of each of the twenty amino acids is determined by the R group. This group may be as simple as a hydrogen atom (in the case of the amino acid glycine) or as complex as a ring-shaped structure (as found in the amino acid phenylalanine). It may be charged, either positively or negatively, or it may be uncharged.

Cells join amino acids together to form peptides (strings of up to ten amino acids), polypeptides (strings of ten to one hundred amino acids), or proteins (single or multiple polypeptides folded and oriented to one another so they are functional). The

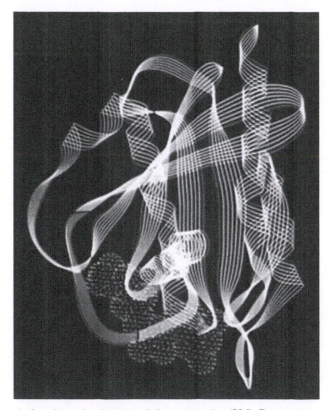

A three-dimensional image of the ras protein. (U.S. Department of Energy Human Genome Program, http://www.ornl.gov/hgmis)

Protein structure. By Holger87 (Own work), via Wikimedia Commons

amino acids are joined together by covalent bonds, called peptide bonds (in the box in the following figure), between the carbon atom of the carboxyl group of one amino acid (—COOH) and the nitrogen atom of the amino group (—NH2) of the next adjacent amino acid.

During the formation of the peptide bond, a molecule of water (H_2O) is lost (an -OH from the carboxyl group and an -H from the amino group), so this reaction is also called a dehydration synthesis. The result is a dipeptide (a peptide made of two amino acids joined by a peptide bond) that has a "backbone" of nitrogens and carbons (N—Cα—C—N—Cα—C) with other elements and R groups protruding from the backbone. An amino acid may be joined to the growing peptide chain by formation of a peptide bond between the carbon atom of the free carboxyl group (on the right of the preceding figure) and the nitrogen atom of the amino acid being added. The end of a polypeptide with an exposed carboxyl group is called the C-terminal end, and the end with an exposed amino group is called the N-terminal end.

The atoms and R groups that protrude from the backbone are capable of interacting with each other, and these interactions lead to higher-order secondary, tertiary, and quaternary structures.

SECONDARY STRUCTURE

The next level of structure is secondary structure, which involves the formation of hydrogen bonds between the oxygen atoms in carboxyl groups with the hydrogen atoms of amino groups from different parts of the polypeptide. Hydrogen bonds are weak bonds that form between atoms that have a very strong attraction for electrons (such as oxygen or nitrogen), and a hydrogen atom that is bound to another atom with a very strong attraction for electrons. Secondary structure does not involve the formation of bonds with R groups or atoms that are parts of R groups, but involves bonding just between amino and carboxyl groups that are in the peptide bonds making up the backbone of polypeptides.

These hydrogen bonds between backbone molecules lead to the formation of two major types of structures: alpha helices and beta-pleated sheets. An alpha helix is a rigid structure shaped very much like a telephone cord; it spirals around as the oxygen of one amino acid of the chain forms a hydrogen bond with the hydrogen atom of an amino acid five amino acids away on the protein strand. The rigidity of the structure is caused by the large number of hydrogen bonds (individually weak but collectively strong) and the compactness of the helix that forms. Many alpha helices are found in proteins that function to maintain cell structure.

Beta sheets are formed by hydrogen bonding between amino acids in different regions (often very far apart on the linear strand) of a polypeptide. The shape of a beta-pleated sheet may be likened to the bellows of an accordion or a sheet of paper that has been folded multiple times to form pleats. Because of the large number of hydrogen bonds in them, beta sheets are also strong structures, and they form planar regions that are often found at the bottom of "pockets" inside proteins to which other molecules attach.

In addition to alpha helices or beta-pleated sheets, other regions of the protein may have no obvious secondary structure; these regions are said to have a "random coil" shape. It is the combinations of random coils, alpha helices, and beta sheets that form the secondary structure of the protein.

TERTIARY STRUCTURE

The final level of protein shape (for a single polypeptide or simple protein) is called tertiary structure. Tertiary structure is caused by the numerous interactions of R groups on the amino acids and of the protein with its environment, which is usually aqueous (water based). Various R groups may either be attracted to and form bonds with each other, or they may be repelled from each other. For example, if an R group has an overall positive electrical charge, it will be attracted to R groups with a negative charge but repelled from other positively charged R groups. For a polypeptide with one hundred amino acids, if amino acid number 6 is negatively charged, it could be attracted to a positively charged amino acid at position 74, thus bringing two ends of the protein that are linearly distant into close proximity. Many of these attractions lead to the formation of hydrogen, ionic, or covalent bonds. For example, sulfur is contained in the R groups of a few of the amino acids, and sometimes a disulfide bond (a covalent bond) will be formed between two of these. It is the arrangement of disulfide bonds in hair proteins that gives hair its physical properties of curly versus straight, for instance. Hair permanent treatments actually break these disulfide bonds and then reform them when the hair is arranged as desired. Many other R groups in the protein will also be attracted to or repelled from each other, leading to an overall folded shape that is most stable. In addition, because most proteins exist in an aqueous environment in the cell, most proteins are folded such that their amino acids with hydrophilic R groups (R groups attracted to water) are on the outside, while their amino acids with hydrophobic R groups (R groups repelled from water) are tucked away in the interior of the protein.

QUATERNARY STRUCTURE

Many polypeptides are nonfunctional until they physically associate with another polypeptide, forming a functional unit made up of two or more subunits. Proteins of this type are said to have quaternary structure. Quaternary structure is caused by interactions between the R groups of amino acids of two different polypeptides. For example, hemoglobin, the oxygen-carrying protein found in red blood cells, functions as a tetramer, with four polypeptide subunits.

Because secondary, tertiary, and quaternary interactions are caused by the R groups of the specific amino acids, the folding is ultimately dictated by the amino acid sequence of the protein. Although there may be numerous possible final conformations that a polypeptide could take, it usually assumes only one of these, and this is the conformation that leads to proper protein function. Many polypeptides

are capable of folding into their final conformation spontaneously. More complex ones may need the assistance of other proteins, called chaperones, to help in the folding process.

IMPACT AND APPLICATIONS

The function of a protein may be altered by changing its shape, because proper function is dependent on proper conformation. Many genetic defects are detrimental because they represent a mutation that results in a change in protein structure. Changes in protein conformation are also an integral part of metabolic control in cells. Normal cellular processes are controlled by "turning on" and "turning off" proteins at the appropriate time. A protein's activity may be altered by attaching a molecule or ion to that protein that results in a change of shape. Because the shape is caused by R group interactions, binding of a charged ion such as calcium to the protein will alter these interactions and thus alter the shape and function of the protein. One molecular "on/off" switch that is used frequently within a cell involves the attachment or removal of a phosphate group to or from a protein. Attachment of a phosphate will significantly alter the shape of the protein by repelling negatively charged amino acids and attracting positively charged amino acids, which will either activate the protein to perform its function (turn it on) or deactivate it (turn it off).

Cancer and diseases caused by bacterial infections or viral infections are often the result of nonfunctional proteins that have been produced with incorrect shapes or that cannot be turned on or off by a molecular switch. The effects may be minor or major, depending upon the protein, its function, and the severity of the structural deformity. Understanding how a normal protein is shaped and how it is altered in the disease process allows for the development of drugs that may block the disease. This may be accomplished by blocking or changing the effect of the protein of interest or by generating drugs or therapies that mimic the normal functioning of the protein. Thus, understanding protein structure is essential for understanding proper protein function and for developing molecular-based disease treatments. For example, in January 2016 a study published in the journal *Nature* outlined the structure of a protein complex believed to be integral in human immune system response. The findings bring the potential to create new types of drugs to treat diseases ranging from cancer to inflammatory conditions such as psoriasis and rheumatoid arthritis.

Sarah Lea McGuire, Ph.D.;
updated by Bryan Ness, Ph.D.

FURTHER READING

Banaszak, Leonard J. *Foundations of Structural Biology.* San Diego: Academic, 2000. Print.

Brändén, Carl-Ivar, and John Tooze. *Introduction to Protein Structure.* 2nd ed. New York: Garland, 1999. Print.

Buxbaum, Engelbert. *Fundamentals of Protein Structure and Function.* New York: Springer, 2007. Print.

Doerr, Allison. "Protein Structure through Time." *Nature Methods.* Macmillan, 30 Dec. 2015. Web. 20 Jan. 2016.

Haggerty, Lauren M. *Protein Structure.* New York: Nova Science, 2011. Digital file.

Johnson, George B. *How Scientists Think: Twenty-One Experiments That Have Shaped Our Understanding of Genetics and Molecular Biology.* Dubuque: Brown, 1996. Print.

Kihara, Daisuke, ed. *Protein Structure Prediction.* 3rd ed. New York: Humana, 2014. Print.

Kyte, Jack. *Structure in Protein Chemistry.* 2nd ed. New York: Garland, 2007. Print.

Lechtenberg, Bernhard C., et al. "Structure of a HOIP/E2~ubiquitin Complex Reveals RBR E3 Ligase Mechanism and Regulation." *Nature.* Macmillan, 20 Jan. 2016. Web. 20 Jan 2016.

Lodish, Harvey, et al. *Molecular Cell Biology.* 7th ed. New York: Freedman, 2013. Print.

McRee, Duncan Everett. *Practical Protein Crystallography.* 2nd ed. San Diego: Academic, 1999. Print.

Maddox, Brenda. *Rosalind Franklin: The Dark Lady of DNA.* New York: Harper, 2002. Print.

Murphy, Kenneth P. *Protein Structure, Stability, and Folding.* Totowa: Humana, 2001. Print.

Rangwala, Huzefa, and George Karypis. *Introduction to Protein Structure Prediction: Methods and Algorithms.* Hoboken: Wiley, 2011. Digital file.

Whitford, David. *Proteins: Structure and Function.* Hoboken: Wiley, 2005. Print.

See also: Central dogma of molecular biology; DNA repair; DNA replication; DNA structure and function; Genetic code; Genetic code, cracking of; Molecular genetics; Protein synthesis; RNA structure and function; RNA transcription and mRNA processing; RNA world; Synthetic genes.

Protein synthesis

CATEGORY: Molecular genetics

SIGNIFICANCE: Cellular proteins can be grouped into two general categories: proteins with a structural function that contribute to the three-dimensional organization of a cell, and proteins with an enzymatic function that catalyze the biochemical reactions required for cell growth and function. Understanding the process by which proteins are synthesized provides insight into how a cell organizes itself and how defects in this process can lead to disease.

KEY TERMS

amino acid: the basic subunit of a protein; there are twenty commonly occurring amino acids, any of which may join together by chemical bonds to form a complex protein molecule

peptide bond: the chemical bond between amino acids in protein

polypeptide: a linear molecule composed of amino acids joined together by peptide bonds; all proteins are functional polypeptides

ribonucleic acid (RNA): a nucleic acid (chain of nucleotides) that serves various functions with respect to DNA, including protein synthesis and gene expression and regulation

translation: the process of forming proteins according to instructions contained in an RNA molecule

THE FLOW OF INFORMATION FROM STORED TO ACTIVE FORM

The cell can be viewed as a unit that assembles resources from its environment into biochemically functional molecules, then organizes these molecules in three-dimensional space in a way that allows for cell growth and replication. In order to carry out this process, a cell must have the biosynthetic means to assemble resources into molecules, and it must contain the information required to produce the biosynthetic and structural machinery. Deoxyribonucleic acid, or DNA, represents the stored form of this information, whereas proteins are the end product. There are thousands of different proteins in cells, either serving a structural role or acting as enzymes that catalyze the biosynthetic reactions of the cell. Following the discovery of the structure of DNA in 1953 by James Watson and Francis Crick, scientists began to study the process by which the information stored in DNA is converted into protein molecules.

BACTERIAL PROTEIN SYNTHESIS

Bacterial DNA transcribed into mRNA and then translated into protein. Proteins are linear, functional molecules composed of a unique sequence of amino acids. About twenty different amino acids are used to synthesize proteins. Although the sequence of amino acids for each protein is present in each DNA molecule, DNA cannot synthesize proteins by itself. Another, similar molecule, called ribonucleic acid (RNA), is necessary to decode the information contained in DNA and do the work of assembling proteins.

There are various types of RNA, each one distinguished by its function. The process of protein synthesis involves three types of RNA. Messenger RNA (mRNA) copies the information contained in a cell's DNA—the sequence of amino acids that makes up a particular protein—and carries it to a part of the cell called the ribosome, where protein synthesis takes place. Transfer RNA (tRNA) decodes the information carried by the mRNA and then transports the required amino acids to the appropriate location during synthesis. Ribosomal RNA (rRNA) acts as the engine that carries out most of the steps during protein synthesis. Together with a specific set of proteins, rRNA forms ribosomes that bind the mRNA, serve as the platform for tRNA to decode the mRNA, and catalyze the formation of peptide bonds between amino acids. Each ribosome is composed of two subunits: a small (40s) and a large (60s) subunit, each of which has its own function. The "s" in 40s and 60s is an abbreviation for Svedberg units, which are a measure of how quickly a large molecule or complex molecular structure sediments (or sinks) to the bottom of a centrifuge tube while being centrifuged. The larger the number, the larger the molecule.

Like all RNA, mRNA is composed of just four types of nucleotides: adenine (A), guanine (G), cytosine (C), and uracil (U). (DNA contains thymine in the place of uracil, but the other three bases are the same.) Each type bonds only with one other type: guanine with cytosine, and adenine with uracil (or, in DNA, thymine). Therefore, when an mRNA molecule temporarily bonds with a DNA molecule, it forms a mirror image of the nucleotide sequence contained in the DNA. This step is called transcription.

Transcription is the first step in the process by which a DNA molecule composed of a linear sequence of nucleotides gives rise to a protein molecule composed of a linear sequence of amino acids.

This process is called translation, since it converts the "language" of nucleotides that make up DNA into the "language" of amino acids that make up a protein. This is achieved by means of three-nucleotide sequences called codons. The four nucleotides—A, G, C, and U—mean that there are sixty-four possible codons. Each codon (save for some exceptions) corresponds to a specific amino acid. As there are only twenty amino acids coded for in DNA, most amino acids correspond to several different codons. For example, six different codons (UCU, UCC, UCA, UCG, AGU, and AGC) specify the amino acid serine, whereas only one (AUG) specifies the amino acid methionine. A molecule of mRNA, therefore, is simply a linear array of codons (that is, three-nucleotide "words" that are "read" by tRNAs together with ribosomes). The region within an mRNA containing this sequence of codons is called the coding region.

Before translation can occur in eukaryotic cells, mRNA molecules undergo processing steps at both ends to add features that will be necessary for translation. (These processing steps do not occur in prokaryotic cells.) Nucleotides are structured such that they have two ends, a 5′ and a 3′ end, that are available to form chemical bonds with other nucleotides. Each nucleotide present in an mRNA has a 5′-to-3′ orientation that gives a directionality to the mRNA, so that the RNA begins with a 5′ end and finishes in a 3′ end. The ribosome reads the coding region of an mRNA in a 5′-to-3′ direction. Following the synthesis of an mRNA from its DNA template, one guanine is added to the 5′ end of the mRNA in an inverted orientation. It is the only nucleotide in the entire mRNA present in a 3′ to 5′ orientation and is referred to as the cap. A long stretch of adenosine is added to the 3′ end of the mRNA to make what is called the poly-A tail.

Typically, mRNAs have a stretch of nucleotide sequence that lies between the cap and the coding region. This is referred to as the leader sequence and is not translated. Therefore, a signal is necessary to indicate where the coding region initiates. The codon AUG usually serves as this initiation codon; however, other AUG codons may be present in the coding region. Any one of three possible codons (UGA, UAG, or UAA) can serve as stop codons that signal the ribosome to terminate translation. Several accessory proteins assist ribosomes in binding mRNA and help carry out the required steps during translation.

THE TRANSLATION PROCESS: INITIATION

Translation occurs in three phases: initiation, elongation, and termination. The function of the 40s ribosomal subunit is to bind to an mRNA and locate the correct AUG as the initiation codon. It does this by binding close to the cap at the 5′ end of the mRNA and scanning the nucleotide sequence in its 5′ to 3′ direction in search of the initiation codon. Marilyn Kozak identified a certain nucleotide sequence surrounding the initiator AUG of eukaryotic mRNAs that indicates to the ribosome that this AUG is the initiation codon. She found that the presence of an A or G three nucleotides prior to the AUG and a G in the position immediately following the AUG were critical in identifying the correct AUG as the initiation codon. This is referred to as the "sequence context" of the initiation codon. Therefore, as the 40s ribosomal subunit scans the leader sequence of an mRNA in a 5′ to 3′ direction, it searches for the first AUG in this context and may bypass other AUGs not in this context.

Nahum Sonenberg demonstrated that the scanning process by the 40s subunit can be impeded by the presence of stem-loop structures present in the leader sequence. These form from base pairing between complementary nucleotides present in the leader sequence. Two nucleotides are said to be complementary when they join together by hydrogen bonds. For instance, the nucleotide (or base) A is complementary to U, and these two can form what is called a "base pair." Likewise, the nucleotides C and G are complementary. Several accessory proteins, called eukaryotic initiation factors (eIFs), aid the binding and scanning of 40s subunits. The first of these, eIF4F, is composed of three subunits called eIF4E, eIF4A, and eIF4G. The protein eIF4E is the subunit responsible for recognizing and binding to the cap of the mRNA. The eIF4A subunit of eIF4F, together with another factor called eIF4B, functions to remove the presence of stem-loop structures in the leader sequence through the disruption of the base pairing between nucleotides in the stem loop.

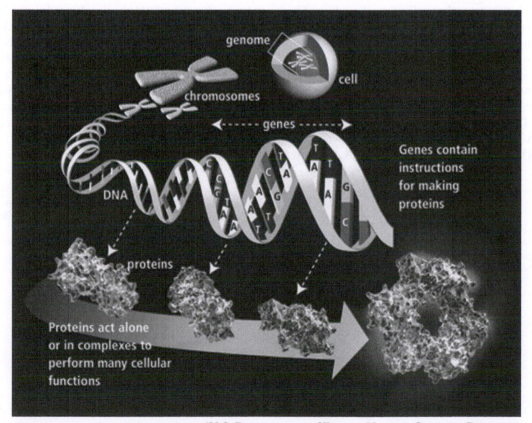

The fundamental steps in protein synthesis. (U.S. Department of Energy Human Genome Program, http://www.ornl.gov/hgmis)

The protein eIF4G is the large subunit of eIF4F, and it serves to interact with several other proteins, one of which is eIF3. It is this latter initiation factor that the 40s subunit first associates with during its initial binding to an mRNA.

Through the combined action of eIF4G and eIF3, the 40s subunit is bound to the mRNA, and through the action of eIF4A and eIF4B, the mRNA is prepared for 40s subunit scanning. As the cellular concentration of eIF4E is very low, mRNAs must compete for this protein. Those that do not compete well for eIF4E will not be translated efficiently. This represents one means by which a cell can regulate protein synthesis. One class of mRNA that competes poorly for eIF4E encodes growth-factor proteins. Growth factors are required in small amounts to stimulate cellular growth. Sonenberg has shown that the overproduction of eIF4E in animal cells leads to a reduction in the competition for this protein, and mRNAs such as growth-factor mRNAs that were previously poorly translated when the concentration of eIF4E was low are now translated at a higher rate when eIF4E is abundant. This in turn results in the overproduction of growth factors, which leads to uncontrolled growth, a characteristic typical of cancer cells.

A protein that specifically binds to the poly-A tail at the 3′ end of an mRNA is called the poly-A-binding protein (PABP). Discovered in the 1970's, the only function of this protein was thought to be to protect the mRNA from attack at its 3′ end by enzymes that degrade RNA. Daniel Gallie demonstrated another function for PABP by showing that the PABP-poly-A-tail complex was required for the function of the eIF4F-cap complex during translation initiation. The idea that a protein located at the 3′ end of an mRNA should participate in events occurring at the opposite end of an mRNA seemed strange initially. However, RNA is quite flexible and is rarely present in a straight, linear form in the cellular environment. Consequently, the poly-A tail can easily approach the cap at the 5′ end. Gallie showed that PABP interacts with eIF4G and eIF4B, two initiation factors that are closely associated with the cap, through protein-to-protein contacts. The consequence of this interaction is that the 3′ end of an mRNA is held in close physical proximity to its cap. The interaction between these proteins stabilizes their binding to the mRNA, which in turn promotes protein synthesis. Therefore, mRNAs can be thought of as adopting a circular form during translation that looks similar to a snake biting its own tail. This idea is now widely accepted by scientists.

One additional factor, called eIF2, is needed to bring the first tRNA to the 40s subunit. Along with the initiator tRNA (which decodes the AUG codon specifying the amino acid methionine), eIF2 aids the 40s subunit in identifying the AUG initiation. Once the 40s subunit has located the initiation codon, the 60s ribosomal subunit joins the 40s subunit to form the intact 80s ribosome. (Svedberg units are not additive; therefore, a 40s and 60s unit joined together do not make a 100s unit.) This marks the end of the initiation phase of translation.

Bacterial DNA transcribed into mRNA and then translated into protein. By Joan L. Slonczewski, John W. Foster (Microbiology: An Evolving Science), via Wikimedia Commons.

The Translation Process: Elongation and Termination

During the elongation phase, tRNAs bind to the 80s ribosome as it passes over the codons of the mRNA, and the amino acids attached to the tRNAs are transferred to the growing polypeptide. Binding of the tRNAs to the ribosome is assisted by an accessory protein called eukaryotic elongation factor 1 (eEF1). A codon is decoded by the appropriate tRNA through base pairing between the three nucleotides that make up the codon in the mRNA and three complementary nucleotides within a specific region (called the anticodon) within the tRNA. The tRNA binding sites in the 80s ribosome are located in the 60s subunit. The ribosome moves over the coding region one codon at a time, or in steps of three nucleotides, in a process known as translocation. When the ribosome moves to the next codon to be decoded, the tRNA containing the appropriate anticodon will bind tightly in the open site in the 60s subunit (the A site). The tRNA that bound to the previous codon is present in a second site in the 60s subunit (the P site). Once a new tRNA has bound to the A site, the ribosomal RNA itself catalyzes the formation of a peptide bond between the growing polypeptide and the new amino acid. This results in the transfer of the polypeptide attached to the tRNA present in the P site to the amino acid on the tRNA present in the A site. A second elongation factor, eEF2, catalyzes the movement of the ribosome to the next codon to be decoded. This process is repeated one codon at a time until a stop codon is reached.

The termination phase of translation begins when the ribosome reaches one of the three termination or stop codons. These are also referred to as "nonsense" codons, as the cell does not produce any tRNAs that can decode them. Accessory factors, called release factors, are also required to assist this stage of translation. They bind to the empty A site in which the stop codon is present, and this triggers the cleavage of the bond between the completed protein from the last tRNA in the P site, thereby releasing the protein. The ribosome then dissociates into its 40s and 60s subunits, the latter of which diffuse away from the mRNA. The close physical proximity of the cap and poly-A tail of an mRNA maintained by the interaction between PABP and the initiation factors (eIF4G and eIF4B) is thought to assist the recycling of the 40s subunit back to the 5´ end of the mRNA to participate in a subsequent round of translation.

Impact and Applications

The elucidation of the process and control of protein synthesis provides a ready means by which scientists can manipulate these processes in cells. In addition to infectious diseases, insufficient dietary protein represents one of the greatest challenges to world health. The majority of people now living are limited to obtaining their dietary protein solely through the consumption of plant matter. Knowledge of the process of protein synthesis may allow molecular biologists to increase the amount of protein in important crop species. Moreover, most plants contain an imbalance in the amino acids needed in the human diet that can lead to disease. For example, protein from corn is poor in the amino acid lysine, whereas the protein from soybeans is poor in methionine and cysteine. Molecular biologists may be able to correct this imbalance by changing the codons present in plant genes, thus improving this source of protein for those people who rely on it for life.

Daniel R. Gallie, Ph.D.

Further Reading

Atkins, John F., Raymond F. Gesteland, and Thomas R. Cech, eds. *RNA Worlds: From Life's Origins to Diversity in Gene Regulation.* Cold Spring Harbor: Cold Spring Harbor Laboratory, 2011. Print.

Bethaz, Carlo, and Vito Li Puma, eds. *New Research on Protein Synthesis.* New York: Nova, 2014. Print.

Crick, Francis H. C. "The Genetic Code: III." *Scientific American* Oct. 1966: 55–62. Print.

Keiler, Kenneth C., ed. *Bacterial Regulatory RNA: Methods and Protocols.* New York: Humana, 2012. Print.

Krebs, Jocelyn E., Elliott S. Goldstein, and Stephen T. Kilpatrick, eds. *Lewin's Genes XI.* 11th ed. Burlington: Jones, 2014. Print.

Lake, James A. "The Ribosome." *Scientific American* Aug. 1981: 84–97. Print.

Liljas, Anders, and Måns Ehrenberg. *Structural Aspects of Protein Synthesis.* 2nd ed. Hackensack: World Scientific, 2013. Print.

Rich, Alexander, and Sung Hou Kim. "The Three-Dimensional Structure of Transfer RNA." *Scientific American* Jan. 1978: 52–62. Print.

Tropp, Burton E. *Molecular Biology: Genes to Proteins.* 4th ed. Sudbury: Jones, 2012. Print.

Whitford, David. *Proteins: Structure and Function.* Hoboken: Wiley, 2005. Print.

See also: Central dogma of molecular biology; DNA repair; DNA replication; DNA structure and function; Genetic code; Genetic code, cracking of; Molecular genetics; Protein structure; RNA structure and function; RNA transcription and mRNA processing; RNA world; Synthetic genes.

Proteomics and genetics

CATEGORY: Molecular genetics; Techniques and methodologies

SIGNIFICANCE: The study of proteomics and its relationship to genomics focuses on the vast family of gene-regulating proteins. These polypeptides and their functions affect the expression of various genetically related diseases, such as Alzheimer's and cancer. By focusing on the interrelated groups of regulator functions, geneticists are learning the connections between structure, abundance within the cell, and how each protein relates to expression.

KEY TERMS

chromatography: a separation technique involving a mobile solvent and a stationary, adsorbent phase

mass spectroscopy: a method of analyzing molecular structure in which sample molecules are ionized and the resulting fragmented particles are passed through electric and magnetic fields to a detector

peripheral proteins: proteins of the chromosome that do not directly affect transcription

protein folding structure: the three-dimensional structure of proteins created by the folding of linked amino acids upon each other; this structure is held together by intermolecular forces, such as hydrogen bonds and ionic attractions

protein marker: a sequence of DNA that chemically attracts a particular regulatory protein sequence or structure

regulators: proteins that control the transcription of a gene

senile plaques: protein sections that are no longer functional and clutter the intercellular space of the brain, disrupting proper processes

transcription: the process by which mRNA is formed using DNA as a template

translation: the process of building a protein by bonding amino acids according to the mRNA marker present

WHAT IS "PROTEOMICS"?

Historically, much of the focus in genetic research was on genes and the completion of the Human Genome Project. However, the focus has shifted to a new and related topic, the proteome. Proteins are known to perform most of the important functions of cells. Therefore, proteomics is, essentially, the study of proteins in an organism and, most important, their function. There are many aspects to the understanding of protein function, including where a particular protein is located in the cell, what modifications occur during its activity, what ligands may bind to it, and its activity. Researchers are seeking to identify all the proteins made in a given cell, tissue, or organism and determine how those proteins interact with metobolites, with themselves, and with nucleic acids. By studying proteomics, scientists hope to uncover underlying causes of disease at the cellular level, invent better methods of diagnosis, and discover new, more efficient medicines for the treatment of disease

BROAD-BASED PROTEOMICS OVERVIEW

This is an overview of broad-based proteomics and how it compares to a more traditional focused perspective when trying to understand proteins.

Proteomics has moved to the forefront of molecular research, especially in the area of drug research. Neither the structure nor the function of a protein can be predicted from the DNA sequence alone. Although genes code for proteins, there is a large difference between the number of messenger (mRNA) molecules transcribed from DNA and the number of proteins in a cell. In addition, two hundred known modifications occur during the stages between transcription and post-translation, including phosphorylation, glycosylation, proteolytic processing, deamidation, sulfation, and nitration. Other factors that affect the expression of proteins include aging, stress, environmental forces, and medications. In addition, changes to the sequence of amino acids may occur during or after translation.

Public domain image from cancer.gov http://visualsonline.cancer.gov/details.cfm?imageid=3483. TECAN Genesis 2000 robot preparing Ciphergen SELDI-TOF protein chips for proteomic pattern analysis. Highly accurate cancer prognosis can be accomplished by ide. See page for author, via Wikimedia Commons

METHODS OF PROTEOMIC RESEARCH

In order to study the functions of a protein, it must be separated from other proteins or contaminants, purified, and structurally characterized. These are the major tasks facing researchers in the field.

In order to obtain a sufficient quantity of a particular protein for study, the coding plasmid can be injected into *Escherichia coli* bacteria and the cells will translate the protein multiple times. Alternatively, it must be extracted from biological tissues. The desired polypeptide must then be separated from cells or tissues that may contain thousands of unique proteins. This can be accomplished by homogenizing the tissue, extracting the proteins with solvents or by centrifugation, and further purifying the protein by various means, including high-pressure liquid chromatography (HPLC, separation by solubility differences) and two-dimensional (2-D) gel electrophoresis (separation of molecules by charge and molecular mass). A relatively recent development in laboratory technique research is three-dimensional (3-D) gel electrophoresis, allowing for further separation and identification of proteins.

Structural characterization begins with establishing the order of linked amino acids in the protein. This can be accomplished by the classical techniques of using proteases to fragment the protein chemically and then analyzing the fragments by

separation and spectroscopic analysis. The molecular mass of small polypeptides can be investigated by employing several techniques involving mass spectrometry (MS). Sequentially coupled mass spectrometers (the "tandem" MS/MS techniques) are being used to analyze the amino acid sequence and molecular masses of isolated larger polypeptides. These MS/MS analyses are sometimes added to a separation method, such as HPLC, to analyze mixtures of polypeptides.

Historically, Linus Pauling used analytical data from x-ray diffraction (or crystallography) to determine the three-dimensional, helical structure of proteins. The method is still being used to investigate the structures of proteins and ligand-protein complexes. Such studies may lead to significant improvements in the design of medicinal drugs. One significant drawback to analyzing protein structure by x-ray diffraction, however, is that the method requires a significant quantity (approximately 1 milligram) of the protein. Transmission electron microscopy (TEM), which uses electron beams to produce images and diffraction patterns from extremely small samples or regions of a sample, is therefore often preferable. The TEM method may involve auxiliary techniques to analyze data, including enhancement of images by means of computer software.

	Broad-based Approach	Focused Approach
Goal	Understand the proteome as a whole	Understand specific protein information
Basic Steps	1) Identify organism 2) Understand sample type and preparation 3) Utilize analytical technology that is compatible with sample type 4) Bioinformatic analysis of the **proteomic** sample 5) Build a **proteomic** model	1) Identify protein 2) Understand sample type and preparation 3) Isolate protein 4) Utilize analytical technology that is compatible 5) Bioinformatic analysis of the **protein** sample 6) Model **protein's** function and/or structure
Pros	• Proteomic information about a specific tissue under certain conditions can be gained • Relationships between many proteins can be understood	• Inexpensive and results can be generated much quicker than a larger proteomic study • Functional and structural information about a protein can be determined
Cons	• Extensive upfront planning • The study will cost more and last longer than a focused study • There is no guarantee quality proteomic data will be generated in the end	• Protein information may not be valuable without a global proteomic understanding • Hard to develop global relationships from many focused experiments taken together
Common Technologies Implemented	• SDS-PAGE Gel Electrophoresis • 2DE-DIGE • HPLC • Mass Spectroscopy (MS) • Proteomic modeling tools (Bioinformatics)	• SDS-PAGE Gel Electrophoresis • HPLC • Mass Spectroscopy (MS) • Molecular modeling tools (Bioinformatics)

This is an overview of Broad-based proteomics and how it compares to a more traditional focused perspective when trying to understand proteins. By Mccrearym (Own work), via Wikimedia Commons

Although such methods provide valuable information in analyzing the structure of proteins, they suffer from the loss of spatial information that occurs when tissues are homogenized, when the protein is obtained from a manufactured, bacterial environment, or when it is otherwise isolated. Matrix-assisted laser desorption/ionization time-of-flight (MALDI-TOF) mass spectrometry is a complementary method of analysis that does not yield structural information but provides protein profiles from intact tissue, allowing comparison of diseased versus normal tissue.

Large databases of mass spectroscopic data are being assembled to assist in future identification of known proteins. Further databases of proteome information include particular molecular masses, charges, and, in some cases, connections to the genes regulated or the parent gene of the peptide in question. Scientists hope to relate regulators and the complex web of peripheral proteins that affect the function of each gene.

CHALLENGES AND LIMITATIONS OF CURRENT METHODS

The amount of data being obtained by proteomics research poses a problem in organizing and processing the information obtained on proteins. The Human Proteome Organization (HUPO) and the European Bioinformatics Institute (EBI) are two organizations whose purposes include the management and organization of proteomics information and databases, and the facilitation of the advancement of this scientific endeavor.

Analyzing MS data from proteins and relating the complex array of proteins within a single cell to the linear genetic material of DNA present challenges to researchers that they are tackling through computer algorithms, programs, and databases. The SWISS-PROT database, for example, is an annotated protein-sequence database maintained by the Swiss Bioinformatics Institute.

Other obstacles to relating proteins to parent genes include the loss of quaternary structure during separation and the presence of post-translation processing, which can alter the amino acid sequence to the extent that it becomes almost unrecognizable from the parent gene. A lack of protein amplification methods—techniques that would produce more copies of a protein to aid in study—requires

sensitive analysis methods and increasingly strong detectors.

DISEASE

Proteins often act as markers for disease. As researchers study proteins, they have found that disease may be characterized by some proteins that are being overproduced, not being produced at all, or being produced at inappropriate times. As the correlation of proteins to disease becomes clearer, better diagnostic tests and drugs are being explored. For example, Alzheimer's disease and Down syndrome are associated with a common protein fragment as the major extracellular protein component of senile plaques.

Researchers are investigating changes in protein expression in heart disease and heart failure, and several hundred cardiac proteins have already been identified. The study of proteomics in immunological diseases has revealed that there is a connection between the human neutrophil α-defensins (HNPs) and human immunodeficiency virus, HIV-1. HNPs are small, cysteine-rich, cationic antimicrobial proteins that are stored in the azurophilic granules of neutrophils and released during phagocytosis to kill ingested foreign microbes.

Similarly, cancer is being studied to find a roster of proteins that are present in cancerous cells but not in normal cells. The Clinical Proteomics Program, a joint effort of the National Cancer Institute (NCI) and the Food and Drug Administration has searched for the differences between cancerous and normal cells, and also for protein "markers." In 2011, NCI started the Clinical Proteomic Tumor Analysis Consortium, which sought to uncover cancers' molecular bases through proteomic research and technology.

POSSIBLE FUTURE DIRECTIONS

Three fields of proteomics have taken the lead in research: glycomics, metabolomics, and metabonomics. Glycomics addresses the importance of the sugar coatings of proteins and cells. This area of study has arisen because of the many roles of sugar coatings in important cellular functions, including the immunological recognition sites, barriers, and sites for attack by pathogens. Metabolomics is the study of the proteins left behind as the cell performs its processes. This field primarily looks at small proteins produced as by-products. Metabonomics is often used inter-changeably with metabolomics but differs in that it examines the change that proteins produce when the cell responds to stresses, such as disease.

Audrey Krumbach, Kayla Williams,
and Massimo D. Bezoari, M.D.;
updated by Kecia Brown, M.P.H.

FURTHER READING

Donev, Rossen, ed. *Proteomics in Biomedicine and Pharmacology.* San Diego: Elsevier, 2014. Print.

Glick, Bernard R., T. L. Delovitch, and Cheryl L. Patten. *Medical Biotechnology.* Washington, DC: ASM, 2014. Print.

Hopker, Hans-Rudolf, et al. *Proteomics in Practice: Guide for Successful Research Design.* 2nd ed. Weinham: Wiley, 2008. Print.

Liebler, David G. *Introduction to Proteomics: Tools for the New Biology.* Totowa: Humana, 2001. Print.

Link, Andrew J., ed. *2-D Proteome Analysis Protocols.* Totowa: Humana, 1999. Print.

Poliseno, Laura. *Pseudogenes: Functions and Protocols.* New York: Humana, 2014. Print.

Twyman, Richard M. *Principles of Proteomics.* 2nd ed. Oxon: Garland, 2013. Print.

See also: Bioinformatics; Genomics; Human genetics; Human Genome Project; Protein structure; Protein synthesis.

Pseudogenes

CATEGORY: Molecular genetics

SIGNIFICANCE: Pseudogenes are DNA sequences derived from partial copies, mutated complete copies of functional genes, or normal copies of a gene that has lost its control sequences and therefore cannot be transcribed. They may originate by gene duplication or retrotransposition. They seem to be nonfunctional regions of the genome that may evolve at a maximum rate, free from the evolutionary constraints of natural selection.

KEY TERMS

introns: noncoding segments of DNA within a gene that are removed from pre-messenger RNA (pre-mRNA) as a part of the process of producing mature mRNA

long interspersed sequences (LINES): long repeats of DNA sequences scattered throughout a genome

neutral theory of molecular evolution: the theory that most DNA sequence evolution is a result of mutations that are neutral with respect to the fitness of the organism

retrotransposon (retroposon): a DNA sequence that is transcribed to RNA and reverse transcribed to a DNA copy able to insert itself at another location in the genome

reverse transcriptase: an enzyme, isolated from retroviruses, that synthesizes a DNA strand from an RNA template

short interspersed sequences (SINES): short repeats of DNA sequences scattered throughout a genome

DEFINITION AND ORIGIN

Pseudogenes are DNA sequences that resemble genes but are not correctly transcribed or translated to a functional polypeptide. If a functional gene is duplicated so that there are two nonhomologous copies of it in the genome, one of the copies can retain the code for the original polypeptide product, while the other is free from such constraints, since one copy of the gene is sufficient to produce the protein. Because mutations in one copy do not destroy the gene's function, they may be retained, and the unneeded copy can evolve more quickly. It may change to produce a different, functional polypeptide (and effectively become a new gene), or it may remain nonfunctional as a pseudogene. There are two types of pseudogenes, defined by how they were produced: nonprocessed and processed.

ARTHROBACTER ARILAITENSIS RE117 GENOME
Patró DE GENS - HIPÒTESI 2R

NONPROCESSED PSEUDOGENES

Nonprocessed (or duplicated) pseudogenes arise when a portion of the original gene is duplicated, with portions necessary for proper functioning missing or altered or when the complete original gene is duplicated. They can be identified by the presence of introns and may have mutations in the promoter that prevent transcription or the correct removal of introns, or they may have other mutations (such as premature stop codons) within exons that result in translation of a nonfunctional polypeptide.

Circle 7 represents the pseudogenes (excluding transposase pseudogenes) By Monnet C, Loux V, Gibrat J-F, Spinnler E, Barbe V, et al., via Wikimedia Commons

A series of tandem duplications of a gene can result in clustered gene families, which can include expressed genes, expressed pseudogenes (which are

Many paralogous genes suffer disabling mutations, become pseudogenes, and are then lost. One could imagine this condition being evidence of a single round of genome duplication followed by significant gene losses. By Dehal P, Boore JL (doi:10.1371/journal. pbio.0030314), via Wikimedia Commons

transcribed but produce no functional polypeptide), and nonexpressed pseudogenes that are not transcribed. The alpha-globulin and beta-globulin clusters are examples of such gene families. Other examples of nonprocessed pseudogenes include members of the immunoglobulin (Ig) and major histocompatibility complex (MHC) gene families.

PROCESSED PSEUDOGENES

Processed pseudogenes originate from transcribed RNA copies of genes that are copied back to DNA by the enzyme reverse transcriptase. Processed pseudogenes are usually integrated into the genome in a different location from the original gene. Reverse transcriptase is an enzyme produced by retroviruses, which have RNA genomes that are reverse transcribed to DNA when the viruses infect host cells. Retrotransposons, which are related to retroviruses, are DNA sequences that transpose or duplicate themselves by reverse transcription of a transcribed RNA copy of the sequence.

Often, retrotransposons will carry alon g a copy of the surrounding host DNA, resulting in the duplication of that sequence—a processed pseudogene. Because the introns of a gene are removed from the RNA transcript, processed pseudogenes are not exact copies of the original DNA sequence; the introns are missing. Copies of protein-coding genes copied by this mechanism are members of a type of repetitive DNA called LINES (for long interspersed sequences) and exist in multiple copies scattered around the genome, each up to several thousand base pairs in length. Short processed pseudogenes are members of another class of repetitive DNA called SINES (short interspersed sequences of up to several hundred base pairs in length) and result from the retrotransposon-mediated copying of tRNA or rRNA genes. SINES of this type are sometimes very abundant in genomes because they may have internal promoters, so that they are more easily transcribed, and therefore transposed. The most prominent of SINES are those that are members of the *Alu* family, which occur an average of once every six thousand base pairs in the human genome.

PSEUDOGENES AND NEUTRAL EVOLUTION

In 2003, Japanese researchers reported the discovery of a mouse pseudogene that is involved in regulating the expression of its related "functional" gene. This discovery suggested that at least some pseudogenes may have important functions. Although pseudogenes are commonly found across genomes, most do not appear to serve any function, and until further research uncovers more functional pseudogenes this assumption appears warranted. Their abundance can be explained by the tendency of duplicated sequences to be further copied. Retrotransposition increases the number of copies of processed pseudogenes, and gene duplication leading to unprocessed pseudogenes favors mechanisms that generate additional copies, leading to clustered gene families. Natural selection does not tend to eliminate these additional copies because their presence does not harm the organism as long as there is at least one functional copy of the original gene. In other words, pseudogenes are selectively neutral.

Because of their selective neutrality, pseudogenes are especially useful for estimating neutral mutation rates in genomes. The neutral theory of evolution predicts that, because of the constraints of selection, functional regions of the genome (such as the exons, or coding sequences, of genes) will evolve more slowly than less critical sequences, such as introns, or nonfunctional sequences like pseudogenes. The number of nucleotide differences between homologous sequences of related species can be used to calculate estimates of evolutionary rates, and such estimates support the neutral theory: the greatest rates of divergence occur within pseudogenes. Using comparisons from several pseudogenes, researchers can establish the baseline neutral mutation rate for a group of species.

Stephen T. Kilpatrick, Ph.D.

Further Reading

Alberts, Bruce, et al. "DNA, Chromosomes, and Genomes." *Molecular Biology of the Cell.* 5th ed. New York: Garland, 2008. Print.

Barrett, Lucy W., Sue Fletcher, and Steve D. Wilton. Untranslated Gene Regions and Other Non-Coding Elements: Regulation of Eukaryotic Gene Expression. New York: Springer, 2013. Print.

Gerstein, Mark, and Deyou Zheng. "The Real Life of Pseudogenes." *Scientific American* 295.2 (2006): 48–55. Print.

Graur, Dan, and Wen-Hsiung Li. *Fundamentals of Molecular Evolution.* 2nd ed. Sunderland: Sinauer, 1999. Print.

Lewin, Benjamin. *Genes IX.* Sudbury: Jones, 2007. Print.

Li, Wen-Hsiung, Takashi Gojobori, and Masatoshi Nei. "Pseudogenes as a Paradigm of Neutral Evolution." *Nature* 292.5820 (1981): 237–39. Print.

Poliseno, Laura. *Pseudogenes: Functions and Protocols.* New York: Humana, 2014.

Roberts, Thomas C., and Kevin V. Morris. "Not So Pseudo Anymore: Pseudogenes ss Therapeutic Targets." *Pharmacogenomics* 14.16 (n.d.): 2023–34. *Biological Abstracts.* Web. 26 Aug. 2014.

Sen, Kamalika, and Tapash Chandra Ghosh. "Pseudogenes and Their Composers: Delving in the 'Debris' of Human Genome." *Briefings in Functional Genomics* 12.6 (2013): 536–47. *Academic Search Alumni Edition.* Web. 26 Aug. 2014.

Zhang, Zhaolei, and Mark Gerstein. "The Human Genome Has Forty-Nine Cytochrome C Pseudogenes, Including a Relic of a Primordial Gene That Still Functions in a Mouse." *Gene* 312 (2003): 61. Print.

See also: Gene families; Repetitive DNA.

Pseudohermaphrodites

Category: Diseases and syndromes

Significance: Pseudohermaphrodites are individuals born with either ambiguous genitalia or external mgenitalia that are the opposite of their chromosomal sex. These individuals need a thorough medical evaluation and appropriate medical intervention to help ensure a healthy, well-adjusted life.

Key terms

ambiguous genitalia: external sexual organs that are not clearly male or female

genotype: the sum total of the genes present in an individual

gonads: organs that produce reproductive cells and sex hormones, for example, testes in males and ovaries in females *karyotype:* the number and kind of chromosomes present in every cell of the body (normal female karyotype is 46,XX and normal male karyotype is 46,XY)

phenotype: the physical appearance and physiological characteristics of an individual, which depend on the interaction of genotype and environment

NORMAL FETAL DEVELOPMENT

Prior to nine weeks in gestational age, a male and a female fetus have identical external genitalia (sexual organs) consisting of a phallus and labioscrotal folds. The phallus develops into a penis in males and a clitoris in females; labioscrotal folds become the scrotum in males and the labial folds in females. Early in development, the gonads can develop into either testes or ovaries. In a fetus with a normal male karyotype (46,XY), the primitive gonads become testes, which produce testosterone. Testosterone in turn causes enlargement of the primitive phallus into a penis. It is the presence of the Y chromosome, and in particular a small, sex-determining region of the Y chromosome termed the *SRY* locus, that drives the formation of the testes. The presence of the *SRY* locus appears to be essential for development of a normal male.

PSEUDOHERMAPHRODITISM

A true hermaphrodite is born with both ovarian and testicular tissue. A male pseudohermaphrodite has a 46,XY karyotype with either female genitalia or ambiguous genitalia (but only testicular tissue); a female pseudohermaphrodite has a 46,XX karyotype with either male genitalia or ambiguous genitalia (but only ovarian tissue). Ambiguous genitalia typically consist of a small, abnormally shaped, phalluslike structure, often with hypospadias (in which urine comes from the base of the penis instead of the tip) and abnormal development of the labioscrotal folds (not clearly a scrotum or labia). A vaginal opening may be present.

Most cases of pseudohermaphroditism result from abnormal exposure to increased or decreased amounts of sex hormones during embryonic development. The most common cause of female pseudohermaphroditism is exposure of a female fetus to increased levels of testosterone during the first half of pregnancy. Maternal use of anabolic steroids can cause this condition, but the most common genetic cause of increased testosterone exposure is congenital adrenal hyperplasia (CAH). CAH results from an abnormality in the

enzymatic pathways of the fetus that make both cortisol (a stress hormone) and the sex steroids (such as testosterone). At several points in these pathways, there may be a nonfunctioning enzyme that results in too little production o f cortisol and too much production of the sex steroids. This will result in partial masculinization of the external genitalia of a female embryo. Females with CAH are usually born with an enlarged clitoris (often mistakenly thought to be a penis) and partial fusion of the labia. Males can also have CAH, but the excess testosterone does not affect their genital development since a relatively high level of testosterone exposure is a normal part of their development.

The most common causes of male pseudohermaphroditism are abnormalities of testosterone production or abnormalities in the testosterone receptor at the cellular level. One example is a deficiency in 5-alpha-reductase, the enzyme that converts testosterone to dihydrotestosterone (DHT). When there is a deficiency of this enzyme, there will be a deficiency of DHT, which is the hormone primarily responsible for masculinization of external genitalia. A male who lacks DHT will have female appearing external genitalia or ambiguous genitalia at birth. Often these individuals are reared as females, but at puberty they will masculinize because of greatly increased production of testosterone. These individuals may actually develop into nearly normal-appearing males. Abnormalities of the testosterone receptor can also result in a range of different conditions in affected males, from normal female appearance (a totally defective receptor) to ambiguous genitalia (partially defective receptor) in a 46,XY male. These individuals will not masculinize at puberty because no matter how much testosterone or DHT they produce, their bodies cannot respond to the hormones. Both male and female pseudohermaphroditism can result from chromosomal abnormalities. The absence or dysfunction of the *SRY* locus produces an individual with normal female genitalia but a 46,XY karyotype. Individuals with a 46,XX karyotype who have the *SRY* locus transposed to one of their X chromosomes will have a normal male appearance.

IMPACT AND APPLICATIONS

Some forms of pseudohermaphroditism are lifethreatening, and so early diagnosis is imperative. Both males and females with CAH are at risk for sudden death caused by low cortisol levels and other hormone deficiencies. Early diagnosis is relatively easy in affected females since their genital abnormalities are noticeable at birth. Affected males are often not recognized until they have a life threatening event, which usually occurs in the first two weeks of life. Treatment of CAH consists of appropriate hormone supplementation that, if instituted early in life, can help prevent serious problems. CAH is inherited in an autosomal recessive manner, so parents of an affected individual have a 25 percent chance of having another affected child with each pregnancy.

The sex of rearing of a child with ambiguous genitalia is usually determined by the child's type of pseudohermaphroditism. Typically, sex of rearing will be based on the chromosomal sex of the child. These children may need sex hormone supplementation or surgery to assist in developing genderappropriate genitalia. Children with pseudohermaphroditism with normal-appearing genitalia at birth may not be recognized until puberty, when abnormal masculinization or feminization may occur. These individuals need medical evaluation and karyotype determination to guide the proper medical treatment.

Patricia G. Wheeler, M.D.

FURTHER READING

Hunter, R. H. F. *Sex Determination, Differentiation, and Intersexuality in Placental Mammals.* New York: Cambridge University Press, 1995. Discusses the genetic determination of sex in mammals. Illustrations (some color), bibliography, index.

Meyer-Bahlburg, Heino. "Intersexuality and the Diagnosis of Gender Identity Disorder." *Archives of Sexual Behavior* 23, no. 1 (February, 1994): 21. Addresses gender identity and its relation to pseudohermaphroditism.

Moore, Keith L., and T. V. N. Persaud. "The Urogenital System." In *The Developing Human: Clinically Oriented Embryology.* 8th ed. Philadelphia: Saunders/Elsevier, 2008. Details embryology from a clinical perspective, providing discussions of the stages of organs and genital system development, discussing pseudohermaphrodites.

Preves, Sharon E. "Medical Sex Assignment." In *Intersex and Identity: The Contested Self.* New Brunswick, N.J.: Rutgers University Press, 2003. Includes a discussion of pseudohermaphrodites.

Simpson, J. L. "Disorders of the Gonads, Genital Tract, and Genitalia." In *Emery and Rimoin's Principles and Practice of Medical Genetics,* edited by David L. Rimoin et al. 5th ed. 3 vols. Philadelphia:

Churchill Livingstone Elsevier, 2007. A detailed account of male and female pseudohermaphroditism. Illustrations, bibliography, index.

Speiser, Phyllis W., ed. *Congenital Adrenal Hyperplasia.* Philadelphia: W. B. Saunders, 2001. Contents address prenatal treatment, newborn screening, new treatments, surgery, gender, sexuality, cognitive function, and pregnancy outcomes. Illustrated.

WEB SITES OF INTEREST

Intersex Society of North America
http://www.isna.org
The society is "devoted to systemic change to end shame, secrecy, and unwanted genital surgeries for people born with an anatomy that someone decidedis not standard for male or female." Its Web site offers information on such conditions as clitoromegaly, micropenis, hypospadias, ambiguous genitals, early genital surgery, adrenal hyperplasia, Klinefelter syndrome, and androgen insensitivity syndrome.

Johns Hopkins University, Division of Pediatric Endocrinology, Syndromes of Abnormal Sex Differentiation
http://www.hopkinschildrens.org/intersex A guide for parents and their families providing information about syndromes of abnormal sex differentiation.

Medline Plus, Intersex
http://www.nlm.nih.gov/medlineplus/ency/article/001669.htm Features information on 46,XX Intersex and other intersex conditions, including the causes, diagnosis, symptoms, and treatment of these conditions. Additional information can be retrieved by using the search engine to search on the word "pseudohermaphroditism."

National Organization for Rare Disorders (NORD)
http://www.rarediseases.org Offers information and articles about rare genetic= conditions and diseases, including XYY syndrome,= in several searchable databases.

See also: Androgen insensitivity syndrome; Biological clocks; Gender identity; Hermaphrodites; Homosexuality; Human genetics; Metafemales; RNA transcription and mRNA processing; Steroid hormones; X chromosome inactivation; XYY syndrome.

Pseudohypoparathyroidism

CATEGORY: Diseases and syndromes
ALSO KNOWN AS: Albright's hereditary osteodystrophy; Types 1A and 1B pseudohypoparathyroidism

DEFINITION

Pseudohypoparathyroidism denotes a group of inherited disorders characterized by deficiency in the end-organ response to parathyroid hormone (PTH) and in some instances because of abnormal PTH receptors. The term "pseudohypoparathyroidism" is used because there is evidence of clinical hypoparathyroidism but serum PTH levels are normal.

RISK FACTORS

A family history of pseudohypoparathyroidism is the primary risk factor for the disease.

ETIOLOGY AND GENETICS

Parathyroid glands assist in the control of calcium use and removal by the body by producing parathyroid hormone, or PTH. PTH helps control calcium, phosphorus, and vitamin D levels within the blood and bone. Individuals with pseudohypoparathyroidism produce the required amount of PTH, but the body is "resistant" to its effect. This causes low blood calcium levels and high blood phosphate levels. Pseudohypoparathyroidism is very rare and is caused by abnormal genes. Type 1A, also called Albright's hereditary osteodystrophy, is an inherited autosomal dominant trait, and therefore only one parent could potentially pass the defective gene to cause the condition. The condition results in short stature, round face, abnormally developed metacarpal and metatarsal bones, and subcutaneous bone ossification. Type 1B is less understood than type 1A and involves resistance to PTH only in the kidneys. Type 2 is very similar to type 1 in its clinical features, but the events that take place in the kidneys are different.

Type 2 pseudohypoparathyroidism also involves low blood calcium and high blood phosphate levels, but persons with this form do not develop the physical characteristics seen in those with Type 1A. Recent studies report the *GNAS* gene encodes the alpha-subunit of the stimulatory G proteins. These proteins are important in intracellular signal transduction of peptide and neurotransmitter receptors. Heterozygous inactivating maternally inherited mutations of *GNAS* lead to a phenotype in which Albright hereditary osteodystrophy is associated with pseudohypoparathyroidism type 1A. Such mutations include translation initiation mutations, amino acid substitutions, nonsense mutations, splice-site mutations, and small insertions or deletions. E. Fernandezrebollo and colleagues found the *GNAS* gene of a five-year-old boy with pseudohypoparathyroidism to have a heterozygous inversion of exon 2 and part of intron 1 of de novo origin. This report demonstrated the first evidence for an inversion at the *GNAS* gene responsible for pseudohypoparathyroidism type 1.

SYMPTOMS

Symptoms of pseudohypoparathyroidism are related to low levels of calcium known as hypocalcemia. Hypocalcemia causes increased irritability of nerves, leading to numbness and tingling of the hands, feet, and lips. Tetany, which is manifested clinically as muscular spasms first affecting the hands and feet, is another symptom of pseudohypoparathyroidism. Laryngeal spasms can occur, leading to obstruction of the respiratory system. Severe hypocalcemia can lead to generalized convulsions in children. Other complications of hypocalcemia associated with pseudohypoparathyroidism may include other endocrine problems, leading to lowered sexual drive and lowered sexual development, lowered energy levels, and increased weight. Individuals with Albright's hereditary osteodystrophy may have symptoms of calcium deposits under the skin and the physical characteristics of a round face and short neck and short stature in children.

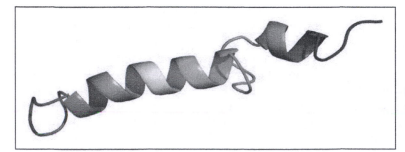

Structure of the PTH protein. Based on PyMOL rendering of PDB 1bwx. By Emw (Own work), via Wikimedia Commons

Gene expression pattern of the GNAS gene. Genomics Institute of the Novartis Research Foundation, via Wikimedia Commons

SCREENING AND DIAGNOSIS

Blood tests are evaluated to determine calcium, phosphorus, and PTH levels. Urine tests are also utilized to determine key endocrine levels. Genetic testing is utilized to determine positive family history of the abnormalities. Magnetic resonance imaging (MRI) creates a detailed picture of the brain and surrounding nerve tissues and is helpful in diagnosing decreased levels of calcium causing increased irritability of nerve tissue.

TREATMENT AND THERAPY

Calcium and vitamin D supplements are prescribed to maintain proper calcium levels. A low-phosphorus diet may be necessary if blood phosphate levels remain higher than normal. Emergency treatment with intravenous calcium is needed if an individual presents an acute hypocalcemia crisis such as tetany, laryngeal spasm, and convulsions.

PREVENTION AND OUTCOMES

Low blood calcium in pseudohypoparathyroidism is usually milder than in other forms of hypoparathyroidism. Proper medical attention and follow-up are important in prevention and treatment of other endocrine problems, as patients with type 1A pseudohypoparathyroidism have an increased occurrence of other endocrine abnormalities to include hypothyroidism and hypogonadism.

Jeffrey P. Larson, P.T., A.T.C.

FURTHER READING

"Albright's Hereditary Osteodystrophy." *A Dictionary of Nursing.* Oxford: Oxford UP, 2008. Print.

Bringhurst, F. R., M. B. Demay, and H. M. Kronenberg. "Disorders of Mineral Metabolism." *Williams Textbook of Endocrinology,* Eds. H. M. Kronenberg, M. Schlomo, K. S. Polansky, and P. R. Larsen. 11th ed. St. Louis: Saunders, 2008. Print.

Chandrasoma, P., and C. Taylor. *Concise Pathology.* 3d ed. Norwalk: McGraw, 2001. Digital file.

Copstead, Lee Ellen. *Perspectives on Pathophysiology.* Philadelphia: Saunders, 1994. Print.

Genetics Home Reference. "*GNAS.*" *Genetics Home Reference.* US NLM, 4 Aug. 2014. Web. 11 Aug. 2014.

Mantovani, G., et al. "Clinical Utility Gene Card for: Pseudohypoparathyroidism." *European Journal of Human Genetics* 21.6 (2013): 5 pp. *MEDLINE with Full Text.* Web. 11 Aug. 2014.

McKusick, Victor A., Cassandra L. Kniffin. "#103580 Pseudohypoparathyroidism, Type 1A; PHP1A." *OMIM.org.* Johns Hopkins U, 28 May 2010. Web. 11 Aug. 2014.

Topiwala, Shehzad. "Pseudohypoparathyroidism." *MedlinePlus.* US NLM/NIH, 19 July 2012. Web. 11 Aug. 2014.

Wysolmerski, J. J. and K. L. Insogna. "The Parathyroid Glands, Hypercalcemia, and Hypocalcemia." *Williams Textbook of Endocrinology.* Eds. H. M. Kronenberg, M. Schlomo, K. S. Polansky, and P. R. Larsen. 11th ed. St. Louis: Saunders, 2008. Print.

See also: Adrenomyelopathy; Androgen insensitivity syndrome; Autoimmune polyglandular syndrome; Congenital hypothyroidism; Diabetes insipidus; Graves' disease; Obesity; Pancreatic cancer; Pancreatitis; Pearson syndrome; Steroid hormones.

Punctuated equilibrium

CATEGORY: Evolutionary biology; Population genetics

SIGNIFICANCE: Punctuated equilibrium is a model of evolutionary change in which new species originate abruptly and then exist through a long period of stasis. This model is important as an explanation of the stepwise pattern of species change seen in the fossil record.

KEY TERMS

allopatric speciation: a theory that suggests that small parts of a population may become genetically isolated and develop differences that would lead to the development of a new species

heterochrony: a change in the timing or rate of development of characters in an organism relative to those same events in its evolutionary ancestors

phyletic gradualism: the idea that evolutionary change proceeds by a progression of tiny changes, adding up to produce new species over immense periods of time

EVOLUTIONARY PATTERNS

Nineteenth-century English naturalist Charles Darwin viewed the development of new species as occurring slowly by a shift of characteristics within populations, so that a gradual transition from one species to another took place. This is now generally referred to as "phyletic gradualism." A number of examples from the fossil record were put forward to support this view, particularly that of the horse, in which changes to the feet, jaws, and teeth seem to have progressed in one direction over a long period of time. Peter Sheldon in 1987 documented gradual change in eight lineages of trilobites over a three-million-year period in the Ordovician period in Wales.

Despite these and other examples (some of which have since been reinterpreted), it is clear that the fossil record more commonly shows a picture of populations that are largely stable through time, separated by abrupt morphological breaks. This pattern was recognized by Darwin but was attributed by him to the sketchy and incomplete nature of the fossil record. So few animals become fossilized, and conditions for fossilization are so rare, that he felt only a fragmentary sampling of gradual transitions was present, giving the appearance of abrupt change.

One hundred years later, the incompleteness of the fossil record no longer seemed convincing as an explanation. In 1972, Niles Eldredge and Stephen Jay Gould published their theory of the evolutionary process, which they called "punctuated equilibrium." This model explains the lack of intermediates by suggesting that evolutionary change occurs only in short-lived bursts in which a new species arises abruptly from a parent species, often with relatively large morphological changes, and thereafter remains more or less stable until its extinction.

THE PROCESS OF PUNCTUATED EQUILIBRIUM

A number of explanations have been put forward to show how this process might take place. One of these, termed allopatric speciation, was first proposed by Ernst Mayr in 1963. Mayr pointed out that a reproductive isolating mechanism is needed to provide a barrier to gene flow and that this could be provided by geographic isolation. Allopatric or geographical isolation could result when the normal range of a population of organisms is reduced or fragmented. Parts of the population become separated in peripheral isolates, and if the population is small, it may become modified rapidly by natural selection or genetic drift, particularly if it is adapting to a new environment. This type of process is commonly called the "founder effect," because the characteristics of a small group of individuals will overwhelmingly determine the possible characteristics of their descendants. As the initial members of the peripheral isolate may be few in number, it might take only a few generations for the population to have changed enough to become reproductively isolated from the parent population. In the fossil record, this will be seen as a period of stasis representing the parent population, followed by a rapid morphological change as the peripheral

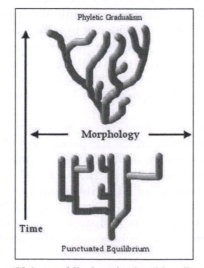

Punctuated equilibrium. public domain via wikimedia commons

population is isolated from it and then replaces it, either competitively or because it has become extinct or has moved to follow a shifting habitat. Because this is thought to take place rapidly in small populations, fossilization potential is low, and unequivocal examples are not common in the fossil record. However, in 1981, Peter Williamson published a well-documented example from the Tertiary period of Lake Turkana in Kenya, which showed episodes of stasis and rapid change in populations of freshwater mollusks. The increases in evolutionary rate were apparently driven by severe environmental change that caused parts of the lake to dry up.

Punctuated changes may also have taken place because of heterochrony, which is a change in the rate of development or timing of appearance of ancestral characters. Paedomorphosis, for example, would result in the retention of juvenile characters in the adult, while its opposite, peramorphosis, would result in an adult morphologically more advanced than its ancestor. Rates of development could be affected by a mutation, perhaps resulting in the descendant growing for much longer than the ancestral form, thus producing a giant version. These changes would be essentially instantaneous and thus would show as abrupt changes of species in the fossil record.

IMPACT AND APPLICATIONS

The publication of the idea of punctuated equilibrium ignited a storm of controversy that still persists. It predicts that speciation can be very rapid, but more important, it is consistent with the prevalence of stasis over long periods of time so often observed in the fossil record. Species had long been viewed as flexible and responsive to the environment, but fossil species showed no change over long periods despite a changing environment. Biologists have thus had to review their ideas about the concept of species and the processes that operate on them. Species are now seen as real entities that have characteristics that are more than the sum of their component populations. Thus the tendency of a group to evolve rapidly or slowly may be intrinsic to the group as a whole and not dependent on the individuals that compose it. This debate has helped show that the fossil record can be important in detecting phenomena that are too large in scale for biologists to observe.

David K. Elliott, Ph.D.

FURTHER READING

Ayala, Francisco J. "Punctuated Equilibrium and Species Selection." *Back to Darwin: A Richer Account of Evolution.* Ed. John B. Cobb Jr. Grand Rapids: Eerdmans, 2008. 185–92. Print.

Chevin, Luis-Miguel. "Genetic Constraints on Adaptation to a Changing Environment." *Evolution* 67.3 (2013): 708–21. *Academic Search Complete.* Web. 20 Jan. 2016.

Eldredge, Niles. *Time Frames: The Rethinking of Darwinian Evolution and the Theory of Punctuated Equilibria.* New York: Simon, 1985. Print.

Eldredge, Niles, and Stephen Jay Gould. "Punctuated Equilibria: An Alternative to Phyletic Gradualism." *Models in Paleobiology.* Ed. Thomas J. M. Schopf. San Francisco: Freeman, 1972. 82–116. Print.

Gould, Stephen Jay. "The Meaning of Punctuated Equilibria and Its Role in Validating a Hierarchical Approach to Macroevolution." *Perspectives on Evolution.* Ed. Roger Milkman. Sunderland: Sinauer, 1982. 83–104. Print.

Gould, Stephen Jay, and Niles Eldredge. "Punctuated Equilibria: The Tempo and Mode of Evolution Reconsidered." *Paleobiology* 3.2 (1977): 115–51. *JSTOR.* Web. 20 Jan. 2016.

Singh, Rama S., Jianping Xu, and Rob J. Kulathinal, eds. *Rapidly Evolving Genes and Genetic Systems.* Oxford: Oxford UP, 2012. Print.

Pennell, Matthew W., Luke J. Harmon, and Josef C. Uyeda. "Is There Room for Punctuated Equilibrium in Macroevolution?" *Trends in Ecology & Evolution* 29.1 (2014): 23–32. Print.

Prothero, Donald R. *Bringing Fossils to Life: An Introduction to Paleobiology.* 3rd ed. New York: Columbia UP, 2013. Print.

Sepkoski, David, and Michael Ruse, eds. *The Paleobiological Revolution: Essays on the Growth of Modern Paleontology.* Chicago: U of Chicago P, 2009. Print.

Somit, Albert, and Steven A. Peterson, eds. *The Dynamics of Evolution: The Punctuated Equilibrium Debate in the Natural and Social Sciences.* Ithaca: Cornell UP, 1992. Print.

See also: Artificial selection; Consanguinity and genetic disease; Evolutionary biology; Genetic load; Hardy-Weinberg law; Inbreeding and assortative mating; Molecular clock hypothesis; Natural selection; Population genetics; Speciation.

Purine nucleoside phosphorylase deficiency

CATEGORY: Diseases and syndromes
ALSO KNOWN AS: PNP-deficiency

DEFINITION

Purine nucleoside phosphorylase (PNP) deficiency is a rare and severe, inherited primary immunodeficiency disease. PNP-deficiency destroys T-cell lymphocytes in the immune system, severely weakening the immune system and decreasing life expectancy.

RISK FACTORS

Family history is the only known risk factor for this disease. It is an autosomal recessive disorder, and symptomatic individuals inherit a defective purine nucleoside phosphorylase gene (*PNP*) gene at chromosomal location 14q11.2 from each parent. Carrier parents have a 25 percent chance of passing this genetic defect to their offspring. Neurological symptoms often accompany this disease, but the route by which they develop is still undiscovered. Risk is evenly distributed between males and females.

ETIOLOGY AND GENETICS

This inherited genetic disease causes the absence or mutation of *PNP*. PNP deficiency is one of several severe combined immunodeficiency (SCID) diseases, which also include adenosine deaminase (ADA) deficiency and X-linked severe combined immunodeficiency (X-SCID). Individuals with X-SCID comprise the majority of SCID cases (Allenspach et al. 2013). PNP deficiency accounts for only about 4 percent of all combined immunodeficiency diseases (CID) and is differentiated by recurring symptoms of chronic and unusual infections resistant to drug therapies, neurological symptoms, lymphopenia, and increased incidences of lymphomas and autoimmune diseases at a young age.

Purines are components necessary in cellular energy systems and for the production of DNA and RNA. Purines are often recycled during catabolism using the purine salvage pathway. When the PNP enzyme is deficient along this pathway, elevated levels of deoxyguanosine triphosphate (dGTP) begins to accumulate in lymph tissues, whose primary function is immunity. Subsequently, the production of

1RCT
Human purine nucleoside phosphorylase PDB1rct. By A2-33 (Own work), via Wikimedia Commons

ribonucleotide reductase necessary for the synthesis of deoxynucleotides, which are used in the genetic code, and mitochondrial DNA repair is inhibited. As a result, T-cell lymphocyte and thymocyte sensitivity increases, leading to T-cell destruction and a decreased ability to fight infection. Unlike ADA deficiency, B-cell lymphocytes in the immune system are not affected.

SYMPTOMS

PNP deficiency is often difficult to diagnosis because of recurring sinopulmonary and urinary tract infections that may also indicate other diseases, such as B-cell immunodeficiency, vitamin B12 deficiency, or interstitial cystitis. But PNP deficiency is distinguished from other diseases by neurological and autoimmune diseases coupled with unusual, recurring, and drug-resistant bacterial, fungal, mycobacterial, protozoal, and viral infections. Drug-resistant pneumonia and oral thrush before one year of age are usually the first indications of a PNP deficiency. Often neurological symptoms precede infections because T-cell immunity declines gradually, thus delaying onset of infections. Ataxia, autoimmune hemolytic anemia, autoimmune neutropenia, behavioral issues, bronchiectasis, central nervous vasculitis,

developmental and motor delays, diarrhea, failure to thrive, herpes infections, hypertonia, idiopathic thrombocytopenia, lupus, malabsorption, mental retardation, neurological symptoms, nodular lymphoid hyperplasia of the gastrointestinal tract, spasticity, recurrent sinopulmonary and urinary tract infections, thyroiditis, and tremors are all symptoms that have been associated with a PNP deficiency.

SCREENING AND DIAGNOSIS

When an immunodeficiency disease is suspected, family and patient history, physical exam, blood screening tests, and skin tests are used to make an accurate diagnosis. A physical exam usually finds absent or underdeveloped lymph glands and tissue. Blood screening tests include complete blood count and manual differential, quantitative serum immunoglobulin levels, antibody response measurement, and complement response.

These blood tests usually show a marked decrease in circulating lymphocytes and serum antibodies. The US National Library of Medicine's *Genetics Home Reference* reported in 2014 that approximately two-thirds of PNP deficient individuals present with neurological symptoms, including muscle spasticity and intellectual disability. Autoimmune hemolytic anemia, immune thrombocytopenia, neutropenia, thyroiditis, and lupus diseases are often found.

CHROMOSOME 14
Human Chromosom 14. public domain via wikimedia commons

Chest x-rays usually show an underdeveloped thymus gland. Average age of diagnosis is six and a half months.

TREATMENT AND THERAPY

PNP deficiency is fatal, but recent treatments can extend life span. Treatment first involves treating any infections with appropriate antibiotic therapies. If failure to thrive is present, then appropriate nutrition interventions are also prescribed. In the case of anemia, red blood cell transfusions improve symptoms for a limited time. Successful bone marrow and stem cell transplantation from a compatible donor cure the underlying immunodeficiency and improve immune system function. However, accompanying neurological disorders or autoimmune diseases are not cured by bone marrow transplantation, and treatment of these disorders depends on the specific disease. Prophylactic precautions include avoiding situations where germs may spread and cause infections, use of good hygiene and nutrition practices, avoidance of live viral immunizations, and treatment with long-term, low-dose antibiotics to prevent and control infections. In vitro studies show gene and intracellular enzyme replacement therapies as well as infusing PNP fusion proteins may resolve PNP deficiency and offer promising treatments in the future. Transplants of stem cells from umbilical cord blood may also resolve neurological symptoms.

PREVENTION AND OUTCOMES

Genetic counseling to assess risk is recommended when there is a family history of PNP deficiency. Prenatal diagnosis is possible in families with a previously affected child.

However, prognosis is generally poor for PNP-deficiency, and life expectancy is usually not more than ten years of age at this time.

Alice C. Richer, RD

FURTHER READING

Allenspach, Eric, David J. Rawlings, and Andrew M. Scharenberg. "X-Linked Severe Combined Immunodeficiency." *GeneReviews.* Ed. Roberta A. Pagon et al. Seattle: U of Washington, Seattle, 1993–2014. *NCBI Bookshelf.* Natl. Center for Biotechnology Information, 24 Jan. 2013. Web. 20 Aug. 2014.

Dror, Yigal, et al. "Purine Nucleoside Phosphorylase Deficiency Associated with a Dysplastic Marrow Morphology." *Pediatric Research* 55.3 (2004): 472–477. Print.

Gates, Robert H. *Infectious Disease Secrets.* 2d ed. Philadelphia: Hanley, 2003. Print.

Genetics Home Reference. "Purine Nucleoside Phosphorylase Deficiency." *Genetics Home Reference.* US NLM, 18 Aug. 2014. Web. 20 Aug. 2014.

Grunebaum, E., A. Cohen, and C. M. Roifman. "Recent Advances in Understanding and Managing Adenosine Deaminase and Purine Nucleoside Phosphorylase Deficiences." *Current Opinion in Allergy and Clinical Immunology* 13.6 (2013): 630–638. *MEDLINE with Full Text.* Web. 20 Aug. 2014.

Janeway, Charles A.. *Immunobiology: The Immune System in Health and Disease.* 7th ed. New York: Garland, 2007. Print.

McKusick, Victor A., and Cassandra L. Kniffin. "#613179 Purine Nucleoside Phosphorylase Deficiency." *OMIM.* Johns Hopkins U, 8 Jan. 2013. Web. 20 Aug. 2014.

MedlinePlus. "Immune System and Disorders." *MedlinePlus.* US NLM/NIH, 20 Aug. 2014. Web. 20 Aug. 2014.

Walker, P. L., et al. "Purine Nucleoside Phosphorylase Deficiency: A Mutation Update." *Nucleosides, Nucleotides & Nucleic Acids* 30.12 (2011): 1243–1247. *MEDLINE with Full Text.* Web. 20 Aug. 2014.

See also: Agammaglobulinemia; Allergies; Antibodies; Anthrax; Ataxia telangiectasia; Autoimmune disorders; Autoimmune polyglandular syndrome; Chediak-Higashi syndrome; Chronic granulomatous disease; Hybridomas and monoclonal antibodies; Immunodeficiency with hyper-IgM; Immunogenetics; Infantile agranulocytosis; Myeloperoxidase deficiency.

Pyloric stenosis

CATEGORY: Diseases and syndromes

ALSO KNOWN AS: Infantile hypertrophic pyloric stenosis; IHPS

DEFINITION

Normally, food passes from the stomach to the small intestine. In pyloric stenosis, food cannot pass freely be cause the entrance between the stomach and the small intestine is abnormally narrow. The narrowing is caused by the enlargement of the pylorus (the muscle at the entrance to the stomach). This leads to a functional obstruction of the gastric outlet. This condition is the most common cause of intestinal obstruction in infancy.

Almost all cases of pyloric stenosis happen in very young babies (usually three to twelve weeks old). This problem happens about two to four times out of every one thousand births. It is much more common in males than in females. The sooner pyloric stenosis is treated, the fewer problems will result and the healthier a baby will be, so parents who think their child has this condition should contact their doctors immediately.

RISK FACTORS

The following risk factors increase a baby's chance of developing pyloric stenosis; parents whose child has any of these risk factors should tell their doctor. Risk factors include prematurity and a family history of pyloric stenosis. Pyloric stenosis is more common in male babies (particularly firstborn males) and more common in Caucasian than in Latino, Asian, or African American babies.

Another important risk factor is exposure to the macrolide antibiotics such as erythromycin and related medicines. Treatment of young infants with macrolide antibiotics has been found to be strongly associated with IHPS and is usually administered if the potential treatment benefits outweigh the risk. Maternal use of macrolides during the first two weeks after birth is also associated with an increased risk of IHPS. A possible association has also been found with use during late pregnancy.

ETIOLOGY AND GENETICS

The etiology of pyloric stenosis is multifactorial, suggesting that there is a broad range of genetic and environmental factors that may contribute to the appearance of this birth defect. While there is no single gene that when mutated will always cause this condition, researchers have identified at least five genes in which mutations may significantly in crease the risk of developing this disorder. Since in put from several genes is probably involved, most cases do not conform to a predictable pattern of inheritance. Be that as it may, a 2010 report from Denmark demonstrated compelling evidence for strong familial aggregation and heritability of IHPS during a 30-year period when a total of 3362 children underwent surgery to correct the condition. The report noted that there was no difference in rate ratios for maternal and paternal relatives of children with pyloric stenosis and no difference according to sex of cohort member or sex of relative. Scattered reports in the literature note rare, isolated families in which pyloric stenosis is in herited as an autosomal dominant condition, but these are exceptions to the norm. In autosomal dominant inheritance, a single copy of the mutation is sufficient to cause full expression of the trait. An affected individual has a 50 percent chance of transmitting the mutation to each of his or her chil dren.

The five genes that are known to be associated with increased susceptibility to the development of pyloric stenosis are known as IHPS1-5, with the gene letters standing for infantile hypertrophic pyloric stenosis. IHPS1 is located on the long arm of chromosome 12, at position 12q24.2-q24.31, and IHPS2 is located on chromosome 16 at position 16p13-p12. The remaining genes are IHPS3 (at position 11q14 q22), IHPS4 (at position Xq23), and IHPS5 (at position 16q24.3). Little is known about the cellular action or interaction of the protein products of these

Horizontal cut 10 days after surgery (Psyloric Stenosis) in a 4 weeks old baby. By Kiu77 (Own work), via Wikimedia Commons

Pyloromyotomy scar (rather large) 30 hrs post-op in a 1 month-old baby. By Sven Teschke, Germany Steschke (Own work), via Wikimedia Commons

SYMPTOMS

Symptoms of pyloric stenosis usually begin when babies are three to five weeks old. They include forceful vomiting of formula or milk (but not mixed with bile as that finding would suggest a different problem); acting hungry most of the time; weight loss; signs of dehydration, such as less urination, dry mouth, and crying with out tears; low activity level; fewer bowel movements; and blood-tinged vomit (which happens when repeated vomiting irritates the stomach, causing mild stomach bleeding).

Physical signs may also include a firm, nontender, and mobile hard lump that is 1-2 cm in diameter, described as an "olive," usually found in the right upper quadrant of the abdomen at the lateral edge of the rectus abdominis muscle. This is most easily found after the infant has vomited and when calm, or when the gastric contents have been removed via a tube placed in the stomach. The palpation of an olive mass has a 99% positive predictive value for IHPS diagnosis.

SCREENING AND DIAGNOSIS

When the above signs and symptoms are noted, it often leads to a suspicion for the presence of IHPS. If the examining clinician finds the "olive" lump noted above, the diagnosis can be confirmed using ultrasound imaging. Older types of x-rays (such as upper GI imaging) are now rarely used. In rare cases, if the diagnosis is not conclusive, a procedure called upper GI endoscopy may be recommended. This procedure involves passing a special scope through the esophagus to the stomach in order to directly visualize the stomach and the junction to the small intestine. If a baby is diagnosed with IHPS, the parents and families are often referred to a pediatric surgeon (a doctor specializing in surgery in children).

TREATMENT AND THERAPY

Pyloric stenosis is treated with a surgery called a pyloromyotomy, with a baby asleep under anesthesia. In a pyloromyotomy, the outside of the pylorus muscle is cut to relieve the blockage. Prior to surgery, fluids and electrolytes will be given intravenously to correct the dehydration and electrolyte imbalances that are common in babies with pyloric stenosis. After the operation, fluids are given by vein until the baby can take all of his or her normal feedings by mouth.

PREVENTION AND OUTCOMES

There are no known ways of preventing pyloric stenosis, although there are some studies that suggest that breast-feeding might have a protective effect and might reduce the risk.

Nathalie Smith, M.S.N, R.N.;
reviewed by Daus Mahnke, M.D. "Etiology and
Genetics" by Jeffrey A. Knight, Ph.D.; updated by Gary M.
Flashner, M.S., M.D.

FURTHER READING

EBSCO Publishing. "Health Library: Pyloric Stenosis." Ipswich, Mass.: Author, 2009. Available through http://www.ebscohost.com.

Kim, S. S., et al. "Pyloromyotomy: A Comparison of Laparoscopic, Circumumbilical, and Right Up per Quadrant Operative Techniques." *Journal of the American College of Surgeons* 201, no. 1 (July, 2005): 66-70.

Pisacane, A., et al. "Breast Feeding and Hypertrophic Pyloric Stenosis: Population-Based Case Control Study." *British Medical Journal* 312, no. 7033 (March 23, 1996): 745-746. Udassin, R. "New Insights in Infantile Hypertrophic Pyloric Stenosis." Israel Medical Association Journal 6, no. 3 (March, 2004): 160-161.

White, J. S., et al. "Treatment of Infantile Hypertro phic Pyloric Stenosis in a District General Hospi tal: A Review of 160 Cases." Journal of Pediatric Sur gery 38, no. 9 (2003): 1333-1336.

Pandya S, Heiss K. Pyloric stenosis in pediatric surgery: an evidence-based review. *Surg Clin North Am.* 2012 Jun. 92(3):527-39, vii-viii.

McAteer JP, Ledbetter DJ, Goldin AB. Role of bottle feeding in the etiology of hypertrophic pyloric stenosis. *JAMA Pediatr.* 2013 Dec. 167(12):1143-9.

Lund M, Pasternak B, Davidsen RB, Feenstra B, Krogh C, Diaz LJ, et al. Use of macrolides in mother and child and risk of infantile hypertrophic pyloric stenosis: nationwide cohort study. *BMJ.* 2014 Mar 11. 348:g1908.

Feenstra B, Geller F, Carstensen L, Romitti PA, Körberg IB, Bedell B, et al. Plasma lipids, genetic variants near APOA1, and the risk of infantile hypertrophic pyloric stenosis. *JAMA.* 2013 Aug 21. 310(7):714-21.

Krogh C, Fischer TK, Skotte L, Biggar RJ, Oyen N, Skythe A. Familial aggregation and heritability of pyloric stenosis. *JAMA.* 2010 Jun 16. 303(23):2393-9.

Takeuchi M, Yasunaga H, Horiguchi H, Hashimoto H, Matsuda S. Pyloromyotomy versus i.v. atropine therapy for the treatment of infantile pyloric stenosis: nationwide hospital discharge database analysis. *Pediatr Int.* 2013 Aug. 55 (4):488-91.

WEB SITES OF INTEREST

American Association of Pediatrics
http://www.aap.org

The American Pediatric Surgical Association
http://www.eapsa.org/parents/pyloric.htm

Caring for Kids, Canadian Paediatric Society
http://www.caringforkids.cps.ca

The Montreal Children's Hospital
http://www.thechildren.com
http://emedicine.medscape.com/article/803489-overview
http://pediatrics.aappublications.org/content/early/2015/02/10/peds.2014-2026

See also: Celiac disease; Colon cancer; Crohn disease; Familial adenomatous polyposis; Hereditary diffuse gastric cancer (HDGC); Hereditary mixed polyposis syndrome; Hirschsprung's disease; Lynch syndrome.

Q

Quantitative inheritance

SIGNIFICANCE: Quantitative inheritance involves metric traits. These traits are generally associated with adaptation, reproduction, yield, form, and function. They are thus of great importance to evolution, conservation biology, psychology, and especially the improvement of agricultural organisms.

KEY TERMS

genotype: the genetic makeup of an organism at all loci that affect a quantitative trait

heritability: the proportion of phenotypic differences among individuals that are a result of genetic differences

metric traits: traits controlled by multiple genes with small individual effects and continuously varying environmental effects, resulting in continuous variation in a population

phenotype: the observed expression of a genotype that results from the combined effects of the genotype and the environment to which the organism has been exposed

THE GENETICS UNDERLYING METRIC TRAITS

An understanding of the genetics affecting metric traits came with the unification of the Mendelian and biometrical schools of genetics early in the 1900s. The statistical relationships involved in inheritance of metric traits such as height in humans were well known in the late 1800s. Soon after that, Gregor Mendel's breakthrough on particulate inheritance, obtained from work using traits such as the color and shape of pea plants, was rediscovered. However, some traits did not follow Mendelian inheritance patterns. For example, Francis Galton crossed pea plants with uniformly large seeds with plants that had uniformly

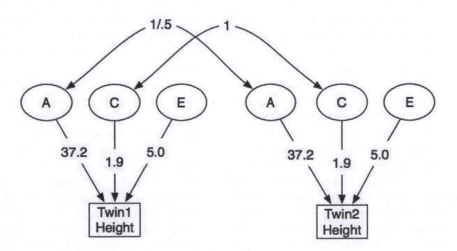

TWIN STUDY STRUCTURAL ACE MODEL
Heritability of adult body height: a comparative study of twin cohorts in eight countries. Tim bates at en.wikipedia, via Wikimedia Commons

HUMAN HEIGHT GROWTH PER MONTH, UNITED STATES (50TH PERCENTILE)
STARTING TIME INTERVAL: 0.5-1.5 MONTHS. STATURE AT 0.5 MONTHS: 52.7 CM (BOYS), 51.7 CM (GIRLS).

HUMAN HEIGHT GROWTH PER MONTH, UNITED STATES

Human height growth per month for the United States, ages 0–20, 50th percentile. Source: *Centers for Disease Control and Prevention. Accessed on February 23, 2013.* By Cantus (Own work), via Wikimedia Commons

small seeds. The seed size of the progeny was neither large nor small but intermediate. However, when the progeny were mated among themselves, seed size formed a distribution from small to large, with many intermediate sizes.

How could particulate genetic factors explain a continuous distribution? The solution was described early in the twentieth century when Swedish plant breeder Herman Nilsson-Ehle crossed red wheat with white wheat. The resulting progeny were light red in color. When matings were made within the progeny, the resulting kernels of wheat ranged in color from white to red. Nilsson-Ehle was able to categorize the wheat into five colors: red, intermediate red, light red, pink, and white. Intermediate colors occurred with greater frequency than extreme colors. Nilsson-Ehle deduced that particulate genetic factors, now known as alleles, were involved, with red wheat inheriting four red alleles, intermediate red inheriting three red alleles, light red inheriting two red alleles, pink inheriting one red allele, and white inheriting no red alleles. These results were consistent with Mendel's findings, except that two sets of factors, now known as loci, were controlling this trait, rather than the single locus observed for the traits considered by Mendel. Further, these results could be generalized to account for additional inheritance patterns controlled by more than two loci. Quantitative

inheritance was mathematically described by British statistician and geneticist Ronald A. Fisher.

Under many circumstances, the environment also modifies the expression of traits. A combination of many loci with individually small effects alone would produce a rough bell-shaped distribution for a quantitative trait. However, environmental effects are continuous and independent of genetic effects, allowing them to blur the boundaries of the genetic categories and potentially make it difficult or even impossible to identify the effects of individual loci for many quantitative traits. The distribution of phenotypes, reflecting combined genetic and environmental effects, is typically a smooth, bell-shaped curve.

Genetic and environmental effects jointly influence the value of most metric traits. The relative magnitudes of genetic and environmental effects are measured using heritability statistics. Heritability has several practical definitions that are essentially equivalent. One definition states that heritability is equal to the proportion of observed differences among organisms for a trait due to genetic differences. For example, if one-quarter of the differences among cows in terms of how much milk they produce are caused by differences in their genotypes, the heritability of milk production is 25 percent, and the remaining 75 percent of differences among the animals are attributed to environmental effects. An alternative definition is that heritability is equal to the proportion of differences among sets of parents that are passed on to their progeny. For example, if the average height of a pair of parents is eight inches (twenty centimeters) more than the mean of their population and the heritability of height is 50 percent, then their progeny would be expected to average four inches (ten centimeters) taller than their peers in the population.

FUNDAMENTAL RELATIONSHIPS OF QUANTITATIVE GENETICS

Two relationships are fundamental to the understanding and application of quantitative genetics. First, there is a tendency toward likeness among related individuals. Although similarities of human stature and facial appearance within families are familiar to most people, the same is true for such traits in all organisms. Correlation among relatives exists for such diverse traits as blood pressure, plant height, grain yield, and egg production. These correlations are caused by relatives sharing a portion of genes in common. The more closely the individuals are related, the greater the proportion of genes that are shared. Identical twins share all of their genes, while full siblings or a parent and offspring are expected to share one-half of their genes. This relationship is commonly used in the improvement of agricultural organisms. Individuals are chosen to be parents based on the performance of their relatives. For example, bulls of dairy breeds are chosen to become widely used as sires based on the milk-producing ability of their sisters and daughters.

The second fundamental relationship is that in organisms that do not normally self-fertilize, vigor is depressed in progeny that result from inbreeding—that is, the mating of closely related individuals. This effect is known as inbreeding depression. It may be the basis of the social taboos regarding incestuous relationships in humans as well as the dispersal systems for some other species of mammals, such as wolves. Physiological barriers have evolved to prevent fertilization between close relatives in many species of plants. Some mechanisms function as an anatomical inhibitor to prevent union of pollen and ova from the same plant; in maize, for example, the male and female flower are widely separated on the plant. Indeed, in some species, such as asparagus

and holly trees, the sexes are separated in different individuals, and all seeds must consequently result from cross-pollination. In other systems, cross-pollination is only required for fertile seeds to result. The pollen must originate from a plant genetically different from the seed parent. These phenomena are known as self-incompatibility and are present in species such as broccoli, radishes, some clovers, and many fruit trees.

The corollary to inbreeding depression is hybrid vigor, a phenomenon of improved fitness that is often evident in progeny resulting from hybridization, or the mating of individuals less related than the average in a population. Hybrid vigor has been used in breeding programs to achieve remarkable productivity of hybrid seed corn as well as crossbred poultry and livestock. Hybrid vigor results in increased reproduction and efficiency of nutrient utilization. The mule, which results from mating a male donkey to a female horse, is a well-known example of a hybrid that has remarkable strength and hardiness compared to the parent species; unfortunately, however, it is also sterile.

QUANTITATIVE TRAITS OF HUMANS

Many traits of humans, like those of other organisms, are quantitatively inherited. Psychological characteristics, intelligence quotient (IQ), and birth weight have been studied extensively. The heritability of IQ has been reported to be high. Other personality characteristics, such as incidence of depression, introversion, and enthusiasm, have also been reported to be highly heritable. Musical ability is another characteristic under some degree of genetic control. These results have been consistent across replicated studies and are thus expected to be reliable; however, some caution must be exercised when considering the reliability of results from individual studies. Most studies of heritability in humans have involved likeness of twins reared together and apart. The difficulty in obtaining such data results in a relatively small sample size, at least relative to similar experiments in animals. One unfortunate response to studies of quantitative inheritance in humans was the eugenics movement.

Birth weight of humans is of interest because it is both under genetic control and subject to influence by well-known environmental factors, such as smoking by the mother. Birth weight is subject to stabilizing selection, in which individuals with intermediate values have the highest rates of survival. This results in genetic pressure to maintain the average birth weight at a relatively constant value.

QUANTITATIVE CHARACTERS IN AGRICULTURAL IMPROVEMENT

The ability to meet the demand for food by a growing world population is dependent on continuously increasing agricultural productivity. Reserves of high-quality farmland have nearly all been brought into production, and a sustainable increase in the harvest of fish is likely impossible. Many countries that struggle to meet the food demands of their populations are too poor to increase agricultural yields through increased inputs of fertilizer and chemicals. Increased food production will, therefore, largely depend on genetic improvement of the organisms produced by farmers worldwide.

Most characteristics of economic value in agriculturally important organisms are quantitatively inherited. Traits such as grain yield, baking quality, milk and meat production, and efficiency of nutrient utilization are under the influence of many genes as well as the production environment. The task of breeders is not only to identify organisms with superior genetic characteristics but also to identify those breeds and varieties well adapted to the specific environmental conditions in which they will be produced. The type of dairy cattle that most efficiently produces milk under the normal production circumstances in the United States, which includes high health status, unlimited access to high-quality grain rations, and protection from extremes of heat and cold, may not be ideal under conditions in New Zealand, where cattle are required to compete with herdmates for high-quality pasture forage. Neither of these animals may be ideal under tropical conditions where extremely high temperatures, disease, and parasites are common.

Remarkable progress has been made in many important food crops. Grain yield has responded to improvement programs. Development of hybrid corn increased yield several fold over the last few decades of the twentieth century. Development of improved varieties of small grains resulted in an increased ability of many developing countries to be self-sufficient in food production. Grain breeder Norman Borlaug won the Nobel Peace Prize in 1970 for his role in developing grain varieties that contributed to the Green Revolution.

Can breeders continue to make improvements in the genetic potential for crops, livestock, and fish to yield enough food to support a growing human population? Tools of biotechnology are expected to increase the rate at which breeders can make genetic change. Ultimately, the answer depends on the genetic variation available in the global populations of food-producing organisms and their wild relatives. The potential for genetic improvement of some species has been relatively untapped. Domestication of fish for use in aquaculture and the use of potential crop species such as amaranth are two possible ways to augment world food reserves. Wheat, corn, and rice provide a large proportion of the calories supporting the world population. The yields of these three crop species have already benefited from many generations of selective breeding. For continued genetic improvement, it is critical that variation not be lost through the extinction of indigenous strains and wild relatives of important food-producing organisms.

IMPACT AND APPLICATIONS

Molecular genetics and biotechnology have also added new tools for analyzing the genetics of quantitative traits. In any organism that has had its genome adequately mapped, genetic markers can be used to determine the number of loci involved in a particular trait. In carefully constructed crosses, geneticists look for statistical correlations between markers and the trait of interest. When a high correlation is found, the marker is said to represent a quantitative trait locus (QTL). Often a percentage effect for each QTL can be determined, and because the location of markers is typically known, the likely location of the gene can also be inferred (that is, it must be somewhere near the marker). A good understanding of the QTLs involved in the expression of a quantitative trait can help researchers determine the best way to improve the organism.

Although QTLs are much easier to discover in organisms where controlled crosses are possible, studies have also been carried out in humans. In humans, geneticists must rely on whatever matings have happened; due to ethical limitations, they cannot set up specific crosses. Studies in humans have attempted to quantify the number of QTLs responsible for such things as IQ and various physical traits. However, ethicists continue to worry that conclusions from such research will be used in a new wave of eugenics. In spite of the risk of misusing an improved understanding of human quantitative traits, human biology and medicine stand to benefit.

William R. Lamberson, Ph.D.;
updated by Bryan Ness, Ph.D.

FURTHER READING

Allendorf, Fred W., Gordon Luikart, and Sally N. Aitken. *Conservation and the Genetics of Populations.* 2nd ed. Hoboken: Wiley, 2013. Print.

Charmantier, Anne, Dany Garant, and Loeske E. B. Kruuk, eds. *Quantitative Genetics in the Wild.* New York: Oxford UP, 2014. Print.

Falconer, Douglas S., and Trudy F. C. Mackay. *Introduction to Quantitative Genetics.* 4th ed. Harlow: Pearson, 1996.Print.

Gillespie, John H. *Population Genetics: A Concise Guide.* 2nd ed. Baltimore: Johns Hopkins UP, 2004. Print.

Hamilton, Matthew B. *Population Genetics.* Hoboken: Wiley, 2009. Print.

Snustad, D. Peter, and Michael J. Simmons. *Principles of Genetics.* 6th ed. Hoboken: Wiley, 2012. Print.

Templeton, Alan R. *Population Genetics and Microevolutionary Theory.* Hoboken: Wiley, 2006. Print.

See also: Artificial selection; Biofertilizers; Consanguinity and genetic disease; Epistasis; Genetic load; Hardy-Weinberg law; Hybridization and introgression; Inbreeding and assortative mating; Mendelian genetics; Polygenic inheritance; Population genetics; Speciation; Twin studies.

R

Race

CATEGORY: Human genetics and social issues

SIGNIFICANCE: Humans typically have been categorized into a small number of races based on common traits, ancestry, and geography. Knowledge of human genomic diversity has increased awareness of ambiguities associated with traditional racial groups. The sociopolitical consequences of using genetics to devalue certain races are profound, and based on the available data, are completely baseless.

KEY TERMS

eugenics: a movement concerned with the improvement of human genetic traits, predominantly by the regulation of mating

Human Genome Diversity Project: an extension of the Human Genome Project in which DNA of native people around the world is collected for study

population: a group of geographically localized, interbreeding individuals

race: a collection of geographically localized populations with well-defined genetic traits

CONFLICTING DEFINITIONS OF RACE

Few ideas have had such a contentious history as the use of the term "race." Categorization relied on consideration of salient traits such as skin color, body form, and hair texture to classify humans into distinct subcategories. The term "race" is currently believed to have little biological meaning, in great part because of advances in genetic research. Studies have revealed that a person's genes cannot define their ethnic heritage and that no gene exists exclusively within one race/ethnocultural group. Biomedical scientists remain divided on their opinion about "race" and how it may be used in treating human genetic conditions. For aracial or subspecies classification scheme to be objective and biologically meaningful, researchers must decide carefully which heritable characteristics (passed to future generations genetically) will define the groups. Several principles are considered. First, the unique traits must be discrete and not continually changing by small degrees between populations. Second, everyone placed within a specific race must possess the selected trait's defining variant. All the selected characteristics are found consistently in each member of the group. For example, if blue eyes and brown hair are chosen as defining characteristics, everyone designated as belonging to that race must share both of those characteristics. Individuals placed in other races should not exhibit this particular combination. Third, individuals of the same race must have descended from a common ancestor, unique to those people. Many shared characteristics present in individuals of a race may be traced to that ancestor by heredity. Based on the preceding defining criteria (selection of discrete traits, agreement of traits, and common ancestry), pure representatives of each racial category should be detectable.

Most researchers maintain that traditional races do not conform to scientific principles of subspecies classification. For example, the traits used to define traditional human races are rarely discrete. Skin color, a prominent characteristic employed, is not a well-defined trait. Approximately eleven genes influence skin color significantly, but fifty or so are likely to contribute. Pigmentation in humans results from a complex series of biochemical pathways regulated by amounts of enzymes (molecules that control chemical reactions) and enzyme inhibitors, along with environmental factors. Moreover, the number of melanocytes (cells that produce melanin) do not differ from one person to another, while their level of melanin production does. Like most complex traits involving many genes, human skin color varies on a continuous gradation. From lightest to darkest, all intermediate pigmentations are represented. Color may vary

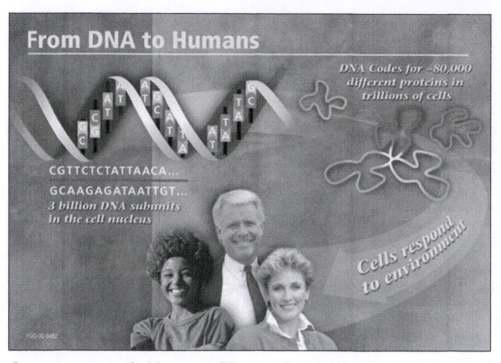

On average, any two people of the same or a different race diverge genetically by a mere 0.2 percent, and only 0.012 percent contribute to traditional racial variations. Allelic variations account for most of the superficial differences perceived as race. (U.S. Department of Energy Human Genome Program, http:// www.ornl.gov/hgmis)

widely even within the same family. The boundary between black and white is an arbitrary, human-made border, not one imposed by nature.

In addition, traditional defining racial characteristics, such as skin color and facial characteristics, are not found in all members of a race. For example, many Melanesians, indigenous to Pacific islands, have pigmentation as dark as any human but are not classified as "black." Another example is found in individuals of the Cherokee Nation that have Caucasoid facial features and very dark skin, yet have no European ancestry. When traditional racial characteristics are examined closely, many groups are left with no conventional racial group. No "pure" genetic representatives of any traditional race exist. Common ancestry must also be considered. Genetic studies have shown that Africans do not belong to a single "black" heritage. In fact, several lineages are found in Africa. An even greater variance is found in African Americans. Besides a diverse African ancestry, on average 13 percent of African American ancestry is Northern

European. Yet all black Americans are consolidated into one race.

The true diversity found in humans is not patterned according to accepted standards of a subspecies. Only at extreme geographical distances are notable differences found. Human populations in close proximity have more genetic similarities than distant populations. Well-defined genetic borders between human populations are not observed, and racial boundaries in classification schemes are most often formed arbitrarily.

HISTORY OF RACIAL CLASSIFICATIONS

Efforts to classify humans into a number of distinct types date back at least to the 19th Dynasty of Ancient Egypt. The sacred text Book of Gates described four distinct groups: "Egyptians," "Asiatics," "Libyans," and "Nubians" were defined using both physical and geographical characteristics. Applying scientific principles to divide people into distinct racial groups has been a goal for much of human history.

In 1758, the founder of biological classification, Swedish botanist Carolus Linnaeus, arranged humans into four principal races: *Americanus, Europeus, Asiaticus,* and *Afer*. Although geographic location was his primary organizing factor, Linnaeus also described the races according to subjective traits such as temperament. Despite his use of archaic criteria, Linnaeus did not give superior status to any of the races.

Johann Friedrich Blumenbach, a German naturalist and admirer of Linnaeus, developed a classification with lasting influence. Blumenbach maintained that the original forms, which he named "Caucasian," were those primarily of European ancestry. His final classification, published in 1795, consisted of five races: Caucasian, Malay, Ethiopian, American, and Mongolian. The fifth race, the Malay, was added to Linnaeus's classification to show a step-by-step change from the original body type.

After Linnaeus and Blumenbach, many variations of their categories were formulated, chiefly by biologists and anthropologists. Classification "lumpers" combined people into only a few races (for example, black, white, and Asian). "Splitters" separated the traditional groups into many different races. One classification scheme divided all Europeans into Alpine, Nordic, and Mediterranean races. Others split Europeans into ten different races. No one scheme of racial classification came to be accepted throughout the scientific community.

Linkage tree for 9 population clusters showing genetic distances (F_{ST})
(Cavalli-Sforza *et al.*, 1994:80)

F_{ST} distance matrix for the 9 clusters shown above
(x10,000 with standard errors obtained by bootstrap analysis)

	AFR	NEC	EUC	NEA	ANE	AME	SEA	PAI	NGA
African	0.0								
Non-European Caucasian	1340.0 ± 301	0.0							
European Caucasian	1655.6 ± 416	154.7 ± 29	0.0						
Northeast Asian	1979.1 ± 452	640.4 ± 134	938.2 ± 217	0.0					
Arctic Northeast Asian	2008.5 ± 387	708.2 ± 160	746.7 ± 210	459.7 ± 98	0.0				
Amerindian	2261.4 ± 434	955.5 ± 204	1038.2 ± 276	746.5 ± 183	577.4 ± 89	0.0			
Southeast Asian	2206.3 ± 529	939.6 ± 262	1240.4 ± 339	630.5 ± 299	1039.4 ± 326	1341.7 ± 418	0.0		
Pacific Islander	2505.4 ± 648	953.7 ± 230	1344.7 ± 354	723.8 ± 262	1181.2 ± 331	1740.7 ± 544	436.7 ± 87	0.0	
New Guinean and Australian	2472.0 ± 536	1179.1 ± 189	1345.7 ± 231	734.4 ± 118	1012.5 ± 257	1457.9 ± 283	1237.9 ± 277	808.7 ± 264	0.0

Linkage tree and Fst distance matrix for 9 population clusters created using data gathered from Cavalli-Sforza, L.L., Menozzi, P. & Piazza, A,. The History and Geography of Human Genes, 1994. By Varoon Arya (Own work), via Wikimedia Commons

GENETICS AND THEORIES OF HUMAN EVOLUTION

Advances in DNA technology have greatly aided researchers in their quest to reconstruct the history of *Homo sapiens* and its diversification. Analysis of human DNA has been performed on both nuclear and mitochondrial DNA. The nucleus is the organelle that contains the majority of the cell's genetic material. Mitochondria are organelles responsible for generating cellular energy. Each mitochondrion contains a single, circular DNA molecule. Research suggests that Africa was the root of all humankind and that humans first arose there 100,000 to 200,000 years ago. Several lines of research, including DNA analysis of humanoid fossils, provide further evidence for this theory.

Many scientists are using genetic markers to decipher the migrations that fashioned past and present human populations. For example, DNA comparisons revealed three Native American lineages. Some scientists believe one migration crossed the Bering Strait, most likely from Mongolia. Another theory states that three separate Asian migrations occurred, each bringing a different lineage.

GENETIC DIVERSITY AMONG RACES

Three primary forces produce the genetic components of a population: natural selection, nonadaptive genetic change, and mating between neighboring populations. The first two factors may result in differences between populations, and reproductive isolation, either voluntary or because of geographic isolation, perpetuates the distinctions. Natural selection refers to the persistence of genetic traits favorable in a specific environment. For example, a widely held assumption concerns skin color, primarily a result of the pigment melanin. Melanin offers some shielding from ultraviolet solar rays. According to this theory, people living in regions with concentrated ultraviolet exposure have increased melanin synthesis and, therefore, dark skin color conferring protection against skin cancer. Individuals with genes for increased melanin have enhanced survival rates and reproductive opportunities. The reproductive opportunities produce offspring that inherit those same genes for increased melanin. This process results in a higher percentage of the population with elevated melanin production genes. Therefore, genes coding for melanin production are favorable and persist in these environments.

The second factor contributing to the genetic makeup of a population is nonadaptive genetic change. This process involves random genetic mutations (alterations). For example, certain genes are responsible for eye color. Individuals contain alternate forms of these genes, or alleles, which result in different eye color. Because these traits are impartial to environmental influences, they may endure from generation to generation. Different populations will spontaneously produce, sustain, and delete them.

The third factor, mating between individuals from neighboring groups, tends to merge traits from several populations. This genetic mixing often results in offspring with blended characteristics.

Several studies have compared the overall genetic complement of various human populations. On average, any two people of the same or a different race diverge genetically by a mere 0.1 percent. It is estimated that only 0.012 percent contributes to traditional racial variations. Hence, most of the genetic differences found between a person of African descent and a person of European descent are also different between two individuals with the same ancestry. The genes do not differ. It is the proportion of individuals expressing a specific allele that varies from population to population.

Upon closer examination, it was found that the continent of Africa is unequaled with respect to cumulative genetic diversity. Numerous races are found in Africa, Khoisan Africans of southern Africa being the most distinct. Therefore two people of different ethnicities who do not have recent African ancestry (for example Northern Europeans and South East Asians) have more similar genetics than any two distinct African ethnic groups. This finding supports theories of early human migration in which humans first evolved in Africa and a subset left the continent, experienced a population bottleneck, and then established the human populations around the world.

HUMAN GENOME DIVERSITY PROJECT AND ADVANCES IN RESEARCH

Many scientists are attempting to reconcile the negativities associated with racial studies. The Human Genome Diversity Project (HGDP), was initiated by Stanford University in 1993 and functions independently from the Human Genome Project. The HGDP aims to collect and store DNA from ethnically diverse populations around the world, creating a library of samples to represent global human diversity. Results of future studies may aid in gene therapy treatments and greater success with organ transplantation. As a result, a more thorough understanding of the genetic diversity and unity in the species *Homo sapiens* will be possible.

At the population level, human diversity is greatest within racial/cultural groups rather than between them. Originally, geneticists who studied genetic diversity of human populations were limited to data from very few genetic loci (locations in the genome that are of interest); however, recent studies are able to simultaneously analyze hundreds to thousands of loci. It is currently estimated that 90 percent of genetic variation in human beings is found within each purported racial group, while differences between the groups only equate to the remaining 10 percent.

A second method of studying human genetic diversity is to compare ethnically diverse individuals and search for similarities and differences in their genomes. Early studies involved only a few dozen genetic loci and as a result did not find individuals to cluster (group together) based on their geographic origin. Recent studies, however, were able to analyze substantially more genetic loci and resulted in data with stronger statistical power. These studies focused on individuals from three distinct geographic areas: Europe, sub-Sahran Africa, and East Asia. Indeed, individuals clustered or shared more genetic similarities with others of the same geographic region. Participants from Africa were found to have the greatest diversity, which is in agreement with population studies. Another cluster consisted exclusively of Europeans, and a third comprised the Asian individuals. However, when individuals from neighboring regions were also analyzed, such as South Indians, the analysis showed similarities to both East Asians and Europeans. This finding may be explained by the numerous migrations between Europe and India during the past ten thousand years. Many individuals did not cluster with their geographic cohorts, demonstrating that individuals are not easily categorizeable into neat groups of races but tend to share more genetic similarities with people from their region.

Race or an individual's ancestry can sometimes provide useful information in medical decision making, as gender or age often do. Certain genetic conditions are more common among ethnocultural groups. For example, hemochromatosis is more prevalent within Northern Europeans and Caucasians, whereas sickle-cell disease is more often found in Africans and African Americans. Meanwhile other genetic diseases are equally prevalent across racial groups, as seen in spinal muscular atrophy (SMA). If a disease-causing gene is common, then it is likely to be relatively ancient and thus shared across ethnicities. Moreover, some genetic conditions remain prevalent in populations because they provide an adaptive advantage to the individual, as seen in sickle-cell disease carriers being protected against malarial infection. Likewise, an individual's response to drugs may be mediated by their genetic makeup. A gene called *CYP2D6* is involved in the metabolism or breakdown of many important drugs such as codeine and morphine. Some individuals have no working copy of this gene whereas others have one or two copies that function properly. The majority of individuals with no working copies are of European heritage (26 percent), whereas fewer Asian (6 percent) and African populations (7 percent) fall into this category. Thus it may be tempting to make medical decisions based on a patient's ethnic heritage; however, this may lead to inaccurate diagnoses (missing sickle-cell disease in an Asian individual) or inappropriate drug administration (prohibiting a Caucasian person from taking codeine). Ideally, each individual should have medical decisions made based on their genetic makeup in lieu of their ethnic heritage. Future patients may be able to first request an analysis of their genome, which would aid their physicians in making some genetically appropriate medical decisions.

SOCIOPOLITICAL IMPLICATIONS

Race is often portrayed as a natural, biological division, the result of geographic isolation and adaptation to local environment. However, confusion between biological and cultural classification obscures perceptions of race. When individuals describe themselves as "black," "white," or "Hispanic," for example, they are usually describing cultural heredity as well as biological similarities. The relative importance of perceived cultural affiliations or genetics varies depending on the circumstances. Examples illustrating the ambiguities are abundant. Nearly all people with African American ancestry are labeled black, even if they have a white parent. In addition, dark skin color designates one as belonging to the black race, including Africans and aboriginal Australians, who have no common genetic lineage. State laws, some on the books until the late 1960s, required a "Negro" designation for anyone with one-eighth black heritage (one black great-grandparent).

Unlike biological boundaries, cultural boundaries are sharp, repeatedly motivating discrimination, genocide, and war. In the early and mid-twentieth century, the eugenics movement, advocating the genetic improvement of the human species, translated into laws against interracial marriage, sterilization programs, and mass murder. Harmful effects include accusations of deficiencies in intelligence or moral character based on traditional racial classification.

The frequent use of biology to devalue certain races and excuse bigotry has profound implications for individuals and society. Blumenbach selected Caucasians (who inhabit regions near the Caucasus Mountains, a Russian and Georgian mountain range) as the original form of humans because in his opinion they were the most beautiful. All other races deviated from this ideal and were, therefore, less beautiful. Despite Blumenbach's efforts not to demean other groups based on intelligence or moral character, the act of ranking in any form left an ill-fated legacy.

In conclusion, race remains a contentious issue both in many fields of science and within the greater society. Recent genomic studies at both the individual and the population level have shown that the majority of human genetic composition is universal and shared across all ethnocultural groups. Shared genetics is most commonly found in individuals who originate from the same geographic region. However, there is no scientific support for the concept of distinct, "pure," and nonoverlapping races. Unfortunately throughout human history, the use and abuse of the term "race" has been pursued for sociopolitical gains or to justify bigotry toward and abuses of individuals. It is now known that human genetic diversity is a continuum, with natural selection, nonadaptive genetic change, and mating as the true driving forces for human genetic diversity.

Stacie R. Chismark, M.S.;
updated by Kayla Mandel Sheets, M.S.

FURTHER READING

Cavalli-Sforza, Luigi L. *The Great Human Diasporas: A History of Diversity and Evolution.* Tr., Serah Thorne. Reading: Addison-Wesley, 1995. Print.

Cavalli-Sforza, Luigi L., et al. *The History and Geography of Human Genes.* Princeton: Princeton UP, 1996. Print.

Fish, Jefferson M., ed. *Race and Intelligence: Separating Science from Myth.* Mahwah: Lawrence Erlbaum, 2002. Print.

Garcia, Jorge J. E. *Race or Ethnicity? On Black or Latino Identity.* Ithaca: Cornell UP, 2007. Print.

Gates, E. Nathaniel, ed. *The Concept of "Race" in Natural and Social Science.* New York: Garland, 1997. Print.

Gibbons, A. "Africans' Deep Genetic Roots Reveal Their Evolutionary Story." *Science* 324 (2009): 575. Print.

Gould, Stephen Jay. *The Mismeasure of Man.* Rev. ed. New York: Norton, 1996. Print.

Graves, Joseph L., Jr. *The Emperor's New Clothes: Biological Theories of Race at the Millennium.* New Brunswick: Rutgers UP, 2001. Print.

Hayden, Erika Check. "Taboo Genetics." *Nature* 502 (2013): 24–26. Print.

Herrnstein, Richard J., and Charles Murray. *The Bell Curve: Intelligence and Class Structure in America.* New York: Free Press, 1994. Print.

Hunt, Linda M., Nicole D. Truesdell, and Meta J. Kreiner. "Genes, Race, and Culture in Clinical Care." *Medical Anthropology Quarterly* 27.2 (2013): 253–71. Print.

Jorde, L. B., and S. P. Wooding. "Genetic Variation, Classification, and 'Race.'" *Nature Genetics* 36.11 (2004): S28. Print.

Kevles, Daniel J. *In the Name of Eugenics: Genetics and the Uses of Human Heredity.* Cambridge: Harvard UP, 1995. Print.

Roberts, Dorothy E. "Race, Gender, and Genetic Technologies: A New Reproductive Dystopia?." *Signs* 40.1 (2014). Print.

Royal, C., and G. Dunston. "Changing the Paradigm from 'Race' to Human Genome Variation." *Nature Genetics* 36 (2004): S5–S7. Print.

Valencia, Richard R., and Lisa A. Suzuki. *Intelligence Testing and Minority Students: Foundations, Performance Factors, and Assessment Issues.* Thousand Oaks: Sage, 2000. Print.

Vogel, Friedrich, and Arno G. Motulsky. *Vogel and Motulsky's Human Genetics: Problems and Approaches.* 3rd ed. Berlin: Springer Science & Business Media, 1997. Print.

See also: Biological determinism; Eugenics; Eugenics: Nazi Germany; Evolutionary biology; Genetic engineering: Social and ethical issues; Heredity and environment; Intelligence; Miscegenation and anti-miscegenation laws; Sociobiology; Sterilization laws.

RB1 gene

CATEGORY: Molecular genetics
SIGNIFICANCE: *RB1*, the retinoblastoma susceptibility gene, was the first tumor-suppressor gene to be discovered as well as the first hereditary cancer gene to be cloned. Study of *RB1* has led to a greater understanding of cancer genes and the development of the "two-hit" model for antioncogene-associated cancers, as a result of retinoblastoma research.

KEY TERMS

allele: one of two or more different genes containing specific inheritable characteristics that occupy corresponding positions (loci) on paired chromosomes

anti-oncogene: tumor-suppressor gene

chromosome: a linear strand of DNA that carries genetic information

deletion: the loss of a portion of a chromosome

exon: one of the coding regions of the DNA of genes

expression: use of a gene to create the corresponding protein

hotspot: DNA positions where genetic recombination occurs with above-average frequency

locus: the position of a gene on a chromosome

mutation: a change in gene, potentially capable of being transmitted to offspring

retinoblastoma: most common intraocular malignancy (eye cancer) in children

GENETICS SUMMARY AND LOCATION

The *RB1* gene is an anti-oncogene (tumor suppressor) and was first recognized and identified in patients with hereditary retinoblastoma by Thaddeus Dryja's laboratory at the Massachusetts Eye and Ear Infirmary at Harvard Medical School, originally isolated using the technique called chromosome walking. The cytogenic location of *RB1* is 13q14.2,

RB1 I, Filip em, via Wikimedia Commons

which means it is on the long arm (q) of chromosome 13 at position 14.2, specifically located from base pair 47,775,911 to base pair 47,954,022. *RB1* is a very large gene, extending over 180 kilobase pairs, containing 27 exons. The promoter region of *RB1* gene is distinctive because it contains binding motifs for transcription factors Sp1 and ATF but no TATA or CAAT box.

The amino acid sequence for *RB1* product is more than 75 percent identical for humans, rats, mice, and frogs. *RB1* exists in all vertebrates, which may indicate that it has a critical biological role that has been maintained through evolution.

RB PROTEIN AND TUMOR SUPPRESSION

RB protein plays an integral role in cell cycle regulation. It controls auxiliary proteins, mediating their replication processes. During the G_1 (resting phase) phase of a cell cycle, RB protein binds to E2F factor and blocks the transcription of S-phase (phase in which DNA synthesis occurs) genes, mediating the G_1-to-S phase checkpoint. A loss of RB protein, due to *RB1* mutation, causes elimination of G_1-to-S phase checkpoint, increasing the odds of unregulated cellular production or cancer.

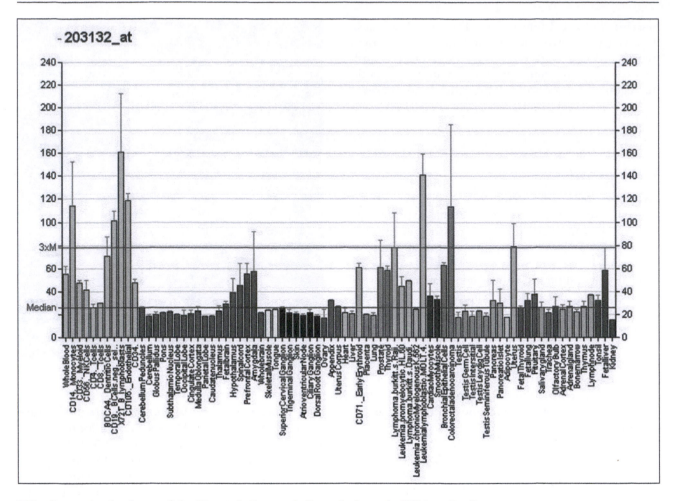

RB1 Genomics Institute of the Novartis Research Foundation, via Wikimedia Commons

There are two distinct types of cancer genes, proto-oncogenes and anti-oncogenes. Proto-oncogenes are easier to identify and involve gene mutations that result in a gain-of-function, motivating cells to become cancerous. Anti-oncogenes are the most frequently mutated genes (except in leukemia and lymphoma) and cause a decreased expression, leading to cancer. *RB1* was the very first of only a few tumor-suppressing anti-oncogenes, that have been discovered and studied, and thus, *RB1* has served as an important model for study of anti-oncogene-associated cancers.

RB1 MUTATIONS
In 1971 Alfred Knudsen described the "two-hit" theory, a mutation model based on retinoblastoma

observations and Mendelian genetics, which can be applied to inherited cancers. The theory states that in hereditary cancers, the predisposed individuals already carry one allele mutation and therefore, oncogenesis only requires one more mutation to occur. In nonhereditary cases, two or more mutational events are required. This hypothesis was validated with the first cloning of the *RB1* gene. Genotyping of retinoblastoma tumors concluded that mutations in both alleles of the *RB1* gene were required for tumor development to begin.

The majority of mutations of *RB1* occur between internal exons 2 and 25. There are more than 930 reported mutations, identified in more than 1000 families. The band of *RB1* mutations is very diverse, and does not demonstrate any distinct hotspots, although certain discrete hotspots of recurrent mutations have been characterized. The majority of these recurrent mutations are associated with C to T transitions in CGA codons. Normally in genetic mutations of large genes, the specific location of the stop codon will influence the phenotypic expression. This is not the case with *RB1*; the precise site of the mutation does not alter the phenotype.

The method of mutation analysis depends on the patient's family history and the specimens (blood or tumor) that are available. The mutations of *RB1* are distributed along almost the entire length of the gene, which suggests that no single analysis method will be fully sensitive. Approximately 90 percent of all *RB1* mutations can be detected by current molecular analysis procedures whereas 10 percent cannot.

RETINOBLASTOMA

Retinoblastoma, in its hereditary or nonhereditary form, is a malignant tumor, or tumors, which develop from the immature retina. In order for tumorgenesis to occur, mutations in both alleles of the *RB1* gene are required. According to the Children's Oncology Group (2011), retinoblastoma occurs in early childhood and affects approximately 1 in 20,000 children. Only 6 to 10 percent of affected children have any previous family history.

As also reported by the Children's Oncology Group, hereditary retinoblastoma is responsible for approximately 40 percent of all cases. It is transmitted in an autosomal dominant fashion and is characterized by multiple tumors in both eyes. Patients with the hereditary form are heterozygous for a mutation of *RB1* that has been inherited from one of their parents or has occurred in embryonic development (*RB1+/RB1-*). Tumors are formed when a single mutation in the functioning *RB1* allele occurs, creating a loss of heterozygosity at the *RB1* locus. The nonhereditary form involves only one eye and a single tumor. These patients are wild-type homozygotes (*RB1+/RB1+*) and require two distinct mutational events to occur, causing a loss of function at both *RB1* loci in order for tumor formation to begin. The incidence of two mutational events occurring is rather low, in contrast to the single mutational event required for heterozygotes in order for tumor formation to be initiated.

If left untreated, retinoblastoma is consistently fatal, but with early diagnosis and current treatment methods, the survival rate is nearly 95 percent, according to the Retinoblastoma Center of Houston (2011). Survivors of hereditary retinoblastoma have a vulnerability toward other cancers, notably osteosarcoma (37 percent) and soft-tissue sarcomas (16.8 percent), melanomas (7.4 percent), brain tumors (4.5 percent), and leukemia (2.4 percent). The incidence of retinoblastoma appears to be increasing as early diagnosis and improved treatment options have improved the survival of patients who have gone on to transmit this autosomal dominant trait to the next generation.

IMPACT

The discovery and characterization of the *RB1* gene, its mutations, and protein product have been fundamental in the understanding of the mechanisms of inherited cancers. Knudsen's "two-hit" theory established a critical model for tumorgenesis, uncovering new mechanisms for cancer origination. Research has concentrated on the structure and function of the *RB1* gene, as well as the regulation of the transcription and translational anti-oncogenic activity of the *RB1* protein. Numerous mutational categories have been established and aligned with phenotypic expression. These findings are significant as they expand the ability of physicians to offer improved diagnostic, prognostic, and genetic counseling to patients, as well as more specialized therapeutic interventions.

April D. Ingram

FURTHER READING

Klintworth, Gordon K., Alec Garner, and J. Godfrey Heathcote. *Garner and Klintworth's Pathobiology of Ocular Disease*. London: Informa Healthcare, 2008. Print.

McKusick, Victor, Marschall Stevens Runge, and Cam Patterson. *Principles of Molecular Medicine*. Totowa: Humana, 2006. Print.

"Retinoblastoma." *Genetics Home Reference*. US Natl. Lib. of Medicine, 4 Aug. 2014. Web. 8 Aug. 2014.

Tan, Dongfeng, and Henry T. Lynch. *Principles of Molecular Diagnostics and Personalized Cancer Medicine*. Philadelphia: Lippincott, 2013. Print.

Vogelstein, Bert, and Kenneth W. Kinzler, eds. *The Genetic Basis of Human Cancer.* 2d ed. New York: McGraw, 2002. Print.

"What Is Retinoblastoma?" *American Cancer Society.* American Cancer Soc., 5 Dec. 2013. Web. 8 Aug. 2014.

See also: *BRAF* gene; *BRCA1* and *BRCA2* genes; *MLH1* gene; *PMS* genes; *RhoGD12* gene; *SCLC1* gene.

Refsum disease

CATEGORY: Diseases and syndromes

ALSO KNOWN AS: Phytanic acid oxidase deficiency; phytanic acid storage disease; heredopathia atactica polyneuritiformis; hereditary motor and sensory neuropathy IV (HMSN IV or HMSN4); classic Refsum disease (CRD); adult Refsum disease (ARD); Disorder of cornification 11 (phytanic acid type); Hereditary sensory and motor neuropathy type 4; Doc 11 (phytanic acid type); Hypertrophic neuropathy of Refsum

DEFINITION

Refsum disease is a very rare, severe, progressive inherited disorder that results in symptoms such as pain, difficulty walking, heart failure, skin issues, and/or loss of the ability to smell, see, and hear. The features of the disease are caused by the harmful buildup of fatty substances in the body and brain.

The feet of the elder sibling showed abnormal second and third toes with a shortened fourth metatarsal. By Hari Jayaram, via Wikimedia Commons

Extensive perivascular "bone spicule" pigmentation seen in both fundi of the younger sibling. By see above, via Wikimedia Commons

RISK FACTORS

Refsum disease is a genetic condition caused by the inheritance of the same nonworking gene that causes Refsum from both parents. Most Refsum disease cases have been reported in the United Kingdom and Norway. The incidence of the condition is very low. In the United Kingdom, the disease is found in 1 in 1,000,000 individuals. This condition is not caused by infections and cannot be transmitted by an affected individual.

ETIOLOGY AND GENETICS

Refsum disease is caused by the buildup of a substance called phytanic acid in the cells of the body. This abnormal buildup is caused by either a lack of an enzyme called phytanoyl-CoA hydroxylase or a decreased quantity of a critical cell part called the peroxisome-targeting signal type 2 receptor. When the enzyme or the receptor is missing, the accumulation of the phytanic acid in the cells, tissues, and body fluids results in the inability of the brain and body to work correctly.

Refsum disease is an autosomal recessive genetic condition, which occurs when a child receives two copies of a nonworking gene. Individuals with only one copy of a nonworking gene for a recessive condition are known as carriers and have no problems related to the condition. In fact, every individual carries between five and ten nonworking genes for harmful, recessive conditions. When two people with the same nonworking recessive gene meet, there is a chance, with each pregnancy, for the child to inherit two copies, one from each parent. That child then has no working copies of the gene and therefore has the signs and symptoms associated with the disease. Defects in two genes have been identified as the cause of Refsum disease: *PHYH* and *PEX7*. More than 90 percent of all cases of Refsum disease result from mutations in the PHYH gene. The remaining cases are caused by mutations in a gene called PEX7.

SYMPTOMS

The symptoms of Refsum disease involve progressive deterioration of motor and neurocognitive function including loss of smell, loss of physical milestones, a type of early-onset blindness called retinitis pigmentosa, nerve disorders (neuropathy), pain, deafness, stumbling gait, enlarged heart, heart arrhythmia, and cardiac failure. However, Refsum disease symptoms vary significantly in severity and time of onset from person to person. It is rare to see all the symptoms of Refsum disease in one individual.

The onset of Refsum disease can occur from seven months of age to mid-adulthood. The most common time of onset is late childhood. Symptoms often start with loss of the sense of smell (anosmia) and progressive loss of vision caused by a specific form retinal degeneration (retinitis pigmentosa). Over the next ten to fifteen years, as the disease progresses, affected individuals will often develop difficulty walking (ataxia), skin issues (ichthyosis), weakness, pain, and numbness from nerve malfunction (peripheral neuropathy), and possibly shortened finger or toe bones. Death most often occurs as a result of cardiac failure.

SCREENING AND DIAGNOSIS

Screening for Refsum disease is not part of routine testing in the prenatal or newborn periods of life. Theoretically, prenatal diagnosis supported by testing of cultured amniocytes is possible. In some cases, all members of a family, including a person with Refsum disease, are screened to reveal presymptomatic cases.

Diagnosis is most often suspected on the basis of disease signs and symptoms such as loss of smell, stumbling gait (ataxia), and early-onset blindness called retinitis pigmentosa. Biochemical testing is available to confirm the diagnosis through a combination of elevated phytanic acid levels in the blood and related chemicals and/or low or missing amounts of phytanoyl-CoA hydroxylase. Although there is often high protein levels found in the cerebrospinal fluid and low level of cholesterol in the blood, these may be found in many other disorders. X-rays and MRI imaging may be recommended to look for characteristic one and brain abnormalities. Molecular genetic testing for nonworking *PHYH* and *PEX7* genes is the most definitive test available.

TREATMENT AND THERAPY

At this time, there is no cure for Refsum disease. Chronic treatment of the condition relies on a special diet that removes phytanic acid intake. This involves elimination of all sources of chlorophyll from the diet. The major dietary exclusions are green vegetables (source of phytanic acid) and animal fat (phytol). Lifelong strict adherence to the diet is usually recommended. A high carbohydrate intake may also be recommended in order to avoid rapid weight loss tissue phytanic acid is metabolized. Periodic monitoring of fat-soluble vitamins, vitamin B-12, copper or selenium, and sodium is often recommended as well. Careful monitoring for cardiac arrhythmias and other heart abnormalities by a cardiologist is often needed. Other symptoms would be treated individually, such as using hydrating creams for skin issues.

If symptoms are severe and the patient is deteriorating, and there is a need for a rapid decrease in symptom causing phytanic acid levels, a treatment called plasmapheresis is sometimes used to quickly reduce the amount of phytanic acid in the blood. Use of ibuprofen must be avoided in individuals affected by Refsum disease as it may interfere with the breakdown of phytanic acid.

In patients with severe hearing loss in both ears, there may be a discussion about the possible benefits of cochlear implants.

A few approaches for treating the underlying lack of enzyme that causes Refsum disease are under investigation, such as enzyme replacement therapy, but these are not yet approved by the Food and Drug Administration (FDA) for use in affected individuals.

PREVENTION AND OUTCOMES

Carrier testing is available for individuals who are interested in learning if they carry a nonworking *PHYH* or *PEX7* gene. Genetic counseling is available for parents who have an affected child or are concerned about being a carrier for a nonworking *PHYH* or *PEX7* gene. As the severity and symptoms of Refsum disease vary from individual to individual, life expectancy depends on the ability to follow the special low-phytanic-acid diet as well as the speed of progression of the disease.

Dawn A. Laney, M.S.; updated by Gary M. Flashner, M.S., M.D.

FURTHER READING

Bompaire F, Marcaud V, Trionnaire EL, Sedel F, Levade T. "Refsum Disease Presenting with a Late-Onset Leukodystrophy." *JIMD Rep.* 2015. 19:7-10.

Gonick, Larry, and Mark Wheelis. *The Cartoon Guide to Genetics.* New York: Harper Perennial, 1991.

Parker, James, and Philip Parker, eds. *The Official Parent's Sourcebook on Refsum Disease: A Revised and Updated Directory for the Internet Age.* San Diego: Icon Health, 2002.

Sá MJ, Rocha JC, Almeida MF, Carmona C, Martins E, Miranda V, et al. "Infantile Refsum Disease: Influence of Dietary Treatment on Plasma Phytanic Acid Levels." *JIMD Rep.* 2015 Aug 25

Schönfeld P, Reiser G. "Brain Lipotoxicity of Phytanic Acid and Very Long-chain Fatty Acids. Harmful Cellular/Mitochondrial Activities in Refsum Disease and X-Linked Adrenoleukodystrophy." *Aging Dis.* 2016 Mar. 7 (2):136-49.

Wanders RJA, Waterham HR, Leroy BP. "Refsum Disease." 2006 Mar 20 [Updated 2015 Jun 11]. In: Pagon RA, Adam MP, Ardinger HH, et al., editors. GeneReviews® [Internet]. Seattle (WA): University of Washington, Seattle; 1993-2017.

Willett, Edward. *Genetics Demystified.* New York: McGraw Hill, 2005.

WEB SITES OF INTEREST

National Institute of Neurological Disorders and Stroke (NINDS): Refsum Disease Information Page http://www.ninds.nih.gov/disorders/refsum/refsum.htm

United Leukodystrophy Foundation

http://www.ulf.org

https://rarediseases.info.nih.gov/diseases/5691/refsum-disease

https://ghr.nlm.nih.gov/condition/refsum-disease

http://emedicine.medscape.com/article/1114720-overview

See also: Adrenoleukodystrophy; Alexander disease; Alzheimer's disease; Amyotrophic lateral sclerosis; Arnold-Chiari syndrome; Ataxia telangiectasia; Canavan disease; Cerebrotendinous xanthomatosis; Charcot-Marie-Tooth syndrome; Chediak-Higashi syndrome; Dandy-Walker syndrome; Deafness; Epilepsy; Essential tremor; Friedreich ataxia; Huntington's disease; Jansky-Bielschowsky disease; Joubert syndrome; Kennedy disease; Krabbé disease; Leigh syndrome; Leukodystrophy; Limb girdle muscular dystrophy; Maple syrup urine disease; Metachromatic leukodystrophy; Myoclonic epilepsy associated with ragged red fibers (MERRF); Narcolepsy; Nemaline myopathy; Neural tube defects; Neurofibromatosis; Parkinson disease; Pelizaeus-Merzbacher disease; Pendred syndrome; Periodic paralysis syndrome; Prion diseases: Kuru and Creutzfeldt-Jakob syndrome; Spinal muscular atrophy; Vanishing white matter disease.

Reiter's syndrome and genetics

CATEGORY: Diseases and syndromes

ALSO KNOWN AS: Reactive arthritis; Post-infectious arthritis; Post-infectious reactive arthropathy; PIRA; Reiter syndrome

DEFINITION

Reiter's syndrome is an inflammatory reaction to an infection somewhere in the body. It usually follows a urogenital or intestinal infection. Symptoms of the disorder primarily involve three body systems: the joints, the eyes, and the urinary or genital tract.

RISK FACTORS

Risk factors include having family members with Reiter's syndrome and inheriting the genetic trait associated with Reiter's syndrome (*HLA-B27*). The disease is more common in males and may be relatively high among patients with AIDS, especially men who are seropositive for HLA-B27. Those between ages twenty and forty seem to be most at risk. As noted under "Definition", the risk is much greater following a urogenital or intestinal infection, the latter causing the majority of uncommon cases in children. About 10% of patients have no preceding symptomatic infection.

ETIOLOGY AND GENETICS

The causes of Reiter's syndrome are not well understood, but it seems clear that both genetic and environmental factors play contributing roles. Approximately 80 percent of affected individuals carry the *HLA-B27* gene, but not all individuals who express this gene will develop the disease. For

A differential diagnosis revealed that the rash on the bottom of this individual's feet, known as keratoderma blennorrhagica, was due to Reiter's syndrome, not a syphilitic infection as was initially suspected. Reiter's syndrome, sometimes referred to as "seronegative spondyloarthropathy" or "reactive arthritis", consists of predominately three symptoms: arthritis, conjunctivitis, and urinary tract infections, or urethritis. More recently, doctors have recognized a fourth major feature, ulcerations of the skin and mouth. By Photo Credit: Content Providers(s): CDC/ Dr. M. F. Rein Transwiki approved by: w:en:User:Dmcdevit, via Wikimedia Commons

example, while 50 percent of the children of an affected parent will inherit the *HLA-B27* gene, only about 25 percent of these will subsequently develop Reiter's syndrome following a triggering event. This gene is one of a family of genes located at the major histocompatability locus on the short arm of chromosome 6 (at position 6p21.3). It encodes a protein that is present on the surface of almost all cells and functions to display protein fragments (peptides) that have been exported from the cell to components of the immune system. If the antigens are recognized as foreign, an inflammatory response is triggered. The conditions under which the HLA-B27 protein initiates an inflammatory response resulting in reactive arthritis are not clear, and theories range from the improper presentation of peptides to the misfolding of the protein itself. This gene variant is also associated with a group of autoimmune disorders known as the seronegative spondarthritides, the most common of which are ankylosing spondylitis and psoriatic of the *HLA-B27* gene variant varies quite widely among different human populations. It is found in about 8 percent of Caucasians and only 3 to 5 percent of African Americans, but it is present in as many as 25 percent of Eskimo populations and 50 percent of Haida Indians. A simple blood test is available to determine if an individual carries this gene.

SYMPTOMS

Symptoms occur in three main areas of the body: the joints, the eyes, and the urinary tract and genitals. Men and women may experience different symptoms. The disease may be milder in women. Symptoms may come and go. In rare cases, heart and kidney problems may develop.

Specific symptoms in the joints include asymmetric swelling, pain, and redness, especially in the knees, ankles, and feet; heel pain; thickening and sausage-shaped deformity of fingers; and back pain and stiffness.

Symptoms in the eyes include redness, pain, irritation, blurred vision, tearing, discharge, and sometimes sun sensitivity or swollen eyelids. Exam may show inflammation affecting anatomic locations in multiple areas of the eye.

Symptoms in the male urinary tract and reproductive system include frequent urination, a burning sensation when passing urine, penile discharge, sores at the end of the penis, fever, and chills. Symptoms in the female urinary tract and reproductive system include a burning sensation when passing urine and an inflamed vagina and cervix. Similar to eye exam findings noted above, examination may show inflammation affecting anatomic locations in multiple areas of the male and female urogenital organs.

Other symptoms include rash, especially on the palms or soles; ulcers in the mouth or on the tongue; changes in fingernails/toenails; weight loss; poor appetite; fatigue; and fever.

Rare complications may include heart problems, such as heart conduction defects, including

SOA-arthritis public domain via wikimedia commons

arrhythmia, a heart murmur (aortic insufficiency), and pericarditis (an inflammation of the outer lining of heart). Other rare complications may include lung problems, such as pneumonia, pulmonary fibrosis, and fluid on the lung (pleural effusion). There may also be nervous system problems, such as neuropathy, which may include a tingling or loss of sensation, and behavior changes.

SCREENING AND DIAGNOSIS

The doctor may ask about a patient's symptoms and medical history and may perform a physical exam. The doctor uses these findings to help make the diagnosis. There is no specific test to check for.

REITER'S SYNDROME

Testing may include blood tests to check for signs of inflammation (sedimentation rate and C-reactive protein), signs of infection and anemia (complete blood count), and the genetic factor associated with Reiter's syndrome (*HLA-B27*). Additional tests may include culture, gram stain, or other tests to look for bacteria that commonly cause infections associated with Reiter's syndrome; HIV testing for those patients at risk; TB skin testing for those at risk; the removal of synovial fluid from around the joints to check for infection; X rays; ultrasound, a test that uses sound waves to examine the inside of the body; a magnetic resonance imaging (MRI) scan, a test that uses magnetic and radio waves to make pictures of the inside of the body; and a computed tomography (CT) scan, a type of X ray that uses a computer to make pictures of the inside of the body.

TREATMENT AND THERAPY

There is no cure for Reiter's syndrome. However, early treatment of the infection may slow or stop the course of the disease. Most patients recover from the initial episode within six months. However, as many as 30% of patients may develop chronic symptoms. Some patients suffer from additional bouts of the disorder.

Treatment aims to relieve symptoms and may include short-term bed rest to take the strain off the joints, and exercise, including gentle range-of-motion exercises to improve flexibility, strengthening to build muscles that can better support the joints, and physical therapy with specific exercises to keep muscles strong and joints moving. Treatment also aims to protect the joints, which may include the use of assistive devices and occupational.

The doctor may prescribe medications, including nonsteroidal anti-inflammatory drugs (NSAIDs), such as aspirin and ibuprofen. Additional medications may include sulfasalazine (Azulfidine), steroid injections into the inflamed joint, topical steroid creams applied to skin lesions, and, in some cases, antibiotics to treat the triggering infection. No dietary limitations are necessary unless the patient is receiving steroid therapy.

Immunosuppressive drugs (drugs that decrease the immune system's ability to function), such as azathioprine (Imuran) and methotrexate, and eye drops may also be prescribed.

Unfortunately, few treatment options exist for HIV-infected patients with severe Reiter's syndrome. Treatment in the setting of HIV infection poses special problems. However, potentially immunosuppressive therapies (eg, cyclosporine, methotrexate, and psoralen plus ultraviolet A [PUVA]) have been used in some cases, with variable success and relatively few severe complications.

No specific surgical interventions are typically recommended; however, in those who develop eye complications, surgical intervention may be needed to prevent permanent loss of vision.

PREVENTION AND OUTCOMES

In most cases, the key to preventing Reiter's syndrome is to avoid the triggering infection. As regards triggers from urogenital infections, safe sex practices are recommended including the use of barrier methods such as condoms. As regards intestinal infections, it is recommended that raw foods be appropriately stored, washed, handled and prepared/cooked. Appropriate hand-washing is also a key component to preventing intestinal infections.

As noted under "Treatment and Therapy", surgical intervention may be needed to prevent permanent visual loss in those who experience eye complications.

Patients who know that they carry the HLA-B27 gene may be advised to be particularly cautious as regards to potential exposure to triggering infections. Debra Wood, R.N.; reviewed by Jill D. Landis, M.D. "Etiology and Genetics" by Jeffrey A. Knight, Ph.D.; updated by Gary M. Flashner, M.S., M.D.

FURTHER READING

Alvarez-Navarro C, Cragnolini JJ, Dos Santos HG, Barnea E, Admon A, Morreale A, et al. "Novel HLA-B27-restricted epitopes from Chlamydia trachomatis generated upon endogenous processing of bacterial proteins suggest a role of molecular mimicry in reactive arthritis." *J Biol Chem.* 2013 Sep 6. 288(36):25810-25.

Carter JD, Hudson AP. "Recent advances and future directions in understanding and treating Chlamydia-induced reactive arthritis." *Expert Rev Clin Immunol.* 2016 Sep 20. 1-10.

EBSCO Publishing. *Health Library: Reiter's Syndrome.*

Fauci, Anthony S., et al., eds. *Harrison's Principles of Internal Medicine.* 17th ed. New York: McGraw-Hill Medical, 2008.

Firestein, Gary S., ed. *Kelley's Textbook of Rheumatology.* 8th ed. Philadelphia: Saunders/Elsevier, 2009. Goldman, Lee, and Dennis Ausiello, eds. *Cecil Medi- cine.* 23d ed. Philadelphia: Saunders Elsevier, 2008.

Goroll, Allan H., and Albert G. Mulley, Jr., eds. *Primary Care Medicine: Office Evaluation and Management of the Adult Patient.* 6th ed. Philadelphia: Wolters Kluwer Health/Lippincott Williams & Wilkins, 2009.

Ipswich, Mass.: Author, 2009. Available through http://www.ebscohost.com.

Kobayashi S, Ichikawa G. "Reactive arthritis induced by tonsillitis: a type of 'focal infection'." *Adv Otorhinolaryngol.* 2011. 72:79-82.

Noble, John, et al. *Textbook of Primary Care Medicine.* 3d ed. St. Louis: Mosby, 2001.

Schmitt SK. Reactive Arthritis. *Infect Dis Clin North Am.* 2017 Mar 11.

Singh AK, Misra R, Aggarwal A. "Th-17 associated cytokines in patients with reactive arthritis/undifferentiated spondyloarthropathy." *Clin Rheumatol.* 2011 Jun. 30(6):771-6

WEB SITES OF INTEREST
American College of Obstetrics and Gynecology: "Why Screen for Chlamydia?"
http://www.acog.org/departments/dept_notice.cfm?recno=7&bulletin=4805

Arthritis Foundation
http://www.arthritis.org

The Arthritis Society
http://www.arthritis.ca

National Institute of Arthritis and Musculoskeletal and Skin Diseases
http://www.niams.nih.gov

Public Health Agency of Canada
http://www.phac-aspc.gc.ca

Spondylitis Association of America
http://www.spondylitis.org
http://emedicine.medscape.com/article/331347-overview#a1
https://rarediseases.info.nih.gov/diseases/5693/reactive-arthritis

See also: Agammaglobulinemia; Allergies; Antibodies; Anthrax; Ataxia telangiectasia; Autoimmune disorders; Autoimmune polyglandular syndrome; Chediak-Higashi syndrome; Chronic granulomatous disease; Hybridomas and monoclonal antibodies; Immunodeficiency with hyper-IgM; Immunogenetics; Infantile agranulocytosis; Myeloperoxidase deficiency; Purine nucleoside phosphorylase deficiency.

Repetitive DNA

CATEGORY: Molecular genetics

SIGNIFICANCE: Eukaryotic nuclei contain repetitive DNA elements of different origin (polymorphisms) that constitute between 20 and 90 percent of the genome, depending on the species. These repetitive DNA sequences are typically moved through DNA by specific DNA interactions (transposons via transposition) or using RNA intermediates (retrotransposons via retrotransposition). The human genome is composed of about 42 percent retrotransposons and 2 to 3 percent transposons. The presence and type of repetitive DNA elements have provided insights into evolution, gene flow, gene mapping, forensic investigation, and various aspects of biomedicine, including disease diagnosis and detection.

KEY TERMS

allele: an alternative form of a gene located at a specific location or locus on a chromosome

nucleotide: a basic unit of DNA, consisting of a five-carbon sugar, a nitrogen-containing base, and a phosphate group *polymorphism:* the existence of different alleles for a particular gene locus among individuals of the same species

retrotransposition: the movement of repetitive DNA sequences within a genome via RNA intermediates

tandem repetitive DNA (TR-DNA): nucleotide sequences that include repeating sections oriented in head-to-tail arrays, such as (GGAAT)

ntransposon: a DNA segment that is able to replicate itself and insert the new DNA sequence either in a new location within the same chromosome or into another chromosome or plasmid

variable number tandem repeat (VNTR): a DNA sequence in which short nucleotide sequences are repeated over and over; chromosomes from different individuals frequently have different numbers of the basic repeat

TYPES OF REPETITIVE DNA

The eukaryotic nuclear genome is characterized by repetitive DNA elements in the form of nucleotide sequences of varying length and base composition, either localized to a particular region of the genome or dispersed throughout it (for example, on different chromosomes). Some of these DNA elements are repeated only a few times, whereas others

may be repeated millions or billions of times; thus, the percentage of the total genome represented by repetitive DNA varies widely among taxa. Tandem repeats are repetitive DNA sequences that are adjacent to each other in a block or array, whereas interspersed repeats are found throughout the genome, surrounded by unique (non-repetitive) DNA sequences.

The two major classes of tandem repetitive DNAs (TR-DNAs) are those that are localized to a particular region or regions of the genome and those that are dispersed throughout the genome. TR-DNAs feature repeating units that are oriented in head-to-tail arrays. The repetitive units of an array may be genes, promoters, or intergenic spacers, or they may be simple nucleotide sequences. For example, in the kangaroo rat, the simple sequence AAG is repeated 2.4 billion times.

Localized TR-DNA is often composed of members of multigene families. For example, in humans, there are 350 copies of the ribosomal RNA (rRNA) genes on five different chromosomes that occur as tandemly repeated arrays. Transfer RNA (tRNA) and immunoglobin genes are other examples of multigene families that are tandemly repeated. However, most localized TR-DNA consists of simple,

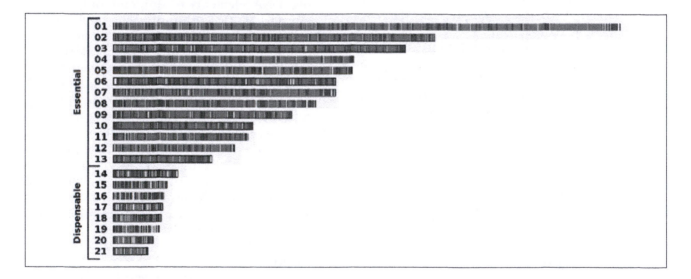

The 21 chromosomes of the Mycosphaerella graminicola genome drawn to scale. Red indicates regions of single-copy sequence; repetitive sequences are in shown blue. Chromosome 1 is almost twice as long as any of the others. The core chromosomes 1–13 are the largest. Dispensable chromosomes 14–21 are smaller than the core chromosomes and have a higher proportion of repetitive DNA as indicated by the blue bands. By Stephen B. *Goodwin, Sarrah Ben M'Barek, Braham Dhillon, Alexander H. J. Wittenberg, Charles F. Crane, James K. Hane, Andrew J. Foster, Theo A. J. Van der Lee, Jane Grimwood, Andrea Aerts, John Antoniw, Andy Bailey, Burt Bluhm, Judith Bowler, Jim Bristo*

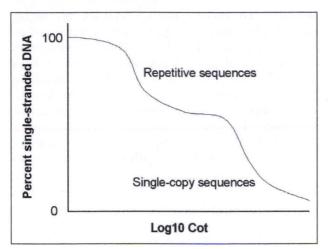

CoT analysis of amount of repetitive DNA sequence By Tim Vickers (Own work), via Wikimedia Commons

noncoding repetitive DNA sequences that often, but not always, can be found in heterochromatic or centromeric regions.

Dispersed TR-DNA sequences are scattered throughout the genome and can be divided into two major groups: short interspersed elements (SINEs) and long interspersed repeats (LINEs). TR-DNA sequences are sometimes referred to as satellite DNA, classified according to length of the repeated unit and length as a whole as either satellites, minisatellites, or microsatellites.

ORIGIN AND EVOLUTION OF DISPERSED REPETITIVE DNA ELEMENTS

Dispersed repetitive DNA is believed to be an evolutionary device that catalyzes the formation of new genes. Within a species, DNA sequences are thought to maintain similarity by gene conversion (a type of DNA repair mechanism that occurs during meiosis and is believed to maintain the DNA coding sequence of the organism being replicated), while repetitive sequences disrupt this process and allow new genes to evolve. SINEs are believed to disrupt gene conversions between chromosomes, while the longer LINE elements disrupt the gene conversions within the chromosome. SINEs are transposable elements, capable of "jumping" from one locus to another via an RNA intermediate. SINEs are called nonviral retropseudogenes because they are derived from mRNA transcripts of DNA sequences. The RNA transcript is reverse transcribed into DNA and then inserted into the genome. Although SINEs resemble the genes

from which they derived, they no longer function properly. The most common and best-characterized SINEs in humans are the highly repetitive *Alu* sequences, so named because they are cleaved multiple times by the restriction endonuclease *Alu*I, derived from the bacterium *Arthrobacter luteus*. An estimated one million *Alu* sequence copies are scattered across the human genome, each one approximately 300 base pairs (bp) in length, constituting as much as 10 percent of the human genome. These *Alu* repeat sequences may have developed by retrotransposition of the 7SL RNA gene sequence. They include an RNA polymerase III promoter sequence that is sometimes transcribed.

LINEs are derived from a viral ancestor and are also capable of transposition. The most common LINE elements in humans, and the only type that still actively transposes, are designated LINE-1, or L1, and make up around 17 percent of the human genome. Full-length, functional (that is, transpositionally competent) L1 elements are approximately 6 kb in length, but most copies of L1 are truncated at the 5' end and incapable of moving. Full-length L1 copies contain two protein-coding regions, or open reading frames (ORFs): Open reading frames (ORFs) ORF-1 and ORF-2. ORF-1 encodes an RNA-binding protein, and ORF-2 codes for reverse transcriptase. The transposition of LINE elements into various parts of the genome is believed to contribute to evolution through the creation of new genes with altered ORFs.

ARE INTERSPERSED REPEATED ELEMENTS "JUNK" DNA?

Repeated DNA elements were once believed to be "selfish" DNA or "junk" DNA, DNA concerned only with their own proliferation within the host cell's genome. Recent studies, however, reveal that repetitive elements interact with the genome with profound evolutionary consequences. For example, satellite DNA found near the centromere may play a role in assembling and fusing chromosomal microtubules during cell division. In addition, transposable genetic elements such as SINEs, LINEs, and *Alu* sequences may have played a significant role in the evolution of particular proteins. For example, *Alu* elements flanking the primordial human growth hormone gene are believed to be responsible for the evolution the chorionic somatomammotropin hormone 1 (*CSH1*) gene. Transposable repeated elements may have contributed substantially to the origin of new gene functions by initiating a copy of an existing gene (which, over time, may acquire a different function) or by creating a "composite" gene composed of domains from two or more previously unrelated genes.

CLASSIFICATION OF SIMPLE TANDEM REPEATS

TR-DNA sequences are classified into four major groups based on three characteristics: the number of nucleotides in the repetitive unit, the number of times the unit is repeated, and whether the element is localized or scattered across the genome. The four groups include satellites, minisatellites, microsatellites, and dispersed *Alu* sequences. Satellite DNA is composed of tandemly repeated basic DNA sequences, ranging from two to hundreds of nucleotides in length and repeated more than one thousand times, locally, in the DNA. Satellite DNA represents an example of a localized simple repeat typically found in the centromeric region of a chromosome. Tandemly repeated basic DNA sequences, ranging from nine to one hundred nucleotides in length, repeated ten to one hundred times, and scattered throughout the genome are known as minisatellites. Microsatellites are also dispersed repetitive sequence elements; however, microsatellites are composed of short DNA sequence repeats of a basic unit one to six nucleotides in length that are tandemly repeated ten to one hundred times at each locus. The most common microsatellite loci in humans are dinucleotide arrays of $(CA)_N$. However, on average, at least one tri- or tetranucleotide microsatellite locus is found in each 10 kilobase pairs (kb) of human genomic DNA. In a separate group, the basic unit of dispersed *Alu* sequences is one to five nucleotides in length, and this unit is repeated ten to forty times per locus.

POLYMORPHISM AT LOCI COMPOSED OF SIMPLE TANDEM REPEATS

For purposes of convenience, the four groups of simple tandem repeats discussed above (satellite DNA, minisatellites, microsatellites, and *Alu* sequences) are sometimes collectively referred to as variable number tandem repeats (VNTRs). Separate VNTR loci are thought of as alleles; therefore, in humans, each VNTR locus will be represented by two alleles, one paternal and the other maternally inherited. All VNTR loci exhibit high rates of mutation. For these reasons, VNTR loci are highly polymorphic, meaning that a large number of alleles exist at any given locus. This polymorphism can be assayed using laboratory techniques such as polymerase chain reaction (PCR) or Southern blotting to examine the differences in the lengths of the alleles (repetitive elements) at a particular DNA locus. Length differences at VNTR loci arise as a result of mispairing of repeats during replication, mitosis, or meiosis, theoretically resulting in the loss or gain of one to many of the repeat units. Empirical studies and computer-based modeling experiments have demonstrated that each mutation usually increases or decreases the number of repeated units of an allele in a "one-step" manner. In other words, most mutations result in the loss or gain of only one repeated unit.

The multiallelic variation arising through this variation in repeat copy number provides useful genetic markers for many different applications. For example, under conditions of random mating and because of high mutation rates at VNTR loci, most individuals within the human population are heterozygous at any selected VNTR locus. This observation directly led to the origin of DNA fingerprinting (or DNA profiling), which is now considered admissible forensic evidence in many judicial systems worldwide. Length variation of VNTRs creates a powerful tool for identity analysis (for example, paternity testing) and is routinely used by population geneticists to examine gene flow among populations. In the fields of genomics and biomedicine, VNTR loci are useful genetic landmarks for mapping the location of other genes of interest, including genes with a particular function or those implicated in disease.

TRANSPOSABLE ELEMENTS AND HUMAN DISEASE

Retrotranspositions of LINEs and SINEs into coding or noncoding genomic DNAs represent major insertional mutations. The effects of such insertions vary but are usually deleterious, leading to debilitating human diseases. Among a growing list of diseases known in some cases to be caused by the insertion of LINEs or SINEs are Duchenne muscular dystrophy, Glanzmann thrombasthenia, hemophilia, hypercholesterolemia, neurofibromatosis, Sandhoff disease, and Tay-Sachs disease. Translocation of repeated sequences has also been demonstrated to "turn on" tumorogenic oncogenes; for example, one type of colon cancer is associated with the insertion of repetitive DNA.

Other studies suggest that "unstable" VNTRs, including minisatellite, microsatellite, and *Alu* loci, can also cause disease. These studies suggest that a threshold number of repeats of the basic nucleotide unit may exist that can be accommodated at a given locus. When this threshold number of repeats is exceeded by over-amplification of the basic repeated unit, serious diseases may arise. Among the diseases attributed to over-amplification of tandem repeats of simple DNA sequences are fragile X syndrome and Huntington's disease.

J. Craig Bailey, Ph.D.;
updated by Joy Frestedt, Ph.D., RAC, CCTI

FURTHER READING

Garrido-Ramos, Manuel A., ed. *Repetitive DNA.* Basel: Karger, 2012. Print. Vol. 7 of *Genome Dynamics.* M. Schmid, gen. ed. 7 vols. to date. 2006–. Korf, Bruce R., and Mira B. Irons. *Human Genetics and Genomics.* 4th ed. Chichester: Wiley, 2013. Print.

Lander, Eric S., et al. "Initial Sequencing and Analysis of the Human Genome." *Nature* 409.6822 (2001): 860–921. Print.

Li, Wen-Hsiung. *Molecular Evolution.* Sunderland: Sinauer, 1997. Print.

Maichele, Andrea J., Nancy J. Farwell, and Jeffrey S. Chamberlain. "A B2 Repeat Insertion Generates Alternate Structures of the Mouse Muscle γ-Phosphorylase Kinase Gene." *Genomics* 16.1 (1993): 139–49. Print.

Maraia, Richard J., ed. *The Impact of Short Interspersed Elements (SINEs) on the Host Genome.* Austin: Landes, 1995. Print.

Meisenberg, Gerhard, and William H. Simmons. *Principles of Medical Biochemistry.* 3rd ed. Philadelphia: Saunders, 2012. Print.

Shapiro, James A. "A 21st Century View of Evolution: Genome System Architecture, Repetitive DNA, and Natural Genetic Engineering." *Gene* 345.1 (2005): 91–100. Print.

Shapiro, James A., and Richard von Sternberg. "Why Repetitive DNA Is Essential to Genome Function." *Biological Reviews* 80.2 (2005): 227–50. Print.

Strachan, Tom, and Andrew P. Read. *Human Molecular Genetics.* 4th ed. New York: Garland, 2011. Print.

See also: Aging; Anthrax; Chromosome structure; Chromosome walking and jumping; DNA fingerprinting; Gene families; Genome size; Genomics; Human genetics; Model Organism: *Neurospora-crassa*; Molecular clock hypothesis; Pseudogenes; RFLP analysis; Telomeres.

Restriction enzymes

CATEGORY: Genetic engineering and biotechnology; Molecular genetics

SIGNIFICANCE: Restriction enzymes are bacterial enzymes that are capable of cutting DNA molecules at specific nucleotide sequences. The discovery of these enzymes was a pivotal event in the development of genetic engineering technology, and they are routinely and widely used in molecular biology.

KEY TERMS

enzyme: a molecule, usually a protein, that is used by cells to facilitate and speed up a chemical reaction

methylation: the process of adding a methyl chemical group (one carbon atom and three hydrogen atoms) to a particular molecule, such as a DNA nucleotide

nuclease: a type of enzyme that breaks down the sugar-phosphate backbone of nucleic acids such as DNA and RNA

nucleotides: the building blocks of nucleic acids, composed of a sugar, a phosphate group, and nitrogencontaining bases

DISCOVERY AND ROLE OF RESTRICTION ENZYMES IN BACTERIA

Nucleases are a broad class of enzymes that destroy nucleic acids by breaking the sugar-phosphate backbone of the molecule. Until 1970, the only known nucleases were those that destroyed nucleic acids nonspecifically—that is, in a random fashion. For this reason, these enzymes were of limited usefulness for working with nucleic acids such as DNA and RNA. In 1970, molecular biologist Hamilton O. Smith discovered a type of nuclease that could fragment DNA molecules in a specific and therefore predictable pattern. This nuclease, HindII, was the first restriction endonuclease, or restriction enzyme. Smith was

The process of cutting DNA with restriction enzymes. (U.S. Department of Energy Human Genome Program, http://www.ornl.gov/hgmis)

working with the bacterium Haemophilus influenzae (H. influenzae) when he discovered this enzyme, which is capable of destroying DNA from other bacterial species but not the DNA of H. influenzae itself. The term "restriction" refers to the apparent role these enzymes play in destroying the DNA of invading bacteriophages

As more restriction enzymes from a wide variety of bacterial species were discovered in the 1970s, it became increasingly clear that these enzymes could be useful for creating and manipulating DNA fragments in unique ways. What was not clear was how these enzymes were able to distinguish between bacteriophage DNA and the bacterial cell's own DNA. A chemical comparison between DNA that could and could not be fragmented revealed that the

DNA molecules differed slightly at the restriction sites (the locations the enzyme recognized and cut). Nucleotides at the restriction site were found to have methyl functional groups (–CH3) attached to them, giving this phenomenon the name DNA methylation.

The conclusion was that the methylation somehow protected the DNA from attack, which could account for Smith's observation that H. influenzae DNA was not destroyed by its own restriction enzyme; presumably the enzyme recognized a specific methylation pattern on the DNA molecule and left it alone. Foreign DNA, such as that from another species, would not have the correct methylation pattern, or might not be methylated at all, and could therefore be fragmented by the restriction enzyme. Hence, restriction enzymes are now regarded as part of a simple yet effective bacterial defense mechanism to guard against foreign DNA, which can enter bacterial cells with relative ease.

MECHANISM OF ACTION

To begin the process of cleaving a DNA molecule, a restriction enzyme must first recognize the appropriate place on the molecule. The recognition site for most restriction enzymes involves a short, usually four- to six-nucleotide palindromic sequence. A palindrome is a word or phrase that reads the same backward and forward, such as "Otto" or "madam"; in terms of DNA, a palindromic sequence is one that reads the same on each strand of DNA but in opposite directions. *Eco*RI, derived from the bacterium *Escherichia coli*, is an example of an enzyme that has a recognition site composed of nucleotides arranged in a palindromic sequence:

——GAATTC——————CTTAAG——

restriction enzyme EcoRI By Tinastella (Own work), via Wikimedia Commons

Whether the top sequence is read from left to right or the bottom sequence is read from right to left, it is always GAATTC.

An additional consideration in the mechanism of restriction-enzyme activity is the type of cut that is made. When a restriction enzyme cuts DNA, it is actually breaking the "backbone" of the molecule, which consists of a chain of sugar and phosphate molecules. This breakage occurs at a precise spot on each strand of the double-stranded DNA molecule. The newly created ends of the DNA fragments are informally referred to as either "sticky ends" or "blunt ends," depending on whether or not single-stranded regions of DNA are generated by the cutting activity of the restriction enzyme. For example, the enzyme *Eco*RI is a sticky-end cutter; when the cuts are made at the recognition site, the result is:

—GAATTC— —G AATTC—
→
—CTTAAG— —CTTAA G—

The break in the DNA backbone is made just after the G in each strand; this helps weaken the connections between the nucleotides in the middle of the site, and the DNA molecule splits into two fragments. The single-stranded regions, where the bases TTAA are not paired with their complements (AATT) on the other strand, are called overhangs; however, the bases in one overhang are still capable of pairing with the bases in the other overhang, as they did before the DNA strands were cut. The ends of these fragments will readily stick to each other if brought close together—hence the name "sticky ends."

Enzymes that create blunt ends make a flush cut and do not leave any overhangs, as demonstrated by the cutting site of the enzyme *Alu*I: *RAB23*

——AGCT—— ——AG CT——
→
——TCGA—— ——TC GA——

Because of the lack of overhanging single-strand regions, these two DNA fragments will not readily rejoin. In practice, either type of restriction enzyme may be used, but enzymes that produce sticky ends are generally favored over blunt-end cutters because of the ease with which the resulting fragments can be rejoined.

IMPACT AND APPLICATIONS

It is no exaggeration to say that the entire field of genetic engineering would have been impossible without the discovery and widespread use of restriction enzymes. On the most basic level, restriction enzymes allow scientists to create recombinant DNA molecules (hybrid molecules containing DNA from different sources, such as humans and bacteria). No matter what the source, DNA molecules can be cut with restriction enzymes to produce fragments that can then be rejoined in new combinations with DNA fragments from other molecules. This technology has led to advances such as the production of human insulin by bacterial cells such as *Escherichia coli*.

The DNA of most organisms is relatively large and complex; in fact, it is usually so large that it becomes difficult to manipulate and study the DNA of some organisms, such as humans. Restriction enzymes provide a convenient way to cut large DNA molecules very specifically into smaller fragments that can then be used more easily in a variety of molecular genetics procedures.

Another area of genetic engineering that is possible because of restriction enzymes is the production of restriction maps. A restriction map is a diagram of a DNA molecule showing where particular restriction enzymes cut the molecule and the molecular sizes of the fragments that are generated. The restriction sites can then be used as markers for further study of the DNA molecule and to help geneticists locate important genetic regions. Use of restriction enzymes has also revealed other interesting and useful markers of the human genome, called restriction fragment length polymorphisms (RFLP). The name refers to changes in the size of restriction fragments caused by mutations in the recognition site for a particular restriction enzyme. The recognition site is mutated so that the restriction enzyme no longer cuts there, resulting in one long fragment where, before the mutation, there would have been two shorter fragments. These changes in fragment length can then be used as markers for the region of DNA in question. Because they result from mutations in the DNA sequence, they are inherited from one generation to the next. Thus, these mutations have been a valuable tool for molecular biologists mapping human DNA and for those scientists involved in "fingerprinting" individuals by means of their DNA.

Because restriction enzymes cannot be used to make specific, chosen cuts in the DNA, scientists continued searching for ways to overcome this obstacle. In 2012, Jennifer Doudna of the University of California, Berkeley, and Emmanuelle Charpentier of the Helmholtz Centre for Infection Research in Germany, first announced that they had invented a new method for editing DNA that they called CRISPR. In subsequent years, they and other researchers used the tool to create molecules that could cut their DNA at points chosen by the researcher, eventually repairing defective DNA in mice.

Randall K. Harris, Ph.D.; updated by Bryan Ness,
Ph.D.

FURTHER READING

Allison, Lizabeth A. *Fundamental Molecular Biology.* 2nd ed. Hoboken: Wiley, 2012. Print.

Drlica, Karl. *Understanding DNA and Gene Cloning: A Guide for the Curious.* 4th ed. Hoboken: Wiley, 2004. Print.

Karp, Gerald. *Cell and Molecular Biology: Concepts and Experiments.* 7th ed. Hoboken: Wiley, 2013. Print.

Krebs, Jocelyn E., Elliott S. Goldstein, and Stephen T. Kilpatrick. *Lewin's Genes XI.* Burlington: Jones, 2014. Print.

Loenen, Wil A. M., and Elisabeth A. Raleigh. "The Other Face of Restriction: Modification-Dependent Enzymes." *Nucleic Acids Research* 42.1 (2014): 56–69. Print.

Pratt, Charlotte W., and Kathleen Cornely. *Essential Biochemistry.* 3rd ed. Hoboken: Wiley, 2014. Print.

Tóth, Eszter, et al. "Restriction Enzyme Body Doubles and PCR Cloning: On the General Use of Type IIS Restriction Enzymes for Cloning." *PLOS ONE* 9.3 (2014): 1–12. Web. 13 Aug. 2014.

Voet, Donald, Judith G. Voet, and Charlotte W. Pratt. *Fundamentals of Biochemistry: Life at the Molecular Level.* 4th ed. Hoboken: Wiley, 2013. Print.

Watson, James D., et al. *Recombinant DNA: Genes and Genomes—A Short Course.* 3rd ed. New York: Freeman, 2007. Print.

Zimmer, Carl. "Breakthrough DNA Editor Borne of Bacteria." *Quanta Magazine.* Simons Foundation, 6 Feb. 2015. Web. 26 Jan. 2016.

See also: Bacterial genetics and cell structure; Bioinformatics; Biopharmaceuticals; Blotting: Southern, Northern, and Western; Cloning; Cloning vectors; DNA fingerprinting; Forensic genetics; Gender identity; Genetic engineering; Genetic engineering: Historical development; Genetic engineering: Social and ethical issues; Genomic libraries; Model organism: Xenopus laevis; Molecular genetics; Population genetics; RFLP analysis; Shotgun cloning; Synthetic genes.

Retinitis pigmentosa

CATEGORY: Diseases and syndromes
ALSO KNOWN AS: RP; Rod-Cone Dystrophy

DEFINITION

Retinitis pigmentosa (RP) is a group of inherited eye diseases that often leads to severe visual problems. The retina is a layer of light-sensitive tissue that lines the back of the eye. It converts visual images that people see into nerve impulses that it sends to the brain. Some types of RP are associated with other inherited conditions. This disorder is named for the irregular clumps of black pigment that usually occur in the retina with this disease.

RISK FACTORS

Having family members with RP and being male are risk factors for the disease.

ETIOLOGY AND GENETICS

Retinitis pigmentosa is an inherited disorder, yet the identification of the genes involved has proven to be an extraordinary challenge. Since retinal cells are so highly specialized, it is not surprising that they depend on a large number of specific genes and their protein products to create vision. Mutations more than sixty different genes have been identified that can cause retinitis pigmentosa.

RP can be passed on by all types of inheritance: approximately 20% of RP is autosomal dominant (ADRP), 20% is autosomal recessive (ARRP), and 10% is X linked (XLRP), while the remaining 50% is found in patients without any known affected relatives. RP is most commonly found in isolation, but it can be associated with systemic disease.

If the the disease is inherited in an autosomal recessive fashion, which means that both copies of a particular gene must be deficient in order for the individual to be afflicted, then typically, an affected child is born to two unaffected parents, both of whom are carriers of the recessive mutant allele. The probable outcomes for children whose parents are both carriers are 75 percent unaffected and 25 percent affected. At least 35 genes have been associated with the autosomal recessive form of the disorder. The most common of these is USH2A; mutations in this gene are responsible for 10 to 15 percent of all cases of autosomal recessive retinitis pigmentosa.

Fundus of patient with retinitis pigmentosa, early stage. Hamel Orphanet Journal of Rare Diseases 2006 1:40 doi:10.1186/1750-1172-1-40 By Christian Hamel (Retinitis pigmentosa by Christian Hamel), via Wikimedia Commons

Photograph of the United States Supreme Court Building, modified to illustrate the effect of visual field loss, tunnel vision, in patients with Retinitis Pigmentosa. By Piksteel SANET STEYN (Own work), via Wikimedia Commons

Other retinitis pigmentosa mutations are inherited in an autosomal dominant manner, meaning that a single copy of the mutation is sufficient to cause full expression of the disease. An affected individual has a 50 percent chance of transmitting the mutation to each of his or her children. Many cases of dominant retinitis pigmentosa, however, result from a spontaneous new mutation, so in these instances affected individuals will have unaffected parents. Mutations in the RHO gene are the most common cause of autosomal dominant retinitis pigmentosa, accounting for 20 to 30 percent of all cases.

Changes in at least six genes are thought to cause the X-linked form of the disorder. Together, mutations in the RPGR and RP2 genes account for most cases of X-linked retinitis pigmentosa. Mothers who carry the mutated gene on one of their two X chromosomes face a 50 percent chance of transmitting this disorder to each of their male children. Female children have a 50 percent chance of inheriting the gene and becoming carriers like their mothers. Affected males will pass the mutation on to all of their daughters but to none of their sons.

Finally, one rare form of retinitis pigmentosa results from mutations in the mitochondrial gene *MT-ATP6*. Each retinal cell contains anywhere from several to more than one hundred copies of mito chondrial DNA (deoxyribonucleic acid) eligible for testing, and each mitochondrial DNA molecule con tains thirteen structural genes that encode protein components of respiratory chain complexes. Inheri tance of mitochondrial DNA follows a pattern of strict maternal inheritance, since all of the mito chondria in a fertilized egg (zygote) come from the egg cell. Thus affected females will transmit the dis ease to all of their offspring, but affected males pro duce unaffected children.

SYMPTOMS

Loss of vision is usually first noted in childhood or early adulthood. The disease gradually worsens. After a number of years, vision loss may become se vere. Symptoms var y, depending on the type of reti nal cell and eye structures affected. Both eyes often experience similar vision loss.

It should be noted that RP is a slowly progressive disease over many years and that most patients never become completely blind. In fact, even though many people with RP are considered "legally blind," it is only because they have very constricted fields of vi sion (poor peripheral vision). Some still maintain excellent central visual acuity.

Other symptoms may include night blindness (the most common symptom); eyes taking longer to adjust to dim lighting; trouble seeing in foggy or rainy weather; eyes being slow to make the adjust ment from bright sun to indoor lighting; and de creased peripheral vision and a narrowing field of vision, often called "tunnel vision." Additional symp toms include a perception of persistent flashes of light; difficulty seeing colors, especially blue; visual loss, partial or complete, usually gradually progressive; and clumsiness from lack of sight, especially in narrow spaces, such as door ways. Blurry vision from cataracts may complicate RP later in the disease.

SCREENING AND DIAGNOSIS

The doctor may ask about a patient's symptoms and medical history and may perform an eye exam. The patient may be referred to an eye specialist, such as an ophthalmologist.

An electroretinogram (ERG) is the most critical diagnostic test for RP because it provides an objective measure of rod and cone function across the retina and is sensitive to even mild photoreceptor impairment. This test is also used to track disease progression. Other tests, may include dark adaptometry (the minimum intensity of light that will stimulate the rods or cones to elicit a subjective response); visual field testing to check peripheral vision, which is how well a patient sees off to his or her side, rather than directly ahead, without moving his or her eyes; and blood tests to rule out other possible disorders.

TREATMENT AND THERAPY

For the most part, there is no effective treatment or cure for retinitis pigmentosa. Treatment aims to help patients function with the vision that they have. The doctor can counsel patients about expected pat terns of vision loss based on the type of RP they have.

Recommendations include the use of beta-carotene and vitamin A. One comprehensive epidemiologic study suggested that large doses of vitamin A can slow the progression of RP by approximately 2 per cent per year. However, the use of this finding is controversial. For one thing, it is a very mild effect given the large dose. Second, there may be side effects of such large doses of vitamin A. Patients should always talk to their doctors before taking any supplements.

Other recommendations include light avoidance. Although no direct link has been established, it is generally recommended that everyone, especially patients with disorders such as RP, wear dark ultravi olet (UV)-protected sunglasses and a wide-brimmed hat in bright, sunny conditions, such as while skiing or at the beach.

Gene therapy is under investigation and holds promise for the future.

Surgical interventions may be considered for appropriate patients. This might include cataract removal. On February 14, 2013, the U.S. Food and Drug Administration approved the Argus II Retinal Prosthesis System, the first implanted device to treat select adult patients with advanced retinitis pigmentosa (RP). The device includes includes a small video camera, transmitter mounted on a pair of eyeglasses, video processing unit (VPU), and an implanted retinal prosthesis (artificial retina). The device replaces the function of degenerated cells in the retina and may improve a patient's ability to perceive images and movement. The VPU transforms images from the video camera into electronic data that is wirelessly transmitted to the retinal prosthesis. Cell transplantation procedures are currently under investigation.

Aids for low vision may include magnifying glasses; electronic magnifiers, which project an enlarged im age onto a screen; night vision scopes, which en large distant objects under conditions of low light; and lenses for distant vision (eyeglasses or contacts).

It may be recommended that patients have annual examinations, including visual field testing and periodic (every 5 year) ERG evaluations. Changes in examination findings can help guide patients in their activities and can help with prognosis.

Some community organizations offer classes to help people with vision loss adjust and learn how to use vision aids. If a patient is considered legally blind, he or she is entitled to many low-vision ser vices at no cost.

PREVENTION AND OUTCOMES

Once RP has been inherited there are no known ways to prevent the disorder from occurring. Individuals who have RP or have a family history of the disorder may consider talking with a genetic counselor when deciding whether to have children.

Debra Wood, R.N.; reviewed by Christopher Cheyer, M.D. "Etiology and Genetics" by Jeffrey A. Knight, Ph.D.; updated by Gary M. Flashner, M.S., M.D.

FURTHER READING

Berson EL, Rosner B, Sandberg MA, Weigel-Difranco C, Willett WC. "Omega-3 Intake and Visual Acuity in Patients With Retinitis Pigmentosa Receiving Vitamin A." *Arch Ophthalmol.* 2012 Feb 13.

da Cruz L, Coley BF, Dorn J, Merlini F, Filley E, Christopher P. "The Argus II epiretinal prosthesis system allows letter and word reading and long-term function in patients with profound vision loss." *Br J Ophthalmol.* 2013 May. 97(5):632-6.

EBSCO Publishing. *Health Library: Retinitis Pig mentosa.* Ipswich, Mass.: Author, 2009. Available through http://www.ebscohost.com.

Fahim AT, Bowne SJ, Sullivan LS, et al. "Allelic Heterogeneity and Genetic Modifier Loci Contribute to Clinical Variation in Males with X-Linked Retinitis Pigmentosa Due to RPGR Mutations." *PLoS One.* 2011. 6(8):e23021

Fauci, Anthony S., et al., eds. *Harrison's Principles of Internal Medicine.* 17th ed. New York: McGraw-Hill Medical, 2008.

Foundation of the American Academy of Ophthalmology. *Retina and Vitreous, Basic and Clinical Science Course, 2008-2009.* San Francisco: American Academy of Ophthalmology, 2008.

Goldman, Lee, and Dennis Ausiello, eds. *Cecil Medicine.* 23d ed. Philadelphia: Saunders Elsevier, 2008.

Hebrard M, Manes G, Bocquet B, et al. "Combining gene mapping and phenotype assessment for fast mutation finding in non-consanguineous autosomal recessive retinitis pigmentosa families." *Eur J Hum Genet.* 2011 Dec. 19(12):1256-63.

Yanoff, Myron, et al. *Ophthalmology.* 3d ed. Edinburgh: Mosby Elsevier, 2009.

WEB SITES OF INTEREST

Canadian Association of Optometrists
http://www.opto.ca/en/public

Canadian National Institute for the Blind
http://www.cnib.ca/en/Default.aspx

Foundation Fighting Blindness
http://www.blindness.org

Genetics Home Reference
https://ghr.nlm.nih.gov/condition/retinitis-pigmentosa

Prevent Blindness America
http://www.preventblindness.org

RP International
http://www.rpinternational.org

https://rarediseases.info.nih.gov/diseases/5694/retinitis-pigmentosa

https://nei.nih.gov/health/pigmentosa/pigmentosa_facts

https://www.aao.org/eye-health/diseases/what-is-retinitis-pigmentosa

https://nei.nih.gov/news/briefs/RP_FDA_approval

https://ghr.nlm.nih.gov/gene/MT-ATP6#conditions

See also: Aniridia; Best disease; Choroideremia; Color blindness; Corneal dystrophies; Glaucoma; Gyrate atrophy of the choroid and retina; Macular degeneration; Norrie syndrome; Progressive external ophthalmoplegia; Retinoblastoma.

Retinoblastoma and genetics

CATEGORY: Diseases and syndromes

DEFINITION

Retinoblastoma is a rare type of childhood cancer of the retina of the eye. It typically develops before the age of 3 years although a few are not found until a child is close to age 5. Most congenital or hereditary retinoblastomas are found during the first year of life, while non-inherited retinoblastomas tend to be diagnosed in 1 and 2-year-olds.

The retina is a layer of light sensitive tissue that lines the back of the eye. It converts visual images into nerve impulses in the brain that allow people to see. If not treated, the tumors will continue growing. The cancer may grow along the optic nerve and reach the brain, or it may travel to other parts of the body.

Cancer occurs when cells in the body (in this case, retina cells) divide without control or order. Normally, cells divide in a regulated manner. If cells keep dividing uncontrollably when new cells are not needed, a mass of tissue forms, called a growth or tumor. Tumors can invade nearby tissue and spread to other parts of the body.

RISK FACTORS

The main risk factor for retinoblastoma is a mutation of the *RB1* gene. A family history of the disease is also a critical risk factor although only about 5% of patients who develop this disease have a positive family history.

If a patient who has been treated for retinoblastoma has been shown to have tumor involvement of the choroid layer of the eye (behind the retina) and/or involvement of the optic nerve, there is a greater risk for recurrence of the tumor.

ETIOLOGY AND GENETICS

The *RB1* gene, found on the long arm of chromosome 13 at position 13q14.1-q14.2, is the single gene that is responsible for almost all cases of retinoblastoma. It specifies a protein known as pRb that normally acts as a tumor-suppressor protein in retinal cells and in several other cell types. Tumor suppressor proteins act in a variety of ways to regulate cell growth by preventing cells from dividing too fast or at inappropriate times. Specifically, the pRb protein represses the transcription of several other genes whose protein products are needed in order to initiate a new round of DNA replication in the cell. When functional pRb is unavailable as a result of mutations in the *RB1* genes, this control of cell growth is lost and tumor formation may develop.

Retinoblastomas are often categorized as being either germinal or nongerminal. In germinal retinoblastomas (55 percent of all cases), the mutated *RB1* genes are found in all body cells. These are the cases that can be inherited and in which there is often a family history of the disease. In nongerminal cases (45 percent), the mutations in *RB1* have been acquired over time in the retinal tissue only, and affected individuals are not at risk of passing them on to their offspring. In germinal retinoblastoma, the inheritance pattern is most often consistent with an autosomal dominant mode of transmission. A single inherited copy of the mutation is sufficient in most cases to cause expression of the disease. An affected individual has a 50 percent chance of transmitting the mutation to each of his or her children. Many cases of germinal retinoblastoma, however, result from a spontaneous new mutation, so in these instances affected individuals will have unaffected parents.

Retinoblastoma See page for author, via Wikimedia Commons

Ocular fundus aspect of retinoblastoma See page for author, via Wikimedia Commons

SYMPTOMS

Signs of retinoblastoma are usually noticed by the parent or caregiver and may include, but are not limited to, eyes that do not look normal, often described as a glazed look or a "cat's eye." Approximately 20-35% of cases affect both eyes.

Another sign may include the pupil looking white rather than red when a light is directed at the eye; this is often noticed on a photograph. An additional sign may be eyes that may appear to be crossed or looking in different directions. Less common signs and symptoms may include eyes that may grow in size, eye pain, redness in the white part of the eye, tearing, a pupil that may not respond to light; white spots on the iris, swelling of the tissue area that directly surrounds one or both eyes; one pupil appearing

dilated; rare pooling or a collection of blood inside the anterior chamber of the eye (the space between the cornea and the iris); nystagmus (rapid, rhythmic, repetitious, and involuntary eye movements); and the iris (colored part of the eye) changing color. In untreated cases, there may develop an abnormal protrusion or displacement of an eye.

SCREENING AND DIAGNOSIS

The doctor may ask about a child's symptoms and family medical history and may perform a physical exam. Many retinoblastomas are found during routine physical exams. If a tumor is suspected, the child is often referred to a specialist for a more complete eye exam. In children with a family history of the disease, eye exams often begin within a day or two of birth. Additional eye exams are scheduled at regular intervals thereafter.

Once a retinoblastoma is found, staging tests are performed to find out if the cancer has spread and, if so, to what extent. Treatment depends on the stage of the cancer. The cancer may be localized to the one or both eyes or it may have spread to tissues around the eye or to other parts of the body.

Tests may include, but are not limited to, an eye exam. In this test, the pupil is dilated with eyedrops; then the inside of the eye is examined with a lighted instrument that allows the examiner to view structures inside the eye.

Other tests may include DNA analysis of the retinoblastoma gene. This may also be recommended for the parents and any siblings.

Imaging tests may include ultra sound, a test that uses sound waves to examine the inner part of the eye; and a magnetic resonance imaging (MRI) scan, which uses magnetic waves to make pictures of the inside of the body. An MRI can be used to check the spread of the cancer to the brain or other tissue. A computed tomography (CT) scan is a type of X ray that uses a computer to make pictures of the eye. CT scans of other areas of the body may be done to check if the cancer has spread. Sedative medications are often used to help the child remain still during close examination and testing.

If spread of the cancer is suspected, then examination of the bone marrow and cerebrospinal fluid may be recommended because the primary mode of spread of retinoblastoma is through the blood stream to the bone marrow and back through the optic nerve into the cerebrospinal fluid that surrounds the brain and spinal cord.

TREATMENT AND THERAPY

The child is often referred to a specialist for treatment. Without treatment, the cancer cells will continue to grow.

Medical therapy is often directed toward complete control of the tumor and the preservation of as much useful vision as possible. Treatment is usually individualized to the specific patient. Options vary, depending on whether the disease is limited to the eye or has spread and how large and where in the eye the tumor is located. Therapies may be used alone or in combination.

Surgical removal of the tumor has been the standard management of very unfavorable retinoblastoma cases. This involves surgical removal of the entire eye and as much of the optic nerve as possible when there is no chance of preserving useful vision in an eye. The optic nerve is the nerve leading from the eye to the brain that is responsible for vision. Surgery may be used for a large tumor in one eye.

Radiation therapy is a form of treatment that involves the use of radiation to kill cancer cells and shrink tumors. Radiation may be external radiation therapy, in which radiation is directed at the tumor from a source outside the body. Incidence of local control is high and retinal late effects are minimal with external beam radiation therapy; however, its use comes with potentially serious long term negative effects. As a result, this form of treatment is reserved only for selected patients. More commonly, internal radiation therapy is used where radioactive materials are placed into the body near the cancer cells.

Cryotherapy, used on small tumors, is the use of cold to freeze and destroy cancer cells. Thermo therapy uses heat to kill cancer cells. In photocoagulation, lasers are used to destroy a small tumor.

Chemotherapy is the use of drugs to kill cancer cells. This treatment may be given in many forms, including pill, injection, and through a catheter. The drugs enter the bloodstream and travel through the body killing mostly cancer cells, but also some healthy cells.

In order to achieve the best outcomes, different treatment approaches are often used either in combination or in sequence. There continues to be ongoing research focused on continual improvements in these various approaches with the hope of continuing to improve outcomes.

PREVENTION AND OUTCOMES

Genetic counseling and close monitoring and screening for people at risk for retinoblastoma may be recommended in order to detect the disease early Early diagnosis and treatment improve the chance of successful treatment.

Early detection techniques include screening. It may be suggested that children born into families with a history of retinoblastoma have regular eye exams to screen for development of the tumor. Genetic counseling may help determine a person's risk of developing retinoblastoma. If a patient has retinoblastoma or has a family history of the disorder, he or she can talk to a genetic counselor when deciding whether to have children.

Patients who have been treated for retinoblastoma require regular medical exams to assess the success of treatment and to check for recurrence of disease. Children with retinoblastoma are at increased risk for other cancers in the body and should be monitored in order to check for other cancers.

Debra Wood, R.N.; reviewed by Christopher Cheyer, M.D. "Etiology and Genetics" by Jeffrey A. Knight, Ph.D.; updated by Gary M. Flashner, M.S., M.D.

FURTHER READING

Abeloff, Martin D., et al., eds. *Abeloff's Clinical Oncology*. 4th ed. Philadelphia: Churchill Livingstone/Elsevier, 2008.

EBSCO Publishing. *Health Library: Retinoblastoma.*

Brinkman TM, Merchant TE, Li Z, Brennan R, Wilson M, Hoehn ME, et al. "Cognitive function and social attainment in adult survivors of retinoblastoma: A report from the St. Jude Lifetime Cohort Study." *Cancer*. 2014 Nov 24

Suzuki S, Yamane T, Mohri M, Kaneko A. "Selective ophthalmic arterial injection therapy for intraocular retinoblastoma: the long-term prognosis." *Ophthalmology*. 2011 Oct. 118(10):2081–7.

Lin HY, Liao SL. "Orbital development in survivors of retinoblastoma treated by enucleation with hydroxyapatite implant." *Br J Ophthalmol*. 2011 May. 95(5):630–3.

Ipswich, Mass.: Author, 2009. Available through http://www.ebscohost.com.

Kleigman, Robert M., et al., eds. *Nelson Textbook of Pediatrics*. 18th ed. Philadelphia: Saunders Elsevier, 2007.

Pizzo, Philip A., and David G. Poplack. *Principles and Practice of Pediatric Oncology*. 5th ed. Philadelphia: Lippincott Williams & Wilkins, 2006.

Yanoff, Myron, et al. *Ophthalmology*. 3d ed. Edinburgh: Mosby Elsevier, 2009.

WEB SITES OF INTEREST

American Cancer Society
http://www.cancer.org

BC (British Columbia) Cancer Agency
http://www.bccancer.bc.ca/default.htm

Cancer Care Ontario
http://www.cancercare.on.ca

Genetics Home Reference
https://ghr.nlm.nih.gov/gene/RB1

National Cancer Institute
http://www.cancer.gov

https://rarediseases.info.nih.gov/diseases/7563/retinoblastoma

http://emedicine.medscape.com/article/1222849-overview

https://aapos.org/client_data/files/2011/311_parulekar_handouts_all.pdf

See also: Aniridia; Best disease; Choroideremia; Color blindness; Corneal dystrophies; Glaucoma; Gyrate atrophy of the choroid and retina; Macular degeneration; Norrie syndrome; Progressive external ophthalmoplegia; Retinitis pigmentosa.

Rett syndrome

CATEGORY: Diseases and syndromes
ALSO KNOWN AS: Rett's disorder

DEFINITION

Rett syndrome is a developmental nervous system disorder. It primarily affects girls. It is uncommon, but not rare. It occurs in 1 out of every 10,000-23,000 female births. Boys with the gene defect that causes this disorder are usually stillborn or die shortly after birth.

Rett syndrome can be classified into classic and atypical, depending on the symptoms.

Many people with Rett syndrome live into adulthood. Most have severe disabilities. While many cannot talk or walk, they usually have a full range of feelings and often communicate through their eyes. People with Rett syndrome usually need daily care throughout their lives.

RISK FACTORS

There are no known risk factors for Rett syndrome, except being female. The mutation that causes the syndrome appears to be sporadic.

ETIOLOGY AND GENETICS

Classic Rett syndrome is caused by mutations in the *MECP2* gene, which is located on the long arm of the X chromosome at position Xq28. The protein encoded by this gene is called the methyl CpG binding protein 2 (MeCP2), and it is normally present at high levels in mature nerve cells. While its exact molecular function remains unclear, it appears to be important for forming the proper synapses, or connections, between adjacent nerve cells so that essential chemical communication between cells can occur. MeCP2 also has a regulatory function, since it has been shown under some conditions to repress several other genes, thus preventing the accumulation of additional proteins when they are not necessary. It is not understood, however, how mutations that result in a missing or defective MeCP2 protein lead to the developmental problems and clinical symptoms of Rett syndrome.

An atypical form of Rett syndrome called the early-onset seizure variant is associated with mutations in another gene on the X chromosome called *CDKL5* (at position Xp22). This gene specifies the enzyme known as cyclin-dependent kinase-like 5. Like MeCP2, it is essential for normal brain development and appears to be involved in the regulation of gene activity of other genes in nerve cells.

The pattern of inheritance for mutations in both of these genes is the same: They are inherited in an X-linked dominant fashion. A single copy of the defective gene is sufficient to cause the severe disease symptoms noted in girls with Rett syndrome. One normal copy of the gene is required in order to have sufficient brain function to be consistent with life. That is why Rett syndrome is found only in girls, since an affected boy would not have a second X chromosome that carried the normal allele. There are only scattered reports in the literature of affected females bearing children and passing the defective gene on to daughters in the next generation. As a consequence, more than 99 percent of Rett syndrome cases are sporadic, in that they result from new mutations in females with no previous family history of the disorder.

SYMPTOMS

A girl with Rett syndrome will start developing normally. She will smile, move, and pick items up with her fingers. However, by eighteen months of age the developmental process seems to stop or reverse itself.

Australian physician Andreas Rett first described the syndrome. By Penarc (Own work), via Wikimedia Commons

Methyl-CpG-binding protein 2, MECP2; Rett Syndrome is caused by mutations in this gene. By Jawahar Swaminathan and MSD staff at the European Bioinformatics Institute, via Wikimedia Commons

The age of onset and the severity of symptoms can vary. There are four stages.

Stage I, the early-onset stage, occurs in children between the ages of six to eighteen months and lasts for months. Symptoms may include less eye contact with parents, less interest in toys and play, hand-wringing, slow head growth, and being a calm and quiet baby.

Stage II, the rapid destructive stage, occurs in children between the ages of one to four years old and lasts for weeks to months. Symptoms may include a small head; mental retardation; a loss of muscle tone; the inability to purposely use hands; the loss of (previous) ability to talk; repeatedly moving hands to mouth; and other hand movements, such as clapping, tapping, or random touching. Hand movements stop during sleep. Additional symptoms may include holding breath, gaps in breathing, or taking rapid breaths; irregular breathing stops during sleep. Teeth grinding, laughing or screaming spells, decreased social interactions, irritability, trouble sleeping, tremors, cold feet, and trouble crawling or walking may also be symptoms.

Stage III, the plateau stage, occurs in children who are in their preschool through school years and lasts for years. Symptoms may include difficulty controlling movement, seizures, and less irritability and crying. Communication may improve.

Stage IV, the late motor deterioration stage, occurs when stage III ceases, which can be anywhere from age five to twenty-five, and its duration lasts up to decades. Symptoms may include a decreased ability to walk, muscle weakness or wasting, stiffness of muscles, spastic movements, and scoliosis (curvature of the spine). Breathing trouble and seizures often decrease with age. Puberty usually begins at the expected age.

SCREENING AND DIAGNOSIS

The doctor will ask a parent about a child's symptoms and medical history, do a physical and neurological exam, and exclude other disorders, such as autism. The doctor can also do genetic testing, which can often confirm the diagnosis. The *MECP2* gene mutation is present in 95 percent of girls with Rett Syndrome and in 50 percent of those with the atypical form. However, not everyone with this mutation will have Rett syndrome. Some females may be normal or have only mild symptoms. However, these women can pass the gene to their daughters, and the daughters may then be more severely affected.

Some of the motor functions of Rett syndrome are similar to those of autism. Children with autism, who are more often boys, do not maintain person-to-person contact. Most girls with Rett syndrome, however, prefer human contact to focusing on inanimate objects. These differences may give the first clue in diagnosing Rett syndrome.

Aside from genetic testing, the diagnosis is confirmed by comparing the physical and developmental findings with those typically found in Rett syndrome. Tests may include a blood test to check for genetic mutation (*MECP2* gene); an electroencephalogram (EEG), a test that records the electrical activity of the brain; and a video EEG, a test that combines EEG with a video to see if some of the child's movements are caused by seizures.

TREATMENT AND THERAPY

There is no cure for Rett syndrome, although animal studies have suggested that the effects may be at least partially reversible using PTP1B inhibitors (PTP1B being an enzyme whose function is usually regulated by the *MECP2* gene). As of late 2015, no human trials of this treatment had been undertaken. Patients with Rett syndrome condition need to be monitored for skeletal problems and heart problems.

Treatment aims to control symptoms and includes medication, such as anticonvulsants to control seizure activity; stool softeners or laxatives, if the patient is constipated; drugs to help with breathing; and drugs to ease agitation. Scientists are investigating a group of medications called histone deacetylase inhibitors as a possible treatment for Rett syndrome.

Patients should eat small, frequent meals and take supplements, and may be tube fed if they are unable to consume enough food. Their diet should also include fluids and high-fiber foods to help control constipation.

Rehabilitation therapies may include occupational therapy to help patients learn to perform daily activities, such as dressing and eating; and physical therapy to help patients improve coordination and movement (can sometimes prolong the ability to walk). The use of braces and splints may be recommended. Speech therapy aides can help build communication skills, and social workers can help a family cope with caring for a child with Rett syndrome.

Parents can use various techniques to try to limit their children's problem behaviors. They can keep a diary of their children's behaviors and activities to help determine the cause of agitation. Other techniques that may help to prevent or control behavior problems include giving children warm baths and massages, playing soothing music, and creating a quiet environment.

PREVENTION AND OUTCOMES

There is no way to prevent Rett syndrome. Individuals who have questions about the risk of Rett syndrome in their families can talk to a genetic counselor.

FURTHER READING

Kazantsev, A. G., and L. M. Thompson. "Therapeutic Application of Histone Deacetlyase Inhibitors for Central Nervous System Disorders." *Nature Reviews. Drug Discovery* 7.10 (2008): 854-68. Print.

Kleigman, Robert M., et al., eds. *Nelson Textbook of Pediatrics.* 18th ed. Philadelphia: Saunders, 2007. Print.

Rett Syndrome." Mayo Clinic. *Mayo* Foundation for Medical Education and Research, 17 Sept. 2015. Web. 1 Dec. 2015.

Rett Syndrome Fact Sheet." *National Institute of Neurological Disorders and Stroke.* Natl. Inst. of Health, 27 July 2015. Web. 1 Dec. 2015.

Singer, H. S., and S. Naidu. "Rett Syndrome: 'We'll Keep the Genes on for You.'" *Neurology* 56.5 (2001): 582-84. Print.

Tarr, Peter. "In Mice, an Experimental Drug Treatment for Rett Syndrome Suggests the Disorder Is Reversible." *Cold Spring Harbor Laboratory.* Cold Spring Harbor Laboratory, 27 July 2015. Web. 1 Dec. 2015.

Tasman, Allan, et al. *Psychiatry.* 3rd ed. Hoboken: Wiley, 2008.

See also: Adrenoleukodystrophy; Alexander disease; Alzheimer's disease; Amyotrophic lateral sclerosis; Arnold-Chiari syndrome; Ataxia telangiectasia; Autism; Canavan disease; Cerebrotendinous xanthomatosis; Charcot-Marie-Tooth syndrome; Chediak-Higashi syndrome; Dandy-Walker syndrome; Deafness; Epilepsy; Essential tremor; Friedreich ataxia; Huntington's disease; Jansky-Bielschowsky disease; Joubert syndrome; Kennedy disease; Krabbé disease; Leigh syndrome; Leukodystrophy; Limb girdle muscular dystrophy; Maple syrup urine disease; Metachromatic leukodystrophy; Myoclonic epilepsy associated with ragged red fibers (MERRF); Narcolepsy; Nemaline myopathy; Neural tube defects; Neurofibromatosis; Parkinson disease; Pelizaeus-Merzbacher disease; Pendred syndrome; Periodic paralysis syndrome; Prion diseases: Kuru and Creutzfeldt-Jakob syndrome; Refsum disease; Spinal muscular atrophy; Vanishing white matter disease.

Reverse transcriptase

CATEGORY: Genetic engineering and biotechnology; Molecular genetics

SIGNIFICANCE: Retroviruses infect eukaryotic cells, using reverse transcriptases (RTs) to turn their RNA genomes to DNA that enables their host to use the DNA to make new virus particles. Retroviral DNA, often dormant for years before new virus particles are released, can be oncogenic, giving infected cells high incidences of cancer. Purified RTs are used to make RNA into DNA for biotechnology.

KEY TERMS

deoxyribonucleoside triphosphate (dNTP): one of four monomers (dATP, dCTP, dGTP, dTTP) incorporated into DNA

DNA polymerase: an enzyme that catalyzes the formation of a DNA strand using a template DNA or RNA molecule as a guide

primer: A short piece of single-stranded DNA that can hybridize to denatured DNA and provide a start point for extension by a DNA polymerase

proofreading activity: enzyme activity in DNA polymerase that fixes errors made in copying templates

retroviruses: viruses that possess RNA genomes with genetic information that flows from RNA to host DNA via reverse transcriptases

GENETIC INFORMATION FLOW AND RETROVIRUSES

The central dogma of molecular genetics states that information flow is from DNA to RNA to proteins. RNA polymerase transcribes RNA using a DNA template. For structural genes, the transcribed RNA is a messenger RNA (mRNA), which is used by ribosomes to produce a protein. To maintain and reproduce its DNA, an organism uses RNA to make DNA, via DNA polymerase. It was long believed by geneticists that there were no exceptions to the central dogma.

Some viruses, retroviruses, possess RNA genomes with genetic information flow from RNA to DNA (via reverse transcriptases), and back, before translation. Retroviruses have been isolated from cancers and cancer tissue cultures from birds, rodents, primates, and humans, and some retroviruses cause a high incidence of certain cancers. Flow of retroviral genetic information from RNA to DNA was proposed in 1964 by Howard Temin (1934-1994) for Rous sarcoma virus. Temin, along with David Baltimore, jointly received the Nobel Prize in Physiology or Medicine in 1975 for independently discovering the enzyme reverse transcriptase (RT).

Rous sarcoma virus causes tumors in birds. Temin's hypothesis was based on effects of nucleic acid synthesis inhibitors on replication of the virus. First, the process was inhibited by actinomycin D, an inhibitor of DNA-dependent RNA synthesis. Furthermore, DNA synthesis inhibition by cytosine arabinoside, early after infection, stopped viral replication. Therefore, a DNA intermediate seemed involved in viral replication. The expected process was termed reverse transcription because RNA becomes DNA instead of DNA becoming RNA.

RT DISCOVERY AND PROPERTIES

Retrovirus infection begins with injection of RT and single-stranded RNA into host cells. RT (an RNA-dependent DNA polymerase) causes biosynthesis of viral DNA using an RNA template from the retrovirus HIV (human immunodeficiency virus), the causative agent of acquired immunodeficiency syndrome (AIDS). RTs have been purified from many retroviruses. Avian, murine, and human RTs have been studied most. All have ribonuclease H (RNase H) activity on the same protein as polymerase activity. Ribonuclease H degrades RNA strands of DNARNA hybrids. A nuclease that degrades DNA is later involved in retrovirus DNA integration into host cell DNA. Most biochemical properties of purified RTs are common to them and other DNA polymerases. For example, all require the following for DNA synthesis: a primer on which synthesis begins, a template that is copied, and a supply of the four dNTPs.

An RT converts a retroviral single-stranded RNA genome to "integrated double-stranded DNA" as follows: First a hybrid (DNA-RNA) duplex is made from viral RNA, as an antiparallel DNA strand is produced. The RNA-directed DNA polymerase activity of RT is primed by host cell transfer RNA, which binds to the viral RNA. Then, the viral RNA strand is destroyed by RNase H, and the first DNA strand now becomes the template for synthesis of a second antiparallel DNA strand. Resultant duplex DNA is next integrated into a host cell chromosome, where it is immediately used to make virus particles or, alternatively, it takes up residence in the host cell's genome, remaining unused—often for years—until it is activated and causes cancer or production of new viruses.

IMPORTANCE OF REVERSE TRANSCRIPTASES

RTs can use almost any RNA template for DNA synthesis. Low RT template specificity allows RT to be used to make DNA copies of a wide variety of RNAs in vitro. This has been very useful in molecular biology, especially in production of exact DNA copies of purified RNAs. Once the copies are made by RT, they can be cloned into bacterial expression vectors, where mass quantities of the gene product can be produced. It has also been shown that RT activity takes part in making telomeres (protective chromosome ends). Telomere formation and maintenance are essential cell processes, related to life span and deemed important to understanding cancer.

RTs are also important in treatment of acquired immunodeficiency syndrome (AIDS). The drugs most useful for AIDS treatment are RT inhibitors such as zidovudine, didanosine, zalcitabine, and stavudine. RTs are also associated with the difficulty in maintaining successful long-term AIDS treatment, due to rapid development of resistant HIV in individual AIDS patients. The resistance is postulated to be due to RT's lack of a proofreading component. Inadequate proofreading in sequential replication of HIV viral particles from generation to generation is believed to cause the rapid mutation of the viral genome.

Sanford S. Singer, Ph.D.

FURTHER READING

Goff, S. P. "Retroviral Reverse Transcriptase: Synthesis, Structure, and Function." *Journal of Acquired Immune Deficiency Diseases* 3, no. 8 (1990): 817-831. A solid, well-illustrated paper.

Joklik, Wolfgang K., ed. *Microbiology: A Centenary Perspective.* Washington, D.C.: ASM Press, 1999. Thoroughly reviews important microbiology issues, including reverse transcriptase papers by Howard Temin and David Baltimore.

Litvack, Simon. *Retroviral Reverse Transcriptases.* Austin, Tex.: R. G. Landes, 1996. Describes discovery, biosynthesis, structure, inhibitors, and action mechanistics of reverse transcriptase. Illustrations and bibliographic references.

Morel, Gérard, and Mireille Raccurt. "Reverse Transcription." In *PCR/RT-PCR In Situ Light and Electron Microscopy.* Boca Raton, Fla.: CRC Press, 2003. Describes how to use the techniques of polymerase chain reaction (PCR) and reverse transcription

PCR (RT-PCR) in order to visualize DNA and RNA in tissues and cell cultures.

O'Connell, Joe, ed. *RT-PCR Protocols*. Totowa, N.J.: Humana Press, 2002. Collects several papers on the use of reverse transcription polymerase chain reaction in analysis of mRNA, quantitative methodologies, detection of RNA viruses, genetic analysis, and immunology. Tables, charts, index.

Shippen-Lentz, D., and E. H. Blackburn. "Functional Evidence for an RNA Template in Telomerase." *Science* 247, no. 4942 (February 2, 1990): 546-552. Points to the RT activity in telomerases. Illustrated.

Skowron, Gail, and Richard Ogden, eds. *Reverse Transcriptase Inhibitors in HIV/AIDS Therapy*. Totowa, N.J.: Humana Press, 2006. Examines how reverse transcriptase inhibitors are being used in drug discovery, pharmacology, development of drug resistance, toxicity, and prevention of mother-to-child transmission of HIV/AIDS. Reviews the role of reverse transcriptase in the life cycle of viruses.

Varmus, Harold. "Retroviruses." *Science* 240, no. 4858 (June 6, 1988): 1427-1435. The discoverer of oncogenes describes properties of different retroviruses, including the mechanism of reverse transcription.

WEB SITES OF INTEREST

Biotechnology Index, Reverse Transcriptases
http://www.vivo.colostate.edu/hbooks/genetics/biotech/enzymes/rt.html
The index, prepared by the department of biomedical sciences at Colorado State University, includes a page about reverse transcriptases.

Cells Alive!
http://www.cellsalive.com/hiv2.htm
Features an explanation of how reverse transcription converts viral RNA into DNA as part of its discussion of the human immunodeficiency virus (HIV).

RCSD Protein Data Bank
http://www.rcsb.org/pdb/static.do?p=education_discussion/molecule_of_the_month/pdb33_1.html
The Research Collaboratory for Structural Bioinformatics (RCSB) Protein Data Bank is an archive of information about proteins, nucleic acids, and "complex assemblies." The site provides an explanation of reverse transcriptases.

See also: cDNA libraries; Central dogma of molecular biology; Model organism: *Chlamydomonas reinhardtii*; Pseudogenes; Repetitive DNA; RNA isolation; RNA structure and function; RNA world; Shotgun cloning.

Reverse transcription polymerase chain reaction (RT-PCR)

CATEGORY: Molecular genetics

SIGNIFICANCE: This technique uses ribonucleic acid (RNA) and a heat-resistant enzyme to produce many copies of deoxyribonucleic acid (DNA). The development of RT-PCR has greatly advanced genetics research and is used in the detection of many inherited disorders and infections.

THE BASICS OF RT-PCR

DNA, the genetic material of most organisms, is used to make a form of nucleic acid called ribonucleic acid (RNA) that provides the blueprint to actually manufacture molecules such as proteins. This process is called transcription. Reverse transcription (RT) involves the use of RNA as the template to make DNA. This involves an enzyme called reverse transcriptase.

KEY TERMS

deoxyribonucleotide the building block of DNA consisting of a nitrogen-containing molecule, deoxyribose containing sugar, and phosphate(s)

enzyme a protein that allows a reaction to proceed more quickly or with less supplied energy, but which is not altered by the reaction

protein a molecule composed of amino acids

primer a fragment of nucleic acid that is used to initiate the replication of DNA

reverse transcriptase enzyme that catalyzes the formation of DNA from RNA

RNA ribonucleic acid: a form of genetic material composed of nucleotides

In RT-PCR, a strand of RNA is reverse transcribed to produce what is called complementary DNA (cDNA) It is the cDNA that is subsequently amplified in number in the PCR reaction.

RT-PCR used to be done by hand. Now, the process is carried out in an automated machine that can produce tens of thousands of copies of the selected sequence of DNA within hours. Organizations such as The Institute for Genomic Research (TIGR) that have dozens of PCR machines are capable of producing millions of copies of DNA in a day.

THE COMPONENTS OF PCR

PCR relies on the presence of a template, deoxyribonucleotides, a pair of primers, and DNA polymerase. The template is the RNA strand.

Deoxyribonucleotides are the building blocks of DNA. There are four deoxyribonucleotides: adenine, thymine, cytosine, and guanine. Their three-dimensional structures are such that adenine will bond with thymine, and cytosine will bond with guanine. In the double strand of DNA that forms the helical structure found in the cell, the two strands will be complementary to one another; thus, a sequence of adenine-thymine-guanine on one strand will be mirrored by thymine-adenine-cytosine on the other strand.

Primers are sequences of deoxyribonucleotides that have been deliberately constructed to be complementary with the sequences of a portion of each DNA strand. This causes the primers to associate with one or the other of the DNA strands. Binding of primer to DNA is important in the PCR process. DNA polymerase is an enzyme that catalyzes the construction of DNA from the building blocks that are supplied. PCR is carried out at an elevated temperature that helps keep the DNA strands separated from each other, so the polymerase must be capable of functioning at the higher temperatures (many proteins including enzymes change their structure at higher temperature, causing lose of function). PCR became possible with the discovery of Taq polymerase, an enzyme made by the thermophilic ("heat-loving") bacterium *Thermus aquaticus*, which naturally lives in hot springs.

THE THREE STEPS OF PCR

Part of the sequence of the targeted DNA has to be known in order to design the primers. In the first step, the targeted double-stranded DNA is heated to more than 90 degrees Celsius (194 degrees Fahrenheit). During this process, the two strands of the targeted DNA separate from each other. Each strand is capable of being a template.

The second step involves a gradual decrease to a temperature at which the two DNA strands would normally reassociate, but primers are also present in the solution at a greater concentration than DNA.

This causes reassociation to occur between the primers and the specific complementary regions on each DNA strand. Complete reassociation of the DNA strands cannot occur. The association between the primers and the DNA will produce a short region of two strands with a longer region having a single strand of the DNA.

The third step, amplification, focuses on these single strands of DNA. In the presence of the necessary deoxyribonucleotides and other compounds, DNA polymerase catalyzes the manufacture of a complementary strand of DNA. At the end of this process, the newly constructed strands can be separated at high temperature to begin the cycle again.

As the cycles are repeated again and again, the number of each target sequence doubles with each cycle (a logarithmic increase).

PCR reactions are carried out in an apparatus called a thermocycler, which is designed to change temperatures automatically. The various conditions of temperature and reaction times can be programmed and the procedure occurs without operator assistance.

IMPACT

American molecular biologist Kary Mullis developed PCR in the 1970's. The ability to quickly amplify DNA revolutionized molecular biology. In 1993, Mullis received the Nobel Prize in Physiology or Medicine. RT-PCR has also greatly advanced genetics research. For example, the technique was invaluable in the sequencing of the human genome. RT-PCR is also widely used in the detection of many inherited disorders.

Brian D. Hoyle, Ph.D.

FURTHER READING

Hodge, Russ. *The Future of Genetics: Beyond the Human Genome Project*. New York: Facts On File, 2009. A consideration of future advancements on human genetics research.

Read, Andrew. *New Clinical Genetics*. Oxfordshire, England: Scion, 2007. Concise summary of human genetics from a clinical standpoint.

Strachan, Tom. *Human Molecular Genetics*. London: Garland Science, 2003. Comprehensive consideration of human genetics.

See also: Ancient DNA; Anthrax; Bioinformatics; Blotting: Southern, Northern, and Western; Central dogma of molecular biology; Cloning vectors; DNA fingerprinting; DNA sequencing technology; Forensic genetics; Genetic engineering: Historical development; Human Genome Project; In vitro fertilization and embryo transfer; Mitochondrial diseases; Molecular genetics; Paternity tests; Polymerase chain reaction (PCR); Repetitive DNA; RFLP analysis; RNA isolation.

RFLP analysis

CATEGORY: Techniques and methodologies

SIGNIFICANCE: RFLP analysis was the first simple method available for distinguishing individuals based on DNA sequence differences. The conceptual basis for this technique is still widely used in genetics, although RFLP analysis has been largely supplanted by faster and more powerful techniques for the comparison of genetic differences.

KEY TERMS

gel electrophoresis: a method for separating DNA molecules by size by applying electric current to force DNA through a matrix of agarose, which inhibits the migration of larger DNA fragments more than small DNA fragments

restriction enzymes: proteins that recognize specific DNA sequences and then cut the DNA, normally at the same sequence recognized by the enzymes

Southern blotting: a method for transferring DNA molecules from an agarose gel to a nylon membrane; once the DNA is on the membrane, it is incubated with a DNA containing an identifiable label and is then used to detect similar or identical DNA sequences on the membrane

THE PROCEDURE

Restriction fragment length polymorphism (RFLP) analysis is a method for distinguishing individuals and analyzing relatedness, based on genetic differences. RFLP analysis relies on small DNA sequence differences that lead to the loss or gain of restriction enzyme sites in a chromosome or to the change in size of a DNA fragment bracketed

by restriction enzyme sites. These sequence differences lead to a different pattern of bands on a gel (reminiscent of a bar code) that varies from individual to individual.

RFLP analysis starts with the isolation of DNA. Typically, DNA isolation requires the use of detergents, protein denaturants, RNA degrading enzymes, and alcohol precipitation to separate the DNA from the other cellular components. This DNA could be isolated from a blood sample provided by an individual, from evidence left at the scene of a crime, or from other sources of cells or tissues.

restriction enzyme is used to break DNA sample into pieces By Ramin Herati, via Wikimedia Commons

This liquid-filled box and attached power supply are used for gel electrophoresis. By Jeffrey M. Vinocur (Own work), via Wikimedia Commons

The purified DNA is then digested with a molecular "scissors" called a restriction enzyme. Restriction enzymes recognize and cut precise sequences, typically six base pairs in length. If one base pair is changed in that recognition sequence, the enzyme will not cut the DNA at that point. However, if a sequence that is not recognized by a restriction enzyme is altered by mutation, so that it now is recognized, the DNA will be cleaved at that point. In other cases, the DNA sequences recognized by the restriction enzymes themselves are not changed, but the length of DNA between two restriction enzyme sites differs between individuals. These types of mutations occur with enough regularity that often even two closely related individuals will have some detectable differences in the sizes of DNA fragments produced from restriction enzyme digestion.

Once the DNA has been digested with a restriction enzyme, it is separated by size in an agarose gel. At this point, the DNA appears, to the eye, to be a smear of molecules of all sizes, and it is not generally possible to differentiate the DNAs from different individuals at this stage. The size-fractioned DNA is next transferred to a nylon membrane in a process called Southern blotting. The result of the transfer is that the location and arrangement of the DNA fragments in the gel is maintained on the membrane, but the DNA is now single-stranded (critical for the next step in the process) and much easier to handle.

The final step in the process is to detect specific DNA fragments on the membrane. This is done by using a DNA fragment that is labeled to act as a probe, to home in on and identify similar DNA sequences on the membrane. Before use, the probe is made single-stranded, so it can bind to the single-stranded DNA on the membrane. The probe DNA can be labeled with radioactivity, in which case it is detected using X-ray film. The probe DNA can also be labeled with molecules that are bound by proteins, and the proteins can then be detected either directly or indirectly.

In a case in which a restriction enzyme site has been added or removed, the probe is normally a DNA fragment that is found in only one location in the genome. In cases in which one is looking at the size of fragments bracketed by restriction enzyme sites, the probe DNA is normally a DNA molecule that is found in several sites in the genome, and the DNA fragments that are identified in this analysis are ones that tend to vary between individuals. In many cases, the probe DNA binds to regions of DNA that consist of variable number tandem repeats (VNTRs). The number of VNTRs tends to vary between different individuals and, consequently, these sequences are useful for identification.

APPLICATIONS

One of the earliest uses of this technique in clinical medicine was in the prenatal diagnosis of sickle-cell disease. Previous work had shown that many individuals with the disease had a mutation in their DNA that eliminated a restriction enzyme site in a gene encoding a hemoglobin protein. This information was used to develop a diagnostic RFLP procedure. A section of the hemoglobin gene is used as a probe. The size of restriction enzyme fragments identified is different in individuals who have sickle-cell disease (and therefore have two mutant alleles) compared with individuals who carry either one mutant allele or have two unmutated hemoglobin alleles. This method allowed for the identification of affected fetuses using DNA from cells isolated from amniotic fluid (a much simpler and safer procedure than the previous method of diagnosis, which required isolating fetal red blood cells).

Another widely reported use of RFLP analysis has been in forensic science. RFLP methods have been critical in helping to identify criminals, and these methods have also helped exonerate innocent people. The first application of RFLP in forensic analysis was in the case of the murders of two young girls in England, in 1983 and 1986. Initially, a seventeen-year-old boy confessed to the murders. RFLP analysis, using DNA from the crime scene, indicated that he was not the murderer. After extensive investigation, including RFLP analysis of DNA from more than forty-five hundred men, a suspect was identified. Confronted with the evidence, the suspect pleaded guilty to both murders and was jailed for life. Since then, RFLP analysis has been used in thousands of criminal cases. Other forensic applications of RFLP include its use as evidence in court cases involving paternity determinations and its role in identifying the bodies of missing persons who otherwise could not be identified.

In addition to the clinical and forensic applications described above, RFLP analysis has been used in many subdisciplines of biology since the early 1980's. The applications of RFLP analysis range from the conservation of endangered species to the identification of strains of bacteria associated with disease outbreaks to basic research involving the classification of organisms.

Although RFLP analysis has been widely used since its inception, it is increasingly being displaced by polymerase chain reaction (PCR) methods, which typically are much faster and require much less DNA. RFLP analysis was, however, an important step in the introduction of modern DNA analysis into the biology laboratory and the courtroom. The guiding principle behind RFLP analysis—identifying individuals, strains, and species, based on DNA sequence differences—remains a part of newer techniques.

Patrick G. Guilfoile, Ph.D.

FURTHER READING

Allison, Lizabeth A. "Recombinant DNA Technology and Molecular Cloning." In *Fundamental Molecular Biology*. Malden, Mass.: Blackwell, 2007. Includes information about RFLP.

Chang, J. C., and Y. W. Kan. "A Sensitive New Prenatal Test for Sickle-Cell Anemia." *New England Journal of Medicine* 307, no. 1 (July 1, 1982): 30-32. A short and readable scientific paper describing one of the first applications of RFLP analysis to clinical medicine. The same issue of the journal also has another, somewhat more detailed, article on the same topic by S. H. Orkin et al.

Guilfoile, P. *A Photographic Atlas for the Molecular Biology Laboratory*. Englewood, Colo.: Morton, 2000. An illustrated guide to molecular biology techniques, including a substantial illustrated section on RFLP analysis.

Hartl, D. L., and Elizabeth W. Jones. "Types of DNA Markers Present in Genomic DNA." In *Genetics: Analysis of Genes and Genomes*. 7th ed. Sudbury, Mass.: Jones and Bartlett, 2009. This excellent introductory genetics textbook devotes a section of chapter 2 to a discussion of RFLP within the broader context of DNA structure and genetic variation.

Jeffreys, A., V. Wilson, and S. L. Thein. "Individual-Specific Fingerprints of Human DNA." *Nature* 316, no. 6023 (July 4-10, 1985): 76-79. A technical article that describes some of the background information that led to the use of RFLP analysis in forensic science.

Karp, Gerald. "Genetic Analysis in Molecular Biology." In *Cell and Molecular Biology: Concepts and Experiments*. 5th ed. Chichester, England: John Wiley and Sons, 2008. Includes information about RFLP.

Orkin, S. H., et al. "Improved Detection of the Sickle Mutation by DNA Analysis: Application to Prenatal Diagnosis." *New England Journal of Medicine* 307, no. 1 (July 1, 1982): 32-36. Appears in the same issue as another article on the topic by J. C. Chang and Y. W. Kan.

See also: Blotting: Southern, Northern, and Western; Chromosome theory of heredity; DNA fingerprinting; Gender identity; Genetic engineering; Genetic testing; Model organism: *Arabidopsis thaliana;* Paternity tests; Polymerase chain reaction; Prenatal diagnosis; Restriction enzymes.

Rh incompatibility and isoimmunization

CATEGORY: Diseases and syndromes
ALSO KNOWN AS: RhD incompatibility

DEFINITION

One of the first tests performed at the beginning of a pregnancy is blood-type. This basic test determines a pregnant woman's blood type and Rh factor. People with different blood types have proteins specific to that blood type on the surface of their red blood cells. There are four blood types (A, B, AB, and O). Each of the four blood types is additionally classified according to the presence of another protein on the surface of the red blood cells that indicates an individual's Rh factor. If an individual carries this protein, he or she is Rh positive. If he or she does not carry the protein, he or she is Rh negative.

Most people, about 85 percent, are Rh positive. However, if a woman who is Rh negative and a man who is Rh positive conceive a baby, there is the potential for incompatibility. The baby growing inside the Rh-negative mother may have Rh-positive blood, inherited from the father. Statistically, at least 50 percent of the children born to an Rh-negative mother and an Rh-positive father will be Rh positive.

If an Rh-negative mother-to-be of her first child is carrying an Rh-positive fetus, exposure to fetal antigens can cause the mother to produce antibodies against those antigens. There is no harm to that first child, and usually, the placenta acts as a barrier to fetal blood entering the maternal circulation. But if there is a "break" in that placental barrier (which can be triggered by a variety of factors), the mother then produces the antibodies. In subsequent pregnancies, the maternal antibodies will attach to fetal red blood cells and destroy them. This leads to fetal anemia and various potentially serious complications for the new-born baby.

RISK FACTORS

Risk factors for Rh incompatibility and isoimmu niza-tion include being a pregnant woman with Rh neg-ative blood who had a prior pregnancy with a fe tus that was Rh positive; being a pregnant woman who had a prior blood transfusion or amniocentesis; and being a pregnant woman with Rh-negative blood who did not receive Rh immunization prophylaxis during a prior pregnancy with an Rh-positive fetus. Other risk factors are those that can cause a "break" in the

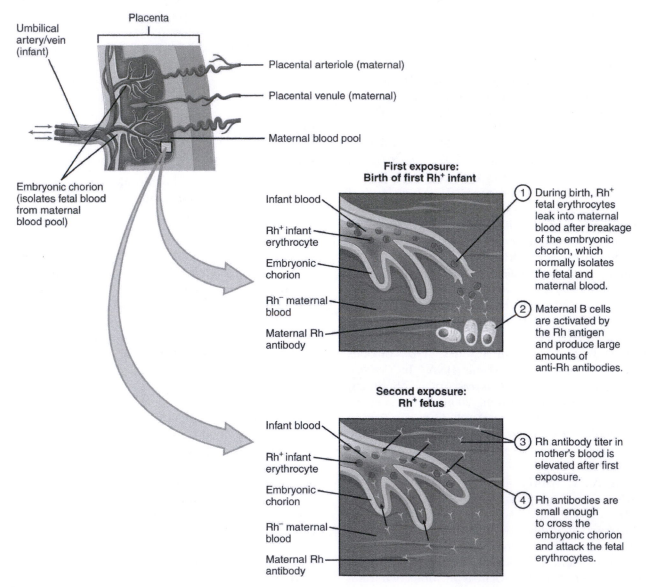

Hemolytic disease of the newborn By OpenStax College, via Wikimedia Commons

placental barrier described under definition. They include, but are not limited to:

- Past abortion or ectopic pregnancy
- Partial molar pregnancy
- Blighted ovum
- Antepartum bleeding
- Procedures (such as amniocentesis or past blood transfusion)
- Abdominal trauma

ETIOLOGY AND GENETICS

The Rh locus on the short arm of chromosome 1 at position 1p36.2-p34 actually consists of two genes, *RHD* and *RHCE*, that are organized in tandem and are so similar in sequence that it is clear that they evolved from the duplication of a common ances tral gene. There are two phenotypes, Rh positive and Rh nega-tive, that are distinguished by the presence or absence of the RhD antigen (the protein product of the *RHD* gene) on the surface of red blood cells. The *RHCE* gene encodes both the RhC and RhE proteins, but since these do not confer antigenic properties on the cell, they do not con tribute to the Rh phenotype. Most individuals who are Rh negative have a deletion of the entire *RHD* gene and retain only the *RHCE* gene.

The Rh-positive allele is dominant to the Rh neg-ative allele, so Rh-positive individuals have either one or two copies of the *RHD* gene. Rh-negative in dividuals lack the *RHD* gene on both of their copies of chromosome 1. Two Rh-positive individuals who are both heterozygous (having only one copy of the *RHD* gene) have a 25 percent chance of having an Rh-negative child and a 75 percent chance of hav-ing an Rh-positive child. In all cases of Rh incom-patability, the mother is Rh negative and both the father and the developing fetus are Rh positive.

SYMPTOMS

Signs and complications affect only the newborn. They occur when standard preventive measures are not taken and can vary from mild to very serious. The mother's health is not affected.

Signs in the newborn baby include anemia and swelling of the body (also called hydrops fetalis), which may be associated with heart failure and respi-ratory problems.

Signs in the early stage include a high biliru-bin level (greater than 18 milligrams/cubic centi meters), extreme jaundice, an absent startle reflex, a poor suck, and lethargy. Symptoms in the interme diate stage include a high-pitched cry, an arched back with neck hyperextended backward (opisthot onos), a bulging fontanel (soft spot), and seizures. Late-stage symptoms include high-pitched hearing loss, mental retardation, muscle rigidity, speech dif ficulties, seizures, and movement disorder.

The late stage signs are due to very high levels of bilirubin causing brain damage, a rare condition called kernicterus.

SCREENING AND DIAGNOSIS

There are no physical symptoms that would prompt a woman to suspect a potential problem with Rh in compatibility. It is very common practice for health care providers to order a blood test that will deter mine whether a mother-to-be is Rh positive or Rh negative.

If the blood test indicates that a patient has devel-oped Rh antibodies, it is common to include identifi-cation of the specific antibody and its titer. There are several classes of antibodies. The two of interest are IgM and IgG. If the antibody can be identified as an IgM, then it does not cross the placenta and there is no risk of hemolysis to the fetus. Anti-K, anti-D, anti-E, anti-Fya , anti-Jka, and antibodies directed against Rh antigens comprise the majority of antibodies respon-sible for hemolytic disease of the newborn.

For the antibody sensitized patient, the blood may be monitored regularly to assess the level of antibod-ies it contains. If the levels are high, an amniocentesis and ultrasound evaluations might be recommended to determine the degree of impact on the fetus.

TREATMENT AND THERAPY

Since Rh incompatibility is almost completely pre-ventable with the use of prophylactic immuniza tion (Rh immune globulin injection or RhoGAM), pre vention remains the best treatment.

An injection of Rho immune globulin is usually given at week twenty-eight to thirty-two of the preg nancy. This desensitizes the blood to Rh-positive blood. Another injection is usually given within seventy-two hours after delivery (or miscarriage, induced abortion, or ectopic pregnancy). This injection further desensitizes their blood for future pregnancies.

Treatment of a pregnancy or newborn depends on the severity of the condition. If the condition is mild, treatment includes aggressive hydration and photo-therapy using bilirubin lights.

Treatment for hydrops fetalis includes amniocentesis to determine severity, an intrauterine fetal transfusion, and early induction of labor. In more severe cases, a direct transfusion of packed red blood cells (compatible with the infant's blood) and exchange transfusion of the newborn may be done to rid the infant's blood of the maternal antibodies that are destroying the red blood cells. Treatment may also include control of heart failure and fluid retention.

Treatment for kernicterus includes exchange transfusion (which may require multiple exchanges) and phototherapy.

Full recovery is expected for mild Rh incompatibility. As noted previously, both hydrops fetalis and kernicterus represent extreme conditions. Both have guarded outcomes; hydrops fetalis has a high risk of mortality. Long-term problems can result from severe cases, including developmental/cognitive delays, movement disorders, hearing loss, and seizures.

PREVENTION AND OUTCOMES

Rh incompatibility is almost completely preventable. Rh-negative mothers should be followed closely by their obstetricians during pregnancy. If the father of the infant is Rh-positive, the mother is given a midterm injection of RhoGAM and a second injection within a few days of delivery. These injections prevent the development of antibodies against Rh-positive blood. This effectively prevents the condition. Routine prenatal care should help identify, manage, and treat any complications of Rh incompatibility.

Rick Alan; reviewed by Jeff Andrews, M.D., FRCSC, FACOG "Etiology and Genetics" by Jeffrey A. Knight, Ph.D.; updated by Gary M. Flashner, M.S., M.D.

FURTHER READING

Available through http://www.ebscohost.com. Moise, K. J., Jr. "Management of Rhesus Alloimmunization in Pregnancy." *Obstetrics and Gynecology* 112, no. 1 (July, 2008): 164–176.

Beers, Mark H., ed. *The Merck Manual of Medical Information.* 2d home ed., new and rev. Whitehouse Station, N.J.: Merck Research Laboratories, 2003. EBSCO Publishing. *Health Library: Rh Incompatibility and Isoimmunization.* Ipswich, Mass.: Author, 2009.

Elalfy MS, Elbarbary NS, Abaza HW. "Early intravenous immunoglobin (two-dose regimen) in the management of severe Rh hemolytic disease of newborn–a prospective randomized controlled trial." *Eur J Pediatr.* 2011 Apr. 170(4):461–7.

Kolialexi A, Tounta G, Mavrou A. "Noninvasive fetal RhD genotyping from maternal blood." *Expert Rev Mol Diagn.* 2010 Apr. 10(3):285–96

Smits-Wintjens, V. E., F. J. Walther, and E. Lopriore. "Rhesus Haemolytic Disease of the Newborn: Postnatal Management, Associated Morbidity, and Long-Term Outcome." *Seminars in Fetal and Neonatal Medicine* 13, no. 4 (August, 2008): 265-271.

WEB SITES OF INTEREST

American College of Obstetricians and Gynecologists
http://www.acog.org

Kids Health from Nemours: Rh Incompatability
http://kidshealth.org/parent/pregnancy
_newborn/pregnancy/rh.html

March of Dimes Foundation: Rh Disease
http://www.marchofdimes.com/professionals/
14332_1220.asp

The Society of Obstetricians and Gynaecologists of Canada
http://www.sogc.org/index_e.asp

Women's Health Matters
http://www.womenshealthmatters.ca/index.
cfmhttps://www.nhlbi.nih.gov/health/
health-topics/topics/rh
http://emedicine.medscape.com/article/
797150-overview

See also: ABO blood types; Chronic myeloid leukemia; Fanconi anemia; Hemophilia; Hereditary spherocytosis; Infantile agranulocytosis; Myelodysplastic syndromes; Paroxysmal nocturnal hemoglobinuria; Porphyria; Sickle-cell disease.

RhoGDI2 gene

CATEGORY: Diseases and syndromes
SIGNIFICANCE: The activity of the *RhoGD12* gene has been linked to stopping cancerous tumors from

spreading to other areas of the body. People with cancer whose *RhoGD12* gene is active have much less chance of a cancer spreading from one part of the body to another. This gene's ability to act seems to be linked to an endothelin inhibitor and may be helped by the *SRC* gene.

Key terms

anti-oncogene: a gene that stops or suppresses uncontrolled cell growth that may lead to cancer

expression: the ability of a gene to influence the body to perform a certain way

metastasis: the spread of a cancer from its original site to other parts of the body

oncogene: a gene that is known to trigger some type of cancer

suppression: "turning off" a gene or suppressing the gene's normal actions

tumor suppression: stopping the spread of a cancerous tumor from one part of the body to another

Tumor Suppression

RhoGD12 is an anti-oncogene, or a gene that may help suppress the growth of cancer. In 2002, researchers discovered a link between *RhoGD12* and tumor suppression. Researchers put *RhoGD12* into some cells that were then injected into mice that had compromised immune systems. When compared to a control group of mice in which every mouse had many tumors that metastasized, only about half of the mice with *RhoGD12* got tumors, and those mice that had tumors had many fewer tumors than the control group. Current thinking is that this gene is able to affect the way cells move about the body, thus influencing the movement of cancerous cells between body systems.

ET-1 and *RhoGD12*

The impact of the *RhoGD12* gene has been studied extensively in the relationship between bladder cancer and lung cancer. According to studies, about half of patients with late-stage bladder cancer end up having a relapse of their cancer where it spreads to the lungs, which is often the cause of death. Researchers believed that this was caused by a suppression of the *RhoGD12* gene that allowed the cancer to spread. They believed that this suppression occurred because of the *RhoGD12* gene's complicated relationship with an endothelin inhibitor called ET-1. ET-1 is known to cause cells to grow and divide, particularly

cells involved in the production of blood vessels. Due to the increased ineffectiveness of the *RhoGD12* gene to stop the spread of the cancer, ET-1 was able to allow tumors to grow in the lungs at an increased rate. Currently, researchers are unsure as to why or how ET-1 stops the *RhoGD12* gene from helping to suppress the spread of cancer throughout the body.

SRC and RhoGD12SRC

RhoGD12SRC is an oncogene, or a gene that has been known to trigger cancer. This gene was commonly thought to help all cancers grow and spread by allowing cells to grow and divide in an uncontrolled way, and many cancers were treated by using therapies that inhibited this gene from expression. Recent research has shown that this gene may work together with or somehow modify the *RhoGD12* gene to help cells use their natural ability to stop tumor growth in bladder cancer, and that the best treatment for bladder cancer may involve allowing SRC gene expression, even though this may not help in treatment for other types of cancer. This research is changing the way some scientists and doctors think about treating cancer—some genes that negatively influence some types of cancers could be a positive influence for other types of cancers, emphasizing the important of individually treating cancers in the way that is best for the patient and the type of cancer that he or she may have.

Impact

This gene seems to be able to stop metastasis or restrain the secondary growth and spread of any type of cancer. In some recent studies of cancer in humans, the presence of this gene seemed to track along with the stage and grade of the cancer. It is possible that this gene can be used as a marker to determine which cancers are likely to spread and which are likely to remain contained. Research currently focuses on discovering the mechanism by which this gene suppresses cancer growth and determining if that mechanism can be manipulated so this gene can be used in treating cancer or keeping it in check. Research is also ongoing on how this gene is influenced by other genes or substances in the body.

Marianne M. Madsen, M.S.

Further Reading

Gildea, J. J., et al. "*RhoGD12* Is an Invasion and Metastasis Suppressor Gene in Human Cancer." *Cancer*

Research 62, no. 22 (November 15, 2002): 6418-6423. The description of the research that led to *RhoGD12* being identified as an anti-oncogene.

Stafford, L. J., K. S. Vaidya, and D. R. Welch. "Metastasis Suppressors Genes in Cancer." *The International Journal of Biochemistry & Cell Biology* 40, no. 5 (2008): 874-891. Provides a discussion of many types of anti-oncogenes.

Titus, B., et al. "Endothelin Axis Is a Target of the Lung Metastasis Suppressor Gene *RhoGD12.*" *Clinical Cancer Research* 65, no. 16 (2005). This article is a generally cited primary research article describing the research linking *RhoGD12* to ET-1.

Wu, Y., et al. "Neuromedin U Is Regulated by the Metastasis Suppressor *RhoGDI2* and Is a Novel Promoter of Tumor Formation, Lung Metastasis, and Cancer Cachexia." *Oncogene* 26 (2007). This article describes further research linking this gene to tumor suppression in a variety of cancers.

See also: *BRAF* gene; *BRCA1* and *BRCA2* genes; *MLH1* gene; *PMS* genes; *RB1* gene; *SCLC1* gene.

RNA interference (RNAi)

CATEGORY: Cell biology; Genetic engineering and biotechnology; Molecular genetics

SIGNIFICANCE: The term RNAi stands for "RNA interference," a newly discovered gene regulatory mechanism that downregulates gene expression in a sequence-specific manner by acting at the post-transcriptional level. This has undoubtedly been one of the biggest advances in genetics in decades, since it has added another perspective to the role of RNA in cells.

BACKGROUND

In the late 1980s to early 1990s, plant biologist Richard Jorgensen was trying to make intense purple petunias by introducing extra copies of the purple pigment gene (Chalcone synthase *chs*A). He was quite surprised when the effort yielded instead white and variegated petunias. It seemed that somehow the introduced gene (the transgenes) had blocked (silenced) its own expression as well the expression

of the endogenous purple pigment genes (termed "cosuppression"). Analysis of transcription rates in these cells using nuclear run-on assays did not indicate a decrease, implying that the phenomenon should be renamed as post-transcriptional gene silencing (PTGS). Following soon thereafter, were reports of "quelling" observed in the fungi *Neurospora crassa*. An effort to boost the orange phenotype *(all+)* shown by wild-type (wt) *Neurospora* by transforming it with a plasmid containing a 1500 bp fragment of the coding sequence of the *all+* gene, generated

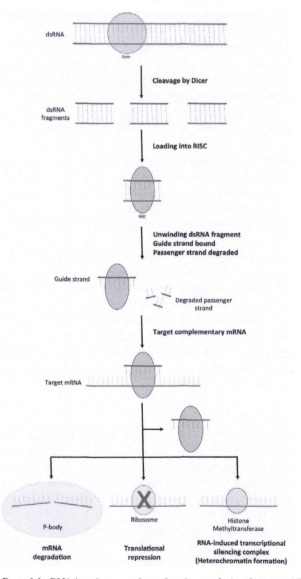

Part of the RNA interference pathway focusing on the involvement of the RNA-induced silencing complex (RISC). By Lonugget (Own work), via Wikimedia Commons

albino *Neurospora.* Once again in these *al1+* quelled strains, it was the level of the mature messenger RNA (mRNA) that was affected in a homology-dependent manner. These findings were better understood when in 1998 Andrew Fire and Craig Mello reported that introduction of double-stranded RNA (dsRNA) corresponding to the *unc-22* gene into a roundworm (*Caenorhabditis elegans*) specifically disrupted the expression of the endogenous *unc-22* gene. *unc-22* in *C. elegans* codes for a nonessential myofilament protein, and a reduction in *unc-22* activity produced a twitching phenotype in these worms. If the dsRNA was introduced into the worm gonads, the phenotype was heritable since the progeny too demonstrated the classic twitching phenotype. This demonstration offered an easy method to generate loss-of-function mutants since the silencing mechanism in *C. elegans* could be initiated simply by soaking the worms in solutions containing dsRNA or by feeding the worms *E. coli* that expressed the dsRNA. The silencing of a functional gene by introduction of exogenous dsRNA, homologous to the target gene was renamed RNA interference (RNAi). Since then RNAi-related events have been identified in a multitude

The major differences between plant and animal gene silencing: natively expressed microRNA or exogenous small interfering RNA is processed by dicer and integrated into the RISC complex, which mediates gene silencing. By Anne Saumet and Charles-Henri Lecellier, via Wikimedia Commons

of eukaryotes ranging from protozoa, parasites, and fruit flies to mouse- and human-derived cell lines.

MOLECULAR MECHANISM

One of the earliest clues into the molecular basis of RNAi was provided by the discovery of short (20–25 nucleotides long) RNAs in the plant cells that matched the silencing target. Around the same time, in vitro RNAi assays using fruit-fly (*Drosophila melanogaster*) extracts revealed that the long dsRNA was being cleaved into 21–23 base pairs (bp) long RNA duplexes with 2 base overhangs at each end. These RNA species were called short interfering RNA (siRNA), and the enzyme responsible for producing these siRNAs from the dsRNA was called Dicer. Soon thereafter, the "sense" strand (sequence is identical to the target mRNA) is destroyed and the fate of the "antisense" strand thereon depends upon the organism. In mammals and fruit flies, the antisense strand is incorporated into the RISC (RNA-induced silencing complex), which is made up of RNA-binding proteins and RNA nucleases such as the Argonaute family of proteins found in the flowering plant *Arabidopsis thaliana*. The activated RISC (with the antisense strand of RNA) can now bind to the target mRNA and cleave it, thereby initiating sequence-specific mRNA degradation. This cleaving activity, whereby the RISC cleaves mRNA as directed by siRNA, is called the "Slicer" activity. In worms and plants, the next set of events following destruction of the siRNA sense strand are somewhat different even though the final outcome—RNA destruction—is similar. In these organisms the antisense strand pairs up with the complementary target mRNA, thus initiating synthesis of a long dsRNA by the enzyme RdRP (RNA dependent RNA polymerase). Then Dicer cleaves the long dsRNA and generates siRNAs which act via the RISC to target mRNAs for destruction, as described earlier.

FUNCTION

Over the years, substantial evidence has been collected that indicates a general role for PTGS (RNAi) in silencing parasitic genes such as viruses, transposons ("jumping genes") and repetitive genes (including transgenes). In plant viruses, the double-stranded RNA intermediate in RNA virus replication has been shown to initiate PTGS/RNAi. These findings were supported by the discovery of virus encoded genes that suppress PTGS by a variety of mechanisms such as reducing target mRNA degradation and counteracting the systemic spread of RNA silencing. In 2005, Courtney Wilkins and her team working with a *C. elegans* infection model (utilizing mammalian vesicular stomatitis virus or VSV) have shown that VSV infection is more potent in RNAi defective worms (*rde-1* and *rde-4* mutants) and vice versa. RNase protection assays to investigate whether RNAi is indeed induced upon viral infection revealed the presence of virus-specific siRNAs only in the virus-infected wild-type cells. Transposon duplication and insertion has long been known to create "junk DNA" and thus destabilize the genome. Experiments wherein worms with mutations in the RNAi pathway genes were shown to be incapable of silencing transposons lead to the idea that RNAi has evolved as a cellular defense mechanism that silences transposable elements in order to maintain genome stability. RNAi has also been shown to limit gene expression in a dosage-dependent manner in plants as well as fruit flies. In both of these instances gene expression is enhanced by adding extra copies of the particular gene but only up to a point. Beyond that point, gene expression (especially transcription) is drastically reduced by modifying proteins that help to package DNA.

IMPACT

Over the years, experiments in *Arabidopsis*, *C. elegans*, and *Drosophila* have shown that besides their usual functions such as maintaining genome stability (by blocking transposition), the proteins involved in the RNAi machinery also play a role in the development of the organism. Research has shown that these genomically encoded short, 21- to 28-nucleotide RNAs that regulate temporal development are in fact members of the microRNA (miRNA) family, whose members have been identified across species as diverse as plants, flies, worms, and humans. Although miRNAs, like the siRNAs, are derived by Dicer activity on the dsRNA precursor and are found to be associated with RISC and their target mRNAs, unlike siRNAs, miRNAs are single-stranded and seem capable of affecting previously unknown, post-transcriptional steps such as RNA splicing, mRNA localization, and RNA turnover. An in-depth understanding of the siRNA-miRNA kinship could provide the key to several technological advancements from understanding gene functions by specific gene silencing (akin to genetic knockouts) to exploiting the therapeutic potential of this innate cellular defense mechanism to treat diseases like macular degeneration, caused by overexpression of certain genes.

Since the mid-ninties, tesearchers have used gene silencing in numerous applications; one of the most notable is to genetically modify crops. Using gene silencing, scientists have been able to alter crops to resist disease. certain insects, and other environmental stresses. There is also the potential—and much ongoing research—for RNAi to be used in gene therapies to cure diseases in humans.

Sibani Sengupta, Ph.D.

FURTHER READING

Agarwal, Neema, et al. "RNA Interference: Biology, Mechanism, and Applications." *Microbiology and Molecular Biology Reviews*, December, 2003, pp. 657-685.

Montgomery, Mary K., SiQun Xu, and Andrew Fire. "RNA as a Target of Double-Stranded RNA Mediated Genetics Interference in *C. elegans*." *Proceedings of the National Academy of Sciences* 95 (December, 1998): 15502–07. Print.

Novina, Carl D., and Philip Sharp. "The RNAi Revolution." *Nature*, 430 (July 8, 2004): 161–164. Print.

"Pocket K No. 34: RNAi for Crop Improvement." *International Service for the Acquisition of Agri-Biotech Applications.* ISAAA, 2015. Web. 30 Nov. 2015.

Wilkins, Courtney, et al. "RNA Interference Is an Antiviral Defence Mechanism in *Caenorhabditis elegans*." *Nature* 436 (August 18, 2005): 1044-1047.

Younis, Adnan, Muhammad Irfan Siddique, Chang-Kil Kim, and Ki-Byung Lim. "RNA Interference (RNAi) Induced Gene Silencing: A Promising Approach of Hi-Tech Plant Breeding." *International Journal of Biological Sciences* 10.10 (2014): 1150–58. Print.

See also: RNA isolation; RNA structure and function; RNA transcription and mRNA processing; RNA world.

RNA isolation

CATEGORY: Molecular genetics

SIGNIFICANCE: All cells in an organism or population of organisms of the same species contain the same (or nearly the same) set of genes. Therefore, understanding which genes are expressed under different conditions is critical to answering many questions in biology, including how cells differentiate into tissues, how cells respond to different environments, and which genes are expressed in tumor cells. The starting point for answering those questions is RNA isolation.

KEY TERMS

cDNA library: a set of copies, or clones, of all or nearly all mRNA molecules produced by cells of an organism

complementary DNA (cDNA): also called copy DNA, DNA that copies RNA molecules, made using the enzyme reverse transcriptase

microarray analysis: a method, requiring isolated RNA, that allows simultaneous determination of which of thousands of genes are transcribed (expressed) in cells

reverse transcription polymerase chain reaction (RT-PCR) a technique, requiring isolated RNA, for quickly determining if a gene or a small set of genes are transcribed in a population of cells

RNA: ribonucleic acid, the macromolecule in the cell that acts as an intermediary between the genetic information stored as DNA and the manifestation of that genetic information as proteins

RNases: ribonucleases, or cellular enzymes that catalyze the breakdown of RNA

CELL LYSIS

RNA isolation is a difficult proposition. RNA has a short life span in cells (as short as minutes in bacteria), and it is somewhat chemically unstable. In addition, enzymes that degrade RNA (RNases) are widespread in the environment, further complicating the task of separating intact RNA from other molecules in the cell.

The first step in RNA isolation is rapidly breaking open cells under conditions where RNA will not be degraded. One method involves freezing cells immediately in liquid nitrogen, then grinding the cells in liquid nitrogen in order to prevent any RNA degradation. Other methods involve lysing cells in the presence of strong protein denaturants so that any RNases present in the cell or the environment will be rapidly inactivated. The difficulty of the cell lysis step depends substantially on the type of cell involved. Bacterial and fungal cells are typically much more difficult to break open than

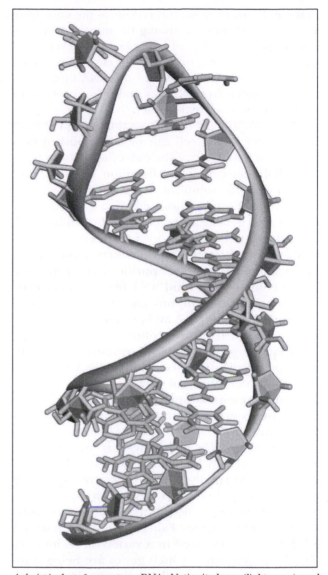

A hairpin loop from a pre-mRNA. Notice its bases (light green) and backbone (sky blue). NMR structure of the central region of the human GluR-B R/G pre-mRNA, from the protein data bank ID 1ysv. Taken from w:PDB ids 1ysv model 1 imaged using w:UCSF Chimera By Vossman (Own work), via Wikimedia Commons

cells from mammals. As a consequence, it is often more difficult to isolate intact RNA from bacteria and fungi.

PROTEIN DENATURATION AND FURTHER PURIFICATION

The next step in RNA isolation is to denature all proteins from the cell, to ensure that RNases will be inactive. In many cases, this is done at the same time as cell lysis. RNases are among the most resilient enzymes known, capable of being boiled or even autoclaved, yet retaining the ability to cleave RNA once they cool down. Consequently, the RNA next needs to be separated from RNases and other proteins to ensure that it will remain intact.

The separation of RNA from the rest of the macromolecules in the cell can be accomplished in a number of ways. One of the older methods for purifying RNA uses ultracentrifugation in very dense cesium chloride solutions. During high-speed centrifugation, these solutions create a gradient, with the greatest density at the bottom of the tube. RNA is the densest macromolecule in the cell, so it forms a pellet in the bottom of the ultracentrifuge tube. A newer technique for RNA purification involves the use of columns that bind RNA but not other macromolecules. The columns are washed to remove impurities, such as DNA and proteins, and then the RNA is eluted from the column matrix. A newer technique is based on the observation that, at an appropriate pH (level of acidity), RNA partitions into the water phase of a water-organic mixture. DNA and proteins either are retained at the boundary of the water-organic mixture or are dissolved in the organic phase.

Once the RNA is isolated, it needs to be handled carefully to ensure that it will not be degraded. Normally this involves resuspending the RNA in purified water, adding an alcohol solution, and storing it at −70 or −80 degrees Celsius (−94 or −112 degrees Fahrenheit). The purified RNA can then be used in a variety of techniques that help determine which genes are being transcribed in particular cells or tissues. These techniques include RT-PCR, Northern hybridization, microarray analysis, and the construction of cDNA libraries.

SPECIAL RNA ISOLATION PROCEDURES

In some cases, a geneticist wants to isolate only RNA from the cytoplasm of the cell, since RNA from the nucleus may be more heterogeneous. In this case, cells are lysed using a gentle detergent that disrupts the cytoplasmic membrane, without disturbing the nuclear membrane. Centrifugation is used to separate the nuclei from the cytoplasm and then the cytoplasmic RNA is further purified as described above.

For some procedures, such as RT-PCR, the RNA sometimes needs to be further purified to ensure that no contaminating DNA is present. In this case, the RNA sample may be treated with the enzyme DNase I, which destroys DNA but leaves RNA intact.

For other procedures, like cDNA library construction, the RNA is often purified to remove ribosomal RNA (rRNA), transfer RNA (tRNA), and other stable RNAs, since the majority of RNA in the cell (typically more than 90 percent) is rRNA and tRNA. In this case, the RNA solution is treated by incubating it with single-stranded DNA containing a chain of eighteen to twenty thymine nucleotides, either on a column or in solution. Messenger RNA (mRNA) from eukaryotes contains runs of twenty to two hundred adenine nucleotides that bind to the single-stranded DNA and allow the mRNA to be purified away from the stable RNAs.

Like most techniques in genetics, RNA isolation methods have improved greatly over the years. With advances in methods for studying gene expression such as microarray analysis, isolating intact RNA is a technique that is more critical than ever in the genetics laboratory.

Patrick G. Guilfoile, Ph.D.

FURTHER READING

Ausubel, Fredrick, et al. *Current Protocols in Molecular Biology.* Hoboken, N.J.: John Wiley and Sons, 1998. Includes RNA isolation protocols from several different laboratories.

Avison, Matthew B. "Isolation and Analysis of RNA." In *Measuring Gene Expression.* New York: Taylor & Francis, 2007. Discusses the properties of different types of RNA and various methods of isolating, purifying, and stabilizing RNA. Describes six protocols for isolating RNA from animal cells and tissues, bacterial and yeast cells, plant and filamentous fungal cells, and tissue culture cells.

Clark, David P. "Nucleic Acids: Isolation, Purification, Detection, and Hybridization." In *Molecular Biology.* Boston: Elsevier Academic Press, 2005. Includes information about RNA isolation.

Farrell, Robert E., Jr. *RNA Methodologies: A Laboratory Guide for Isolation and Characterization.* 3d ed. Boston: Elsevier/Academic Press, 2005. Probably the definitive book on RNA techniques, including RNA isolation. Includes a substantial amount of background information, as well as detailed protocols.

Liu, Dongyou, ed. *Handbook of Nucleic Acid Purification*. Boca Raton, Fla.: CRC Press, 2009. Describes various nucleic acid isolation methods, with sections focusing on techniques to analyze viruses, bacteria, fungi, parasites, insects, mammals, and plants.

O'Connell, Joe, ed. *RT-PCR Protocols*. Totowa, N.J.: Humana Press, 2002. Collects several papers on the use of reverse transcription polymerase chain reaction in analysis of mRNA, quantitative methodologies, detection of RNA viruses, genetic analysis, and immunology. Tables, charts, index.

Sambrook, J., and D. W. Russell, eds. *Molecular Cloning: A Laboratory Manual*. 3d ed. Cold Spring Harbor, N.Y.: Cold Spring Harbor Laboratory Press, 2000. One of the most popular guides to molecular biology protocols. Includes several RNA isolation procedures.

See also: cDNA libraries; DNA isolation; DNA structure and function; Polymerase chain reaction; Reverse transcriptase; RNA structure and function; RNA transcription and mRNA processing.

RNA structure and function

CATEGORY: Molecular genetics

SIGNIFICANCE: Ribonucleic acid (RNA), a molecule that plays many roles in the storage and transmission of genetic information, exists in several forms, each with its own unique function. RNA acts as the messenger between genes in the DNA and their protein product, directing the assembly of proteins. RNA is also an integral part of ribosomes, the site of protein synthesis, and some RNAs have been shown to have catalytic properties. Understanding the structure and function of RNA is important to a fundamental knowledge of genetics; in addition, many developing medical therapies will undoubtedly utilize special RNAs to combat genetic diseases.

KEY TERMS

messenger RNA (mRNA): a type of RNA that carries genetic instructions, copied from genes in DNA, to the ribosome to be decoded during translation

retrovirus: a special type of virus that carries its genetic information as RNA and converts it into DNA that integrates into the cells of the virus's host organism

ribosomal RNA (rRNA): a type of RNA that forms a major part of the structure of the ribosome

ribosomes: organelles that function in protein synthesis and are made up of a large and a small subunit composed of proteins and ribosomal RNA (rRNA) molecules

ribozyme: an RNA molecule that can function catalytically as an enzyme

RNAi: abbreviation for "interference RNA," which hampers mRNA translation

small RNA: a class of RNA in which several subspecies are only twenty to twenty-five base pairs long and involved in the degradation or regulation of mRNA

transcription: the synthesis of an RNA molecule directed by RNA polymerase using a DNA template

transfer RNA (tRNA): a form of RNA that acts to decode genetic information present in mRNA, carries a particular amino acid, and is vital to translation

translation: the synthesis of a protein molecule directed by the ribosome using information provided by an mRNA

THE CHEMICAL NATURE OF RNA

Ribonucleic acid (RNA) is a complex biological molecule that is classified along with DNA as a nucleic acid. Chemically, RNA is a polymer (long chain) consisting of subunits called ribonucleotides linked together by phosphodiester bonds. Each ribonucleotide consists of three parts: the sugar ribose (a five-carbon simple sugar), a negatively charged phosphate group, and a nitrogen-containing base. There are four types of ribonucleotides, and the differences among them lie solely in which of four possible bases each contains. The four bases are adenine (A), guanine (G), cytosine (C), and uracil (U).

The structures of DNA and RNA are very similar, with the following differences. The sugar found in the nucleotide subunits of DNA is deoxyribose, which differs slightly from the ribose found in the ribonucleotides of RNA. In addition, while DNA nucleotides also contain four possible bases, there is no uracil in DNA; instead, DNA nucleotides contain a different base called thymine (T). Finally, while DNA exists as a double-stranded helix in nature, RNA is almost always single-stranded. Like DNA, a single

3D structure of the 5S ribosomal RNA component (PDB file 1JJ2), with gray lines for base pairs and ribbon arrows for double-helical regions, colored blue to red from 5' to 3' end of the chain. Shown in the Mage kinemage graphics program and rendered in Raster3D. By Jane Richardson (Dcrjsr) (Own work), via Wikimedia Commons

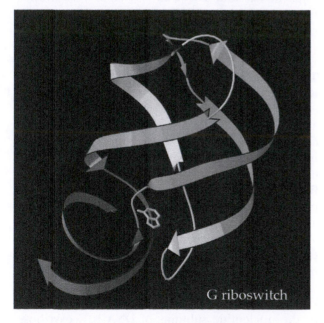

3D structure of G riboswitch RNA molecule (PDB file 1U8D); ribbon arrows for double-helical regions, colored blue to red from 5' to 3' ends of the chain. Shown in Mage. By Jane & David Richardson (Dcrjsr (own work (joint)), via Wikimedia Commons

RNA strand has a 5'-to-3' polarity. These numbers are based on which carbon atom is exposed at the end of the polymer, each of the carbon atoms being numbered around the sugar molecule.

THE FOLDING OF RNA MOLECULES

The function of an RNA molecule is determined by its nucleotide sequence, which represents information derived from DNA. This nucleotide sequence is called the primary structure of the molecule. Many RNAs also have an important secondary structure, a three-dimensional shape that is also important for the function of the molecule. The secondary structure is determined by hydrogen bonding between parts of the RNA molecule that are complementary. Complementary pairing is always between A and U ribonucleotides and C and G ribonucleotides. Hydrogen bonding results in double-stranded regions in the secondary structure.

Since RNA is single-stranded, it was recognized shortly after the discovery of some of its major roles that its capacity for folding is great and that this folding might play an important part in the functioning of the molecule. Base pairing often represents local interactions, and a common structural element is a "hairpin loop" or "stem loop." A hairpin loop is formed when two complementary regions are separated by a short stretch of bases so that when they fold back and pair, some bases are left unpaired, forming the loop. The net sum of these local interactions is referred to as the RNA's secondary structure and is usually important to an understanding of how the RNA works. All transfer RNAs (tRNAs), for example, are folded into a secondary structure that contains three stem loops and a fourth stem without a loop, a structure resembling a cloverleaf in two dimensions.

Finally, local structural elements may interact with other elements in long-range interactions, causing more complicated folding of the molecule. The full three-dimensional structure of a tRNA molecule from yeast was finally confirmed in 1978 by several groups independently, using X-ray diffraction. In this process, crystals of a molecule are bombarded with X-rays, which causes them to scatter; an expert can tell by the pattern of scattering how the different atoms in the molecule are oriented with respect to one another. The cloverleaf arrangement of a tRNA undergoes further folding so that the entire molecule takes on a roughly *L*-shaped appearance in three dimensions. An understanding of the three-dimensional shape of an RNA molecule is crucial to understanding its function. By the late 1990s, the three-dimensional structures of many tRNAs had been worked out, but it had proven difficult to do X-ray diffraction analyses on most other RNAs because of technical problems. More advanced computer programs and alternate structure-determining techniques like mass spectroscopy, nuclear magnetic resonance and cryo electron microscopy are enabling research in this field to proceed, with the RNA structures catalogued online in the Nucleic Acid Database and Protein Data Bank.

SYNTHESIS AND STABILITY OF RNA

RNA molecules of all types are continually being synthesized and degraded in a cell; even the longest-lasting ones exist for only a day or two. Shortly after the structure of DNA was established, it became clear that RNA was synthesized using a DNA molecule as a template, and the mechanism was worked out shortly thereafter. The entire process by which an RNA molecule is constructed using the information in DNA is called transcription. An enzyme called RNA polymerase is responsible for assembling the ribonucleotides of a new RNA complementary to a specific DNA segment (gene). Only one strand of the DNA is used as a template (the sense strand), and the ribonucleotides are initially arranged according to the base-pairing rules. A DNA sequence called the "promoter" is a site RNA polymerase can bind initially and allows the process of RNA synthesis to begin. At the appropriate starting site, RNA polymerase begins to assemble and connect the nucleotides according to the complementary pairing rules, such that for every A nucleotide in the DNA, RNA polymerase incorporates a U ribonucleotide into the RNA being assembled. The remaining pairing rules stipulate that a T in DNA denotes an A in RNA and that a C in DNA represents a G in RNA (and vice versa). This process continues until another sequence, called a "terminator," is reached. At this point, the RNA polymerase stops transcription, and a new RNA molecule is released.

Much attention is rightfully focused on transcription, since it controls the rate of synthesis of each RNA. It has become increasingly clear, however, that the amount of RNA in the cell at a given time is also strongly dependent on RNA stability (the rate at which it is degraded). Every cell contains several enzymes called ribonucleases (RNases) whose job it is to cut up RNA molecules into their ribonucleotides subunits. Some RNAs last only thirty seconds, while others may last up to a day or two. It is important to remember that both the rates of synthesis (transcription) and degradation ultimately determine the amount of functional RNA in a cell at any given time.

THREE CLASSES OF RNA

While all RNAs are produced by transcription, several classes of RNA are created, and each has a unique function. By the late 1960s, three major classes of RNAs had been identified, and their respective roles in the process of protein synthesis had been identified. In general, protein synthesis refers to the assembly of a protein using information encoded in DNA, with RNA acting as an intermediary to carry information and assist in protein building. In 1956, Francis Crick, one of the scientists who had discovered the double-helical structure of DNA, referred to this information flow as the "central dogma," a term that continues to be used, although exceptions to it are now known.

A messenger RNA (mRNA) carries a complementary copy of the DNA instructions for building a particular protein. Making up about 5 percent of the three RNA classes, in eukaryotes mRNA typically represents the information from a single gene and carries the information to a ribosome, the site of protein synthesis. The information must be decoded to make a protein. Nucleotides are read in groups of three (called codons). In addition, mRNAs contain signals that tell a ribosome where to start and stop translating.

Ribosomal RNA (rRNA) is part of the structure of the ribosome and makes up about 80 percent of the total RNA in a cell. Four different rRNAs interact with many proteins to form functional ribosomes that direct the events of protein synthesis. One of the rRNAs interacts with mRNA to orient it properly so translation can begin at the correct location. Another rRNA acts to facilitate the transfer of the growing polypeptide from one tRNA to another (peptidyl transferase activity).

Transfer RNA (tRNA) accounts for 15 percent of the three RNA categories and serves the vital role of decoding the genetic information. There are at least twenty and usually more than forty different tRNAs in a cell. On one side, tRNAs contain an "anticodon" loop, which can base-pair with mRNA codons according to their sequence and the base-pairing rules. On the other side, each contains an amino acid binding site, with the appropriate amino acid for its anticodon. In this way, tRNAs recognize the codons and supply the appropriate amino acids. The process continues until an entire new polypeptide has been constructed.

The attachment of the correct amino acids is facilitated by a group of enzymes called tRNA amino acyl synthetases. Each type of tRNA has a corresponding synthetase that facilitates the attachment of the correct amino acid to the amino acid binding site. The integrity of this process is crucial to translation; if only one tRNA is attached to an incorrect amino acid, the resulting proteins will likely be nonfunctional.

SPLIT GENES AND mRNA PROCESSING IN EUKARYOTES

In bacterial genes, there is colinearity between the segment of a DNA molecule that is transcribed and the resulting mRNA. In other words, the mRNA sequence is complementary to its template and is the same length, as would be expected. In the late 1970s, several groups of scientists made a seemingly bizarre discovery regarding mRNAs in eukaryotes (organisms whose cells contain a nucleus, including all living things that are not bacteria): the sequences of mRNAs isolated from eukaryotes were not collinear with the DNA from which they were transcribed. The coding regions of the corresponding DNA were interrupted by seemingly random sequences that served no apparent function. These "introns," as they came to be known, were apparently transcribed along with the coding regions (exons) but were somehow removed before the mRNA was translated. This completely unexpected observation led to further investigations that revealed that mRNA is extensively processed, or modified, after its transcription in eukaryotes.

After a eukaryotic mRNA is transcribed, it contains several introns and is referred to as immature, or a "pre-mRNA." Before it can become mature and functional, three major processing events must occur: splicing, the addition of a 5 cap, and a "tail." The process of splicing is complex and occurs in the nucleus with the aid of "spliceosomes," large complexes of RNAs and proteins that identify intervening sequences and cut them out of the pre-mRNA. In addition, spliceosomes rejoin the exons to produce a complete, functional mRNA. Splicing must be extremely specific, since a mistake causing the removal of even one extra nucleotide could change the final protein, making it nonfunctional. During splicing, capping and the addition of a poly-A tail

take place. A so-called cap, which consists of a modified G nucleotide, is added to the beginning (5 end) of the pre-mRNA by an unconventional linkage. The cap appears to function by interacting with the ribosome, helping to orient the mature mRNA so that translation begins at the proper end. A tail, which consists of many A nucleotides (often two hundred or more), is attached to the 3 end of the pre-mRNA. This so-called poly-A tail, which virtually all eukaryotic mRNAs contain, seems to be one factor in determining the relative stability of an mRNA. These important steps must be performed after transcription in eukaryotes to produce a functional mRNA.

RIBOZYMES

The traditional roles of RNA in protein synthesis were originally considered its only roles. RNA in general, while considered an important molecule, was thought of as a "helper" in translation. This all began to change in 1982, when the molecular biologists Thomas Cech and Sidney Altman, working independently and with different systems, reported the existence of RNA molecules that had catalytic activity. This means that RNA molecules can function as enzymes; until this time, it was believed that all enzymes were protein molecules. The importance of these findings cannot be overstated, and Cech and Altman ultimately shared the 1989 Nobel Prize in Chemistry for the discovery of these RNA enzymes, or "ribozymes." Both of these initial ribozymes catalyzed reactions that involved the cleavage of other RNA molecules, which is to say they acted as nucleases. Subsequently, many ribozymes have been found in various organisms, from bacteria to humans. Some of them are able to catalyze different types of reactions, and there are new ones reported every year. Thus ribozymes are not a mere curiosity but play an integral role in the molecular machinery of many organisms. Their discovery also gave rise to the idea that at one point in evolutionary history, molecular systems composed solely of RNA, performing many roles, existed in an "RNA world."

RNAi PATHWAY AND SMALL RNAs

At around the same time as these momentous discoveries, still other classes of RNAs were being discovered, each with its own specialized functions. In 1981, Jun-ichi Tomizawa discovered interference RNA whereby RNA has the ability to interfere with protein production. This hindering RNA is known as "antisense RNA" because it is the opposite complement of, and thus can bind to, the "sense" strand of protein-coding mRNA, resulting in the prevention or regulation of the mRNA's translation.

In 1990, the power of antisense RNA showed itself in the form of an unexpected white flower. Researcher Richard Jorgensen was hoping to intensify the color of petunias with the introduction of a transgene to overexpress the pigmentation enzyme when instead he produced a white flower. This tipped off scientists to the existence of the post-transcriptional gene silencing (PTGS) cellular mechanism and the idea that adding genes to an organism can affect its phenotype.

In 1998, Craig Mello and Andrew Fire uncovered another significant use of interference RNA, for which they were awarded the 2006 Nobel Prize in Physiology or Medicine. The researchers noticed that the addition of mRNA and antisense RNA did not turn off their targeted gene in *Caenorhabditis elegans* roundworms as effectively as an injection of double-stranded RNA (dsRNA). Putting the current name to this interference phenomenon, RNAi, the duo had uncovered a crucial piece of a cell's regulation capability and immune response known as the RNAi pathway. When dsRNA enters the cell, the Dicer enzyme chops it into small nucleotides of 20 to 25 bases. These small pieces, known as small interfering RNA (siRNA), are separated and fed into the RNA-induced silencing complex (RISC) where they are bound to their complementary mRNA for the pairs' dismantled demise.

Much excitement and attention toward these protein-regulating small RNAs has unveiled numerous different subspecies and the varying methods in which they are initiated within a cell. siRNA are generated in the cytoplasm from dsRNA and match almost completely to their doomed mRNA. Another small RNA, microRNA (miRNA), is also termed "noncoding RNA" because it initiates from the cell's own gene, but is not created for the traditional purpose of protein-coding, but instead with the intent to restrain protein production. Once made, miRNA gets enzymatically processed before being sent into the cytoplasm where it is transported into the RISC mechanism. In humans, miRNA tend to only moderately complement their targeted mRNA, resulting in a partial restriction of the mRNA's protein translation. This class of small RNA is practically absent

in cancerous cells, and a recent study showed that its addition can profoundly reverse cancer cell growth.

This power to subdue out-of-control cells has revolutionized the search for therapeutic treatments of several human diseases and disorders. By delivering synthetic small RNA to trigger the RNAi pathway or fulfill other policing roles, researchers hope to silence genes that cause not only cancer but also neurodegenerative diseases, diabetes, asthma, and even infectious diseases such as hepatitis, influenza, and HIV. The act of delivering these nuggets of authority is easier said than done; nucleases and immune responses are always at the ready to pounce on these foreign nucleotides. Studies are being conducted to fuse them to delivery vehicles like lipids, antibodies, or polymers in order to transport small RNAs across the cellular membrane.

Other Important Classes of RNA and Specialized Functions

Another major class of RNAs, the small nuclear RNAs (snRNAs), was also discovered in the early 1980's. Molecular biologist Joan Steitz was working on the autoimmune disease systemic lupus when she began to characterize the snRNAs. There are six different snRNAs, now called U1-U6 RNAs. These RNAs exist in the nucleus of eukaryotic cells and play a vital role in mRNA splicing. They associate with proteins in the spliceosome, forming so-called ribonucleoprotein complexes (snRNPs, pronounced "snurps"), and play a prominent role in detecting proper splice sites and directing the protein enzymes to cut and paste at the proper locations.

It has been known since the late 1950's that many viruses contain RNA, and not DNA, as their genetic material. This is another fascinating role for RNA. The viruses that cause influenza, polio, and a host of other diseases are RNA viruses. Of particular note are a class of RNA viruses known as retroviruses. Retroviruses, which include human immunodeficiency virus (HIV), the virus that causes acquired immunodeficiency syndrome (AIDS) in humans, use a special enzyme called reverse transcriptase to make a DNA copy of their RNA when they enter a cell. The DNA copy is inserted into the DNA of the host cell, where it is referred to as a "provirus," and never leaves. This discovery represents one of the exceptions to the central dogma. In the central dogma, RNA is always made from DNA, and retroviruses have reversed this flow of information. Clearly, understanding the structures and functions of the RNAs associated with these viruses will be important in attempting to create effective treatments for the diseases associated with them.

An additional role of RNA was noted during the elucidation of the mechanism of DNA replication. It was found that a small piece of RNA, called a "primer," must be laid down by the enzyme primase, an RNA polymerase, before DNA polymerase can begin. RNA primers are later removed and replaced with DNA. Also, it is worth mentioning that the universal energy-storing molecule of all cells, adenosine triphosphate (ATP), is in fact a version of the RNA nucleotide containing adenine (A).

IMPACT AND APPLICATIONS

The discovery of the many functions of RNA, especially its catalytic ability, has radically changed the understanding of the functioning of genetic and biological systems and has revolutionized the views of the scientific community regarding the origin of life. The key to understanding how RNA can perform all of its diverse functions lies in elucidating its many structures, since structure and function are inseparable. Much progress has been made in establishing the three-dimensional structure of hundreds of RNA molecules.

Extensive research has been conducted on RNA folding, degradation, and regulation, as it has become clear that it plays a vital role in genetic disease, cancer, and retroviral infections. The revelation of the RNAi pathway has ignited hope for treatments of ailments ranging from AIDS to Parkinson disease. One of the first RNAi remedies, Macugen, to pass human trials involved the eye disease wet macular degeneration. This occurs when too many blood vessels are grown due to an overactive gene, and the vessels' leakiness damages vision. The eye has a low population of nucleases, so when naked siRNAs are directly injected into the vitreous cavity, they successfully stunt the overactive gene, and vision is restored.

Additionally, plants, bacteria, and animals have been genetically engineered to alter the expression of some of their genes, in many cases making use of the new RNA technology. An example is a genetically engineered tomato that does not ripen until it is treated at the point of sale. This tomato was created by inserting an antisense RNA gene; when it is expressed, it inactivates the mRNA that codes for the enzyme involved in production of the ripening hormone.

One thing is clear: RNA is one of the most structurally interesting and functionally diverse of all the biological molecules.

Matthew M. Schmidt, Ph.D., and Bryan Ness, Ph.D.;
updated by Cherie Dewar

FURTHER READING

Cech, Thomas R. "The RNA Worlds in Context." *Cold Spring Harbor Perspectives in Biology.* Cold Spring Harbor Laboratory P, 2012. Web. 3 Sept. 2014.

Eckstein, Fritz, and David M. J. Lilley, eds. *Catalytic RNA.* New York: Springer, 1996. Print.

Erickson, Robert P., and Jonathan G. Izant, eds. *Gene Regulation: Biology of Antisense RNA and DNA.* New York: Raven Press, 1992. Print.

Hudgins, Louanne, et al., eds. *Signs and Symptoms of Genetic Conditions: A Handbook.* New York: Oxford UP, 2014. Print.

Leontis, Neocles, and Eric Westhof. *RNA 3D: Structure Analysis and Prediction.* Vol. 27. Heidelberg: Springer-Verlag, 2012. Print.

Murray, James A. H., ed. *Antisense RNA and DNA.* New York: Wiley-Liss, 1992. Print.

Nelson, David L., and Michael M. Cox. *Lehninger Principles of Biochemistry.* 5th ed. New York: W. H. Freeman, 2009. Print.

Robertson, Michael p., and Gerald F. Joyce. "The Origins of the RNA World." *Cold Spring Harbor Perspectives in Biology.* Cold Spring Harbor Laboratory P, 2012. Web. 4 Sept. 2014. Shrivastava, Neeta, and Anshu Srivastava. "RNA Interference: An Emerging Generation of Biologicals." *Biotechnology Journal,* March, 2008, 339–53.Print.

Simons, Robert W., and Marianne Grunberg-Manago, eds. *RNA Structure and Function.* Cold Spring Harbor, N.Y.: Cold Spring Harbor Laboratory Press, 1997. Print.

Watson, James D., et al. *Molecular Biology of the Gene.* 5th ed. Menlo Park, Calif.: Benjamin Cummings, 2003. Print.

See also: cDNA libraries; DNA isolation; Polymerase chain reaction; Reverse transcriptase; RNA isolation; RNA structure and function; RNA transcription and mRNA processing.

RNA transcription and mRNA processing

CATEGORY: Molecular genetics

SIGNIFICANCE: Translation of messenger RNA molecules (mRNAs) occurs even while transcription is taking place in prokaryotes. In eukaryotes the process is much more complex, with transcription occurring in the nucleus, followed by multiple processing steps before a mature mRNA is ready to be translated. All of these extra steps are required for mRNAs to be transported out of the nucleus and for recognition by ribosomes in the cytoplasm.

KEY TERMS

messenger RNA (mRNA): the form of RNA that contains the coding instructions used to make a polypeptide by ribosomes

RNA polymerase: the enzyme that transcribes RNA using a strand of DNA as a template

transcription: the process that converts DNA code into a complementary strand of RNA (mRNA) containing code that can be interpreted by ribosomes

translation: the process, mediated by ribosomes, in which the genetic code in an mRNA is used to produce a polypeptide, the ultimate product of structural genes

RNA POLYMERASE

Transcription is the process whereby the directions for making a protein are converted from DNA-based instructions to RNA-based instructions. This step is required in the process of expressing a gene as a polypeptide, because ribosomes, which assemble polypeptides, can read only RNA-based messages. Although transcription is complicated and involves dozens of enzymes and proteins, it is much simpler in prokaryotes than in eukaryotes. Because prokaryotes lack a nucleus, transcription and translation are linked processes both occurring in the cytoplasm. In eukaryotes, transcription and translation occur as completely separate processes, transcription occurring in the nucleus and translation occurring in the cytoplasm. (It is now known that some translation also occurs in the nucleus, but apparently only a small amount, probably less than 10 percent of the translation occurring in a cell.)

In eukaryotes there are three different types of RNA polymerase that transcribe RNA using a strand of DNA as a template (there is a single type of RNA polymerase in prokaryotes). Two of them, called RNA polymerase I (pol I) and RNA polymerase III (pol III), specialize in transcribing types of RNA that are functional products themselves, such as ribosomal RNA (rRNA) and transfer RNA (tRNA). These RNAs are involved in translation. RNA polymerase II (pol II) transcribes RNA from structural genes, that is, genes that code for polypeptides. Pol II therefore is the primary RNA polymerase and the one that will be the focus of this article when discussing transcription in eukaryotes.

TRANSCRIPTION IN PROKARYOTES

The first step in transcription is for RNA polymerase to identify the location of a gene. In prokaryotes many genes are clustered together in functional groups called operons. For example, the lactose (*lac*) operon contains three genes, each coding for one of the enzymes needed to metabolize the sugar lactose. At the beginning of each operon are two control sequences, the operator and the promoter. The promoter is where RNA polymerase binds, in preparation for transcription. The operator is a control region that determines whether RNA polymerase will be able to bind to the promoter. The operator interacts with other proteins that determine when the associated operon should be expressed. They do this by either preventing RNA polymerase from binding to the promoter or by assisting it to bind.

RNA polymerase recognizes promoters by the specific base-pair sequences they contain. Assuming all conditions are correct, RNA polymerase binds to the promoter, along with another protein called the sigma factor (σ). The beginning of genes are detected with the aid of σ. Transcription begins at a leader sequence a little before the beginning of the first gene and continues until RNA polymerase reaches a termination signal. If the operon contains more than one gene, all of the genes are transcribed into a single long mRNA, each gene separated from its neighbors by a spacer region. The mRNA is put together by pairing ribonucleotides with their complementary nucleotides in the DNA template. In place of thymine (T), RNA uses uracil (U); otherwise the same bases are present in RNA and DNA, the others being adenine (A), guanine (G), and cytosine (C). The pairing relationships are as

A depiction of the process of RNA transcription. Messenger RNA (mRNA) moves the DNA's template or instructions for protein synthesis (genetic code, or arrangement of bases) from the cell nucleus out into the cytoplasm, where it binds to a ribosome, the cell's "protein factory." Transfer RNA molecules then synthesize amino acids by linking to a codon on the mRNA and transferring the resulting amino acid to a growing chain of amino acids, the protein molecule. (U.S. Department of Energy Human Genome Program, http://www.ornl.gov/hgmis)

The process of transcript elongation facilitated by disassembly of nucleosomes. By Edk006 (Own work), via Wikimedia Commons

follows, the DNA base listed first in each pair: A-U, T-A, G-C, and C-G.

RNA polymerase catalyzes the joining of ribonucleotides as they pair with the DNA template. Each mRNA is constructed beginning at the 5′ end (the phosphate end) and ending with the 3′ end (the hydroxyl end). Even while transcription is taking place, ribosomes begin binding to the mRNA to begin translation. As soon as RNA polymerase has completed transcribing the genes of an operon, it releases from the DNA and soon binds to another promoter to begin the process all over again.

TRANSCRIPTION IN EUKARYOTES

Transcription in eukaryotes differs from the process in prokaryotes in the following major ways: (1) Genes are transcribed individually instead of in groups; (2) DNA is complexed with many proteins and is highly compacted, and therefore must be "unwound" to expose its promoters; (3) transcription occurs in a separate compartment (the nucleus) from translation, most of which occurs in the cytoplasm; and (4) initially transcription results in a pre-messenger RNA (pre-mRNA) molecule that must be processed before it emerges as a mature mRNA ready for translation. Additionally, mRNAs are much longer-lived in eukaryotes.

The first step in transcription is for RNA polymerase to find a gene that needs to be transcribed. Only genes occurring in regions of the DNA that have been unwound are prepared for potential transcription. RNA polymerase binds to an available promoter, which is located just before a gene and has a region in it called the TATA box (all promoters have the consensus sequence TATAAAA in them). RNA polymerase is unable to bind to the promoter without assistance from more than a dozen other proteins, including a TATA-binding protein, several transcription factors, activators, and coactivators. There are other DNA sequences farther upstream than the promoter that control transcription too, thus accounting for the fact that some genes are transcribed more readily, and therefore more often, than others.

Once RNA polymerase has bound to the promoter, it begins assembling an RNA molecule complementary to the DNA code in the gene. It starts by making a short leader sequence, then

mRNA By Mtov (Own work), via Wikimedia Commons

transcribes the gene, and finishes after transcribing a short trailer sequence. Transcription ends when RNA polymerase reaches a termination signal in the DNA. The initial product is a pre-mRNA molecule that is much longer than the mature mRNA will be.

mRNA Processing in Eukaryotes

Pre-mRNAs must be processed before they can leave the nucleus and be translated at a ribosome. Three separate series of reactions play a part in producing a mature mRNA: (1) intron removal and exon splicing, (2) 5 capping, and (3) addition of a poly-A tail. Not all transcripts require all three modifications, but most do.

The reason pre-mRNAs are much longer than their respective mature mRNAs has to do with the structure of genes in the DNA. The coding sequences of almost all eukaryotic genes are interrupted with noncoding regions. The noncoding regions are called introns, because they represent "intervening" sequences, and the coding regions are called exons. For an mRNA to be mature it must have all the introns removed and all the exons spliced together into one unbroken message. Special noncoding RNA complexes called small nuclear ribonucleoprotein particles, or snRNPs (pronounced as "snurps" by geneticists), carry out this process. The RNAs in the snRNPs are called small nuclear RNAs or snRNAs. Several snRNPs grouped together form a functional splicing unit called a spliceosome. Spliceosomes are able to recognize short signal sequences in pre-mRNA molecules that identify the boundaries of introns and exons. When a spliceosome has found an intron, it binds correctly, and through formation of a lariat-shaped structure, it cuts the intron out and splices the exons that were on each side of the intron to each other. Genes may have just a few introns, or they may have a dozen or more. Why eukaryotes have introns at all is still an open question, as introns, in general, appear to have no function.

While intron removal and exon splicing are taking place, both ends of maturing mRNAs must also be modified. At the 5′ end (the end with an exposed phosphate) an enzyme adds a modified guanosine nucleotide called 7-methylguanosine. This special nucleotide is added so that ribosomes in the cytoplasm can recognize the correct end of mRNAs, and

it probably also prevents the 5 end of mRNAs from being degraded.

At the 3 end of maturing mRNAs, another enzyme, called polyadenylase, adds a string of adenine nucleotides. Polyadenylase actually recognizes a special signal in the trailer sequence, at which it cuts and then adds the adenines. The result is what is called a poly-A tail. Initially geneticists did not understand the function of poly-A tails, but now it appears that they protect mRNAs from enzymes in the cytoplasm that could break them down. Essentially, poly-A tails are the main reason mRNAs in eukaryotes survive so much longer than mRNAs in prokaryotes.

Once the modifications have been completed, mRNAs are ready to be exported from the nucleus and will now travel through nuclear pores and enter the cytoplasm, where awaiting ribosomes will translate them, using the RNA code to build polypeptides.

Transcription and Disease

Ordinarily transcription works like a well-oiled machine, and only the right genes are transcribed at the right time so that just the right amount of protein product is produced. Unfortunately, due to the great complexity of the system, problems can occur that lead to disease. It has been estimated that about 15 percent of all genetic diseases may be due to improper intron removal and exon splicing in pre-mRNA molecules. Improper gene expression accounts for many other diseases, including many types of cancer.

Beta-thalassemia, a genetic disorder causing Cooley's anemia, is caused by a point mutation (a change in a single nucleotide) that changes a cutting and splicing signal. As a result, the mature mRNA has an extra piece of intron, making the mRNA longer and causing a reading frame shift. A reading frame shift causes everything from the mutation forward to be skewed, so that the code no longer codes for the correct amino acids. Additionally, as in the case of Cooley's anemia, a reading frame shift often introduces a premature stop codon. The gene involved codes for the beta chain of hemoglobin, the protein that carries oxygen in the blood, and this mutation results in a shortened polypeptide that does not function properly.

A single point mutation in a splicing site can have even more far-reaching consequences. In 2000, researchers in Italy discovered an individual who was genetically male (having one X and one Y chromosome) but was phenotypically female. She had no uterus or ovaries and only superficial external female anatomy, making her a pseudohermaphrodite. This condition can be caused by defects either in androgen production or in the androgen receptor. In this case, the defect was a simple point mutation in the androgen receptor gene that led to one intron being retained in the mature mRNA. Within the intron was a stop codon, which meant when the mRNA was translated, a shorter, nonfunctional polypeptide was formed. The subject did show a very small response to androgen, so apparently some of the pre-mRNAs were being cut and spliced correctly, but not enough to produce the normal male phenotype.

The same kinds of mutations as those discussed above can lead to cancer, but mutations that change the level of transcription of proto-oncogenes can also lead to cancer. Proto-oncogenes are normal genes involved in regulating the cell cycle, and when these genes are overexpressed they become oncogenes (cancer-causing genes). Overexpression of proto-oncogenes leads to overexpression of other genes, because many proto-oncogenes are transcription factors, signal proteins that interact with molecules controlling intracellular growth and growth factors released by cells to stimulate other cells to divide.

Overexpression can occur when there is a mutation in one of the control regions upstream from a gene. For example, a mutation in the promoter sequence could cause a transcription factor, and thus RNA polymerase, to bind more easily, leading to higher transcription rates. Other control regions, such as enhancer sequences, often far removed from the gene itself, may also affect transcription rates.

Anything that causes the transcription process to go awry will typically have far-reaching consequences. Geneticists are just beginning to understand some of the underlying errors behind a host of genetic diseases, and it should be no surprise that some of them involve how genes are transcribed. Knowing what the problem is, unfortunately, does not usually point to workable solutions. When the primary problem is an excessive rate of transcription, specially designed antisense RNA molecules (RNA molecules that are complementary to mRNA molecules) might be designed that will bind to the overexpressed mRNAs and disable them. This approach is still being tested. In the case of point mutations that derail the cutting and splicing process, the only solution may be gene therapy, a technique still not considered technically possible and not expected to be feasible for some time to come.

Bryan Ness, Ph.D.

FURTHER READING

Alberts, Bruce, et al. *Essential Cell Biology.* 4th ed. New York: Garland, 2014. Print.

Courey, Albert J. "RNA Polymerases and the Transcription Cycle." *Mechanisms in Transcriptional Regulation.* Malden: Blackwell, 2008. Print.

Hampsey, Michael. "Molecular Genetics of the RNA Polymerase II General Transcriptional Machinery." *Microbiology and Molecular Biology Reviews* 62.2 (1998): 465–503. Print.

Hartmann, Roland K., et al., eds. *Handbook of RNA Biochemistry.* Weinheim: Wiley, 2005. Print.

Latchman, David S. "RNA Polymerases and the Basal Transcription Complex." *Eukaryotic Transcription Factors.* 5th ed. Boston: Elsevier, 2008. Print.

Latchman, David S. "Transcription-Factor Mutations and Disease." *The New England Journal of Medicine* 334.1 (1996): 28–33. Print.

Macfarlane, W. M. "Transcription Demystified." *Journal of Clinical Pathology: Molecular Pathology* 53 (2000): 1–7. Print.

Papantonis, Argyris, et al. "TNF-alpha Signals through Specialized Factories Where Responsive Coding and miRNA Genes Are Transcribed." *EMBO Journal* 31.23 (2012): 4404–414. Print.

Ptashne, Mark, and Alexander Gann. *Genes and Signals.* Cold Spring Harbor: Cold Spring Harbor Laboratory P, 2002. Print.

Raven, Peter H. *Biology.* 9th ed. Dubuque: McGraw, 2011. Print.

Shatkin, Aaron J., and James L. Manley. "The Ends of the Affair: Capping and Polyadenylation." *Nature Structural Biology* 7.10 (2000): 838–42. Print.

White, Robert J. *Gene Transcription: Mechanisms and Control.* Malden: Blackwell, 2001. Print.

See also: Ancient DNA; Antisense RNA; Cancer; Chromosome structure; DNA isolation; DNA repair; DNA replication; DNA structure and function; Genetic code; Genetic code, cracking of; Molecular genetics; Noncoding RNA molecules; One gene-one enzyme hypothesis; Protein structure; Protein synthesis; Pseudohermaphrodites; Repetitive DNA; RNA isolation; RNA structure and function; RNA world.

RNA world

CATEGORY: Evolutionary biology; Molecular genetics

SIGNIFICANCE: The RNA world is a theoretical time in the early evolution of life, during which RNA molecules played important genetic and enzymatic roles that were later taken over by molecules of DNA and proteins. Ideas about RNA's ancient functions have led to new concepts of the origin of life and have important implications for the use of gene therapy to treat diseases.

KEY TERMS

ribosomal RNA (rRNA): a type of RNA that forms a major part of the structure of the ribosome

ribosome: an organelle that functions in protein synthesis, containing a large and a small subunit composed of proteins and ribosomal RNA molecules

ribozyme: an RNA molecule that can function catalytically as an enzyme

THE CENTRAL DOGMA AND THE MODERN GENETIC WORLD

Soon after the discovery of the double-helical structure of DNA in 1953 by James Watson and Francis Crick, Crick proposed an idea regarding information flow in cells that he called the "central dogma of molecular biology." Crick correctly predicted that in all cells, information flows from DNA to RNA to protein. DNA was known to be the genetic material, the "library" of genetic information, and it had been clear for some time that the enzymes that actually did the work of facilitating chemical reactions were invariably protein molecules. The discovery of three classes of RNA during the 1960s seemed to provide the link between the DNA instructions and the protein products.

In the modern genetic world, cells contain three classes of RNA that act as helpers in the synthesis of proteins from information stored in DNA, a process called translation. A messenger RNA (mRNA) is transcribed from a segment of DNA (a gene) that contains information about how to build a particular protein and carries that information to the cellular site of protein synthesis, the ribosome. Ribosomal RNA (rRNA) interacting with many proteins make up the ribosome, whose major job is to coordinate and facilitate the protein-building procedure. Transfer RNA (tRNA) acts as decoding molecules, reading the mRNA information and correlating it

with a specific amino acid. As the ribosome integrates the functions of all three types of RNA, polypeptides are built one amino acid at a time. These polypeptides, either singly or in aggregations, can then function as enzymes, ultimately determining the capabilities and properties of the cell in which they act.

While universally accepted, the central dogma led many scientists to question how this complex, integrated system came about. It seemed to be a classic "chicken and egg" dilemma: proteins could not be built without instructions from DNA, but DNA could not replicate and maintain itself without help from protein enzymes. The two seemed inextricably mutually dependent on each other. An understanding of the origins of the modern genetic system seemed far away.

THE DISCOVERY OF RIBOZYMES

In 1983, a discovery was made that seemed so radical it was initially rejected by most of the scientific community. Molecular biologists Thomas Cech and Sidney Altman, working independently and in

Guanine and Adenine are corrected according to their respective articles in this version. Redrew using Inkscape. By Users Antilived, Fabiolib, Turnstep, Westcairo on en.wikipedia (http://www.accessexcellence.org/RC/VL/GG/rna2.html), via Wikimedia Commons

different systems, announced the discovery of RNA molecules that possessed catalytic activity. This meant that RNA itself could function as an enzyme, obliterating the idea that only proteins could function catalytically.

Cech had been working with the protozoan *Tetrahymena*. In most organisms except bacteria, the coding portions of DNA genes (exons) are interrupted by noncoding sequences (introns), which are transcribed into mRNA but must be removed before translation. Protein enzymes called nucleases are usually responsible for cutting out the introns and joining together the exons in a process called splicing. The molecule with which Cech was working was an rRNA molecule that contained introns but could apparently remove them and rejoin the coding regions without any help. It was a self-splicing RNA molecule, which clearly indicated its enzymatic capability. Altman was working with the enzyme ribonuclease (RNase) P in bacteria, which is responsible for cutting mature tRNA molecules out of an immature RNA segment. RNase P thus also acts as a nuclease. It was known for some time that RNase P contains both a protein and an RNA constituent, but Altman was ultimately able to show that it was the RNA rather than the protein that actually catalyzed the reaction.

The importance of these findings cannot be overstated, and Cech and Altman ultimately shared the 1989 Nobel Prize in Chemistry for the discovery of these RNA enzymes, or ribozymes (joining the terms "ribonucleic acid" and "enzymes"). Subsequently, many ribozymes have been found in various organisms, from bacteria to humans. Some of them are able to catalyze different types of reactions, and new ones are periodically reported. Ribozymes have thus proven to be more than a mere curiosity, playing an integral role in the molecular machinery of many organisms.

At around the same time as these important discoveries, still other functions of RNA were being identified. While perhaps not as dramatic as the ribozymes, antisense RNAs, small nuclear RNAs, and a variety of others further proved the versatility of RNA. While understanding the roles of ribozymes and other unconventional RNAs is important to the understanding of genetic functioning in present-day organisms, these discoveries were more intriguing to many scientists interested in the origin and evolution of life. In a sense, the existence of ribozymes was a violation of the central dogma, which implied that information was ultimately utilized solely in the form of proteins. While the central dogma was not in danger of becoming obsolete, a clue had been found that might possibly allow a resolution, at least in theory, to questions about whether the DNA or the protein came first. The exciting answer: perhaps neither.

A hairpin loop from a pre-mRNA. Notice its bases (light green) and backbone (sky blue). NMR structure of the central region of the human GluR-B R/G pre-mRNA, from the protein data bank ID 1ysv. Taken from w:PDB ids 1ysv model 1 imaged using w:UCSF Chimera By Vossman (Own work), via Wikimedia Commons

THE RNA WORLD THEORY AND THE ORIGIN OF LIFE

Given that RNA is able to store genetic information (as it certainly does when it functions as mRNA) and the new discovery that it could function as an enzyme, there was no longer any need to invoke the presence of either DNA or protein as necessities in the first living system. The first living molecule would have to be able to replicate itself without any help, and just such an "RNA replicase" has been proposed as the molecule that eventually led to life as it is now known. Like the self-splicing intron of *Tetrahymena*, this theoretical ribozyme could have worked on itself, catalyzing its own replication. This RNA would therefore have functioned as both the genetic material and the replication enzyme, allowing it to make copies of itself without the need for DNA or proteins. Biologist Walter Gilbert coined the term "RNA world" for this interesting theoretical period dominated by RNA. Modern catalytic RNAs can be thought of as molecular fossils that remain from this period and provide clues about its nature.

How might this initial RNA have come into being in the first place? Biologist Aleksandr Oparin predicted in the late 1930s that if simple gases thought to be present in Earth's early atmosphere were subjected to the right conditions (energy in the form of lightning, for example), more complex organic molecules would be formed. His theory was first tested in 1953 and was resoundingly confirmed. A mixture of methane, ammonia, water vapor, and hydrogen gas was energized with high-voltage electricity, and the products were impressive: several amino acids and aldehydes, among other organic molecules. Subsequent experiments have been able to produce ribonucleotide bases. It seems reasonable, then, that nucleotides could have been present on the early Earth and that their random linkage could lead to the formation of an RNA chain.

After a while, RNA molecules would have found a way to synthesize proteins, which by their very nature are able to act as more efficient and diverse enzymes than ribozymes. Why are proteins better enzymes than ribozymes? Since RNA contains only four bases, which are fundamentally similar in their chemical properties, the range of different configurations and functional capabilities is somewhat limited. Proteins, on the other hand, can be constructed from a pool of at least twenty different amino acids, whose functional groups differ widely in terms of their chemical makeup and potential reactivity. It is logical to suppose, therefore, that proteins eventually took over most of the roles of RNA enzymes because they were simply better suited to doing so. Several of the original, efficient ribozymes would have been retained, and those are the ones that still can be observed.

How could a world composed strictly of RNAs, however, be able to begin protein synthesis? While it seems like a tall order, scientists have envisioned an early version of the ribosome that was composed exclusively of RNA. Biologist Harry Noller reported in the early 1990s that the activity of the modern ribosome that is responsible for catalyzing the formation of peptide bonds between amino acids is in fact carried out by rRNA. This so-called peptidyl-transferase activity had always been attributed to one of the ribosomal proteins, and rRNA had been envisioned as playing a primarily structural role. Noller's discovery that the large ribosomal RNA is actually a ribozyme allows scientists to picture a ribosome working in roughly the same way that modern ones do, without containing any proteins. As proteins began to be synthesized from the information in the template RNAs, they slowly began to assume some of the RNA roles and probably incorporated themselves into the ribosome to allow it to function more efficiently.

The transition to the modern world would not be complete without the introduction of DNA as the major form of the genetic material. RNA, while well suited to diverse roles, is actually a much less suitable genetic material than DNA for a complex organism, even one only as complex as a bacterium. This is because the slight chemical differences between the sugars contained in the nucleotides of RNA and DNA cause the RNA to be more reactive and much less chemically stable, which is good for a ribozyme but bad if the genetic material is to last for any reasonable amount of time. Once DNA came into existence, therefore, it is likely that the relatively complex organisms of the time quickly adopted it as their genetic material; shortly thereafter, it became double-stranded, which facilitated its replication immensely. This left RNA, the originator of it all, relegated to the status it now enjoys; molecular fossils exist that uncover its former glory, but it functions mainly as a helper in protein synthesis.

This still leaves the question of how DNA evolved from RNA. At least two protein enzymes were probably necessary to allow this process to begin. The first, ribonucleoside diphosphate reductase, converts

RNA nucleotides to DNA nucleotides by reducing the hydroxyl group located on the 2 carbon of ribose. Perhaps more important, the enzyme reverse transcriptase would have been necessary to transcribe RNA genomes into corresponding DNA versions. Examples of both of these enzymes exist in the modern world.

Some concluding observations are in order to summarize the evidence that RNA, and not DNA, was very likely the first living molecule. No enzymatic activity has ever been attributed to DNA; in fact, the 2 hydroxyl group that RNA possesses and DNA lacks is vital to RNA's ability to function as a ribozyme. Furthermore, ribose is synthesized much more easily than deoxyribose under laboratory conditions. All modern cells synthesize DNA nucleotides from RNA precursors, and many other players in the cellular machinery are RNA-related. Important examples include adenosine triphosphate (ATP), the universal cellular energy carrier, and a host of coenzymes such as nicotinamide adenine dinucleotide (NAD), derived from B vitamins and vital for energy metabolism.

IMPACT AND APPLICATIONS

The discovery of ribozymes and the other interesting classes of RNA has dramatically altered the understanding of genetic processes at the molecular level and has provided compelling evidence in support of exciting new theories regarding the origin of life and cellular evolution. The RNA world theory, first advanced as a radical and unsupported hypothesis in the early 1970s, has gained widespread acceptance by scientists. It is the solution to the evolutionary paradox that has plagued scientists since the discovery and understanding of the central dogma: Which came first, DNA or proteins? Since they are inextricably dependent on each other in the modern world, the idea of the RNA world proposes that, rather than one giving rise to the other, they are both descended from RNA, that most ancient of genetic and catalytic molecules. Unfortunately, the RNA world model is not without its problems.

In the mid- to late 1990s, several studies on the stability of ribose, the sugar portion of ribonucleotides, showed that it breaks down relatively easily, even in neutral solutions. A study of the decay rate of ribonucleotides at different temperatures also caused some concern for the RNA world theory. Most current scenarios see life arising in relatively hot conditions,

at least near boiling, and the instability of ribonucleotides at these temperatures would not allow for the development of any significant RNA molecules. Ribonucleotides are much more stable at 0 degrees Celsius (32 degrees Fahrenheit), but evidence for a low-temperature environment for the origin of life is limited. Consequently, some evolutionists are suggesting that the first biological entities might have relied on something other than RNA, and that the RNA world was a later development. Therefore, although the RNA world seems like a plausible model, another model is now needed to establish the precursor to the RNA world.

Apart from origin-of-life concerns, the discoveries that led to the RNA world theory are beginning to have a more practical impact in the fields of industrial genetic engineering and medical gene therapy. The unique ability of ribozymes to find particular sequences and initiate cutting and pasting at desired locations makes them powerful tools. Impressive uses have already been found for these tools in theoretical molecular biology and in the genetic engineering of plants and bacteria. Most important to humans, however, are the implications for curing or treating genetically related disease using this powerful RNA-based technology.

Gene therapy, in general, is based on the idea that any faulty, disease-causing gene can be replaced by a genetically engineered working replacement. While theoretically a somewhat simple idea, in practice it is technically very challenging. Retroviruses may be used to insert DNA into particular target cells, but the results are often not as expected; the new genes are difficult to control or may have adverse side effects. Molecular biologist Bruce Sullenger pioneered a new approach to gene therapy that seeks to correct the genetic defect at the RNA level. A ribozyme can be engineered to seek out and replace damaged sequences before they are translated into defective proteins. Sullenger has shown that this so-called trans-splicing technique can work in nonhuman systems, and in 1996 he began trials to test his procedure in humans.

Many human diseases could be corrected using gene-therapy technology of this kind, from inherited defects such as sickle-cell disease to degenerative genetic problems such as cancer. Even pathogen-induced conditions such as acquired immunodeficiency syndrome (AIDS), caused by the human immunodeficiency virus (HIV), could be amenable to this approach. It is ironic and gratifying that an understanding of the ancient RNA world holds promise for helping scientists to solve some of the major problems in the modern world of DNA-based life.

Matthew M. Schmidt, Ph.D.;
updated by Bryan Ness, Ph.D.

FURTHER READING

Atkins, John F., Raymond F. Gesteland, and Thomas R. Cech, eds. *RNA Worlds: From Life's Origins to Diversity in Gene Regulation.* Cold Spring Harbor: Cold Spring Harbor, 2011. Print.

Bernhardt, Harold S. "The RNA World Hypothesis: The Worst Theory of the Early Evolution of Life (except for All the Others)." *Biology Direct* 7.23 (2012):1–10. Web. 14 Aug. 2014.

de Duve, Christian. "The Beginnings of Life on Earth." *American Scientist* Sept./Oct. 1995: 428–37. Print.

Elliott, David, and Michael Ladomery. *Molecular Biology of RNA.* New York: Oxford UP, 2011. Print.

Hart, Stephen. "RNA's Revising Machinery." *BioScience* 46.5 (1996): 318–21. Print.

Hazen, Robert M. *Genesis: The Scientific Quest for Life's Origin.* Washington: Henry, 2005. Print.

Horgan, John. "The World according to RNA." *Scientific American* Jan. 1996: 27–30. Print.

Luisi, Pier Luigi. *The Emergence of Life: From Chemical Origins to Synthetic Biology.* New York: Cambridge UP, 2006. Print.

Miller, Stanley L. *From the Primitive Atmosphere to the Prebiotic Soup to the Pre-RNA World.* Washington: Natl. Aeronautics and Space Administration, 1996. Print.

Rauchfuss, Horst. *Chemical Evolution and the Origin of Life.* Trans. Terence N. Mitchell. Berlin: Springer, 2008. Print.

Szostak, Jack W. "The Eightfold Path to Non-Enzymatic RNA Replication." *Journal of Systems Chemistry* 3.2 (2012): 1–14. Web. 14 Aug. 2014.

Watson, James D., et al. *Molecular Biology of the Gene.* 7th ed. San Francisco: Benjamin, 2014. Print.

Yang, Lin, John E. Froberg, and Jeannie T. Lee. "Long Noncoding RNAs: Fresh Perspectives into the RNA World." *Trends in Biochemical Sciences* 39.1 (2014): 35–43. Print.

See also: Ancient DNA; Antisense RNA; Chromosome structure; DNA isolation; DNA repair; DNA replication; DNA structure and function; Genetic code; Genetic code, cracking of; Molecular genetics; Noncoding RNA molecules; One gene-one enzyme hypothesis; Protein structure; Protein synthesis; Repetitive DNA; RNA isolation; RNA structure and function; RNA transcription and mRNA processing.

Robert syndrome

CATEGORY: Diseases and syndromes

ALSO KNOWN AS: Roberts syndrome; Roberts-SC phocomelia syndrome; pseudothalidomide syndrome; SC-phocomelia syndrome; Appelt-Gerken-Lenz syndrome; hypomelia hypotrichosis facial hemangioma syndrome; RBS; SC syndrome; tetraphocomelia-cleft palate syndrome

DEFINITION

Robert syndrome is a developmental disorder that affects multiple organ systems, prenatal and postnatal growth, and mental development. It is an autosomal recessive condition caused by mutations in the gene *ESCO2*.

RISK FACTORS

Since Robert syndrome is a rare condition, carrier frequency and prevalence are unknown. Approximately 150 cases have been reported in individuals of a variety of ethnic backgrounds. Couples who are consanguineous or have a family history of Robert syndrome are at increased risk for having an affected child.

ETIOLOGY AND GENETICS

Robert syndrome is an autosomal recessive genetic condition. When both parents are carriers of a single mutation *ESCO2*, there is a 25 percent chance in each pregnancy that the child will inherit both mutation and will be affected with Robert syndrome.

In individuals with Robert syndrome, cytogenetic abnormalities have been noted in the process of cell division. Typically, during metaphase the two sister chromatids of each chromosome are bound closely together. The proteins that bind them together are broken down during anaphase and the sister chromatids separate into sister chromosomes. In individuals with Robert syndrome, the centromeres of the sister chromatids separate during metaphase rather than in anaphase, which is referred to as premature

Roberts syndrome By Hirst B.C., Piersol G.A., via Wikimedia Commons

centromere separation. This gives the chromosomes in a metaphase spread a "railroad track" appearance due to the absence of the primary constriction at the centromere. In addition, there is a lack of cohesion in the heterochromatic (dense, genetically inactive) regions of the sister chromatids. This results in "heterochromatin repulsion" or "puffing" around the centromere and in heterochromatic regions, such as in the acrocentric chromosomes and the long arm of the Y chromosome.

Premature centromere separation and separation of the heterochromatic regions are thought to trigger activation of the mitotic spindle checkpoint in metaphase, which delays mitosis and impairs cell proliferation. This impaired proliferation is thought to cause the growth failure associated with Robert syndrome. The congenital anomalies characteristic of Robert syndrome may result from the loss of progenitor cells during embryogenesis.

The gene *ESCO2* (Establishment of Cohesion 1 homolog 2) is located at 8p21.1. It codes for the protein N-acetyltransferase ESCO2. This enzyme has been found to have autoacetylation activity in vitro. Most of the *ESCO2* mutations that have been described in families with Robert syndrome create a premature stop codon that would result in a

truncated protein or instability in mRNA. However, a point mutation that disrupts autoacetylation activity has also been described in an affected individual. Therefore, the inability of this protein to transfer acetyl groups from one compound to another in affected individuals is thought to be involved in the pathogenesis of Robert syndrome. It is thought that *ESCO2* is involved in regulating the establishment of sister chromatid cohesion during the S phase of the cell cycle.

Symptoms

Robert syndrome commonly affects the growth and development of the limbs and midface. Affected individuals are born with hypomelia, or incomplete development of the limbs, which is typically more severe in the upper limbs. They may also have cleft lip with or without cleft palate, prenatal onset growth deficiency, intellectual disability, and other congenital anomalies.

Screening and Diagnosis

A diagnosis of Robert syndrome can be made with a routine chromosome analysis using Giemsa or C-banding. Chromosomes have a characteristic appearance due to premature centromere separation and separation of the heterochromatic regions.

In addition, molecular genetic testing for Robert syndrome is available. Sequence analysis of *ESCO2* can confirm a diagnosis in an affected individual. Since carrier status cannot be determined from cytogenetic testing, molecular genetic testing must be used for carrier testing. Prenatal diagnosis can be

Case of so called Roberts' syndrome, By John B. Roberts, via Wikimedia Commons

performed on an amniocentesis or chorionic villus sampling with either molecular genetic testing or cytogenetic testing.

TREATMENT AND THERAPY

Following an initial diagnosis, evaluations may include X rays and assessments of the limbs, hands, and face; ophthalmologic evaluation; cardiac evaluation; renal ultrasound; and developmental assessment. Treatment would be based on an individual's specific needs. Limb abnormalities may require reconstructive surgery or prostheses. Facial clefting may require multiple surgeries, speech therapy, and management of recurrent ear infections. Developmental delays may result in a need for special education. Growth and development should be closely monitored.

PREVENTION AND OUTCOMES

The prognosis for an affected individual depends of the severity of the condition. Many severely affected pregnancies result in stillbirth or early infant death. Mildly affected individuals may survive to adulthood. Although prenatal diagnosis is available for pregnancies at risk based on ultrasound findings or family history, there is no effective means of preventing Robert syndrome. Genetic counseling should be made available to the families of affected individuals.

Laura Garasimowicz, M.S.

FURTHER READING

Canepa, G., Pierre Maroteaux, and V. Pietrogrande. *Dysmorphic Syndromes and Constitutional Disease of the Skeleton.* Padova: Piccin, 2001. Print.

Gardner, R. J. McKinlay, Grant R. Sutherland, and Lisa G. Shaffer. *Chromosome Abnormalities and Genetic Counseling.* 4th ed. New York: Oxford UP, 2012. Print.

Gordillo, Miriam. "Roberts Syndrome." *GeneReviews.* Ed. Roberta A. Pagon et al. Seattle: U of Washington, Seattle, 1993–2014. *NCBI Bookshelf.* Natl. Center for Biotechnology Information, 14 Nov. 2013. Web. 15 Aug. 2014.

Gorlin, Robert J., Michael M. Cohen, Jr., and Raoul C. M. Hennekam. *Syndromes of the Head and Neck.* 4th ed. New York: Oxford UP, 2001. Print.

Jones, Kenneth Lyons. *Smith's Recognizable Patterns of Human Malformation.* 7th ed. Philadelphia: Elsevier, 2013. Print.

See also: Apert syndrome; Brachydactyly; Carpenter syndrome; Cleft lip and palate; Congenital defects; Cornelia de Lange syndrome; Cri du chat syndrome; Crouzon syndrome; Down syndrome; Edwards syndrome; Ellis-van Creveld syndrome; Holt-Oram syndrome; Ivemark syndrome; Meacham syndrome; Opitz-Frias syndrome; Patau syndrome; Polydactyly; Rubinstein-Taybi syndrome.

Rubinstein-Taybi syndrome and genetics

CATEGORY: Diseases and syndromes

ALSO KNOWN AS: Rubinstein syndrome; broad thumbs and great toes; broad thumb-hallux syndrome

DEFINITION

Rubinstein-Taybi syndrome (RSTS) is a congenital anomaly and cognitive impairment syndrome with multisystem effects. It was first described as a syndrome by Jack Rubinstein and Hooshang Taybi in 1963 after examining multiple similar cases. RSTS is a dominant genetic condition displaying consistent physical and neurological findings. Some varying attributes are also reported in the literature.

RISK FACTORS

The occurrence of RSTS is approximately 1 in 100,000 newborns. The incidence increases to 50 percent of offspring of affected individuals. Various phenotypical penetrance is reported in families. Other than familial cases, there are no known risk factors.

ETIOLOGY AND GENETICS

RSTS is caused by a heterozygous germline (oocyte, spermatocyte) mutation. Approximately 55 percent of cases of RSTS are caused by mutations in one of two genes, the CREB binding protein (*CREBBP*) gene located on chromosome 16p13.3 and the *EP300* gene located on chromosome 22q12.2. Both genes encode histone acetyltransferases (HAT), which affect cellular signaling pathways and are important in cell growth and differentiation. HAT plays an important

Rubinstein-Taybi Syndrome By see above, via Wikimedia Commons

An Egyptian patient with Rubinstein-Taybi syndrome An Egyptian patient with Rubinstein-Taybi syndrome. Facial features (A), left hand and feet showing broad thumb and big toes (B, C) and X-ray of both hands showing short broad thumbs (D). (Limb Malformations & Skeletal Dysplasia Clinic, MSU, NRC). By see above, via Wikimedia Commons

role in activation of transcription. HAT blocks the restricted access to deoxyribonucleic acid (DNA). In translation, DNA gives ribonucleic acid (RNA) orders to produce a certain needed protein. RNA then produces the requested protein in a process called transcription. These proteins are utilized for cellular processes and development. CREBBP also plays a part in long-term memory formation, and its mutation may result in the cognitive deficits seen in individuals with RSTS. Mutations of these genes are usually point mutations, although translocations, inversions, missense mutations, mosaic microdeletions, and large deletions have been reported. Most mutations are dominant de novo events. The expected recurrence rate in future pregnancies is 0.1 percent. The genetic etiology of the remaining 45 percent of cases has not yet been determined.

SYMPTOMS

RSTS is characterized by neurological and physical features. Neurologically, failure to achieve developmental milestones and mental retardation are common. Later, children exhibit short attention span and self-stimulatory behaviors such as rocking or spinning. Physically, broad great toes and thumbs are hallmarks of the syndrome. In addition, distinct facial features include downslanting palpebral fissures, hypertelorism, higharched eyebrows, prominent beaked nose with the nasal septum extending below the nares, a grimacing mouth, and hypoplastic maxilla. On dental exam, 90 percent of affected individuals exhibit talon cusps. Failure to thrive may follow feeding difficulties in infancy and gastroesophageal reflux is common.

SCREENING AND DIAGNOSIS

Diagnosis is by two methods. Clinically, it includes family history, and patient history and physical examination findings. In the absence of positive genetic tests the diagnosis is based on clinical and radiological findings which include dysmorphological facial features, broad thumbs and first toes, and mental and physical growth delay. Genetic testing now allows confirmation of suspicion in approximately 55 percent of cases using fluorescence in situ hybridization (FISH), DNA sequence analysis, and polymerase chain reaction (PCR) testing. Currently there are no genetic tests that can detect the syndrome in the remaining 45 percent of affected individuals.

TREATMENT AND THERAPY

Early diagnosis permits treatment of medical issues as well as the provision of genetic counseling including information about RSTS, recurrence risks, and prenatal diagnosis. In addition to genetic evaluation, the individual should be screened for cardiac, renal, ophthalmologic, auditory, endocrine, and orthopedic issues. Because of the high incidence of dental problems, referral and follow-up by a pediatric dentist is needed. Because of feeding difficulties, growth and nutrition counseling is beneficial. Individuals with *CREBBP* and *EP300* gene mutations are at risk for future malignancies due to an imbalance of alleles implicated in malignancies such as hematologic, breast, ovarian, hepatic, and colorectal cancer and require close monitoring for development of these tumors.

PREVENTION AND OUTCOMES

No identifiable prevention strategy is currently known to prevent the majority of cases as they are primarily due to a de novo mutation. Only one known case has been detected prior to birth by ultrasound technique. Thus, clinicians must perform thorough physical examinations on newborns and be alert to the dysmorphic and neurological features of this syndrome. The prognosis is dependent on the nature and severity of defects as well as early, consistent medical, dental, and development care for children with this syndrome.

Wanda Todd Bradshaw, R.N., M.S.N.

FURTHER READING

Bloch-Zupan, Agnes, Heddie O. Sedano, and Crispian Scully. *Dento/Oro/Craniofacial Anomalies and Genetics.* Waltham: Elsevier, 2012. Print.

Cassidy, Suzanne B. *Management of Genetic Syndromes.* Hoboken: Wiley, 2010. Print.

Foley, Patricia, et al. "Further Case of Rubinstein-Taybi Syndrome Due to a Deletion in *EP300.*" *American Journal of Medical Genetics,* Part A 149A (2009): 997–1000. Print.

Greco, Elena, Gabriella Sglavo, and Dario Paladini. "Prenatal Sonographic Diagnosis of Rubinstein-Taybi Syndrome." *Journal of Ultrasound Medicine* 28 (2009): 669–72. Print.

Hennekam, Raoul C. M. "Practical Genetics: Rubinstein-Taybi Syndrome." *European Journal of Human Genetics* 14 (2006): 981–85. Print.

Jones, Kenneth Lyons. *Smith's Recognizable Patterns of Human Malformation.* 7th ed. Philadelphia: Elsevier, 2013. Print.

Schorry, Elizabeth, et al. "Genotype-Phenotype Correlations in Rubinstein-Taybi Syndrome." *American Journal of Medical Genetics,* Part A 146A (2008): 2512–519. Print.

Stevens, Cathy A., Jill Pouncey, and Darcy Knowles. "Adults with Rubinstein-Taybi Syndrome." *American Journal of Medical Genetics* 155.7 (2011): 1680–684. Print.

Wiley, Susan, et al. "Rubinstein-Taybi Syndrome Medical Guidelines." *American Journal of Medical Genetics* 119-A (2003): 101–10. Print.

See also: Apert syndrome; Brachydactyly; Carpenter syndrome; Cleft lip and palate; Congenital defects; Cornelia de Lange syndrome; Cri du chat syndrome; Crouzon syndrome; Down syndrome; Edwards syndrome; Ellis-van Creveld syndrome; Holt-Oram syndrome; Ivemark syndrome; Meacham syndrome; Opitz-Frias syndrome; Patau syndrome; Polydactyly; Robert syndrome.

S

Saccharomyces cerevisiae

CATEGORY: Techniques and methodologies

SIGNIFICANCE: *Saccharomyces cerevisiae* is a highly tractable yeast organism. Historically valued for its role in fermentation, it has also played an important role in science as the first eukaryote to have its DNA completely sequenced. Yeast genetic research has been at the forefront of scientists' efforts to identify the genes and processes required for cell growth and division and is now an important tool for nonyeast research to identify proteins that physically interact with one another in the cell.

KEY TERMS

ascus: the cellular structure that results from meiosis in yeast, containing four recombinant spores that are fully capable of growing into haploid yeast cells

budding: the asexual method of duplication used by yeast to create a clone of the original cell

diploid cell: a cell that contains two copies of each chromosome

haploid cell: a cell that contains one copy of each chromosome

mating type: one of two types of yeast cell, depending on a soluble factor that each cell secretes

model organism: an organism well suited for genetic research because it has a well-known genetic history, a short life cycle, and genetic variation between individuals in the population

THE ORGANISM

Saccharomyces cerevisiae (*S. cerevisiae*, or baker's yeast) has been used for millennia as a leavening agent in bread products and for fermentation in beer and wine. Yeast is a simple, one-celled eukaryote with six thousand genes on sixteen chromosomes. It was the first eukaryote to have its entire DNA sequenced.

Yeast can produce offspring using two different methods, a sexual life cycle and an asexual life cycle. In the asexual life cycle, the yeast cell produces the next generation by a process called budding. All genetic components of the mother cell are duplicated, and a small "bud" begins to grow from the mother cell. The bud continues to grow until it is nearly the size of the mother cell. The DNA and other duplicated cellular components are then partitioned into the new bud. The cells undergo cytokinesis and are now separate entities able to grow and continue reproducing independently of one another.

To produce offspring that are not clones of the mother cell, yeast use a sexual life cycle. A yeast cell exists stably as either a diploid or a haploid organism, but only the haploid organism is able to mate and exchange genetic information. Haploid yeast can contain either the *MATa* or *MATalpha* gene. These genes produce soluble factors that distinguish them as one of two mating types. An "a" cell (*MATa*) and an "alpha" cell (*MATalpha*) mate by sequentially fusing their cell walls, their cytoplasms, and finally their nuclei. This diploid cell now contains two copies of each chromosome that can undergo recombination during meiosis. When all environmental signals are ideal, the diploid yeast will undergo meiosis, allowing exchange and recombination of genetic information brought to the diploid by both haploid cells. The result of meiosis is an ascus that contains four recombinant spores that will grow into haploid yeast cells when environmental conditions are ideal.

A MODEL ORGANISM

Researchers choose yeast as a model organism to study specific areas of interest for many different reasons. *Saccharomyces cerevisiae* is nonpathogenic to humans, allowing manipulation in a laboratory with

Saccharomyces cerevisiae By Bob Blaylock (Own work), via Wikimedia Commons

Saccharomyces cerevisiae By Masur (Own work), via Wikimedia Commons

little or no containment required. At a temperature of 30 degrees Celsius (86 degrees Fahrenheit), the yeast population can double in ninety minutes, allowing many experiments to be completed in one day. Among the primary reasons for selection of yeast as a model system is that they offer the possibility of studying the genes and proteins that are required for basic growth functions and cell division. Yeast use many of the same genes and proteins to govern the same processes that animal and plant cells use for growth and division. Each single cell has to take in nutrients, grow, and pass along information to its progeny. In many ways, yeast can be considered a simplified version of a plant or animal cell, in that it lacks all the genes that provide the determinants that are expressed as differences between plants and animals. Another important reason for using yeast is that yeast is amenable to investigation using both genetic and biochemical approaches. This allows for correlation of findings from both approaches and a better understanding of a specific process or activity.

Yeast is also ideal for use as a model system due to at least four well-established techniques and procedures. First, genetics in yeast takes advantage of well-established auxotrophic markers. These markers are usually mutations in biosynthetic pathways that are used to synthesize required cellular components such as amino acids and nucleotides. By using these marker genes, researchers can follow genes and their associated chromosomes from one generation to the next.

Second, yeast is readily transformed by plasmids that function as artificial chromosomes. All that is needed is an auxotrophic marker to follow the plasmid through succeeding generations, a yeast origin of replication to allow replication of the plasmid DNA, and a region into which the gene of interest can be inserted in the plasmid DNA. This allows the researcher to move genes easily from yeast strain to yeast strain and quickly examine the effect of the gene in combination with many other genes.

Third, yeast is easily mutated by chemicals and can be grown in a small space, which allows the researcher quickly to identify mutations in genes that result in a specific phenotype. For example, to define all the genes in the adenine biosynthetic pathway, a researcher would mutate a yeast strain with one of many available mutagenic chemicals, resulting in changes within the DNA. The mutated yeast strains would then be checked to see if the strain was able to grow on media lacking adenine. All of the strains mutant for growth on adenine would be collected and could identify a number of genes involved in the adenine biosynthetic pathway. Further research could establish whether each of these mutations in the yeast identified one gene or many genes.

Fourth, yeast is the model system of choice when examining and identifying proteins that interact with one another in the cell. This technique is called the two-hybrid system.

TWO-HYBRID SYSTEM

The two-hybrid system takes advantage of scientists' understanding of transcription at the *GAL1* gene in yeast. The promoter region of *GAL1* contains a binding site for the Gal4p transcription factor. When the cell is grown on the sugar galactose, Gal4p binds to the promoter of *GAL1* and activates transcription of the *GAL1* gene. Gal4p can be essentially divided into two functional regions: one region that binds to DNA and another region that activates transcription.

The two-hybrid system uses the *GAL1*-Gal4p transcription system to identify previously unknown proteins that interact with a protein of interest. The system consists of a reporter gene under the control of the *GAL1* promoter and two plasmids that produce fusions with the Gal4p transcription factor. The first plasmid contains a gene of interest fused to a DNA-binding domain. This plasmid expresses a protein that is able to bind to the DNA-binding site in the *GAL1* promoter of the reporter gene. This plasmid is unable to activate transcription of the reporter gene, since the Gal4p fragment does not contain the information to activate transcription. The second plasmid is provided from a collection of plasmids that consist of unknown or random genes fused to the transcription activation domain of Gal4p. This plasmid by itself is unable to bind to the DNA-binding site in the *GAL1* promoter and thus is unable to activate transcription of the reporter gene. If both plasmids contain genes whose protein products physically interact in the cell, the complex is able to bind to the DNA-binding region of the

GAL1 promoter, and since the activation domain of Gal4p is also present in this complex, activation of the reporter gene will occur. The production of the reporter gene serves as a signal that both of the gene products interact in the cell. The yeast strain containing the active reporter gene is then selected and further examined to determine the unknown DNA that resides on the second plasmid by sequence analysis.

CELL CYCLE MUTANTS

The isolation, characterization, and identification of conditional mutations in *Saccharomyces cerevisiae* has

led to great advances in our understanding of the genes involved in the cell cycle. Because cell division is an essential process, null mutations in cell cycle genes are lethal. Thus, an approach to isolate temperature-sensitive mutants, cells that grow at room temperature but not at 36 degrees Celsius (96.8 degrees Fahrenheit), was taken. The observation that the formation of the yeast bud occurs at the beginning of the cell cycle and the bud continues to grow through cell cycle progression facilitated analysis of defects in cell division cycle (CDC). At the permissive temperature (room temperature), cell cultures are asynchronous; however, when the culture is switched to the restrictive temperature, cells with mutations in genes affecting cell cycle progression become synchronously arrested, which can be visualized microscopically. Temperature-sensitive mutants with defects in budding, DNA synthesis, nuclear division cytokinesis, and cell division were analyzed. This approach led to the isolation and characterization of the cell division cycle mutants, each of which undergoes growth arrest at specific points in the cell cycle and essentially represents all the key regulators of cell cycle progression. A fundamental observation that arose from this work was that cell cycle progression is controlled by cell-cycle checkpoints, whereby progression of the cell cycle is dependent upon the successful completion of upstream events. These checkpoints maintain cellular integrity by causing the cell cycle to arrest and initiate repair processes before errors are passed on to daughter cells. One of the genes thought to be most important that was identified using this approach is *CDC28*, which, like all of the CDCs, has homologues in all eukaryotes, including humans. Cdc28p, a cyclin-dependent kinase, initiates two pathways that lead to cell division. The identification of the *CDC* genes in yeast and mammalian homologues has led to important insights into defects in cell-cycle checkpoints that ultimately lead to cancer.

RESEARCH AND IMPLICATIONS

The years of work on yeast as a model system have provided many insights into how genes and their protein products interact to coordinate the many cellular mechanisms that take place in all cells from simple yeast to complicated humans. It is impossible to exhaustively list the different areas of research currently being examined or completely list the new understandings that have come to light through the use of the *S. cerevisiae* model system. Every major area of cellular research has at one time or another used yeast to ask some of the more difficult questions that could not be asked in other systems. Work in yeast has aided identification of genes and elucidated the mechanism of many different areas of research, including cell-cycle regulation, mechanisms of signal transduction, the process of secretion, DNA replication, transcription of DNA, translation of messenger RNA into proteins, biosynthetic pathways of amino acids and other basic building blocks of cells, and regulation and progression of cells through mitosis and meiosis. Despite all these advances, there is still much to learn from yeast, and it will continue to provide information for years to come.

Outside of its value in genetic research, *S. cerevisiae* continues to be an important resource in other ways. As implied by its common name of baker's yeast, it is still used as the chief leavening agent for the production of bread products. A different strain of the yeast is also an important factor in the fermentation process used in winemaking and beer brewing. As the craft beer market has expanded, greater attention has been paid to the specific processes used in producing different types and flavors of beer; *S. cerevisiae* belongs to the group of yeasts often referred to as top fermenting. In 2013 the government of Oregon named *S. cerevisiae* as the state's official microbe in recognition of its role in the history of brewing and the state's close association with the craft brew movement.

John R. Geiser, Ph.D.;
updated by Pauline M. Carrico, Ph.D.

FURTHER READING

Aggarwal, Monika, and Robert M. Brosh. "Functional Analyses of Human DNA Repair Proteins Important for Aging and Genomic Stability Using Yeast Genetics." *DNA Repair* 11.4 (2012): 335–48. Print.

Amberg, D., D. Burke, and J. Strathern. *Methods in Yeast Genetics: A Cold Spring Harbor Laboratory Course Manual, 2005 Edition*. Cold Spring Harbor: Cold Spring Harbor Laboratory P, 2005. Print.

Broach, J., J. Pringle, and E. Jones, eds. *The Molecular and Cellular Biology of the Yeast Saccharomyces*. 3 vols. Cold Spring Harbor: Cold Spring Harbor Laboratory P, 1991–97. Print.

Feldmann, Horst. *Yeast: Molecular and Cell Biology*. Wenheim: Wiley, 2010. Print.

Fields, S., and O. Song. "A Novel Genetic System to Detect Protein-Protein Interactions." *Nature* 340 (1989): 245–46. Print.

Hartwell, L. "Yeast and Cancer." *Bioscience Reports* 24 (2004): 523–44. Print.

Lodolo, E. J., et al. "The Yeast Saccharomyces Cerevisiae: The Main Character in Beer Brewing." *FEMS Yeast Research* 8.7 (2008): 1018–36. *PubMed*. Web. 3 Mar. 2015.

McInerny, Christopher J. "Cell Cycle Regulated Gene Expression in Yeasts." *Advances in Genetics*. Ed. Theodore Friedmann, Jay C. Dunlap, and Stephen F. Goodwin. Vol. 73. San Diego: Elsevier, 2011. 51–86. Print.

See also: Cloning vectors; Extra chromosomal inheritance; Linkage maps; Model organisms; Noncoding RNA molecules; Plasmids.

Sandhoff disease

CATEGORY: Diseases and syndromes
ALSO KNOWN AS: Beta-hexosaminidase-beta-subunit deficiency; GM2 gangliosidosis, Type II; hexosaminidase A and B deficiency disease; Sandhoff-Jatzkewitz-Pilz disease; total hexosaminidase deficiency

DEFINITION

Sandhoff disease is a rare, inherited disorder that causes abnormal accumulation of particular types of fats inside nerve cells, which eventually kills them. This disease culminates in a gradual and progressive deterioration of the nervous system.

RISK FACTORS

Anyone whose biological parents both carry mutations in the *HexB* gene is at risk for Sandhoff disease. This genetic disease equally affects males and females but more commonly occurs in the Creole population of northern Argentina; Metis Indians in Saskatchewan, Canada; and Christian Marionite communities from Cyprus.

ETIOLOGY AND GENETICS

Sandhoff disease is an autosomal recessive hereditary disease caused by mutations in the *HexB* gene. The *HexB* gene is located on the long arm of chromosome 5, in band region 13. People must inherit two copies of a mutant form of the *HexB* gene in order to have Sandhoff disease. Children whose parents both carry a mutant copy of the *HexB* gene have a 25 percent chance of being born with Sandhoff disease. The *HexB* gene encodes the information for the synthesis of a protein called hexosaminidase B.

Cells are bordered by the plasma membrane, which is composed of phosphate-containing lipids, proteins, and another groups of lipids called sphingolipids. Many sphingolipids have chains of sugars attached to them and are collectively called glycolipids. Glycolipids are very common in the membranes of nerve cells, but cells must constantly produce new glycolipids and degrade old ones in order to keep their plasma membranes in good working condition.

Once made, membrane lipids are loaded into spherical vesicles that fuse with the membrane. Membrane lipids are removed from the membrane by being loaded into vesicles that pinch off the membrane and fuse with a waiting vesicle called a lysosome. Lysosomes serve as the garbage disposal of cells, and they contain a cadre of enzymes called acid hydrolases that degrade the components brought to the lysosome. Hexosaminidase B is one of the lysosomal acid hydrolases that degrade glycolipids.

Hexosaminidase B is part of two different acid hydrolases. It forms a complex with another protein called hexosaminidase A to form an acid hydrolase called β-hexosaminidase A. Hexosaminidase A is encoded by the *HexA* gene, and mutations in *HexA* cause Tay-Sachs disease, which is clinically very similar to Sandhoff disease. β-hexosaminidase A degrades a glycolipid called the GM ganglioside. Hexosaminidase B also forms a complex with itself to make an acid hydrolase called β-hexosaminidase B, which degrades so called "neutral glycolipids."

Mutations in the *HexB* gene that inactivate hexosaminidase B abrogate the enzymatic activities of β-hexosaminidase A and B. Cells accumulate GM gangliosides and neutral glycolipids, which kills the cells. Because nerve cells make such extensive use of complex glycolipids, they are among the most sensitive to an inability to degrade them. Gradual death of nerve cells causes an inexorable and progressive deterioration of nerve functions.

Sandhoff disease belongs to a larger group of genetic diseases called lysosomal storage diseases, in which the activity of lysosomal acid hydrolases is compromised.

SYMPTOMS

With the classical infantile form of Sandhoff disease, infants begin showing symptoms by six months. They lose muscle tone and movement (motor control) and show an exaggerated startle response to loud noises. As the nervous

The HEXB gene is located on the long (q) arm of chromosome 5 at position 13. By Genetics Home Reference (http://ghr.nlm.nih.gov/gene=hexb), via Wikimedia Commons

system deteriorates, babies suffer from seizures; loss of sight, hearing, and the ability to swallow; and paralysis.

In the juvenile form, symptoms start between three to ten years of age and include muscle weakness, loss of coordination (ataxia) and speech, and mental problems.

The adult-onset form occurs in older people, and the symptoms (muscle weakness) are milder and vary.

SCREENING AND DIAGNOSIS

Biochemical tests on blood or biopsied tissues are required to distinguish Sandhoff disease from Tay-Sachs disease. The absence of β-hexosaminidase A and B activity is diagnostic for Sandhoff disease.

Genetic tests for prenatal or preimplantation diagnoses are available for Sandhoff disease. Prenatal diagnoses use tissue derived from amniocentesis, chorionic villus sampling, placental biopsy, umbilical cord blood sampling, or fetal skin biopsy to screen unborn babies. Preimplantation genetic diagnosis screens individual blastomeres from embryos formed by in vitro fertilization.

TREATMENT AND THERAPY

No cure exists for Sandhoff disease. Antiseizure medication can mitigate seizures, and feeding tubes can prevent food aspiration into the lungs. Experimental treatments with stem cells and gene therapy are ongoing.

PREVENTION AND OUTCOMES

Genetic screening of prospective parents can reduce the rates of Sandhoff disease.

The infantile form of Sandhoff disease usually causes death before the age of four, while the juvenile-onset form causes death by age fifteen. Adult-onset patients experience severe lifestyle restrictions.

Michael A. Buratovich, Ph.D.

FURTHER READING

Mehta, Atul B., and Bryan Winchester. *Lysosomal Storage Disorders: A Practical Guide.* Chichester: Wiley, 2013. Print.

Milunsky, Aubrey, and Jeff M. Milunsky. *Genetic Disorders and the Fetus: Diagnosis, Prevention, and Treatment.* 6th ed. Chichester: Wiley, 2010. Print.

Nelson, David L., and Michael M. Cox. *Lehninger Principles of Biochemistry.* 5th ed. New York: Freeman, 2008. Print.

Noggle, Chad A., Raymond S. Dean, and Arthur MacNeill Horton. *The Encyclopedia of Neuropsychological Disorders.* New York: Springer, 2012. Print.

Parker, James N., and Philip M. Parker. *The Official Parent's Sourcebook on Sandhoff Disease: A Revised and Updated Directory for the Internet Age.* San Diego: Icon Health, 2002. Print.

See also: Fabry disease; Gaucher disease; Gm1-gangliosidosis; Hereditary diseases; Hunter disease; Hurler syndrome; Inborn errors of metabolism; Jansky-Bielschowsky disease; Krabbé disease; Metachromatic leukodystrophy; Niemann-Pick disease; Pompe disease; Sanfilippo syndrome; Tay-Sachs disease.

Sanfilippo syndrome

CATEGORY: Diseases and syndromes

ALSO KNOWN AS: Mucopolysaccharidosis type III; MPS III

DEFINITION

Sanfilippo syndrome is a progressive disorder that primarily affects the central nervous system. In individuals with Sanfilippo syndrome, gene mutations cause a deficiency of an enzyme needed for breakdown of heparan sulfate. There are four subtypes of Sanfilippo syndrome: A, B, C, and D.

RISK FACTORS

A family history of Sanfilippo syndrome is the most significant risk factor. The parents of a child with Sanfilippo syndrome have a 25 percent chance to have another child with the condition. Unaffected siblings of an individual with Sanfilippo syndrome have a 67 percent chance to be a carrier of the condition. There is a high incidence of Sanfilippo syndrome in individuals from the Cayman Islands.

ETIOLOGY AND GENETICS

Sanfilippo syndrome is an autosomal recessive condition. Humans typically have twenty-three pairs of chromosomes. The first twenty-two pairs are the autosomes, and are numbered 1 through 22. The twenty-third pair consists of the sex chromosomes, which are called X and Y. Each chromosome contains many genes. Humans have two copies of most genes. Individuals affected with an autosomal recessive condition have a mutation in both copies of a given gene. In autosomal recessive conditions, individuals with a mutation in one copy of a gene are considered carriers. Mutations in one of four genes (*SGSH, NAGLU, HGSNAT, GNS*) cause each type of Sanfilippo syndrome (A, B, C, D, respectively). *SGSH* and *NAGLU* are both located on chromosome 17. *HGSNAT* is located on chromosome 8, and the *GNS* gene is located on chromosome 12.

Each of the four genes for Sanfilippo syndrome provides instructions for a single enzyme, which is partially responsible for the breakdown of heparan sulfate. Heparan sulfate is a type of mucopolysaccharide, which are complex chains of sugar molecules. Because heparan sulfate is broken down in the lysosome of the cell, Sanfilippo syndrome is considered a lysosomal storage disease.

In individuals with Sanfilippo syndrome, heparan sulfate is stored in the body's tissues. However, the majority of heparan sulfate is stored in the brain. It is also believed that the storage of heparan sulfate interferes with the breakdown of a component of cell membranes, gangliosides. The combination of heparan sulfate and ganglioside accumulation causes the symptoms of Sanfilippo syndrome.

SYMPTOMS

Type A, B, C, and D of Sanfilippo syndrome have similar symptoms, and the type cannot be determined based on symptoms. Sanfilippo syndrome is a progressive disorder that primarily affects the central nervous system. As the condition progresses, the neurological symptoms gradually change. The symptoms of Sanfilippo syndrome have been divided into three phases. The timing and severity of each phase vary from one individual to the next. Phase one is characterized by developmental delay, which is typically identified between twelve months and twenty-four months of age. The delay is typically most significant in speech. The second phase is usually from age three to age ten and is characterized by hyperactivity and behavioral problems. A need for very little sleep may develop during phase two. The third phase typically begins at the end of the first decade. Individuals slowly lose motor skills and eventually are no longer able to walk. Swallowing problems may also develop during the third phase.

SCREENING AND DIAGNOSIS

Mucopolysaccharides are also known as glycosaminoglycans (GAGs). Quantification of GAGs in urine is a screening test for all mucopolysaccharidoses. Thin-layer chromotography (TLC) separation is another screening test that may identify a specific mucopolysaccharidosis. However, if quantification of GAGs and TLC separation is abnormal, then confirmatory enzyme analysis is necessary.

TREATMENT AND THERAPY

Unfortunately, there is currently not a therapy or treatment for Sanfilippo syndrome. However, several potential treatments are currently being researched. Replacing the missing enzyme is a potential treatment; however, the enzyme is unable to get through the protective coating around the brain. Because the symptoms of Sanfilippo syndrome are primarily neurological, the enzyme must be administered directly into the brain. Substrate deprivation therapy (SDT) is a pharmaceutical approach to reduce the amount of GAGS or gangliosides produced by the body. Two SDTs, miglustat and genistein, have been trialed in patients with Sanfilippo syndrome, with some stabilization of neurological symptoms. Gene therapy is another potential treatment and is currently being researched in animal models.

PREVENTION AND OUTCOMES

Genetic testing is available for all four types of Sanfilippo syndrome. If gene mutations are identified in an individual with Sanfilippo syndrome, then preimplantation genetic diagnosis, chorionic villus sampling, and amniocentesis are available to the parents for prevention. Individuals with Sanfilippo syndrome do not typically survive past their late twenties or early thirties.

Beth M. Hannan, M.S.

FURTHER READING

Fernandes, John, Jean-Marie Saudubray, Georges van den Berghe, and John H. Walter. *Inborn Metabolic Diseases.* 4th ed. Germany: Springer, 2006. Print.

Heldermon, C. D., et al. "Disease Correction by Combined Neonatal Intracranial AAV and Systemic

Lentiviral Gene Therapy in Sanfilippo Syndrome Type B Mice." *Gene Therapy* 20.9 (2013): 913–21. Print.

Jakobkiewicz-Banecka, Joanna, Alicja Wegrzyn, and Grzegorz Wegrzyn. "Substrate Deprivation Therapy: A New Hope for Patients Suffering from Neuronopathic Forms of Inherited Lysosomal Storage Diseases." *Journal of Applied Genetics* 48.4 (2007): 383–88. Print.

Mehta, Atul B., and Bryan Winchester. *Lysosomal Storage Disorders: A Practical Guide.* Chichester: Wiley, 2013. Print.

Milunsky, Aubrey, and Jeff M. Milunsky. *Genetic Disorders and the Fetus: Diagnosis, Prevention, and Treatment.* 6th ed. Chichester: Wiley, 2010. Print.

Nussbaum, Robert L., Roderick R. McInnes, and Huntington F. Willard. *Thompson and Thompson Genetics in Medicine.* 7th ed. New York: Saunders, 2007. Print.

Valstar, M. J., et al. "Sanfilippo Syndrome: A Mini Review." *Journal of Inherited Metabolic Disease* 31 (2008): 240–52. Print.

See also: Fabry disease; Gaucher disease; Gm1-gangliosidosis; Hereditary diseases; Hunter disease; Hurler syndrome; Inborn errors of metabolism; Jansky-Bielschowsky disease; Krabbé disease; Metachromatic leukodystrophy; Niemann-Pick disease; Pompe disease; Sandhoff disease; Tay-Sachs disease.

Schizophrenia Spectrum And Other Psychotic Disorders

CATEGORY: Diseases and syndromes

DEFINITION

Schizophrenia is a chronic, severe, disabling brain disorder that interferes with the way a person interprets reality. People with schizophrenia sometimes hear voices or see things that others do not, become paranoid that people are plotting against them, and experience cognitive deficits and social withdrawal. These and other symptoms make it difficult for them to have positive relationships with others. Schizophrenia is different from split or multiple personality disorders. It affects many different areas of the brain, causing a wide range of behavioral, emotional, and intellectual symptoms.

RISK FACTORS

Factors that appear to increase an individual's risk of schizophrenia are very variable. Research has found the following trends and associations:

Family history of schizophrenia and/or epilepsy is definitely a risk factor. Men tend to develop schizophrenia between the ages of 15 – 24. The onset in women is usually slightly later, between ages 25 – 34. There also seems to be a lower risk in those who experience menarche earlier in life. Those with schizophrenia span the full range of intelligence, and no cultural or geographic group appears immune from the disease. Schizophrenia occurs twice as often in unmarried and divorced people as in married or widowed individuals. Those in poorer socioeconomic groups appear to have more severe disease; however, most agree that this is due to severe limitations in available resources to help manage the disease. The rate of left-handedness or mixed-handedness is significantly higher among patients with schizophrenia than the general population. This suggests that an underlying neurologic problem may put these individuals at higher risk. According to some studies, the older a father is when a child is born, the greater the risk is for schizophrenia in his offspring, perhaps because of a greater chance of genetic mutations in the sperm that can be passed on. In one study, children of fathers who were 50 years old or more faced a three-fold risk for schizophrenia compared to children of fathers who were 25 or younger. Other factors include being born during winter months and being born in the city. Additional risk factors include oxygen deprivation during labor and delivery and issues such as premature rupture of membranes, gestational age shorter than 37 weeks, and use of resuscitation and/or an incubator.

Loss of a parent during childhood is another possible risk factor.

In rare cases (about 1 in 40,000 children), schizophrenia is diagnosed in those under age 13.

ETIOLOGY AND GENETICS

Schizophrenia is an extraordinarily complex and variable clinical condition, and its etiology no doubt depends on a host of both genetic and environmental

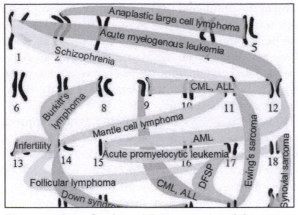

Chromosomal translocations, giving an overview of chromosomes involved. Precise locations within the chromosomes are not specified. Most are cancer forms, but also other conditions, e.g. t(1;11), which is is associated with schizophrenia[1]. Chromosomes are arranged in standard karyogram order.

Abbreviations:

ALL - Acute lymphoblastic leukemia
AML - Acute myeloid leukemia
CML - Chronic myelogenous leukemia
DFSP - Dermatofibrosarcoma protuberans

flowchart By Shawncho (Own work), via Wikimedia Commons

factors. It is safe to assume that there are many genes that contribute either to the susceptibility or the pathology of schizophrenia, but there is no single gene or mutation that exerts an overriding or self-sufficient effect in determining the development of the disease. Over 100 genetic loci scattered throughout the human genome that may be associated with susceptibility to schizophrenia.

In the summer of 2009, three research consortia reported results of their genome wide association studies on the genetics of schizophrenia, and all identified a region of particular importance on the short arm of chromosome 6 (at position 6p22.1). This region is known to contain a large cluster of genes (the major histocompatibility complex) that helps determine immunity and that also codes for proteins that are important for turning other genes on and off. Since mutations in this region are known to influence susceptibility to several autoimmune diseases, it may be likely that schizophrenia has an autoimmune component as well. Genetic variation in the control of such regulatory mechanisms might also account for the environmental component that has been repeatedly shown to contribute to disease susceptibility.

Evidence from additional molecular studies has suggested that large structural changes in DNA (deoxyribonucleic acid) called copy number variants (CNVs) may play a critical role in the development of schizophrenia. These CNVs are usually duplications or deletions of anywhere from hundreds to millions of base pairs in the DNA, and the largest deletions appear only in people with schizophrenia.

With so many genes possibly acting as contributing factors, it is not surprising that there is no predictable inheritance pattern regarding the development of schizophrenia. Many new cases appear in families with one or more other affected members, yet the majority of new cases appear in families in which there is no previous history of the disease.

SIGNS AND SYMPTOMS

Signs of the disease usually start in adolescence or early adulthood. Onset of signs and symptoms may be very variable.

Symptoms include hallucinations—seeing or hearing things/voices that are not there, and delusions—strong but false personal beliefs that are not based in reality. Disorganized thinking; disorganized speech and a lack of ability to speak in a way that makes sense or to carry on a conversation; catatonic behavior, such as slow movement, repeating rhythmic gestures, pacing, walking in circles, negativism, and repetitive speech; emotional flatness, including flat speech, lack of facial expression, and general disinterest and withdrawal; paranoia, a psychosis characterized by systematized delusions of persecution or grandeur; inappropriate laughter; and poor hygiene and self-care are also characteristic signs. Schizophrenia may be present at the same time as other psychiatric disorders such as obsessive-compulsive disorder, substance abuse (of drugs, alcohol, caffeine, or nicotine), and self-injury, including suicide.

SCREENING AND DIAGNOSIS

According to the *Diagnostic and Statistical Manual of Mental Disorders, Fifth Edition, (DSM-5),* to meet the criteria for diagnosis of schizophrenia, the patient must have experienced at least 2 of the following symptoms:

- Delusions
- Hallucinations
- Disorganized speech
- Disorganized or catatonic behavior
- Negative symptoms (diminished emotional expression and or avolition [severe lack of initiative or motivation])

At least 1 of the symptoms must be the presence of delusions, hallucinations, or disorganized speech.

Continuous signs of the disturbance must persist for at least 6 months, during which the patient must experience at least 1 month of active symptoms (or less if successfully treated), with social or occupational deterioration problems occurring over a significant amount of time. These problems must not be attributable to another condition (such as that caused by substance abuse).

Early diagnosis is extremely important. Patients who are diagnosed early and receive ongoing effective management are able to stabilize signs and symptoms, decrease the risk of suicide, decrease alcohol and substance abuse, and reduce the chance of relapse and/or hospitalization.

TREATMENT AND THERAPY

Schizophrenia is not curable, but it is highly treatable. Hospitalization may be required during acute episodes. Treatment of schizophrenia requires integration of medical, psychological, and psychosocial inputs. The bulk of care occurs in an outpatient setting and probably is best carried out by a multidisciplinary team, including some combination of the following: a psychopharmacologist, a counselor or therapist, a social worker, a nurse, a vocational counselor, and a case manager. Clinical pharmacists and internists can also be valuable members of the team because these patients often have common underlying medical problems (such as diabetes, high blood pressure, and various lung diseases) that need to be evaluated and managed.

Symptoms are usually controlled with antipsychotic medications. These medications work by blocking certain chemicals in the brain, which helps control the abnormal thinking that occurs in people with schizophrenia. Determining a medication plan can be a complicated process. Often medications or dosages need to be changed until the right balance is found. This can take months or even years. Examples of medications include haloperidol (Haldol), thioridazine, or fluphenazine.

Relapse is always a challenging issue. Approximately 80% of patients relapse within 1 year if antipsychotic medications are stopped, whereas only 20% relapse if treated. Children, pregnant or breastfeeding women, and elderly patients present special challenges. In all of these cases, medications must be used with particular caution. Treatment compliance can be a challenge, since people often stop taking their medication when they are feeling better. The side effects of traditional antipsychotics can also cause patients to discontinue treatment. The most common are physical side effects, such as slow and stiff movements, restlessness, facial tics, and protruding tongue.

Newer medications, called atypical antipsychotics, have fewer side effects and are better tolerated over long periods of time. However, they may cause weight gain, elevated blood sugar, and elevated serum cholesterol. Examples of these medications include aripiprazole (Abilify), clozapine (Clozaril), risperidone (Risperdal), olanzapine (Zyprexa), pali-peridone (Invega), quetiapine (Seroquel), and ziprasidone (Geodon).

Medications may also be prescribed for coexisting conditions. Conditions often associated with schizophrenia include depression and anxiety. They may be treated with antidepressants, anxiolytic drugs, lithium, and anticonvulsants. Electroconvulsive therapy may be used to treat severe depression, suicidal ideation, or severe psychosis.

Schizophrenia is a lifelong condition. It can be confusing and frightening for the person with the disease and for family members. Individual and family therapy can address social skills, vocational guidance, community resources, coping with the family, living arrangements, general emotional support, and working with the family to help family members deal with the patient.

PREVENTION AND OUTCOMES

There are no guidelines for preventing schizophrenia. However, studies show that early, aggressive treatment leads to better outcomes. The North American Prodrome Longitudinal Study is exploring whether the incorporation of biologic measures into prediction algorithms can provide more accurate identification of young people who are at greatest risk for developing a psychotic disorder. The goal of this study is to establish objective criteria that can be used to develop preventive approaches.

Julie Riley, M.S., RD; reviewed by Theodor B. Rais, M.D. "Etiology and Genetics" by Jeffrey A. Knight, Ph.D.; updated by Gary M. Flashner, M.S., M.D.

FURTHER READING

EBSCO Publishing. *Health Library: Schizophrenia.* Ipswich, Mass.: Author, 2009. Available through http://www.ebscohost.com.

Frith, Christopher D., and Eve C. Johnstone. *Schizophrenia: A Very Short Introduction.* Oxford, En gland: Oxford University Press, 2003.

Moore, David P., and James W. Jefferson. *Handbook of Medical Psychiatry.* 2d ed. Philadelphia: Elsevier Mosby, 2004.

Temes, Roberta. *Getting Your Life Back Together When You Have Schizophrenia.* Oakland, Calif.: New Harbinger, 2002.

Torrey, E. Fuller. *Surviving Schizophrenia: A Manual for Families, Consumers, and Providers.* 4th ed. New York: Quill, 2001.

American Psychiatric Association. *Diagnostic and Statistical Manual of Mental Disorders*: Rev. 5 ed. Washington, D.C.: 2013.

Harrison PJ. "Recent genetic findings in schizophrenia and their therapeutic relevance". Pratt J, ed. *Journal of Psychopharmacology (Oxford, England).* 2015; 29(2): 85-96. doi: 10.1177/0269881114553647.

Marneros A , Pillmann F , Wustmann T : "Delusional disorders—are they simply paranoid schizophrenia?" Schizophr Bull 38(3): 561–568, 2012

Abel KM , Drake R , Goldstein JM : "Sex differences in schizophrenia". International Review of Psychiatry 22(5): 417–428, 2010

Álvarez-Jiménez M, Gleeson JF, Henry LP, et al: "Road to full recovery: longitudinal relationship between symptomatic remission and psychosocial recovery in first-episode psychosis over 7.5 years". Psychol Med 42(3): 595–606, 2012

Gochman P, Miller R, Rapoport JL. "Childhood-Onset Schizophrenia: The Challenge of Diagnosis". Current Psychiatry Reports. 2011; 13(5): 321–322. doi: 10.1007/s11920-011-0212-4.

WEB SITES OF INTEREST

American Psychiatric Association
http://www.psych.org
Canadian Psychiatric Association
http://www.cpa-apc.org
Cochrane Reviews: "Electroconvulsive Therapy for Schizophrenia"
http://www.cochrane.org/reviews/en/ab000076.html
Mayo Clinic. com: Schizophrenia
http://www.mayoclinic.com/health/schizophrenia/DS00196
Mental Health Canada
http://www.mentalhealthcanada.com
National Institute of Mental Health
http://www.nimh.nih.gov
Schizophrenia.com
http://www.schizophrenia.com/index.html
World Fellowship for Schizophrenia and Allied Disorders
http://world-schizophrenia.org
http://emedicine.medscape.com/article/288259-overview
https://pdfs.semanticscholar.org/b6df/6b113345da78988d707d753feb44bf50683d.pdf

See also: Attention deficit hyperactivity disorder (ADHD); Autism; Bipolar affective disorder; Dyslexia; Fragile X syndrome; Tourette syndrome.

SCLC1 gene

CATEGORY: Molecular genetics

SIGNIFICANCE: The *SCLC1* gene is expressed in cells and tissues of individuals with lung cancer, particularly small-cell cancer of the lung. Interactions between cigarette smoking and acquired chromosomal abnormalities facilitate expression of this gene.

KEY TERMS

allele: one member of a pair of different forms of a gene at a specific locus

autosomal dominant: the presence of one abnormal gene allows expression of that gene

chromosomal deletion: chromosomal abnormality in which part of the chromosome is missing or deleted

heterozygosity: different alleles of a given gene at a locus

locus: location on a chromosome occupied by one or more genes

loss of heterozygosity: loss of alleles at numerous chromosomal loci

oncogene: transforms a normal cell into a tumor cell when mutated or expressed

tumor-suppressor gene: a gene that inhibits tumor cell growth

SMALL-CELL LUNG CARCINOMA

According to the American Lung Association, lung cancer is the most common cancer worldwide and the most common cause of cancer deaths in the United States. There are two main types of lung cancer: small-cell lung cancer (SCLC) and non-small-cell lung cancer (NSCLC), with the distinction based primarily on the appearance of the cancer cells under the microscope. SCLC accounts for approximately 14 percent of all lung cancer diagnoses. It is highly aggressive and is associated with poor prognosis, as metastases are generally already present at the time of diagnosis. In 2014 the American Cancer Society reported that the five-year survival rate for SCLC cases diagnosed between 2003 and 2009 was only 6 percent, compared to 18 percent for NSCLC. Tobacco smoke is the most common carcinogen associated with SCLC, with only a vanishingly small percentage of cases occurring in patients who have never smoked.

CHROMOSOME LOCATION AND INHERITANCE

The *SCLC1* gene, also known as *SCLC* or *SCCL*, is located on chromosome 3, between bands 21 and 23 of the short arm of this chromosome (denoted 3p23–p21). Inheritance of this gene is autosomal dominant. Individuals who carry the *SCLC1* gene are predisposed to develop lung cancer, although a combination of several genetic defects and environmental factors is required before cancer develops. SCLC and other types of lung cancer are examples of cancer induced by external factors, such as carcinogens in cigarette smoke, but associated with specific chromosomal changes.

MOLECULAR ABNORMALITIES ASSOCIATED WITH SCLC

Although SCLC is strongly tied to cigarette smoking, with an estimated 90 percent of lung cancers caused by smoking, a number of genetic abnormalities are also observed in lung cancer cells. Some are markers of disease progression, while others play direct roles in lung cancer development. Lung cancers are characterized by multiple gene alterations, such as amplification of oncogenes and deletions or mutations in tumor-suppressor genes during disease progression. Common chromosomal abnormalities associated with lung cancer include deletions on the short arms of chromosomes 3 [del(3p)] and 9 [del(9p)]. The most frequent genetic mutation associated with SCLC is deletion of a region on the short arm of chromosome 3 in an area that contains several genes potentially associated with lung cancer. Specifically, deletion of alleles located on bands 14 through 25—that is, 3p(14–25)—are associated with lung cancer development.

LOSS OF HETEROZYGOSITY AND TUMOR-SUPPRESSOR GENES

In hereditary cancer syndromes that give individuals a predisposition to certain forms of cancer, individuals are heterozygous, which means they have at least one gene pair with different alleles. The other allele of that pair is normal, so the disease phenotype is not immediately expressed. If the normal suppressive gene that inhibits expression of the disease phenotype is lost, such as through chromosomal deletion, a condition called loss of heterozygosity occurs. Loss of heterozygosity at multiple chromosomal loci has been identified in lung cancer, along with changes in tumor-suppressor genes and oncogenes. Most small-cell lung carcinomas are associated with large deletions in segments of 3p, leading to loss of heterozygosity at numerous loci, including many potential tumor-suppressor genes.

IMPACT

The *SCLC1* gene is associated with lung cancer development and is known as a cancer-predisposing gene. A specific acquired chromosomal abnormality, a deletion on the short arm of chromosome 3, is associated with SCLC. Many inherited cancer syndromes exhibit intricate interactions with environmental factors. Interactions between cigarette smoking and a predisposition to developing lung cancer are documented. Susceptibility to many inherited cancer syndromes is now detectable through genetic screening, and advances in molecular genetics associated with some forms of lung cancer can lead to new approaches to diagnosis, treatment, and prognosis.

C. J. Walsh, Ph.D.

Further Reading

American Cancer Society. *Cancer Facts & Figures 2014.* Atlanta: Amer. Cancer Soc., 2014. PDF file.

American Cancer Society. "Lung Cancer (Small Cell)." *American Cancer Society.* Amer. Cancer Soc., 11 Feb. 2014. Web. 15 Aug. 2014.

Cooper, David N. *The Molecular Genetics of Lung Cancer.* Berlin: Springer, 2005. Print.

Driscoll, Barbara, ed. *Molecular Pathology Methods and Reviews.* Vol. 1 of *Lung Cancer.* Totowa: Humana, 2003. Print.

Kantarjian, Hagop M., Robert A. Wolff, and Charles A. Koller. *The MD Anderson Manual of Medical Oncology.* 2nd ed. New York: McGraw, 2011. Print.

Kaye, Frederic J., and Akihito Kubo. "Molecular Genetics of Lung Cancer." *Molecular Genetics of Cancer.* Ed. John K. Cowell. 2nd ed. Oxford: BIOS, 2001. 485–517. Print.

Whang-Peng, Jacqueline, et al. "Specific Chromosome Defect Associated with Human Small-Cell Lung Cancer: Deletion 3p(14–23)." *Science* 215. 4529 (1982): 181–82. Print.

Xu, Zhaolin. "Genomics and Molecular Profiling of Lung Cancer." *Cancer Genomics: From Bench to Personalized Medicine.* Ed. Graham Dellaire, Jason Berman, and Robert Arceci. Waltham: Academic, 2014. 194–211. Print.

See also: *BRAF* gene; *BRCA1* and *BRCA2* genes; Cancer; Chromosome mutation; *DPC4* gene testing; Harvey ras oncogene; *HRAS* gene testing; *MLH1* gene; Mutation and mutagenesis; Oncogenes; Tumor suppressor genes.

Severe combined immunodeficiency syndrome

CATEGORY: Diseases and syndromes

ALSO KNOWN AS: SCID; boy in the bubble syndrome; XSCID; SCIDX1; X-SCID; SCIDX; Athabascan SCID; Swiss agammaglobulinemia; X-linked SCID; Severe combined immunodeficiency, X-linked; SCID, X-linked; Severe combined immunodeficiency T B+ due to gamma chain deficiency; Severe combined immunodeficiency, X-linked, T cell-negative, B cell-positive, NK cell-negative

Definition

Severe combined immunodeficiency syndrome (SCID) is a group of severe, rare (1 in 100,000), congenital conditions defined by a deficiency of the immune response. A mutation in one of several possible genes causes a defect in the specialized white blood cells (lymphocytes) that defend against infection. Patients are prone to repeated and persistent infections, rarely surviving past their first year unless treated within the first three to four months of life with bone marrow transplantation.

Risk Factors

All forms of SCID are inherited. The most common form of SCID (approximately half of reported cases) occurs only in males as it is caused by mutations in the X chromosome (XSCID).

Though the *Artemis* form of SCID is very rare in the general population, it has a high incidence (1 in 2,000) in Navajo and Apache Native Americans. This form of SCID is also known as Athabascan SCID (SCIDA), after the Athabascan linguistic group of Native Americans.

Etiology and Genetics

The immune system is a network of organs, tissues, cells, and protein substances that work together, defending the body against attack by bacteria, viruses, fungi, parasites, or other foreign substances. When a major component of the immune system is not functioning correctly, the body cannot ward off infections. Lymphocytes (T, B, and NK [natural killer] cells) and the proteins they produce make up key components of the immune system. T cells are crucial in identifying invading agents and in activating and regulating other cells of the immune system.

SCID is the prototype of the primary immunodeficiency diseases and is caused by numerous molecular defects that lead to severe compromise in the number and function of T cells, B cells, and occasionally natural killer (NK) cells. All forms are characterized by in the numbers and/or function of T cells. The different genetic forms of SCID vary as to the presence of defects in NK and B cells.

SCID results from mutations in any of more than 15 known genes encoding components involved in lymphocyte development. Since these various genetic causes of SCID account for approximately 90 percent of cases, there are probably additional genetic forms of SCID. Note that, in certain very rare cases, SCID is just one component of the features and defects of the presenting disorder, and inheritance is autosomal recessive. One example is reticular dysgenesis which is defined clinically by the combination of SCID, agranulocytosis and sensorineural deafness. Mutations in the gene encoding Adenylate Kinase 2 (AK2) have been identified as the cause of this disorder. Another is Omenn syndrome. In this disorder, SCID is associated with low IgG, IgA, and IgM and the virtual absence of B cells. There is an elevated number of T cells, but their function is impaired. Omenn syndrome has been found to be caused by mutations in the RAG1 or RAG2 genes. Additional causative genes have also been identified.

XSCID results from mutations in the interleukin-2 receptor gamma gene (*IL2RG*; cytogenetic location: Xq13.1). Defective IL receptors prevent the normal development of T cells.

As noted previously, SCID may also result from autosomal recessive gene defects. Mutations found on autosomal chromosomes have been identified in multiple other genetic forms. Along with reticular dysgenesis and Omenn syndrome, autosomal recessive manifestations are seen with defects in 100 Janus kinase 3 (*JAK3*; cytogenetic location: 19p13.1); IL-7 receptor alpha chain (*IL-7R* : cytogenetic location: 5p13); Artemis (cytogenetic location: 10p13); ligase 4 (*LIG4*; cytogenetic location: 13q33-q34); CD3 delta, epsilon, and zeta chain (CD3δ, CD3ε, and CD3ζ; cytogenetic locations: 11q23, 11q23, and 1q22-q23); and CD45 (cytogenetic location: 1q31-q32). These various components of the immune system are critical in T, B, and/or NK cell development or function via their role in toxic byproduct disposal, DNA repair, signal transduction, or VDJ (variable (V), diversity (D) and joining (J) recombination (a form of genetic recombination which assembles pieces of genes encoding specific proteins that have key roles in the immune system).

ADA (adenosine deaminase) deficiency is the second most common form of SCID, accounting for about one-sixth of reported cases. Mutations in the ADA gene lead to a deficiency in the enzyme and accumulation of toxic by products. Though ADA is present in all cell types, immature lymphocytes in the thymus normally have the highest level of ADA in the body and are thus particularly sensitive to the toxic effects of these by products. Without ADA, immature lymphocytes fail to reach maturity and die.

For example, *Pneumocystis jiroveci* and Cytomegalovirus, both of which are found in healthy people, can cause a fatal pneumonia or hepatitis in SCID children. Similarly, adenovirus usually produces a sore throat and cold in people in the general population but can cause a fatal hepatitis in SCID children. SCID children may also develop severe fungal infections such as thrush (a Candida fungal infection of the mouth). Additionally, they are at risk from the live viruses used in certain vaccines.

Physical findings may involve many organ systems. The abnormal findings are primarily related to the various superimposed infections or to graft-versus-host disease (GVHD) rather than to SCID itself. The patient may show one or more of the following:

- Failure to thrive, manifesting as decreased weight, height, and head circumference
- Dehydration from chronic diarrhea
- Recurrent middle ear infections. It is common that these may be more severe than what is typically seen.
- Various diverse skin rashes, outbreaks and infections associated with bacterial, fungal, and viral diseases.
- Increased respiratory rate and effort and abnormal lung sounds secondary to pneumonia
- Fever from sepsis, systemic fungal infections, or widespread herpes
- Absent lymphatic tissue, including tonsils
- Lymphadenopathy and hepatosplenomegaly in Omenn syndrome or another form known as "bare lymphocyte syndrome"
- Developmental delays.
- Abdominal findings, including tenderness secondary to gastrointestinal (GI) infections and hepatomegaly from viral hepatitis
- Candidiasis and other fungal infections
- Sparse hair, abnormal dentition, and osteopetrosis (bones that are hyperdense and abnormally prone to breaking.

Other symptoms include persistent diarrhea (not necessarily infection related), various rashes, and symptoms associated with autoimmunity.

SCREENING AND DIAGNOSIS

Though SCID is considered rare, some experts believe it may be more common than thought. Great advances in testing and screening have been made over the past 10 years. Now, in many states, testing for X-SCID is now frequently part of newborn screening.

SIGNS AND SYMPTOMS

A baby with SCID often develops serious and life-threatening infections. Bacteria or viruses that typically cause little to no illness in normal children may cause serious illness in SCID children. For exam-Currently, 32 states and the District of Columbia currently screen for SCID. Screening for SCID may also be performed if there is a known family history of the disease or the baby exhibits suggestive symptoms (such as persistent and recurrent infections).

Different US states may use different newborn screening methods. Current screening These may include custom resequencing DNA microarray technology; polymerase chain reaction (PCR) of DNA from universally collected, dried blood spots; and the identification of T-cell receptor excision circles (TRECs).

If SCID is suspected, the following tests may aid diagnosis: complete blood counts (low lymphocyte counts in SCID); T, B, and NK cell counts (T cells are absent or dysfunctional in all forms of SCID; NK and B cells may be absent depending on the form of SCID); and antibody levels (low in SCID; may be artificially high during the first three to four months of life due to maternal antibodies that cross the placenta during pregnancy). Specific genetic testing to identify underlying genetic defects is possible in about 90 percent of cases.

TREATMENT AND THERAPY

In circumstances where a baby is suspected of having the diagnosis, clinicians often act quickly. SCID is a pediatric emergency and usually must be addressed expeditiously. Initially, infections are usually treated with antibiotics, antifungal and antiviral drugs, and intravenous immunoglobulin (IVIg). However, the restoration of a functional immune system is necessary. The preferred treatment is bone marrow transplantation from a healthy donor. If performed within the first three to four months of life it is effective in the majority of patients. Blood-forming stem cells from the bone marrow of a healthy donor provide a functioning immune system that can protect the patient against infection. These stem cells can renew themselves as needed and produce a continuous supply of healthy immune cells.

Additional treatments that may be considered include, but are not limited to, prophylactic antibiotics and antiviral medications; administration of certain non-live vaccines; and regular administration of IVIg.

In the ADA deficiency form of SCID, enzyme replacement therapy with weekly injections of poly-ethylene glycol-modified bovine ADA allows the immune cells to recover. This treatment is effective in the majority of cases.

Gene therapy is still a considered an experimental treatment option for SCID, and studies are ongoing. In this treatment, researchers correct the DNA mutation in a sample of the patient's T cells and then return these corrected T cells to the patient. Though this therapy has been successful in some patients, serious complications, such as a leukemia like disorder, have occurred in others.

In view of the propensity for various forms of infection, customary hygiene practices, such as strict hand washing, are usually recommended. Former interventions of reverse isolation (in a "bubble") as well as special diets are no longer recommended.

PREVENTION AND OUTCOMES

The various forms of SCID cannot be prevented; however, early diagnosis and treatment can greatly reduce the morbidity and mortality associated with untreated disease. Even for those receiving early, successful, curative allogeneic hematopoietic stem cell transplantation (HCST), the long-term outcome in a 90-patient cohort followed for 2-34 years showed that almost half experienced one or more significant clinical events, including persistent chronic GVHD, autoimmune and inflammatory manifestations, opportunistic and non-opportunistic infections, and a requirement for nutritional support.

Genetic counseling is generally recommended if there is a family history of the disease, and there is a desire to have more children.

Anita P. Kuan, Ph.D.; updated by Gary M. Flashner, M.S., M.D.

FURTHER READING

Immune Deficiency Foundation. IDF *Patient and Family Handbook: For Primary Immunodeficiency Diseases.* 4th ed. Towson, Md.: Author, 2007.

"Newborn Screening for Severe Combined Immunodeficiency (SCID): A Review." *Frontiers in Bio science* 10 (May 1, 2005): 1024-1039.

Allenspach E, Rawlings DJ, Scharenberg AM. *X-Linked Severe Combined Immunodeficiency.* 2003 Aug 26 [Updated 2016 Apr 14]. In: Pagon RA, Adam MP, Ardinger HH, et al., editors. GeneReviews® [Internet]. Seattle (WA): University of Washington, Seattle; 1993-2017.

Tasher D, Dalal I. "The genetic basis of severe combined immunodeficiency and its variants". *The Application of Clinical Genetics.* 2012; 5: 67-80. doi: 10.2147/TACG.S18693.

Kwan A, Abraham RS, Currier R, et al. "Newborn Screening for Severe Combined Immunodeficiency in 11 Screening Programs in the United States". *JAMA.* 2014; 312(7): 729-738. doi: 10.1001/jama. 2014. 9132.

WEB SITES OF INTEREST

Biology News Net: "First SCID Gene Chip to Be Introduced at Academy Meeting on Immunodeficiencies"
http://www.biologynews.net/archives/2006/04/22/first_scid_gene_chip_to_be_introduced_at_academy_meeting_on_immunodeficiencies.html
Immune Deficiency Foundation
http://www.primar yimmune.org
National Institutes of Health: Office of Rare Disease Research
https://rarediseases.info.nih.gov/diseases/5618/x-linked-severe-combined-immunodeficiency https://www.cdc.gov/newbornscreening/scid.html
https://ghr.nlm.nih.gov/condition/adenosine-deaminase-deficiency#inheritance
http://www.bloodjournal.org/content/early/2017/03/22/blood-2016-11-745638?sso-checked=true
https://rarediseases.info.nih.gov/diseases/8198/omenn-syndrome
SCID Self-Help Support Group and Resource Guide
http://www.scid.net

See also: Agammaglobulinemia; Allergies; antibodies; Anthrax; Ataxia telangiectasia; Autoimmune disorders; Autoimmune polyglandular syndrome; Chediak-Higashi syndrome; Chronic granulomatous disease; Hybridomas and monoclonal antibodies; Immunodeficiency with hyper-IgM; Immunogenetics; Infantile agranulocytosis; Myeloperoxidase deficiency; Purine nucleoside phosphorylase deficiency.

Shotgun cloning

CATEGORY: Genetic engineering and biotechnology

SIGNIFICANCE: Shotgun cloning is the random insertion of a large number of different DNA fragments into cloning vectors. A large number of different recombinant DNA molecules are generated, which are then introduced into host cells, often bacteria, and amplified. Because a large number of different recombinant DNAs are generated, there is a high likelihood one of the clones contains a fragment of DNA of interest.

KEY TERMS

cloning vector: a plasmid or virus into which foreign DNA can be inserted to amplify the number of copies of the foreign DNA

marker: a gene that encodes an easily detected product that is used to indicate that foreign DNA is in an organism

recombinant DNA: a novel DNA molecule formed by the joining of DNAs from different sources

restriction endonuclease: an enzyme that recognizes a specific nucleotide sequence in a piece of DNA and causes cleavage of the DNA; often simply called a restriction enzyme

RECOMBINANT DNA CLONING AND SHOTGUN CLONING

Before the development of recombinant DNA cloning, it was very difficult to study DNA sequences. Cloning a DNA fragment allows a researcher to obtain large amounts of that specific DNA sequence to analyze without interference from the presence of other DNA sequences. There are many uses for a cloned DNA fragment. For example, a DNA fragment can be sequenced to determine the order of its nucleotides. This information can be used to determine the location of a gene and the amino acid sequence of the gene's protein product. Cloned pieces of DNA are also useful as DNA probes. Because DNA is made of two strands that are complementary to each other, a cloned piece of DNA can be used to probe for copies of the same or similar DNA sequences in other samples. A cloned gene can also be inserted into an expression vector where it will produce the gene's protein product.

Shotgun cloning begins with the isolation of DNA from the organism of interest. In separate test tubes, the DNA to be cloned and the cloning vector DNA are digested (cut) with a restriction endonuclease that cuts the vector in just one location and the foreign DNA many times. Many restriction endonucleases create single-stranded ends that are complementary, so the end of any DNA molecule cut with that endonuclease can join to the end of any other DNA cut with the same endonuclease. When the digested vector and foreign DNA are mixed, they join randomly and are then sealed using DNA ligase, an enzyme that seals the small gap between two pieces of DNA. This creates recombinant DNA molecules composed of a copy of the vector and a random copy of foreign DNA. The recombinant DNA molecules are then introduced into host cells where the cloning vector can replicate each time the cell divides, which is approximately every twenty minutes in the case of *Escherichia coli*. The resulting collection of clones, each containing a potentially different fragment of foreign DNA, is called a genomic library. If a large collection of clones is produced, it is likely that every part of the genome from which the DNA came will be represented somewhere in the genomic library.

The presence of the cloning vector in host cells is determined by selecting for a marker gene in the cloning vector. Most vectors have two marker genes, and often both are different antibiotic resistance genes. A common example is the plasmid pBR322, which has a tetracycline and an ampicillin resistance gene. A restriction endonuclease cuts once somewhere in the tetracycline resistance gene, and if a foreign DNA fragment becomes incorporated, the resulting recombinant plasmid will have a nonfunctional tetracycline resistance gene. A bacterial cell transformed with a recombinant plasmid will therefore be resistant to ampicillin but will be sensitive to tetracycline. Many plasmids will not incorporate any foreign DNA and will be nonrecombinant. Cells that are transformed with a nonrecombinant plasmid will be resistant to both tetracycline and ampicillin. After the bacterial cells have been transformed, they are grown on a medium with ampicillin. The only cells that will survive will be those that have received a plasmid vector. To determine which cells have received a recombinant plasmid, the colonies are carefully transferred onto a new medium that has both ampicillin and tetracycline. On this medium, only cells with nonrecombinant plasmids will survive. Thus, colonies that grew on the first medium, but not on the second, contain recombinant plasmids. Cells from these colonies are collected and grown, each in a separate tube, and these constitute a genomic library.

Once a genomic library has been produced, the DNA fragments contained in it can be screened and analyzed in various ways. Using the right techniques, specific genes can be found, which can then be used in future analyses and experiments.

ALTERNATIVES TO SHOTGUN CLONING

In shotgun cloning, many different DNA fragments from an organism are cloned, and then the specific DNA clone of interest is identified. The number of clones can be reduced, making the search easier, if the DNA of interest is known to be in a restriction endonuclease fragment of a specific size. DNA can be size-selected before cloning using gel electrophoresis, in which an electric current carries DNA fragments through the pores or openings of an agarose gel. DNA migrates through the gel based on DNA fragment size, with the smaller fragments traveling more rapidly than the larger fragments. DNA of a specific size range can be isolated from the gel and then used for cloning. Finally, to clone a piece of DNA known to code for a protein, scientists can use an enzyme called reverse transcriptase to make DNA copies (called a complementary DNA or cDNA) of isolated messenger RNA (mRNA). The cDNA is then cloned, in a similar manner to that already discussed, to produce what is called a cDNA library. One of the advantages of this approach is that the number of clones is greatly reduced.

Susan J. Karcher, Ph.D.; updated by Bryan Ness, Ph.D.

FURTHER READING

Glick, Bernard R. *Molecular Biotechnology: Principles and Applications of Recombinant DNA*. 4th ed. Washington: ASM, 2010. Print.

Environmental Shotgun Sequencing (ESS). (A) Sampling from habitat; (B) filtering particles, typically by size; (C) DNA extraction and lysis; (D) cloning and library; (E) sequence the clones; (F) sequence assembly. By John C. Wooley, Adam Godzik, Iddo Friedberg, via Wikimedia Commons

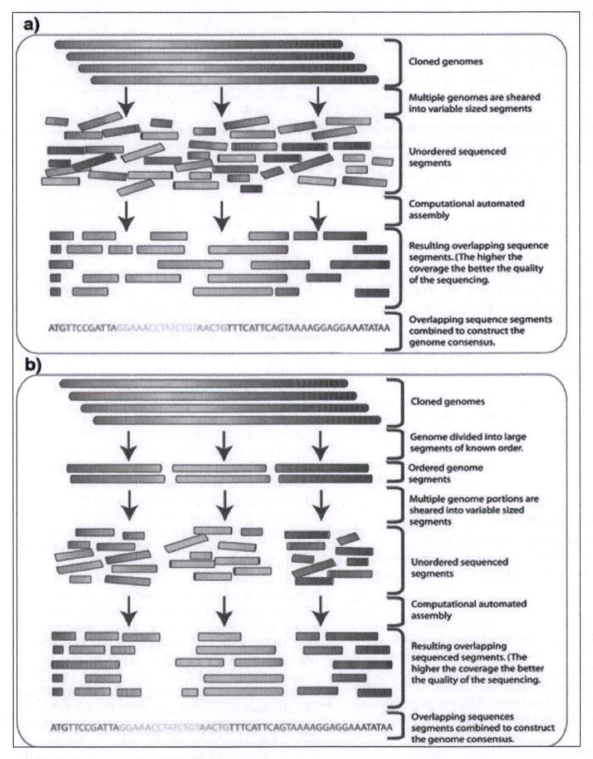

In whole genome shotgun sequencing (top), the entire genome is sheared randomly into small fragments (appropriately sized for sequencing) and then reassembled. In hierarchical shotgun sequencing (bottom), the genome is first broken into larger segments. After the order of these segments is deduced, they are further sheared into fragments appropriately sized for sequencing. By Commins, J., Toft, C., Fares, M. A., via Wikimedia Commons

Godiska, Ronald, et al. "Beyond pUC: Vectors for Cloning Unstable DNA." *DNA Sequencing: Optimizing the Process and Analysis.* Ed. Jan Kieleczawa. Sudbury: Jones, 2005. Print.

Graham, Colin A., and Alison J. M. Hill, eds. *DNA Sequencing Protocols.* 2nd ed. Totowa: Humana, 2001. Print.

Kreuzer, Helen, and Adrianne Massey. *Recombinant DNA and Biotechnology: A Guide for Students.* 3rd ed. Washington: ASM, 2008. Print.

Kreuzer, Helen, and Adrianne Massey. *Recombinant DNA and Biotechnology: A Guide for Teachers.* 3rd ed. Washington: ASM, 2008. Print.

Micklos, David, Greg A. Freyer, and David A. Crotty. *DNA Science: A First Course.* 2nd ed. Cold Spring Harbor: Cold Spring Harbor Laboratory Press, 2003. Print.

Sambrook, Joseph, and David W. Russell. "DNA Sequencing." *Molecular Cloning: A Laboratory Manual.* 4th ed. Cold Spring Harbor: Cold Spring Harbor Laboratory Press, 2012. Print.

Watson, James D., et al. *The Molecular Biology of the Gene.* 7th ed. San Francisco: Pearson, 2014. Print.

See also: cDNA libraries; Cloning; Cloning vectors; Genomic libraries; Genomics; Human Genome Project; Restriction enzymes.

Sickle-cell disease

CATEGORY: Diseases and syndromes
ALSO KNOWN AS: Sickle-cell anemia; hemoglobin S/S disease; sickle-hemoglobin C disease; sickle-beta thalassemia; SCD

DEFINITION

Sickle-cell disease (SCD), also known as sickle-cell anemia, is a hereditary blood disorder that affects red blood cells. Red blood cells undergo hemolysis (breakage) and change shape, which causes vascular occlusive crises (small blood vessel blockages). This results in acute and chronic pain, as well as multi-organ dysfunction.

RISK FACTORS

Individuals of African, Mediterranean, Middle Eastern, Indian, Central American, and Caribbean ancestry have the greatest chance of having a mutation in the beta globin gene (*HBB*). Approximately 1 in 12 individuals of African American ancestry have sickle-cell trait, which means approximately 1 in 600 babies born in the United States to African American parents have sickle-cell disease.

ETIOLOGY AND GENETICS

Sickle-cell disease was the very first example of a genetic disease being traced to its precise origin at the molecular level. The *HBB* gene, located on chromosome 11, encodes the main type of adult hemoglobin (hemoglobin A). Hemoglobin is the major protein in red blood cells whose properties allow it to bind with oxygen in the lungs and transport it to other parts of the body.

Sickle-cell anemia occurs when there is a single point mutation with one nucleotide (thymine instead of adenine) of the *HBB* gene. This causes a substitution of amino acids: Glutamic acid in the sixth codon is replaced by valine. The change of amino acids causes an absence in normal hemoglobin A production. Consequently, a structurally abnormal hemoglobin S is produced. For individuals with sickle-cell anemia, the mutation causes the hemoglobin molecules to stick to one another and changes the normally smooth and flexible, donut shaped appearance of the red blood cell to a characteristic sickled crescent moon shape. This prevents red blood cells from traveling through tiny capillaries, especially under conditions of oxygen deprivation. On average, the life span of red blood cells of healthy individuals is 120 days before they are replaced by new cells. In individuals with sickle-cell disease, the red blood cells have a reduced life span of only 16 days.

Sickle-cell disease is inherited in an autosomal recessive manner. One mutation in the *HBB* gene means that a person is a carrier for sickle-cell disease, which is also known as having sickle-cell trait (hemoglobin A/S). If both parents have sickle-cell trait, then there is a 25 percent risk for each child to have sickle-cell disease because both parents may pass the trait on to a pregnancy (hemoglobin S/S). There is a 50 percent risk for each child to have sickle-cell trait because only one parent may pass on sickle-cell trait and the other parent may pass on the unaffected allele. Lastly, there is a 25 percent chance that the child will be unaffected and not have the

Sickle Cell Disease

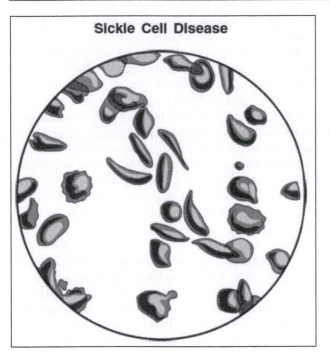

The red blood cells are sickle-shaped rather than round, which causes blockage of capillaries. (Hans & Cassidy, Inc.) (Hans & Cassidy, Inc.)

Sickle-cell disease is a genetic blood disorder with over dominance, characterized by red blood cells that assume an abnormal, rigid, sickle shape By Dr Graham Beards (Own work), via Wikimedia Commons

Figure A shows normal red blood cells flowing freely in a blood vessel. The inset image shows a cross-section of a normal red blood cell with normal hemoglobin. Figure B shows abnormal, sickled red blood cells blocking blood flow in a blood vessel. The in Sickle-cell disease: This image shows normal red blood cells flowing freely in a blood vessel. The inset image shows a cross-section of a normal red blood cell with normal hemoglobin. Figure B shows abnormal, sickled red blood cells blocking blood flow in a blood vessel. The inset image shows a cross-section of a sickle cell with abnormal (sickle) hemoglobin forming abnormal strands. By The National Heart, Lung, and Blood Institute (NHLBI), via Wikimedia Commons

trait because neither parent passes on sickle-cell trait (hemoglobin A/A). If only one parent has sickle-cell trait and the other parent is found to not be a carrier, then there is no chance to have an affected child but there does remain a 50 per cent risk that the child may have sickle-cell trait.

Sickle-cell disease may occur in classical form, as described above for sickle-cell anemia, or may occur as other forms of the blood disorder. Hemoglobin S/S occurs in 60 to 70 percent of affected individuals. There are many mutations that have been reported in the beta globin gene which can interact with sickle-cell trait and cause abnormal hemoglobin to be produced, such as mutations for hemoglobin C trait or beta thalassemia trait. If an individual inherits sickle-cell trait from one parent and hemoglobin C trait from another, for example, then the sickle-Cell Anemia the disease, and people who have sickle cell disease have an increased risk for early death because of anemia and other complications. However, when the red blood cells of individuals with sickle-cell trait are invaded by the malarial parasite, the red blood cells adhere to blood vessel walls, become deoxygenated, and assume a sickle shape, prompting both their de struction and that of their parasitic in vader for malaria. This provides a sickle cell carrier with a natural resistance to malaria and explains the relatively high frequency of the sickle-cell gene in such environments. This is an important phenomenon from an evolutionary stand point because it provides a mechanism by which genetic diversity in a population may be preserved.

SIGNS AND SYMPTOMS

Individuals with sickle-cell trait typically display no symptoms, although some have been known to become ill under extreme circumstances, such as high altitudes with decreased oxygen supply. Symptoms of sickle-cell disease typically appear about six to twelve months after birth, when the last of fetal hemoglobin pregnancy is at 25 percent risk for sickle-hemoglobin C disease, which is often less severe than classical sickle-cell anemia but may show similar symptoms. HbVar, a database of hemoglobin variants, lists more than a thousand entries for globin gene mutations. These mutations may lead to hundreds of clinically significant blood disorders.

Sickle-cell disease is one of the best-documented examples of an evolutionary process known as "heterozygote advantage," in which carriers have a greater probability of surviving or reproducing than either an affected or unaffected, noncarrier individual. In most cases, hereditary diseases with such significant symptoms as those associated with sickle cell disease are kept at low frequencies in populations by natural selection. However, having sickle cell trait provides an advantage in environments such as Africa were malaria is prevalent. Malaria is a deadly, mosquito-borne disease which uses human red blood cells as hosts for part of its life cycle. Individuals who have hemoglobin A/A are vulnerable to (hemoglobin F), a type of hemoglobin that increases the oxygen supply of blood in pregnancy, decreases and

hemoglobin S increases. The severity of the illness varies widely among individuals.

Individuals have varying degrees of red cell breakdown, which may cause a decrease in the amount of red blood cells (hemolytic anemia), jaundice, and physical weakness. The change in the red blood cell shape leads to a critical blockages of blood vessels (sickle-cell crisis), which causes a lack of oxygen to be delivered to the body's tissues. These painful crises are the most distinguishing clinical feature of the disease. Subsequently, this causes organ dysfunction and often causes severe pain in joints and bones. The organs that are most often involved include the spleen, lungs, brain, kidneys, and genitalia. Individuals typically have an enlarged spleen, and the compromised function predisposes mostly children but also adults to infections. The lungs may have significant life-threatening complications (acute chest syndrome), as well as a constriction of blood supply to the lungs (pulmonary hypertension). Other significant complications include the possibility of a stroke or blindness. Individuals may have priapism, a sustained and painful erection, as well as delayed growth and puberty. Despite the many treatments that exist, there remains an increased risk for medical problems and mortality particularly from overwhelming infection. With continued advancements in monitoring and treatment, some patients are now surviving into their fifties.

Specific signs, symptoms and complications may include one or more of the following:

- Bone pain: The long bones of the extremities are often involved, often due to bone marrow infarction
- Anemia: Universally present, chronic, and hemolytic in nature
- Transient aplastic crisis: Serious complication due to infection with Parvovirus B19V. The numbers of all blood cells become dangerously low.
- Infection: Organisms that pose the greatest danger include encapsulated respiratory bacteria, particularly *Streptococcus pneumonia*; adult infections are predominately with gram-negative organisms, especially *Salmonella*
- Growth retardation, delayed sexual maturation, being underweight

- Hand-foot syndrome: This is a dactylitis presenting as bilateral painful and swollen hands and/or feet in children
- Acute chest syndrome: Young children present with chest pain, fever, cough, tachypnea, leukocytosis, and pulmonary infiltrates in the upper lobes; adults are usually afebrile, dyspneic with severe chest pain, with multilobar/lower lobe disease
- Avascular necrosis of the femoral or humeral head: This is due to vascular occlusion
- CNS involvement: Most severe manifestation is stroke
- Ophthalmologic involvement: Ptosis, retinal vascular changes, proliferative retinitis
- Cardiac involvement: Dilation of both ventricles and the left atrium
- GI involvement: Presence of gallstones is common in children, and the liver may become involved
- GU involvement: Kidneys lose concentrating capacity
- Dermatologic involvement: Leg ulcers are a chronic painful problem

Triggers of vaso-occlusive crisis include the following:

- Hypoxemia: May be due to acute chest syndrome or respiratory complications
- Dehydration: Acidosis results in a shift of the oxygen dissociation curve
- Changes in body temperature (eg, an increase due to fever or a decrease due to environmental temperature change)

SCREENING AND DIAGNOSIS

The diagnosis of sickle-cell disease may be made by several different laboratory techniques. High performance liquid chromatography (HPLC), isoelectric focusing (IEF), hemoglobin electrophoresis, and peripheral blood smear are all available testing options. Almost all cases of sickle-cell disease are diagnosed at birth. All fifty states currently provide newborn screening for sickle-cell disease by one of these methods. Molecular genetic testing is available to detect mutations in the HBB gene associated with sickle-cell disease. Mutation analysis is typically reserved for when sickle-cell trait is suspected to be inherited with another hemoglobin variant or for purposes of diagnosing a fetus in pregnancy.

Any individual planning a pregnancy or who is currently pregnant and is from the aforementioned ethnic backgrounds may be offered screening for sickle-cell disease. If a pregnancy is found to be at 25 percent risk for sickle-cell disease, then prenatal diagnosis is available. Prenatal diagnosis includes testing options of a chorionic villus sampling (CVS) at eight to twelve weeks of gestation or amniocentesis at approximately fifteen to twenty weeks of gestation. In CVS, a sample from the placenta is obtained, and in amniocentesis a sample of fetal cells from amniotic fluid is withdrawn. Both diagnostic testing options provide a more than 99 percent detection rate of sickle-cell disease.

For those with diagnosed sickle cell disease, ongoing monitoring and screening may be recommended as regards certain complications the disease. For example, transcranial near-infrared spectroscopy or cerebral oximetry is increasingly being used as a screening tool for low cerebral venous oxygen saturation in children with sickle cell disease. In addition, measurement of blood flow velocity by transcranial Doppler ultrasound (TCD) has proved a good predictor of stroke risk and is considered the gold standard for stroke risk prediction in children.

Genetic counseling is available for individuals at risk for having a pregnancy with sickle-cell disease or for individuals who are diagnosed by new born screening with sickle-cell disease. Genetic counselors may review testing options and participate in the multidisciplinary management and education of children or adults with the diagnosis.

TREATMENT AND THERAPY

The goals of treatment in SCD are symptom control and management of disease complications. Treatment strategies include the following goals:

- Management of vaso-occlusive crisis
- Management of chronic pain syndromes
- Management of chronic hemolytic anemia
- Prevention and treatment of infections
- Management of the complications and the various organ damage syndromes associated with the disease
- Prevention of stroke

- Detection and treatment of pulmonary hypertension

SCD may be treated with the following medications:

- Antimetabolites: Hydroxyurea
- Opioid analgesics
- Nonsteroidal analgesics
- Antibiotics specific to the type of infection present.
- Vaccines (eg, PCV7, PPV23, meningococcal, influenza, recommended scheduled childhood/adult vaccinations)
- Vitamins (eg, folic acid)
- L-glutamine oral powder. Approved by the FDA in 2017 for patients age 5 and older who experience two or more painful crises per year. This was the first new approved therapy for SCD in 20 years. L-glutamine was shown to reduce the number of severe complications (particularly acute chest syndrome) and reduce the number of sickle crises and hospitalizations.

Other approaches to managing SCD include the following:

- Stem cell transplantation: possibly curative
- Transfusions: For sudden, severe anemia due to acute splenic sequestration, parvovirus B19 infection, or hyperhemolytic crises
- Physical therapy
- Heat and cold application
- Acupuncture and acupressure
- TENS
- Combining medications with non-pharmacological treatments, including, but not limited to:
  - Vigorous hydration (plus analgesics): For vaso-occlusive crisis
  - Oxygen, antibiotics, analgesics, incentive spirometry, simple transfusion, and bronchodilators: For treatment of acute chest syndrome

PREVENTION AND OUTCOMES

Despite advancing treatments, there still exists no cure for sickle-cell disease. Stem cell transplantation, whereby an individual receives stem cells from an unaffected individual, has the potential to cure symptoms of sickle-cell disease. Unfortunately, this treatment is only applicable to a small percentage of children with severe disease who fit very specific selection criteria. These criteria include that an individual donating stem cells must be related to the affected individual and be an immunological match. There are significant risks with this procedure that put the individual at risk for developing complications, such as rejection, infection, bleeding, and possible death. Be that as it may, for those who are candidates and receive this treatment, the outcomes are very good with an event-free survival rate of approximately 84% and a mortality rate of less than 6%.

Much early research on sickle-cell disease was performed by Linus Pauling (right), with George Beadle, c. 1952. (California Institute of Technology)

Janet Ober Berman, M.S., C.G.C.; updated by Gary M. Flashner, M.S., M.D.

FURTHER READING

ACOG Committee on Obstetrics "Hemoglobinopathies in Pregnancy." *Obstetrics and Gynecology* 109 (2007): 229–237. Practice recommendations for carrier screening for sickle-cell disease and other blood disorders in or prior to pregnancy. Illustrations for testing algorithm.

MacMillin, M., ed. *Ancestry Based Carrier Screening.* Chicago: National Society of Genetic Counselors, 2005. A guide for which populations should be offered screening for sickle-cell disease and other genetic disorders. Tables for carrier frequency.

Pack-Mabien, A. "A Primary Care Provider's Guide to Preventative and Acute Care Management of Adults and Children with Sickle-Cell Disease." *Journal of the American Academy of Nurse Practitioners* 21 (2009): 250-257. In-depth coverage for symptoms and management of sickle-cell disease as well as new treatment options.

Serjeant, Graham R., and Beryl E. Serjeant. *Sickle Cell Disease.* 3d ed. New York: Oxford University Press, 2001. Discusses the biology of sickle-cell disease and the disease's management. Illustrations, maps, bibliography, index.

Steinberg, Martin H., et al., eds. *Disorders of Hemoglobin: Genetics, Pathophysiology, and Clinical Management.* Foreword by H. Franklin Bunn. New York: Cambridge University Press, 2001. Covers the dis eases' molecular and genetic bases, epidemiology and genetic selection, and diagnoses and treatments. Illustrations (some color), bibliography, index.

Strouse J. Sickle cell disease. *Handb Clin Neurol.* 2016. 138:311–24

Parent F, Bachir D, Inamo J, et al. "A hemodynamic study of pulmonary hypertension in sickle cell disease". *N Engl J Med.* 2011 Jul 7. 365(1):44–53.

Yawn BP, Buchanan GR, Afenyi-Annan AN, Ballas SK, Hassell KL, James AH, et al. "Management of sickle cell disease: summary of the 2014 evidence-based report by expert panel members". *JAMA.* 2014 Sep 10. 312(10):1033–48

McGann PT, Ware RE. "Hydroxyurea therapy for sickle cell anemia". *Expert Opin Drug Saf.* 2015 Sep 14. 1–10.

Wang WC, Ware RE, Miller ST, et al. "Hydroxycarbamide in very young children with sickle-cell anaemia: a multicentre, randomised, controlled trial (BABY HUG)". *Lancet.* 2011 May 14. 377(9778):1663–72.

Gladwin MT, Kato GJ, Weiner D, et al. "Nitric oxide for inhalation in the acute treatment of sickle cell pain crisis: a randomized controlled trial". *JAMA.* 2011 Mar 2. 305(9):893–902.

WEB SITES OF INTEREST

American Sickle Cell Anemia Association
www.ascaa.org
Dolan DNA Learning Center, Your Genes Your Health
http://www.ygyh.org
Gene Reviews
http://www.ncbi.nlm.nih.gov/bookshelf/br.fcgi?book=gene&part=sickle
HbVar
http://globin.cse.psu.edu/hbvar/menu.html
Sickle Cell Disease Association of America
www.sicklecelldisease.org
Sickle Cell Information Center
http://www.scinfo.org
https://rarediseases.info.nih.gov/diseases/8614/sickle-cell-anemia
http://emedicine.medscape.com/article/205926-overview
https://www.ncbi.nlm.nih.gov/books/NBK22238/
https://www.cdc.gov/ncbddd/sicklecell/data.html
https://www.nhlbi.nih.gov/health-pro/guidelines/sickle-cell-disease-guidelines/

See also: ABO blood types; Amniocentesis; Biopharmaceuticals; Chorionic villus sampling; Chronic myeloid leukemia; Fanconi anemia; Genetic engineering; Genetic screening; Genetic testing; Hardy Weinberg law; Hemophilia; Hereditary spherocytosis; Incomplete dominance; Infantile agranulocytosis; Mutation and mutagenesis; Myelodysplastic syndromes; Paroxysmal nocturnal hemoglobinuria; Porphyria; RFLP analysis; Rh incompatibility and isoimmunization; Shotgun cloning; Von Willebrand disease.

Signal transduction

CATEGORY: Molecular genetics
SIGNIFICANCE: Signal transduction consists of all of the molecular events that occur between the arrival of a signaling molecule at a target cell and its response. A significant proportion of the genome in animals consists of genes involved in cell signaling. The protein products of these genes allow cells to communicate with each other in order to coordinate their metabolism, movements, and reproduction. Failure of cells to communicate properly can lead to cancer, defects in embryological development, and many other disorders.

KEY TERMS

cell cycle: the orderly sequence of events by which a cell grows, duplicates its chromosomal DNA, and partitions the DNA into two new cells
cell signaling: communication between cells that occurs most commonly when one cell releases a specific signaling molecule that is received by another cell
receptors: molecules in target cells that bind specifically to a particular signaling molecule
target cell: the cell that receives and responds to a signaling molecule

SIGNAL TRANSDUCTION PATHWAYS
Signal transduction can occur by a number of different, often complex sequences of molecular events called signal transduction pathways, which result in several kinds of target cell response: activating genes or metabolic pathways, affecting the cell cycle, et cetera. Among the signaling molecules found in higher organisms are hormones, local mediators that produce local physiological effects, growth factors that act locally to promote growth, and survival factors that act locally to repress cell suicide (apoptosis). Growth factors

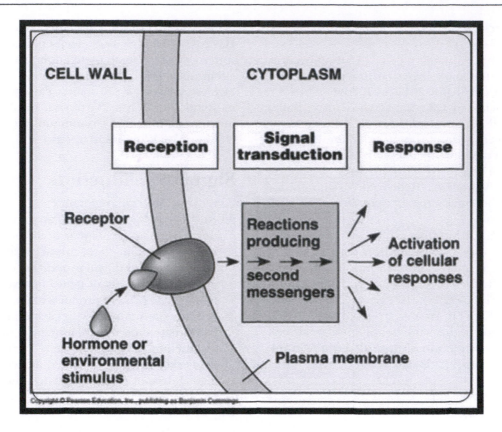

Signal transduction pathways. By Yaneeporn (Own work), via Wikimedia Commons

and survival factors are particularly important during embryological development, when they orchestrate the changes in cell types, positions, and numbers that give rise to the new organism.

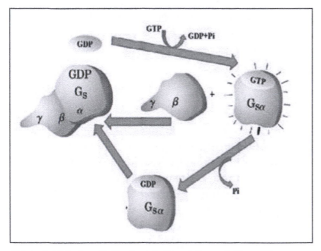

It is a sketch to describe the dessociation and association of α subunit of G protein. By Haoliulh (Own work), via Wikimedia Commons

TYPES OF RECEPTORS

Most signal transduction pathways begin with the binding of signaling molecules to specific receptors in target cells. Signaling molecules are often referred to as receptor ligands. The binding of the ligand to its receptor initiates a signal transduction pathway. A cell can respond to a particular signaling molecule only if it possesses a receptor for it.

Receptors are protein molecules. There are two categories of them, based on location in the cell: receptors that are intracellular and receptors that are anchored in the cell's surface membrane. The membrane-anchored receptors can be further divided based on the steps of the signal transduction pathway that they initiate: receptors that bind to and activate GTP-binding proteins (G proteins), receptors that are enzymes, and receptors that are ion channels. Ion-channel receptors bind neurotransmitters or hormones and increase or decrease the flow of specific ions into the cell, leading to a physiological response by the cell. These receptors generally do not have a direct effect on gene expression, although changes in a cell's calcium-ion concentrations can influence gene expression. Each of the other receptor types stands at the head of a signal transduction pathway that is characteristic for each receptor type and can lead to gene expression.

INTRACELLULAR RECEPTORS

Intracellular receptors include the receptors for lipid-soluble hormones such as steroid hormones. Some of these receptors are in the cell's cytoplasm, and some are in the nucleus. Hormone molecules enter the cell by first diffusing across the membrane and then binding to the receptor. Before the hormones enter the cell, the receptors are attached to "chaperone" proteins, which hold the receptor in a configuration that allows hormone binding but prevents it from binding to DNA. Hormone molecules displace these chaperone molecules, enabling the receptor to bind to DNA. If the receptor is a cytoplasmic receptor, the hormone-receptor complex is first transported into the nucleus, where it binds to a specific DNA nucleotide sequence called a hormone response element (HRE) that is part of the promoter of certain genes. In most cases the receptors bind as dimers; that is, two hormone-receptor complexes bind to the same HRE. The hormone-receptor complex functions as a transcription factor, promoting transcription of the gene and production of a protein that the cell was not previously producing. The hormone hydrocortisone, for example, triggers the synthesis of the enzymes aminotransferase and tryptophan oxygenase. A single hormone such as hydrocortisone can turn on synthesis of two or more proteins if each of the genes for the proteins contains an HRE. In some cases, when hormone-receptor complexes bind to an HRE, they suppress transcription rather than promote it.

G PROTEIN-COUPLED RECEPTORS

Many hormones, growth factors, and other signaling molecules bind to membrane receptors that can associate with and activate heterotrimeric G proteins when a signaling molecule is bound to the receptor. Heterotrimeric G proteins are a family of proteins that are present on the cytoplasmic surface of the cell membrane. Many cell types in the body contain one or more of these family members, and different cell types contain different ones. All heterotrimeric G proteins are made up of three subunits, designated alpha, beta, and

gamma. The alpha subunit has a binding site for GTP (guanosine triphosphate) or GDP (guanosine diphosphate)—hence the name "G proteins"—and is the principal part of the protein that differs from one heterotrimeric G protein family member to another. When the receptor is empty (no signal molecule attached), these G proteins have GDP bound to the alpha subunit, and the G protein is not bound to the receptor.

However, when a signaling molecule binds to the receptor, the cytoplasmic domain of the receptors changes shape so that it now binds to the G protein. In binding to the receptor, the G protein also changes shape, causing the GDP to leave and the GTP to bind instead. Simultaneously, the alpha subunit detaches from the beta-gamma subunit, and both the alpha subunit and the beta-gamma subunit detach from the receptor. Depending on the particular G protein family member involved and the cell type, either the alpha subunit or the beta-gamma subunit then activates (or, with some G protein family members, inhibits) one of several enzymes, most commonly adenylate cyclase or phospholipase C. Alternatively, they can open or close a membrane ion channel, altering the electrical properties of the cell; for example, potassium ion channels in heart muscle cells can be opened by G proteins in response to the neurotransmitter.

ACETYLCHOLINE

In cases where adenylate cyclase or phospholipase C is activated, these enzymes catalyze reactions that produce molecules called second messengers, which, through a series of steps, activate proteins that may lead to a physiological response (such as contraction of smooth muscle), a biochemical response (such as glycogen synthesis), or a genetic response (such as activating a gene).

Activation of adenylate cyclase causes it to catalyze the conversion of adenosine triphosphate (ATP) to the second messenger cyclic adenosine monophosphate (cAMP), which in turn activates a protein called protein kinase A, which, in some cells, moves into the nucleus and phosphorylates and activates transcription factors such as CREB (CRE-binding protein). CREB binds to a specific DNA sequence in the promoter of certain genes called the CRE (cAMP-response element), as well as to other transcription factors, to activate transcription of the gene.

In other cells, protein kinase A activates enzymes or other proteins involved in physiological or metabolic responses.

Activation of phospholipase C catalyzes the breakdown of a glycolipid component of the cell membrane called phosphatidylinositol bisphosphate (PIP2) into two second messengers, inositol triphosphate (IP3) and diacylglycerol (DAG). DAG activates a protein called protein kinase C (PK-C), which in turn activates other proteins, leading to various cell responses, including, in certain cells of the immune system, activation of transcription factors that turn on genes involved in the body's immune response to infection. IP3 causes the release of calcium ions stored in the endoplasmic reticulum. These ions bind and activate the protein calmodulin, which activates a variety of proteins, leading in most cases to a physiological response in the cell.

CATALYTIC RECEPTORS

Catalytic receptors are receptors that function as enzymes, catalyzing specific reactions in the cell. The part of the receptor that is in the cytoplasm (the cytoplasmic domain) has catalytic capability. Binding of a signaling molecule to the external domain of the receptor activates the catalytic activity of the cytoplasmic domain. There are several kinds of catalytic receptors based on the type of reaction they catalyze; these include receptor tyrosine phosphatases, receptor guanylate cyclases, receptor serine/threonine kinases, and receptor tyrosine kinases. Receptor tyrosine kinases (RTKs) are the most common of these.

RTKs are the receptors for many growth factors and at least one hormone. For example, they are the receptors for fibroblast growth factor (FGF), epidermal growth factor (EGF), platelet-derived growth factor (PDGF), nerve growth factor (NGF), and insulin. RTKs play a role in regulating many fundamental processes, such as cell metabolism, the cell cycle, cell proliferation, cell migration, and embryonic development. In most cases, when a ligand binds to this type of receptor, a conformational (shape) change occurs in the receptor so that it binds to another identical receptor-ligand complex to produce a double, or dimeric, receptor. The dimeric receptor then catalyzes a cytoplasmic reaction in which several tyrosine amino acids in the cytoplasmic domain of the receptor itself are phosphorylated. The phosphorylated tyrosines then function as docking sites for several other proteins,

each of which can initiate one of the many branches of the RTK signal transduction pathway, leading to the various cell responses. One of the major branches of the RTK pathway that in many cases results in gene expression begins with the binding of the G protein Ras (which is not one of the trimeric G proteins discussed above) to the activated RTK receptor via adapter proteins. Binding Ras to the adapter proteins activates it by allowing it to bind GTP instead of GDP. Activated Ras then activates a mitogen-activated protein kinase kinase kinase (MAP3K, or MEKK) known as c-Raf, which phosphorylates the enzyme mitogen-activated protein kinase kinase (MAP2K, or MEK), which phosphorylates and activates a mitogen-activated protein kinase (MAPK), an enzyme of the MAP kinase family. This process is known as the MAP kinase cascade. In cases where the final MAPK enzyme is MAP kinase itself, the enzyme dimerizes, moves into the nucleus, and activates genes, usually many genes, by phosphorylating and activating their transcription factors.

SIGNAL TRANSDUCTION AND THE CELL CYCLE

The biochemical machinery that produces the cell cycle consists of several cyclins whose concentrations rise and fall throughout the cycle. Cyclins activate cyclin-dependent kinases (CDKs), which activate the proteins that carry out the events of each stage of the cell cycle. In higher organisms, control of the cell cycle is carried out primarily by growth factors. In the absence of growth factors, many cells will stop the cycle at a point known as the G_1 checkpoint and cease dividing. The cell cycle is started when the cells are exposed to a growth factor. For example, some growth factors start cell division by binding to a membrane receptor and initiating the Ras/MAP kinase signal transduction pathway. The activated transcription factor that results from this pathway activates a gene called *MYC*. The protein that is produced from this gene is itself a transcription factor that activates the cyclin D genes (*CCND1*, *CCND2*, and *CCND3*), which produce cyclin D, an important component of the cell cycle biochemical machinery. Cyclin D activates the enzyme cyclin-dependent kinase 4 (CDK4), which drives the cell into the G_1 phase of the cell cycle. CDK4 also causes an inhibiting molecule called retinoblastoma protein (pRB) to be removed from a transcription factor for the cyclin E gene. Cyclin E is then produced and activates cyclin-dependent kinase 2 (CDK2), which drives the cell into the S phase of the cell cycle, during which chromosomal DNA is replicated, leading to cell division by mitosis.

SIGNAL TRANSDUCTION AND CANCER

Cancer is caused primarily by uncontrolled cell proliferation. Since many signal transduction pathways lead to cell proliferation, it is not surprising that defects in these pathways can lead to cancer. For example, as described above, many growth factors promote cell proliferation by activating the Ras/MAP kinase signal transduction pathway. In that pathway, a series of proteins is activated (Ras, MAP kinase, and so on). If a mutation occurred in the gene for one of these, *ras* for example, such that the mutant Ras protein is always activated rather than being activated only when it binds to the receptor, then the cell would always be dividing and cancerous growth could result. Another example would be if *RB1*, the gene that produces pRB, were mutated such that the pRB could never bind to and inhibit the cyclin E transcription factor; then the cell would divide continuously. Mutations in both the *ras* and *RB1* genes are in fact known to cause cancer in humans.

Robert Chandler, Ph.D.

FURTHER READING

Alberts, Bruce, et al. *Molecular Biology of the Cell*. 5th ed. New York: Garland, 2008. Print.

Cantley, Lewis C., et al., eds. *Signal Transduction: Principles, Pathways, and Processes*. Cold Spring Harbor: Cold Spring Harbor, 2014. Print.

Cell Signaling, Disease and Stem Cells. Spec. issue of *Cell Research* 22.1 (2012): 1–275. Print.

Gomperts, Bastien D., Ijsbrand M. Kramer, and Peter E. R. Tatham. *Signal Transduction*. 2nd ed. Burlington: Academic, 2009. Print.

Hoch, James A., and Thomas J. Silhavy, eds. *Two-Component Signal Transduction*. Washington: ASM, 1995. Print.

Krauss, Gerhard. *Biochemistry of Signal Transduction and Regulation*. 5th rev. ed. Weinheim: Wiley, 2014. Print.

Lodish, Harvey, et al. *Molecular Cell Biology*. 7th ed. New York: Freeman, 2013. Print.

Marks, Friedrich, Ursula Klingmüller, and Karin Müller-Decker. *Cellular Signal Processing: An Introduction to the Molecular Mechanisms of Signal Transduction*. New York: Garland, 2009. Print.

Nelson, John. *Structure and Function in Cell Signalling*. Hoboken: Wiley, 2008. Print.

Special Signaling Issue. Spec. issue of *Cell* 103.2 (2000): 181–361. Print.

See also: Burkitt's lymphoma; Cancer; Cell cycle; Cell division; DNA replication; Gene regulation: Bacteria; Model organism: *Saccharomyces cerevisiae*; Oncogenes; One gene-one enzyme hypothesis; Steroid hormones; Tumor-suppressor genes.

Small-cell lung cancer

CATEGORY: Diseases and syndromes
ALSO KNOWN AS: Oat cell carcinoma; small-cell anaplastic carcinoma; undifferentiated small-cell carcinoma; intermediate cell type; and mixed small cell/large-cell carcinoma.

DEFINITION

Small-cell lung cancer (SCLC) is one of the two major types of lung cancer, the other being non small-cell lung cancer (NSCLC). SCLC originates from nerve cells or hormone-producing cells in the lungs, whereas NSCLC originates from epithelial cells that make up the lining of the lungs.

RISK FACTORS

Smoking is the greatest risk factor for SCLC, with an estimated 87 percent of lung cancers caused by smoking. Other risk factors are exposure to radon, asbestos, beryllium, cadmium, silica, vinyl chloride, nickel or chromium-containing compounds, coal products, mustard gas, chloromethyl esters, diesel exhaust, radiation to the chest, arsenic, air pollution, radioactive substances like uranium, hormone replacement therapy, second-hand smoke, history of lung disease, and genetic factors. Most individuals diagnosed with SCLC are elderly between the ages of 60 and 80 and have a smoking history.

ETIOLOGY AND GENETICS

SCLC accounts for about 10–15 percent of lung cancer cases. Cancer in general is considered to be a genetic disease because cancer is associated with genetic changes in somatic cells that lead

Micrograph of small cell carinoma of the lung, also small cell lung cancer Micrograph of a squamous carcinoma, a type of non-small-cell lung carcinoma. FNA specimen. Pap stain. By Nephron (Own work), via Wikimedia Commons

Micrograph of squamous carcinoma, also squamous cell carcinoma. FNA specimen of a lung lesion. Pap stain. Clinicoradiological findings in the case suggested it was a lung primary, i.e. lung cancer. By Nephron (Own work), via Wikimedia Commons

to uncontrolled cell growth. Lung cancer is not caused by a single gene, but rather several genes with somatic mutation. The human genome is made up of pairs of chromosomes. When tissue from the lungs of smokers is genetically analyzed, several areas of the DNA that makes up chromosomes and contain the genes are found to be damaged, duplicated, or missing. However, not all smokers with genetic dam age in their lung tissue have lung cancer, suggesting that multiple sites of DNA damage must accumulate before lung cancer develops. Not every SCLC case has the same set of mutated genes present, but dam age to specific regions on chromosomes 1, 3, 4, 5, 8, 9, 10, 11, 13,

15, 16, 17, 18, and 20 occurs frequently in SCLCs. In SCLC the most commonly acquired mutated genes are TP53 and RB1. TP53 is a gene that usually causes damaged cells to undergo programmed cell death, known as apoptosis or activates other genes to fix damaged cells. When the TP53 gene is mutated, the damaged cells do not die or restore and can go on to become malignant cells. The RB1 gene makes pRB protein that stops other proteins from DNA replication and helps prevent the growth of tumors. The protein also regulates cell survival, function, and maturation. Loss of these two tumor suppressor genes is common in SCLC.

Other somatic mutations in TP73, CREBBP, EP300, MLL, PTEN, SLIT2, SOX family of genes, and EPHA7, as well as focal amplification of the FGFR1 are also implicated. Findings related to kinase gene mutations (EGFR) and NOTCH family genes provide possible therapeutic opportunities for individual patients.

While 85 percent of all lung cancers occur in former or current smokers, fewer than 20 percent of long-term smokers develop lung cancer, suggesting that genetic factors make some people more susceptible to lung cancer. In 2009, researchers identified two sites of genetic variation on chromosome 15 that people can inherit from a parent that are associated with an increased risk of lung cancer in smokers and former smokers. This happens in an autosomal dominant manner. Inherited mutations increase the risk of the disease, not the disease itself. These genetic variations, called single nucleotide polymorphisms (SNPs), are places in the human genome that vary by a single DNA nucleotide. People who have one or two copies of either of these SNPs and who have ever smoked have increased risks of 28 percent to 81 percent of developing lung cancer. The two SNPs identified are near five genes on chromosome 15. Interestingly, three of these five genes encode proteins that serve as docking sites for nicotine, the addictive agent in tobacco. These findings suggest that nicotine, in addition to several known carcinogens present in tobacco smoke, may be involved in lung cancer development. Another of the genes near the SNPs encodes a component of the proteasome, an important organelle in cells that degrades other proteins. The function of the fifth gene is unknown. Researchers continue to examine which inherited faulty DNA repair mechanisms and environmental exposures increase the risk for SCLC.

Symptoms

In early-stage SCLC, patients often do not have symptoms. Symptoms of lung cancer include a cough that does not go away; chest pain that often gets worse with deep breathing, coughing, or laughing; hoarseness; unexplained weight loss or lack of appetite; bloody or rust-colored spit or phlegm (also called sputum); shortness of breath; recurrent infections like bronchitis and pneumonia; and new onset of wheezing. Small-cell lung cancer commonly spreads or metastasizes to other organs. Symptoms of cancer that has spread include bone pain; weakness or numbness in the limbs; headache, dizziness, or seizure; jaundice; and lumps near the surface of the body such as lymph nodes in the neck. Those who experience these symptoms should see a physician right away.

Screening and Diagnosis

Chest X rays and checking sputum under a microscope to look for cancer cells was studied as a screening tool for lung cancer for several years. Un fortunately, this kind of screening is not very effective, with very few lung cancers found early enough to improve a person's chances for a cure. Because this kind of screening is not very effective, it is not done routinely, even in smokers who are at high risk.

The USPSTF recommends annual screening for lung cancer with low-dose computed tomography (LDCT) in adults aged 55 to 80 years who have a 30 pack-year smoking history and currently smoke or have quit within the past 15 years. Screening should be discontinued once a person has not smoked for 15 years or develops a health problem that substantially limits life expectancy or the ability or willingness to have curative lung surgery.

Physical exam, medical history, imaging tests and biopsy are often done to diagnose SCLC. Additional tests including phlegm cytology, bronchoscopy, needle aspiration and biopsy, thoracentesis, thoracoscopy, mediastinoscopy, and thoracotomy may be performed for further diagnosis and staging.

Treatment and Therapy

Small-cell lung cancer has usually spread or metastasized to other organs before it is diagnosed; therefore, it is usually not treated with surgery, but may be performed in early stage disease. Patients with advanced-stage disease are usually treated with platinum-based chemotherapy (cisplatin or carbo platin), which may be combined with the drugs etoposide or irinotecan. Patients whose tumors respond very well to chemotherapy may also be offered radiation therapy.

The following therapies may be recommended: laser therapy to burn away tumors, medications to treat pain and other symptoms, steroids to reduce inflammation, oxygen to assist with breathing, and nutritional supplements and appetite stimulants.

All patients are encouraged to quit smoking.

Prevention and Outcomes

The most important prevention for SCLC is to not smoke, or to quit smoking. After quitting smoking, it takes about ten years to reduce the risk of lung cancer in former smokers, but the risk never drops to the level of those who never smoked.

Nancy E. Price, Ph.D.; updated by Deanna M. Neff, M.P.H.

Further Reading

Broderick, Peter, et al. "Deciphering the Impact of Common Genetic Variation on Lung Cancer Risk: A Genome-Wide Association Study." *Cancer Research* 69 (2009): 6633–6641. Discusses the research that identified the two inherited SNPs on chromosome 15 that make some people more susceptible to lung cancer.

Cascone T, Gold KA, Glisson BS. *Small Cell Carcinoma of the Lung.* Kantarjian H, Wolff R, eds. The MD Anderson Manual of Medical Oncology. 3rd ed. New York, NY: McGraw-Hill Education. 2016; 323–42.

George, J., Lim, J. S., Jang, S. J., et al. "Comprehensive genomic profiles of small cell lung cancer". Nature. 2015; 524: 47–53.

Girard, L., et al. "Genome-Wide Allelotyping of Lung Cancer Identifies New Regions of Allelic Loss, Differences Between Small Cell Lung Cancer and Non-small Cell Lung Cancer, and Loci Clustering." *Cancer Research* 60 (2000): 4894–4906. Discusses differences in the locations of chromosomal damage in SCLC and NSCLC, and lists the most frequent sites of damage in both lung cancer types.

Hansen, Heine H., and Paul Bunn. *Lung Cancer Therapy Annual* 4. New York: Taylor and Francis, 2005. Discusses recent developments in the diagnosis and treatment of lung cancer.

Rudin CM, Ismaila N, Hann CL, Malhotra N, Movsas B, Norris K, et al. "Treatment of Small-Cell

Lung Cancer: American Society of Clinical Oncology Endorsement of the American College of Chest Physicians Guideline". *J Clin Oncol.* 2015;33 (34):4106–11.

Travis, William D., Elizabeth Brambilla, H. Konrad Müller-Hermelink, and Curtis C. Harris, eds. *World Health Organization Classification of Tumours: Pathology and Genetics Tumours of the Lung, Pleura, Thymus, and Heart.* Lyon, France: IARC Press, 2004. A reference on the histological and genetic typing of tumors of the lung.

WEB SITES OF INTEREST

American Cancer Society: Learn About Lung Cancer— Small Cell
http://www.cancer.org/docroot/lrn/lrn_0. aspLungevity
https://www.lungevity.org/about-lung-cancer/lung-cancer-101/treatment-options/treatment-options-for-non-small-cell-lung-cancer
Management of Small Cell Lung Cancer: ACCP Evidence-Based Clinical Practice Guidelines (2d ed.)
http://www.guideline.gov/summary/summary. aspx?doc_id=11420
National Cancer Institute: General Information About Small Cell Lung Cancer
http://www.cancer.gov/cancertopics/pdq/treatment/small-cell-lung/patient
OMIM® Online Mendelian Inheritance in Man
http://www.omim.org/about

See also: Bloom syndrome; BRAF gene; BRCA1 and BRCA2 genes; Breast cancer; Burkitt's lymphoma; Chemical mutagens; Chromosome mutation; Chronic myeloid leukemia; Colon cancer; Cowden syndrome; DPC4 gene testing; Familial adenomatous polyposis; Gene therapy; Harvey rasoncogene; Hereditary diffuse gastric cancer; Hereditary diseases; Hereditary leiomyomatosis and renal cell cancer; Hereditary mixed polyposis syndrome; Hereditary non-VHL clear cell renal cell carcinomas; Hereditary papillary renal cancer; Homeotic genes; HRAS gene testing; Hybridomas and monoclonal antibodies; Li Fraumeni syndrome; Lynch syndrome; Mutagenesis and cancer; Multiple endocrine neoplasias; Mutation and mutagenesis; Nondisjunction and aneuploidy; Oncogenes; Ovarian cancer; Pancreatic cancer; Prostate cancer; Tumor-suppressor genes; Wilms' tumor aniridia-genitourinary anomalies-mental retardation (WAGR) syndrome.

Smallpox and genetics

CATEGORY: Diseases and syndromes; Viral genetics

DEFINITION

Smallpox is a poxvirus, any of the family of viruses that produce pustules on the surface of the skin. It is a disease of humans existing in two forms. The more virulent and frequently lethal form is *Variola major*, and a milder form is *Variola minor*. Smallpox is very contagious, requiring strict quarantine measures and aggressive vaccination programs to contain and eradicate outbreaks.

Smallpox is a member of the *Poxviridae* family of viruses, which are the largest and most complex of all known viruses. Poxviruses are named for the characteristic rash or pox lesions that occur during most poxvirus infections. The poxviruses include a number of familiar diseases, such as smallpox, cowpox, rabbitpox, sheeppox, and fowlpox. Two subfamilies of poxviruses are recognized based on their hosts. The orthopoxvirus subfamily comprises viruses that affect vertebrates and includes smallpox; the poxviruses of the subfamily parapoxviruses infect invertebrates, primarily insects. There are two types of variola, the poxvirus that causes smallpox: *V. major* causes the more virulent and lethal form of smallpox in humans, and *V. minor* causes a milder form of smallpox. Both varieties infect only humans and monkeys. Other names or synonyms for smallpox include alastrim, amaas, Kaffir mil pox, West Indian modified smallpox, and para-smallpox. Humans have had a long and unfortunate history of association with smallpox. The disease apparently originated in India and spread westward into the Middle East and northern Africa several thousand years ago. An Egyptian mummy of the Twentieth Dynasty shows the characteristic scarring associated with smallpox. Warriors returning from the Crusades brought the disease back with them. In the following centuries, smallpox became endemic throughout much of Europe and became a rite of passage for much of the population—those who contracted smallpox and survived were marked by its scars throughout life. In time, the population built up a partial immunity to the disease. Smallpox was carried by Europeans to the New World and to Australia during the age of exploration. It was spread to the immunologically defenseless Amerindians of North America and Aboriginals of Australia with devastating effect and may have contributed to the ease of European settlement, as it caused widespread death and devastation among the indigenous populations and was at least partly responsible for the depopulation of natives in the newly discovered lands. Before its eradication, smallpox was endemic throughout the world, with major centers of the disease in Africa, Asia, and the Middle East.

Risk Factors

Smallpox is a highly contagious disease, and therefore anyone who comes in contact with it is susceptible to it. Patients who have weak immune systems—such as those with human immunodeficiency virus (HIV) or cancer and organ transplant recipients—are at risk for severe cases of smallpox and would have higher mortality rates. People born after 1971 who did not receive primary immunization would also be highly susceptible.

CA44-271-2 *Face of a man with smallpox. Copy negative. World War 2. El Kettar Civilian Hospital, Algiers.* By Otis Historical Archives of "National Museum of Health & Medicine" (OTIS Archive 1), *via Wikimedia Commons*

Etiology and Genetics

The poxviruses are the largest and most complex of all the viruses that have so far been identified in animals. The variola virus that causes smallpox has a brick-shaped outer envelope and a dumbbell-shaped core that contains the smallpox genome. The smallpox genome is composed of linear, double-stranded DNA containing more than two hundred genes. Chemically, the smallpox virion consists of 90 percent protein, 3 percent DNA, and

5 percent lipid. The DNA genome codes for several hundred polypeptides, including several transcriptases responsible for replication of the virus within the cells of the host.

Replication of smallpox begins when the virus attaches to the surface of a host cell. After binding to receptors on the plasma membrane of the host cell, the host cell passes the virus into the cytoplasm by endocytosis. Once inside the cell, the virus becomes trapped in a lysosome vesicle in the cytoplasm. The first step in removing its viral coat probably occurs at this stage, as host cell enzymes dissolve the viral envelope. The viral core, containing the DNA, then exits the lysosome and enters the cytoplasm, where the viral genome can be expressed. One of the first steps involves the production of enzymes that degrade the proteins of the viral core, which releases the naked viral DNA into the cytoplasm. Additional transcription takes place, initially producing structural proteins and enzymes, including DNA polymerase, which promotes the replication of the viral DNA. Finally, the late messenger RNA (mRNA) is transcribed, producing additional structural proteins and assembly enzymes that complete virion construction. During viral replication, most host-cell protein synthesis is blocked, because transport of host-cell mRNA molecules though the nuclear envelope into the cytoplasm is prevented.

Newly completed virions exit the host cell through microvilli on the cell surface or fuse with the cell membrane, after which they exit the cell by the process of exocytosis. Once in the tissue, fluids, and bloodstream, the newly released and highly infectious viral particles can invade and replicate in other host cells.

Smallpox is transmitted from one human to another, either by direct contact or via droplets released into the air during sneezing and coughing fits. The virus does not live long outside the human body and does not reproduce outside the human body. No natural animal carriers of variola other than monkeys, which are also susceptible, are known for the smallpox disease. In extremely rare cases, smallpox is transmitted by carriers that are themselves immune to the disease but can transmit the disease to others. Still, only a few droplets settling on another person are sufficient to transmit smallpox. Because of the virulence and mode of transmission, public health regulations specify decontamination procedures. Living quarters, bedding, clothes, and other articles of infected persons must be thoroughly cleansed by heat or with formaldehyde, or destroyed altogether.

SYMPTOMS

Historically one of the most devastating and lethal of all human diseases, smallpox is named for the small pustules that occur as a rash over the skin of the victim. Smallpox symptoms include a rash that spreads over the entire body, high fever, chills, aches and pains, and vomiting. The most lethal form, black or hemorrhagic smallpox, results in death within two to six days. The fatality rate varies with health and previous exposure of the local population but ranges from 30 to 90 percent.

Infection occurs when the variola virus enters the respiratory mucosa of the nasal or pharyngeal region of the upper respiratory tract of humans. Apparently, only a few viral particles are needed to produce an infection. After a few hours or a few days, the virus migrates to and invades cells in the lymph nodes of the nasopharyngeal region, where it enters the cells, following which rapid reproduction occurs. After a few days, it enters the bloodstream, a condition called viremia. At this time, symptoms of smallpox appear. The virus spreads into lymph nodes, spleen, and bone marrow, where reproduction continues rapidly. By the eighth day of infection, the virus is contained in white blood cells or leukocytes, which transmit it to the small blood vessels in the dermis of the skin as well as in the mucosa that lines the mouth and pharynx.

Following an incubation period of about two weeks (the range is between seven and seventeen days), symptoms appear, including high fever, headache, nausea, malaise, and often backache. Accompanying these symptoms is a rash that begins in the mouth and spreads across the face, forearms, trunk, and legs. The rash is first confined to a reddish or purplish swelling of the blood vessels but soon becomes pustular as little round nodules appear on the surface of the body. If the patient recovers, the pustules crust over and the resultant scabs eventually split, which causes scarring of the face.

Death occurs within a few days following the appearance of the rash, most commonly from toxemia caused by variola antigens and various immune complexes circulating in the blood. In some cases the disease is followed by encephalitis. Smallpox fatalities typically occur because of complications such as pneumonia, septicemia, and nephritis (kidney failure). Survivors often suffer from general scarring, ulcers, scarring of the cornea leading to blindness, and skin abscesses. Treatment of survivors with chemotherapy has reduced the severity of many of these complications.

The considerably less virulent form of smallpox, *Variola minor*, produces a much less severe illness characterized by fever, chills, and a milder rash. The same conditions are sometimes seen in patients who have previously been vaccinated or even as a response to vaccinations.

SCREENING AND DIAGNOSIS

The Centers for Disease Control and Prevention (CDC) or a CDC Laboratory Response Network–designated variola testing facility can conduct a definitive examination for smallpox by testing a tissue sample from a lesion on the skin of an infected person. Even a single confirmed case of smallpox would be deemed an international emergency because of the devastating nature of the disease and concern that it may be used as a biological weapon.

TREATMENT AND THERAPY

Despite decades of research, there is no specific treatment for smallpox other than bed rest and application of antibiotics to prevent secondary infections. Therefore, only prevention of spread by quarantine of infected persons prevents epidemics. Immediate recognition of the disease remains the strongest control measure, followed by vaccination of all health care personnel and others who may come in contact with infected persons.

Widespread and aggressive inoculation programs conducted during the first half of the twentieth century eradicated smallpox from most regions of the world, including North America, Eurasia, and Oceania, largely as a result of the success of the vaccination process originally developed by Edward Jenner. By 1967 smallpox was found only in thirty-three countries and had an annual infection rate of 10 million to 15 million cases. In that year the World Health Organization (WHO) initiated a campaign to eliminate smallpox completely as a human disease, concentrating in Africa, India, and Indonesia. The last case of smallpox in Asia was reported in Bangladesh in 1975, and the last known smallpox victim was recorded in

Somalia in October 1977. Smallpox eradication was considered accomplished by 1979. The cost of the eradication campaign was $150 million.

Most researchers conclude that the effective eradication of smallpox was made possible for several reasons: smallpox cases could be quickly and positively identified; there are no natural carriers that serve as disease reservoirs; humans were the only carriers; individuals who survived did not continue to harbor the virus; and the smallpox vaccine proved highly effective.

Vaccinia viruses (the active ingredient of the smallpox vaccine) can absorb comparatively large amounts of foreign DNA without losing their ability to replicate, giving rise to the idea that they may provide a vehicle for providing immunity for other viral diseases of humans. One of several ongoing investigations involves insertion of twenty-two to twenty-five kilobase pairs into vaccinia. Experiments using this technique have produced vaccinia strains that encode surface proteins (antigens) of a number of important viruses, including influenza, hepatitis B, and herpesvirus. One possible outcome of these recombinant DNA experiments is the production of vaccinia strains that can serve as vaccines for several viral diseases simultaneously.

PREVENTION AND OUTCOMES

Although smallpox was eradicated globally in 1979, at least two research stocks exist, and there is concern that clandestinely held stocks of the virus may be used as weapons of bioterrorism, the use of living organisms as instruments of terror, such as the deliberate introduction of diseases into civilian populations.

Since 1979, only two stocks of smallpox officially remain: one stock is held at the Centers for Disease Control in Atlanta, Georgia, and the other is kept at VECTOR, Novosibirsk, in central Russia. However, there remains the possibility that clandestine stocks still exist, and these stocks may serve as potential bioterrorism weapons, either to be used against military or civilian populations or to be mounted as international threats. The use of smallpox as a bioterrorism weapon would be classed as an international crime, but prevention of its use is difficult unless all existing stocks can be identified and destroyed.

Smallpox is a potential bioterrorism weapon because of its transmissibility, its known lethality, and the general lack of immunity of much of the global population. Because of its bioterrorism potential, research is now centered on rapid identification methods that enable the early detection of smallpox, as well as aggressive vaccination programs for individuals most at risk, who have been identified as health care workers. In addition, smallpox vaccinations were reinstated in 2002 for some US military personnel and some health care workers, essentially those considered at highest risk. The vaccine is made from live but weakened vaccinia virus that is pricked into the skin. The characteristic blisters scab over within three weeks. During this time it is possible to transmit the virus to other parts of the body and to other people. Reactions to the vaccine range from a mild soreness around the vaccination site to more severe effects that may include brain inflammation and a rare and progressive bacterial inflammation called vaccinia that is sometimes fatal. For these reasons, mass vaccinations of the general public have been discouraged.

Dwight G. Smith, PhD.

FURTHER READING

Anderson, R. M., and R. M. May. *Infectious Diseases of Humans: Dynamics and Control.* Oxford: Oxford UP, 1992. Print.

Brooks, George F., et al. *Jawetz, Melnick, and Adelberg's Medical Microbiology.* 26th ed. New York: McGraw, 2013. Print.

Fenner, F., et al. *Smallpox and Its Eradication.* Geneva: WHO Report, 1988. Print.

Henderson, D. A. *Smallpox: The Death of a Disease— the Inside Story of Eradicating a Worldwide Killer.* Amherst: Prometheus, 2009. Print.

Miller, Judith, Stephen Engelberg, and William Broad. *Germs: Biological Weapons and America's Secret War.* New York: Simon, 2001. Print.

Preston, R. *The Demon in the Freezer: A True Story.* New York: Random. 2002. Print.

"Smallpox." *Health Library.* EBSCO Information Services, 20 June 2013. Web. 27 Aug. 2014.

"Smallpox." *MedlinePlus.* Natl. Lib. of Medecine, 13 Aug. 2014. Web. 27 Aug. 2014.

Tucker, Jonathan B. *Scourge: The Once and Future Threat of Smallpox.* New York: Grove, 2001. Print.

US Dept. of Defense. *Twenty-First Century Bioterrorism and Germ Weapons: US Army Field Manual for the Treatment of Biological Warfare Agent Casualties (Anthrax, Smallpox, Plague, Viral Fevers, Toxins, Delivery Methods, Detection, Symptoms, Treatment, Equipment).*

Washington: US Dept. of Defense Manual, 2002. Print.

World Health Organization. *Future Research on Smallpox Virus Recommended.* Geneva: WHO, 1999. Print.

See also: Anthrax; Bacterial resistance and super bacteria; Biological weapons; Emerging and reemerging infectious diseases; Gene regulation: Viruses; Hereditary diseases; Viral genetics.

Smith-Lemli-Opitz syndrome

CATEGORY: Diseases and syndromes
ALSO KNOWN AS: 7-Dehydrocholesterol reductase deficiency; RSH syndrome; SLOS; SLO syndrome

DEFINITION

Smith-Lemli-Opitz syndrome (SLOS) is a developmental disorder that affects multiple organ systems, prenatal and postnatal growth, and mental development. It is caused by mutations in the *DHCR7* gene that result in deficiency of the enzyme 7-dehydrocholesterol reductase.

RISK FACTORS

A pregnancy is at risk for SLOS when both parents are carriers of mutations in the *DHCR7* gene. SLOS is most common in individuals of northern or central European ancestry and is less common among individuals of African or Asian ancestry.

ETIOLOGY AND GENETICS

SLOS is an autosomal recessive genetic condition. When both parents are carriers of a single mutation in the *DHCR7* gene, there is a 25-percent chance in each pregnancy that the child will inherit both mutations and will be affected with SLOS.

The *DHCR7* gene is located at 11q12-13. It codes for the enzyme 7-dehydrocholesterol (7-DHC) reductase, which normally catalyzes the conversion of 7-DHC to cholesterol. Mutations in the *DHCR7* gene result in a loss of function of 7-DHC reductase. This blocks the final step in the cholesterol biosynthesis pathway.

Individuals who have a mutation in one copy of the *DHCR7* gene may have slightly increased 7-DHC levels but do not experience any clinical consequences. Individuals who have mutations in both copies of the

DHCR7 gene are affected with SLOS. Affected individuals have abnormally low cholesterol levels and elevated levels of the cholesterol precursors 7-DHC and 8-DHC.

Cholesterol deficiency is thought to be the cause of the developmental defects seen in SLOS. During fetal life, very little cholesterol is transported across the placenta from the mother. The fetus relies primarily on biosynthesis of cholesterol. Cholesterol is a major structural component of cell membranes and mitochondrial membranes. It is needed for bile acid, steroid hormone, and vitamin D metabolism. Cholesterol has also been found to bind to hedgehog proteins, a family of signaling proteins that direct embryonic development.

syndactyly of second and third toes is a common charactgeristic of Smith-Lemli-Opitz By AzaToth (Own work), via Wikimedia Commons

Clinical severity of SLOS can be variable and is inversely associated with cholesterol levels. Mortality is highest in individuals with the lowest cholesterol levels. The variability in severity is partially due to the more than 120 disease-causing mutations that have been described in the *DHCR7* gene. The twelve most common mutations account for approximately 69 percent of the alleles found in affected individuals.

Historically, SLOS was classified as type II, which is more severe and often lethal in the neonatal period, and classic type I. However, it is now clear that the difference in severity is related to the genotype. The most severely affected individuals typically have two mutations that result in very little residual 7-DHC reductase activity. Individuals with classic SLOS often

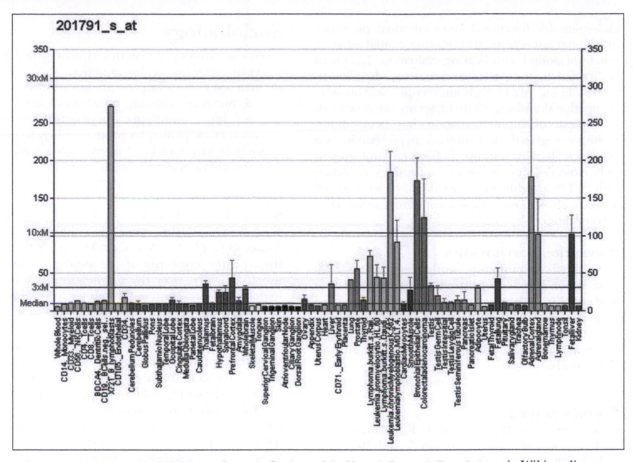

Gene expression pattern of the DHCR7 gene. Genomics Institute of the Novartis Research Foundation, via Wikimedia Commons

have one of these severe mutations and a second missense mutation that results in higher levels of residual 7-DHC reductase activity. Individuals who have two copies of less severe missense mutations may be mildly affected.

SYMPTOMS

Individuals with SLOS have moderate to severe intellectual disability, developmental delays, multiple congenital anomalies, and behaviors characteristic of autism. Birth defects are often seen involving the heart, lungs, kidneys, gastrointestinal tract, genitalia, palate, fingers, and toes.

SCREENING AND DIAGNOSIS

A diagnosis of SLOS can be made by checking blood or tissues for an elevated concentration of 7-DHC. Most affected individuals have low cholesterol levels as well, but some affected individuals have cholesterol

levels that are within the normal range. Sequencing of the *DHCR7* gene is able to identify disease-causing mutations in approximately 96 percent of affected individuals.

Prenatal testing for SLOS should be considered when there is a family history of SLOS, ultrasound findings are suggestive of SLOS, or maternal serum unconjugated estriol levels are low. Prenatally, a diagnosis of SLOS can be made by detecting an elevated concentration of 7-DHC in amniotic fluid or in tissue obtained from chorionic villus sampling (CVS). Enzyme testing can also be performed on cultured cells from an amniocentesis or CVS to confirm the diagnosis.

TREATMENT AND THERAPY

Following an initial diagnosis, evaluations may include a developmental assessment, ophthalmologic evaluation, cardiac evaluation, genitourinary examination, evaluation for functional gastrointestinal problems, nutritional assessment, MRI or other cranial imaging, renal ultrasound, and hearing evaluation. Treatment is directed to the particular problems identified in each child with SLOS. Early intervention and physical, occupational, and speech therapies are often needed.

Cholesterol supplementation has been shown to improve growth and increase nerve conduction velocities. It may improve behavioral problems as well. However, since many of the findings associated with SLOS are due to embryologic developmental defects, cholesterol supplementation cannot cure this condition.

PREVENTION AND OUTCOMES

Stillbirth is common, and approximately 20 percent of affected children die within the first year of life. Although prenatal screening and diagnosis is available, there is no effective means of preventing SLOS. Genetic counseling should be made available to the families of affected individuals.

Laura Garasimowicz, M.S.

FURTHER READING

Cassidy, Suzanne B., and Judith E. Allanson, eds. *Management of Genetic Syndromes.* 3rd ed. Hoboken: Wiley, 2011. Print.

Jones, Kenneth Lyons. *Smith's Recognizable Patterns of Human Malformation.* 7th ed. Philadelphia: Elsevier, 2013. Print.

Parker, Philip M. *Smith-Lemli-Opitz Syndrome: A Bibliography and Dictionary for Physicians, Patients, and Genome Researchers.* San Diego: Icon Group Intl., 2007. Print.

"Smith-Lemli-Opitz/RSH Syndrome Overview." *Smith-Lemli-Opitz/RSH Foundation.* Smith-Lemli-Opitz/RSH Foundation, 2014. Web. 27 Aug. 2014.

See also: Apert syndrome; Brachydactyly; Carpenter syndrome; Cleft lip and palate; Congenital defects; Cornelia de Lange syndrome; Cri du chat syndrome; Crouzon syndrome; Down syndrome; Edwards syndrome; Ellis-van Creveld syndrome; Holt-Oram syndrome; Ivemark syndrome; Meacham syndrome; Opitz-Frias syndrome; Patau syndrome; Polydactyly; Robert syndrome; Rubinstein-Taybi syndrome.

Sociobiology

CATEGORY: History of genetics; Human genetics and social issues; Population genetics

SIGNIFICANCE: Sociobiology attempts to explain social interactions among members of animal species from an evolutionary perspective. The application of the principles of sociobiology to human social behavior initiated severe criticism and accusations of racism and sexism.

HISTORY

Sociobiology is best known from the works of Edward O. Wilson, especially his 1975 book *Sociobiology: The New Synthesis.* This work both synthesized the concepts of the field and initiated the controversy over the application of sociobiological ideas to humans. However, the concepts and methods of sociobiology did not start with Wilson; they can be traced to Charles Darwin and others who studied the influence of genetics and evolution on behavior. Sociobiologists attempt to explain the genetics and evolution of social activity of all types, ranging from flocking in birds and herd formation in mammals to more complex social systems such as eusociality. "The new synthesis" attempted to apply genetics, population biology, and evolutionary theory to the study of social systems.

1. Geospiza magnirostris   2. Geospiza fortis
3. Geospiza parvula   4. Certhidea olivacea

Finches from Galapagos Archipelago

Darwin's finches; his theory of natural selection figures largely in sociobiology. Darwin observed that beak shape varies among finch species. He postulated that the beak of an ancestral species had adapted over time to equip the finches to acquire different food sources. By John Gould (14.Sep.1804 - 3.Feb.1881), via Wikimedia Commons

Edward O. Wilson By Jim Harrison (PLoS), via Wikimedia Commons

When sociobiological concepts were applied to human sociality, many scientists, especially social scientists, feared a return to scientific theories of racial and gender superiority. They rebelled vigorously against such ideas. Wilson was vilified by many of these scientists, and some observers assert that the term "sociobiology" generated such negative responses that scientists who studied in the field began using other names for it. At least one scientific journal dropped the word "sociobiology" from its title, perhaps in response to its negative connotations. However, the study of sociobiological phenomena existed in the social branches of animal behavior and ethology long before the term was coined. Despite the criticism, research has continued under the name sociobiology as well as other names, such as "behavioral ecology." The study of sociobiology also led to the field of evolutionary psychology, a theoretical psychology that examines the evolutionary reasons and advantages to the development of the way that humans think and behave.

SOCIOBIOLOGY AND THE UNDERSTANDING OF ALTRUISM

Sociobiologists have contributed to the understanding of a number of aspects of social behavior, such as altruism. Illogical in the face of evolutionary theory, apparently altruistic acts can be observed in humans and other animal groups. Darwinian evolution holds that the organism that leaves the largest number of mature offspring will have the greatest influence on the characteristics of the next generation. Under this assumption, altruism should disappear from the population as each individual seeks to maximize its own offspring production. If an individual assists another, it uses energy, time, and material it might have used for its own survival and reproduction and simultaneously contributes energy, time, and material to the survival and reproductive effort of the recipient. As a result, more members of the next generation should be like the assisted organism than like the altruistic one. Should this continue generation after generation, altruism would decrease in the population and selfishness would increase. Yet biologists have cataloged a number of altruistic behaviors.

When a prairie dog "barks," thus warning others of the presence of a hawk, the prairie dog draws the hawk's attention. Should it not just slip into its burrow, out of the hawk's reach? When a reproductively mature acorn woodpecker stays with its parents to help raise the next generation, the woodpecker is bypassing its own reproduction for one or more years. Should it not leave home and attempt to set up its own nest and hatch its own young? Eusocial species, such as honeybees and naked mole rats, actually have many members who never reproduce; they work their entire lives to support and protect a single queen, several reproductive males, and their offspring. It would seem that all these altruistic situations should produce a decrease in the number of members of the next generation carrying altruistic genes in favor of more members with "selfish" genes.

Sociobiologists have reinterpreted some of these apparently altruistic acts as camouflaged selfishness. The barking prairie dog, for example, may be notifying the hawk that it sees the predator and that it is close to its burrow and cannot be caught; therefore, the hawk would be better off hunting someone else. Perhaps the young acorn woodpecker learns enough from the years of helping to make its fewer reproductive years more successful than its total reproductive success without the training period.

It is difficult, however, to explain the worker honeybee this way. The worker bee never gets an opportunity to reproduce. Sociobiologists explain this and other phenomena by invoking kin selection. Since the worker bees are closely related to the queen (as sisters or daughters), to reproductive males, and to other workers they help feed and protect, they share a large number of genes with them. If they help raise enough brothers and sisters (especially males and queens) to more than make up for the offspring they do not produce themselves, they will actually increase the proportion of individuals similar to themselves more than if they "selfishly" reproduced.

The prairie dog's behavior might be explained this way as well. The organisms the prairie dog is warning are primarily relatives. By warning them, the prairie dog helps preserve copies of its own genes in its relatives. If the cost of the behavior (an occasional barking prairie dog being captured by a hawk because the warning call drew the hawk's attention) is more than compensated for by the number of relatives saved from the hawk by the warning, kin selection will preserve the behavior. The helper acorn woodpecker's behavior may be explained in similar ways, not as an altruistic act but as a selfish act to favor copies of the helper's genes in its relatives. Another explanation of altruism set forth by sociobiologists is reciprocity or reciprocal altruism: If the prairie dog is sometimes warned by others and returns the favor by calling out a warning when it sees a predator, the prairie dog town will be safer for all prairie dogs.

OPPOSITION TO THE APPLICATION OF SOCIOBIOLOGY TO HUMANS

Wilson's new synthesis attempted to incorporate biology, genetics, population biology, and evolution into the study and explanation of social behavior. When the analyses turned to human sociality, critics feared that they would lead back to the sexist, racist, and determinist viewpoints of the early twentieth century. The argument over the relative importance of heredity or environment (nature or nurture) in determining individual success had been more or less decided in favor of the environment, at least by social scientists. Poor people were not poor because they were inherently inferior but because the environment they lived in did not give them an equal chance. Black, Hispanic, and other minority people were not inordinately represented among the poor because they were genetically inferior but because their environment kept them from using their genetic capabilities.

Sociobiologists entered the fray squarely on the side of an appreciable contribution from genetic and evolutionary factors. Few, if any, said that the environment was unimportant in the molding of racial, gender, and individual characteristics; rather, sociobiologists claimed that the genetic and evolutionary history of human individuals and groups played an important role in determining their capabilities, just as they do in other animals. Few, if any, claimed that this meant that one race, gender, or group was superior to another. However, many (if not all) sociobiologists were accused of promoting racist, sexist, and determinist ideas with their application of sociobiological concepts to humans.

Extremists on both sides of the question have confused the issues. Such extremists range from opponents of sociobiological ideas who minimize genetic or evolutionary influence on the human cultural condition to sociobiologists who minimize the role of environmental influences. In at least some minds, extremists in the sociobiological camp have done as much damage to sociobiology as its most ardent opponents. Sociobiology (by that or another name) will continue to contribute to the understanding of the social systems of animals and humans. The biological, genetic, and evolutionary bases of human social systems must be studied. The knowledge obtained may prove to be as enlightening as has sociobiology's contribution to the understanding of social systems in other animals.

FURTHER READING

Alcock, John. *The Triumph of Sociobiology*. 2001. New York: Oxford UP, 2003. Print.

Baxter, Brian. *A Darwinian Worldview: Sociobiology, Environmental Ethics, and the Work of Edward O. Wilson*. Burlington: Ashgate, 2007. Print.

Blackmore, Susan J. *The Meme Machine*. Foreword by Richard Dawkins. New York: Oxford UP, 1999. Print.

Cartwright, John. *Evolution and Human Behavior: Darwinian Perspectives on Human Nature*. 2d ed., updated and expanded ed. Cambridge: MIT P, 2008. Print.

Cronk, Lee. *That Complex Whole: Culture and the Evolution of Human Behavior*. Boulder: Westview, 1999. Print.

Cziko, Gary. *The Things We Do: Using the Lessons of Bernard and Darwin to Understand the What, How, and Why of Our Behavior*. Cambridge: MIT, 2000. Print.

Powell, Alvin. "'Search until You Find a Passion and Go All out to Excel in Its Expression;' For E. O. Wilson, Wonders Never Cease." *Harvard Gazette.* Harvard U, 15 Apr. 2014. Web. 30 Nov. 2015.

Richerson, Peter J., and Robert Boyd. *Not by Genes Alone: How Culture Transformed Human Evolution.* Chicago: U of Chicago P, 2005. Print.

Segerstrale, Ullica. *Defenders of the Truth: The Battle for Science in the Sociobiology Debate and Beyond.* New York: Oxford UP, 2000. Print.

Van der Dennen, Johan M. G., David Smillie, and Daniel R. Wilson, eds. *The Darwinian Heritage and Sociobiology.* Westport: Praeger, 1999. rint.

Wilson, Edward O. "The Biological Basis of Morality." *Atlantic Monthly* Apr. 1998: 53–70. Print.

Wilson, Edward O. *On Human Nature.* 1978. Cambridge.: Harvard UP, 2004. Print.

Wilson, Edward O. *Sociobiology: The New Synthesis.* 1975. Cambridge: Belknap , 2000. Print.

See also: Aggression; Alcoholism; Altruism; Behavior; Biological clocks; Biological determinism; Criminality; Developmental genetics; Eugenics; Gender identity; Genetic engineering: Medical applications; Genetic engineering: Social and ethical issues; Genetic screening; Genetic testing; Genetic testing: Ethical and economic issues; Heredity and environment; Homosexuality; Human genetics; Inbreeding and assortative mating; Intelligence; Klinefelter syndrome; Knockout genetics and knockout mice; Miscegenation and antimiscegenation laws; Natural selection; Twin studies; XY Y syndrome.

Speciation

CATEGORY: Population genetics

SIGNIFICANCE: Speciation, the biological formation of new species, has produced the wide variety of living things on Earth. Although speciation can be caused by other forces or events, natural selection is considered by many researchers to be one of the primary mechanisms promoting speciation.

KEY TERMS

allopatric speciation: the genetic divergence of populations caused by separation from each other by a geographic barrier such as a mountain range or an ocean

population: a group of organisms of the same species in the same place at the same time with the potential ability to mate; the basic unit of speciation

reproductive isolating mechanism: a characteristic that prevents an individual of one species from interbreeding (hybridizing) with a member of another species

species: a class of organisms with common attributes; individuals are usually able to produce fertile offspring only when mating with members of their own species

sympatric speciation: the genetic divergence of populations that are not separated geographically

SPECIES CONCEPTS

Before the time of Charles Darwin, physical appearance was the only criterion for classifying an organism. This "typological species concept" was associated with the idea that species never change (fixity of species). This way of defining a species causes problems when males and females of the same species look different, as with peacocks and peahens, or when there are several different color patterns among members of a species, as with many insects. Variability within species, whether it is a visible part of their anatomy, an invisible component of their biochemistry, or another characteristic such as behavior, is an important element in understanding how species evolve.

The "biological species concept" uses reproduction to define a species. It states that a species is composed of individuals that can mate and produce fertile offspring in nature. This concept cannot be used to classify organisms such as bacteria, which do not reproduce sexually. It also cannot be used to classify dead specimens or fossils. This definition emphasizes the uniqueness of each individual (variability) in sexually reproducing species. For example, in the human species (*Homo sapiens*), there are variations in body build, hair color and texture, ability to digest milk sugar (lactose), and many other anatomical, biochemical, and behavioral characteristics. All of these variations are the result of genetic mutations, or changes in genes.

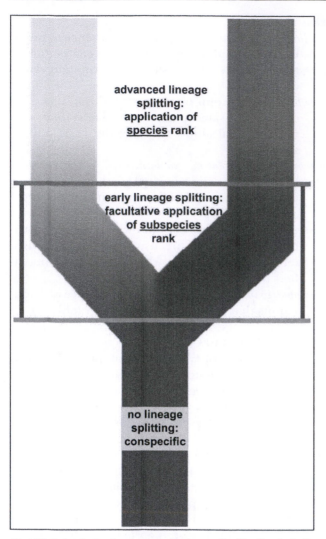

advanced lineage
splitting:
application of
<u>species</u> rank

early lineage splitting:
facultative application
of <u>subspecies</u>
rank

no lineage
splitting:
conspecific

Simplified sketch showing a speciation event. By Hawlitschek O, Nagy ZT, Glaw F (2012), via Wikimedia Commons

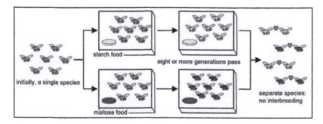

An experiment demonstrating allopatric speciation in the fruit fly (Drosophila pseudoobscura) conducted by Diane Dodd. A single population of flies was divided into two, with one of the populations fed with starch-based food and the other with maltose-based food. After the populations had diverged over many generations, the groups were again mixed; it was observed that the flies would mate only with others from their adapted population. (Public Domain - Wikimedia Commons)

According to evolutionary scientist Ernst Mayr, to a "population thinker," variation is reality and type is an abstraction or average; to a "typological thinker," variation is an illusion and type is the reality. Typological thinking is similar to typecasting or stereotyping, and it cannot explain the actual variability seen in species, just as stereotyping does not recognize the variability seen in people. Additional definitions, such as the "evolutionary species concept," include the continuity of a species' genes through time and other factors not addressed by the biological species concept.

ISOLATION AND DIVERGENCE OF POPULATIONS

Species are composed of unique individuals that are nevertheless similar enough to be able to mate and produce fertile offspring. However, individuals of a species are infrequently in close enough proximity to be able to choose a mate from all opposite-sex members of the same species. Groups of individuals of the same species that are at least potential mates because of proximity are called populations.

The basic type of speciation in most sexually reproducing organisms is believed to be allopatric, in which geographic isolation (separation) of the species into two or more populations is followed by accumulation of differences (divergence) between the populations that eventually prevent them from interbreeding. These differences are caused primarily by natural selection of characteristics advantageous to populations in different environments. If both populations were in identical environments after geographic isolation, they would be much less likely to diverge or evolve into new species.

Subforms of allopatric speciation have been proposed based on the type or degree of separation occurring between two populations. Peripatic speciation involves a minority of a population entering a new environmental niche that then becomes isolated. New genetic traits may then arise in the niche population; many researchers believe that genetic drift likely is an important factor in peripatic speciation. Parapatic speciation occurs when a population reaches a new niche but never becomes totally isolated from the parent population. While a new species forms in the new environment, hybridization may occur as the new and parent species interact.

Another type of speciation is sympatric, in which populations are not separated geographically but reproduction between them cannot occur (reproductive isolation) for some other reason. For example, one population may evolve a mutation that makes the fertilized egg (zygote) that results from interbreeding with the other population incapable of surviving. Another possibility is a mutation that changes where or when individuals are active so that members of the different populations never encounter one another.

Darwin thought that divergence, and thus speciation, occurred gradually, by the slow accumulation of many small adaptations "selected" by the environment. Geneticists now recognize that a very small population, or even a "founder" individual, may be the genetic basis of a new species that evolves more rapidly. This process, called genetic drift, is essentially random. For example, which member of an insect species is blown to an island by a storm is determined not by genetic differences from other members of the species but by a random event—in this case, the weather. This individual (or small number of individuals) is highly unlikely to contain all of the genetic diversity of the entire species. Thus the new population begins with genetic differences that may be enhanced by its new environment. Speciation proceeds according to the allopatric model, but faster. However, extinction of the new population may also occur.

Plants are able to form new species by hybridization (crossbreeding) more often than are animals. When plants hybridize, postmating incompatibility between the chromosomes of the parents and the offspring may immediately create a new, fertile species rather than a sterile hybrid as in animals (such as the mule). A frequent method of speciation in plants is polyploidy, in which two or more complete sets of chromosomes end up in the offspring. (Usually, one complete set is made up of half of each parent's chromosomes.)

Many species reproduce asexually (without the exchange of genes between individuals that defines sexual reproduction), including bacteria and some plants, fish, salamanders, insects, rotifers, worms, and other animals. In spite of the fact that reproductive isolation has no meaning in these organisms, they are species whose chromosomes and genes differ from those of their close relatives.

Speciation may also be created artificially, sometimes with the intention of benefiting humans but also inadvertently due to human impact on ecosystems, such as introducing invasive species that may then hybridize with native ones. The domestication of animals through husbandry practices has created numerous species, as has the agricultural manipulation of plants, though in many cases the details of the divergence are undocumented and subject to much speculation. Humans have also developed new species in laboratory settings, including for the purpose of testing theories of speciation.

Impact and Applications

Environmentalists and scientists recognize that the biodiversity created by speciation is essential to the functioning of Earth's life-support systems for humans as well as other species. Some practical benefits of biodiversity include medicines, natural air and water purification, air conditioning, and food.

The impact of understanding the genetic basis of evolving species cannot be underestimated. Artificial selection (in which humans decide which individuals of a species survive and reproduce) of plants has produced better food crops, such as modern corn from teosinte, and alleviated hunger in developing nations by creating new varieties of existing species such as rice. Hybridization of animals has resulted in mules and beefalo for the farm, both of which are sterile hybrids rather than species. Artificial selection of domesticated animals has produced many different breeds of horses, dogs, and cats, each of which is still technically one species. Genetic engineering promises to create crops that resist pests, withstand frost or drought, and contain more nutrients. Finally, understanding the genetics of the evolving human species has broad implications for curing disease and avoiding birth defects.

Barbara J. Abraham, Ph.D.

Further Reading

Ayala, Francisco J., and John C. Avise, eds. *Essential Readings in Evolutionary Biology*. Baltimore: Johns Hopkins UP, 2014. Print.

Boyd, Robert, and Joan Silk. *How Humans Evolved*. 6th ed. New York: Norton, 2012. Print.

Coyne, Jerry A., and H. Allen Orr. *Speciation*. Sunderland: Sinauer, 2004. Print.

Crow, Tim J., ed. *The Speciation of Modern* Homo sapiens. Oxford: Oxford UP, 2002. Print.

Giddings, Luther Val, Kenneth Y. Kaneshiro, and Wyatt W. Anderson, eds. *Genetics, Speciation, and the Founder Principle*. New York: Oxford UP, 1989. Print.

Hey, Jody. *Genes, Categories, and Species: The Evolutionary and Cognitive Causes of the Species Problem.* New York: Oxford UP, 2001. Print.

Hey, Jody, Walter M. Fitch, and Francisco J. Ayala, eds. *Systematics and the Origin of Species: On Ernst Mayr's 100th Anniversary.* Washington: Natl. Acads., 2005. Print.

Margulis, Lynn, and Dorion Sagan. *Acquiring Genomes: A Theory of the Origins of Species.* New York: Basic, 2003. Print.

Mayr, Ernst. *One Long Argument: Charles Darwin and the Genesis of Modern Evolutionary Thought.* Cambridge: Harvard UP, 1991. Print.

Miller, G. Tyler, and Scott Spoolman. *Living in the Environment.* Stamford: Cengage Learning, 2015. Print.

Nosil, Patrik. *Ecological Speciation.* New York: Oxford UP, 2012. Print.

Serrelli, Emanuele, and Nathalie Gontier. *Macroevolution: Explanation, Interpretation, and Evidence.* New York: Springer, 2015. Print.

See also: Artificial selection; Evolutionary biology; Hardy-Weinberg law; Hybridization and introgression; Lateral gene transfer; Natural selection; Polyploidy; Population genetics; Punctuated equilibrium.

Spinal muscular atrophy

CATEGORY: Diseases and syndromes

ALSO KNOWN AS: Infantile Werdnig-Hoffmann disease; Kugelberg-Welander disease; spinobulbar muscular atrophy (SBMA); Kennedy disease

DEFINITION

Spinal muscular atrophy (SMA) is a progressive neurodegenerative disorder caused by the loss of function of motor neurons, which leads to muscular atrophy. There are five clinical subtypes that range in age of onset and the severity of disease. SMA Type I is the most common subtype, accounting for 50 to 70 percent of SMA children.

RISK FACTORS

SMA has a purely genetic etiology and can occur with or without a family history of the disorder since parents may be an asymptomatic carriers. SMA affects all ethnicities at a similar rate with slightly higher incidence in Caucasian and Jewish populations, and an estimated 1 in 40 being asymptomatic carriers. It affects 1 in 10,000 live births. There are no environmental risk factors reported.

ETIOLOGY AND GENETICS

SMA types I through IV are transmitted in an autosomal recessive pattern whereby a person simultaneously inherits two copies of the disease-causing gene (called SMN1, for survival motor neuron) at conception. Carriers remain symptom-free because one working copy of SMN1 (located at 5q13.2) produces sufficient SMN protein for motor neuron cells to function. The second gene implicated with SMA is called SMN2 (survival motor neuron 2) also located at 5q13.2. This gene can range in copy number from zero to five copies in each cell. SMN1 and SMN2 are very similar in their composition, differing by only one nucleotide. This nucleotide difference does not change the amino acid generated but does alter the gene splicing (paring down mRNA by editing out noncoding regions of DNA). Usually the protein produced by SMN1 is longer than SMN2, but splicing is not a perfect process, and at times an equally long protein is produced from SMN2 and functions much like SMN1 protein. Thus, a person with SMA that has a high copy number of SMN2 genes is predicted to have a less severe case than someone who does not have any SMN2 genes.

SMA type V is caused by mutation in the DNAJB2 gene on chromosome 2q35. The mutation is also inherited in an autosomal recessive pattern.

Another type of SMA called spinal muscular atrophy lower extremity-predominant (SMA-LED1), or Finkel type, is a late-onset form caused by VAPB gene mutations. SMA-LED2 is caused by heterozygous mutation in the BICD2 gene. Both mutations are inherited in an autosomal dominant pattern, which means one copy of the altered gene in each cell from a single parent causes the disease.

Males are affected more frequently in yet another form of SMA, X-linked spinal muscular atrophy. Mutation in the UBA1 gene is located on the X chromosome, which is one of the two sex chromosomes. Having only one X chromosome, males are more likely to get the disorder, while females would have to obtain two copies of the mutation. Fathers cannot pass X-linked traits to their sons.

SYMPTOMS

There is a tremendous range of severity. Generally earlier onset is predictive of a worse prognosis; thus, Type I is most severe, while Type IV is comparatively mild. Type I symptoms begin between birth and six months of age and include hypotonia (low muscle tone and strength), paralysis, and mild joint contractures which result in difficulty sitting without support, breathing, and swallowing. Death occurs most commonly before two years of age, typically caused by complications such as respiratory infections. X-linked SMA is similar to type I. Type II (onset from six to twelve months) symptoms include an inability to sit, but standing or walking unaided is possible. Type III occurs in childhood (over one year of age) and is considerably more mild. Type IV and Finkel type have adult onset of symptoms typically after age 30 that include muscle weakness, tremor, and twitching. Type V presents during young adulthood and displays progressive muscle weakness and atrophy causing gait impairment and loss of reflexes. All forms of SMA have normal cognition and a high rate of mortality and morbidity.

SCREENING AND DIAGNOSIS

Screening and diagnostic testing for SMA are readily available through commercial laboratories. Carrier screening involves evaluating the SMN1 gene for mutations and determining the number of SMN2 genes via sequencing and quantitative polymerase chain reaction (PCR), respectively. Diagnostic testing is recommended if an individual is symptomatic and can help confirm a clinical diagnosis. Confirmation of a mutation may also aid in determining if extended family members should pursue carrier screening. Prenatal diagnosis requires testing fetal cells and thus performing an amniocentesis to sample the amniotic fluid or a chorionic villus sampling (CVS) to biopsy a small portion of the placenta. Signs of prenatal SMA include lack of fetal movement at thirty to thirty-six weeks gestation.

TREATMENT AND THERAPY

There is no cure for SMA, but treatment is available to ease symptoms. Treatment of recurrent pulmonary infections, as well as tracheotomies, may be necessary. Alternative therapies include long-term ventilation, tube feeding, and physical therapy, which can help in prolonging survival. Wheelchairs are often needed. SMA Type I is a fatal condition; thus, palliative care is also provided.

Mouse with spinal muscular atrophy By US National Institute of Health (US National Institute of Health), via Wikimedia Commons

Structure of the SMN1 protein. Based on PyMOL rendering of PDB 1g5v. By Emw (Own work), via Wikimedia Commons

PREVENTION AND OUTCOMES

SMA is best prevented by carrier screening and other testing services. With two carrier parents, the risk is 25 percent for future pregnancies also being affected with SMA. There is also a 50 percent risk of having a future child that is an asymptomatic carrier. Lastly, there is a 25 percent chance of having a future child that is completely unaffected.

Prenatal diagnosis is available with the option of ending the pregnancy should it be affected. Preimplantation genetic diagnosis (PGD) is available to diagnose embryos prior to implantation if pursuing invitro fertilization; however, the procedure is rarely pursued because insurance coverage is extremely limited.

The long term outcomes vary by subtype and severity within each type. Adult onset types have a normal life span.

Kayla Mandel Sheets, M.S.; updated by Deanna M. Neff, M.P.H.

FURTHER READING

Arnold WD, Kassar D, Kissel JT. "Spinal muscular atrophy: diagnosis and management in a new therapeutic era". *Muscle Nerve.* 2015; 51 (2): 157–67.

Cummings, Michael. *Human Heredity: Principles and Issues.* 8th ed. Pacific Grove, Calif.: Brooks/ Cole,

2008. A comprehensive text for referencing basic concepts of human genetics.

Eckart M, Guenther UP, Idkowiak J, Varon R, Grolle B, Boffi P, et al. "The natural course of infantile spinal muscular atrophy with respiratory distress type 1 (SMARD1)". *Pediatrics.* 2012; 129(1): e148–56.

Firth, Helen V., and Jane A. Hurst. *Oxford Desk Reference: Clinical Genetics.* Oxford, England: Oxford University Press, 2005. An overview of human genetic conditions, testing, and treatment.

Harper, Peter S. *Practical Genetic Counseling. 6th ed.* London: Hodder Arnold, 2004. A human genetics reference written by a professor of medical genetics.

WEB SITES OF INTEREST

Families of Spinal Muscular Atrophy www.fsma.org

International support group and resource center for this disease. Includes current research. Genetic and Rare Diseases Information Center
https://rarediseases.info.nih.gov/diseases
GARD provides the public with access to current, reliable, and easy to understand information about rare or genetic diseases in English or Spanish. Genetics Home Reference
https://ghr.nlm.nih.gov/condition

Consumer-friendly information about the effects of genetic variation on human health. SMA Foundation
www.smafoundation.org

Mission of the spinal muscular atrophy (SMA) foundation is to accelerate the development of a treatment or cure for spinal muscular atrophy.

NINDS: Spinal Muscular Atrophy Information Page
www.ninds.nih.gov/disorders/sma/sma.htm

Spinal muscular atrophy (SMA) information page compiled by the National Institute of Neurological Disorders and Stroke (NINDS).

See also: Adrenoleukodystrophy; Alexander disease; Alzheimer's disease; Amyotrophic lateral sclerosis; Arnold-Chiari syndrome; Ataxia telangiectasia; Canavan disease; Cerebrotendinous xanthomatosis; Charcot-Marie-Tooth syndrome; Chediak-Higashi syndrome; Dandy-Walker syndrome; Deafness; Epilepsy; Essential tremor; Friedreich ataxia; Huntington's disease; Jansky-Bielschowsky disease; Joubert syndrome; Kennedy disease; Krabbé disease; Leigh syndrome; Leukodystrophy; Limb girdle muscular dystrophy; Maple syrup urine disease; Metachromatic leukodystrophy; Myoclonic epilepsy associated with ragged red fibers (MERRF); Narcolepsy; Nemaline myopathy; Neural tube defects; Neurofi bromatosis; Parkinson disease; Pelizaeus-Merzbacher disease; Pendred syndrome; Periodic paralysis syndrome; Prion diseases: Kuru and Creutzfeldt-Jakob syndrome; Refsum disease; Vanishing white matter disease.

Spinocerebellar ataxia

CATEGORY: Diseases and syndromes

ALSO KNOWN AS: SCA; SCA1 (SCA2; etc.); spinocerebellar degeneration; olivopontocerebellar atrophy (OPCA); Machado-Joseph disease (SCA3)

DEFINITION

The spinocerebellar ataxias are hereditary movement disorders characterized by ataxia, or loss of coordination, with variable ages of onset and possible development of other neurological features. There are approximately thirty recognized distinct types of spinocerebellar ataxias—though there may be more, given the disorder's great variance—typically labeled as SCA1, SCA2, and so on. Each has a unique genetic cause leading to cell loss in the cerebellum and possibly the spine and brain stem. Dentatorubralpallidalluysian atrophy (DRPLA) may also be categorized as a subtype of SCA, as the symptoms and genetics of this condition are similar.

RISK FACTORS

The only risk factors are a known gene mutation or a family history of SCA. The SCAs can occur in all ethnicities, although some occur at a higher frequency among certain ethnic backgrounds, possibly due to a founder effect. Some SCAs are incredibly rare and have been identified only in a single family of one particular ethnic background. Men and women are equally likely to be affected. There is an average age of onset for each type of SCA, with onset in childhood or young adulthood, while others may not occur until late in life.

Fundus of a 34 year-old patient with cone rod dystrophy due to Spinocerebellar Ataxia Type 7 (SCA7). Note that the macular area, and also the mid periphery, are atrophic. By Christian P Hamel, via Wikimedia Commons

ETIOLOGY AND GENETICS

Each of the numerous SCAs is inherited in an autosomal dominant manner and has a distinct genetic cause, although the exact gene has not been identified for all. First-degree relatives of an affected individual are at a 50 percent risk to develop the same type of SCA. Some SCAs result from single point mutations, but many are trinucleotide repeat expansion disorders causing variation in age of onset, severity, and disease course exhibited among family members with the same disorder. Certain genes have a set number of repeating trinucleotides, but in some SCAs, the number of these repeated trinucleotides has

expanded, causing an unstable gene. For those individuals who have a number of trinucleotide repeats within the reduced penetrance range, it is not possible to predict whether or not SCA will develop. Anticipation is common with some of the SCAs, meaning the number of trinucleotide repeats in an already unstable gene will continue to expand in future generations into the full mutation range. The condition will likely develop if the individual with a full mutation lives long enough. Signs and symptoms may occur at earlier ages of onset and with greater severity in succeeding generations due to anticipation. Family history may appear negative because of reduced penetrance, late onset, or early death of relatives. New gene mutations that are not inherited are also possible but rare.

MACHADO-JOSEPH DISEASE

(SCA3) is the most common SCA, and combined with SCA1, 2, and 6 is responsible for at least 50 percent of all autosomal dominant ataxias. It is estimated that 1 to 5 in 100,000 individuals are affected with an SCA.

While the exact function of each gene and its associated protein is unknown, it appears that the abnormal protein causes nerve cell damage in the brain and spinal cord. Current research focuses on understanding the effect of these gene mutations on the brain and further characterization of each SCA.

SYMPTOMS

All types of SCAs include ataxia. Loss of coordination leads to difficulty with balance and walking, and to clumsiness of the hands. Speech may become slurred, and swallowing may become increasingly difficult. Visual disturbances and eye movement abnormalities are possible. Some SCAs have characteristic features that may aid in diagnosis, such as cognitive impairment, neuropathy, hearing loss, seizures, parkinsonism, other abnormal movements, or specific neurological signs detected on exam. It is essential to see a physician when symptoms interfere with daily activities, injury occurs after a fall, or swallowing becomes difficult.

SCREENING AND DIAGNOSIS

Family history, neurological exam, brain MRI, and genetic testing are all useful in diagnosis.

The MRI may reveal cerebellar atrophy, or loss of tissue, common to all SCAs, in addition to spinal cord or brain stem atrophy. Only genetic testing can establish a diagnosis of a specific SCA, although testing is not available for every known type. Other clinical studies may be necessary to detect neurological findings characteristic of some SCAs.

TREATMENT AND THERAPY

There are no cures or specific treatments, although assistive devices and therapy may be beneficial. Medications may help alleviate some features, but individual response varies.

PREVENTION AND OUTCOMES

Diagnostic genetic testing can help to provide an accurate diagnosis in affected individuals. With a known familial mutation, predictive genetic testing is available to determine whether an unaffected individual has inherited the gene mutation and will develop SCA.

There is no known prevention. Prenatal diagnosis and preimplantation genetic diagnosis may be possible with known familial mutations.

Some SCAs have a slowly progressive course and normal life span, but many progress more rapidly, with ten to twenty years passing from onset until extensive assistance with activities of daily living is required.

Katherine L. Howard, M.S.

FURTHER READING

Ashizawa, Tetsuo, et al. "Clinical Characteristics of Patients with Spinocerebellar Ataxias 1, 2, 3, and 6 in the US; A Prospective Observational Study." *Orphanet Journ. of Rare Diseases* 8.1 (2013): 1–22. Print.

Di Gregorio, Eleonora, et al. "ELOVL5 Mutations Cause Spinocerebellar Ataxia 38." *American Journ. of Human Genetics* 95.2 (2014): 209–17. Print.

Manto, Mario, et al. *Handbook of the Cerebellum and Cerebellar Disorders.* New York: Springer, 2013. Print.

Nussbaum, Robert L., Roderick R. McInnes, and Huntington F. Willard. *Thompson and Thompson Genetics in Medicine.* 7th ed. New York: Saunders, 2007. Print.

Pulst, Stefan. *Genetics of Movement Disorders.* San Diego: Elsevier Science, 2003. Print.

Watts, Ray, and William C. Koller. *Movement Disorders: Neurologic Principles and Practices.* 2d ed. New York: McGraw, 2004. Print.

See also: Adrenoleukodystrophy; Alexander disease; Alzheimer's disease; Amyotrophic lateral sclerosis; Arnold-Chiari syndrome; Ataxia telangiectasia; Canavan disease; Cerebrotendinous xanthomatosis; Charcot-Marie-Tooth syndrome; Chediak-Higashi syndrome; Dandy-Walker syndrome; Deafness; Epilepsy; Essential tremor; Friedreich ataxia; Huntington's disease; Jansky-Bielschowsky disease; Joubert syndrome; Kennedy disease; Krabbé disease; Leigh syndrome; Leukodystrophy; Limb girdle muscular dystrophy; Maple syrup urine disease; Metachromatic leukodystrophy; Myoclonic epilepsy associated with ragged red fibers (MERRF); Narcolepsy; Nemaline myopathy; Neural tube defects; Neurofibromatosis; Parkinson disease; Pelizaeus-Merzbacher disease; Pendred syndrome; Periodic paralysis syndrome; Prion diseases: Kuru and Creutzfeldt-Jakob syndrome; Refsum disease; Sandhoff disease; Sanfilippo syndrome; Spinal muscular atrophy; Vanishing white matter disease.

SRY gene

CATEGORY: Classical transmission genetics; Molecular genetics

SIGNIFICANCE: The *SRY* gene is on the Y chromosome and encodes a transcription factor that triggers development of the male phenotype. The absence of this protein results in development of the female phenotype. Most mutations in *SRY* that disable the protein's DNA-binding domain result in XY females.

Key terms

sex determination: the biological mechanism that determines the sex of an individual

sex reversal: an XY female or XX male

XO chromosome constitution: an individual with one X chromosome and no corresponding X or Y chromosome

XXY chromosome constitution: an individual with two X chromosomes and one Y chromosome

SRY and Sex Determination

The biological mechanisms of sex determination vary widely throughout the animal and plant kingdoms, ranging from purely nongenetic to fully genetic mechanisms. The XX-XY genetic system, in which females have a pair of homomorphic X chromosomes and males a pair of heteromorphic X and Y chromosomes, was investigated most extensively in *Drosophila melanogaster* in the early part of the twentieth century. In 1925, Calvin Bridges published abundant evidence that the ratio of X chromosomes to autosomes determines sex in *Drosophila.* Of particular note was the observation that XXY flies are fertile females, and XO flies are infertile males. The *Drosophila* Y chromosome plays no role in sex determination although it is essential for male fertility.

In 1921, Theophilus Painter identified the Y chromosome in human and opossum males, and demonstrated that it pairs with and segregates from the X chromosome during meiosis. These discoveries suggested an evolutionarily ancestral XX-XY system for both eutherian (placental) and metatherian (marsupial) mammals, which has since been confirmed.

The observation that both *Drosophila* and humans have XX-XY systems of sex determination led most geneticists to assume that the mechanism of sex determination in humans was the same as in *Drosophila.* This assumption persisted until 1959, when C. E. Ford and K. W. Jones found that a woman with Turner syndrome had an XO chromosome constitution, while P. A. Jacobs and J. A. Strong showed that a man with Klinefelter syndrome had an XXY chromosome constitution. That same year, W. J. Welshons and L. B. Russell demonstrated that XO mice are female. The evidence from these and subsequent studies

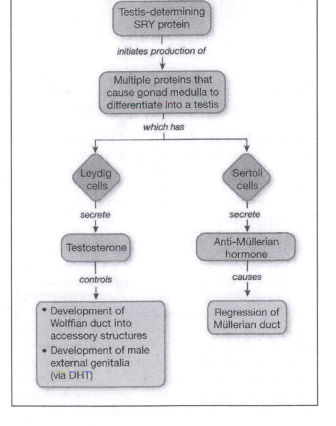

The Wolffian System Pathway By Silverthorn, Dee (Human Physiology: an integrated approach), via Wikimedia Commons

pointed to the presence or absence of the Y chromosome as the principal sex-determining factor in mammals.

People with sex-reversal phenotypes (XY females and XX males) offered clues regarding the molecular mechanism of sex determination in humans. Most XX males had a portion of the Y chromosome translocated onto one of their X chromosomes. The translocated region of the Y chromosome apparently triggered development of the male phenotype and was named the testis determining factor, or *TDF.*

Gene expression pattern of the SRY gene. Genomics Institute of the Novartis Research Foundation, via Wikimedia Commons

Analysis by Peter Good fellow and coworkers of these Y-derived translocated sequences in XX males narrowed the region on the Y chromosome containing *TDF* to a 35-kilobase (kb) segment. Within this segment is an open-reading frame, which they named *SRY*, for sex-determining region Y. Evidence that *SRY* is *TDF* in humans accumulated as numerous XY females were found to have mutations in the region of *SRY* encoding the DNA-binding domain. Moreover, Good fellow and coworkers provided powerful evidence that *SRY* is the testis determining factor when they recovered a phenotypically male XX mouse that was transgenic for the region containing the mouse orthologue *Sry*. The accumulated evidence points to *SRY* as the initial trigger that determines male phenotypic development, although other genes on the Y chromosome, the X chromosome, and autosomes are essential for development of male and female phenotypes and for fertility.

MOLECULAR GENETICS AND EVOLUTION

SRY is a relatively small (3.8-kb) intronless gene that encodes a transcription factor with an HMG (high mobility group) DNA-binding domain. This region encoding this domain is highly conserved in all therian mammals. The sequences within the gene on either side of this conserved region, however, are highly variable among species, indicative of very rapid evolution. The platypus, by contrast, has a different sex-determination mechanism, governed by five X chromosomes and five Y chromosomes. These chromosomes are most closely related to the bird Z chromosome. The therian X and Y chromosomes probably evolved from an ancient autosomal pair of chromosomes ancestral to

platypus chromosome 6 after the divergence of therian mammals and monotremes, approximately 166 million years ago.

IMPACT

The most significant clinical effect of mutations in *SRY* is sex reversal. Nearly all nonsynonymous mutations within the region that encodes the HMG domain result in complete sex reversal, observed as an XY individual with an unambiguous female phenotype. However, a particular mutation in this region has been associated with true hermaphroditism and has also been found in fully fertile male relatives, indicating that it is not fully penetrant.

Daniel J. Fairbanks, Ph.D.

FURTHER READING

Carlson, Elof Axel. *The 7 Sexes: Biology of Sex Determination.* Bloomington: Indiana UP, 2013. Print.

Coward, Kevin, and Dagan Wells. *Textbook of Clinical Embryology.* New York: Cambridge UP, 2013. Print.

Goodfellow, Peter N., and Robin Lovell-Badge. "*SRY* and Sex Determination in Mammals." *Annual Review of Genetics* 27 (1993): 71–92. Print

Richardson, Sarah S. *Sex Itself: The Search for Male and Female in the Human Genome.* Chicago: U of Chicago P, 2013. Print.

Sinclair, A. H., et al. "A Gene from the Human Sex-Determining Region Encodes a Protein with Homology to a Conserved DNA-Binding Motif." *Nature* 346 (1990): 240–45. Print.

Veyrunes, F., et al. "Bird-Like Sex Chromosomes of Platypus Imply Recent Origin of Mammal Sex Chromosomes." *Genome Research* 18 (2008): 965–73. Print.

See also: also: Androgen insensitivity syndrome; Gender identity; Hermaphrodism; Homosexuality; Klinefelter syndrome; Metafemales; Pseudohermaphrodites; Steroid hormones; Turner syndrome; X inactivation; XYY syndrome.

Stargardt's disease

CATEGORY: Diseases and syndromes
ALSO KNOWN AS: Fundus flavimaculatus

DEFINITION

Stargardt's disease is the most common form of inherited juvenile macular degeneration, an eye disorder that causes vision loss. An abnormal collection of fatty yellow pigment called lipfuscin damages the cells of the macula, an area of the retina. It is al most always inherited through an autosomal recessive mode of inheritance, but up to 10 percent of cases may be inherited in an autosomal dominant mode.

RISK FACTORS

Stargardt's disease is an inherited disease; there are no steps that can be taken to avoid developing the disease. Men and women are affected with Stargardt's disease equally. It affects 1 in 8,000 to 10,000 individuals worldwide.

ETIOLOGY AND GENETICS

Stargardt's disease is usually diagnosed after the age of six but before the age of twenty; however, in some cases, the vision loss may not be noticed until age thirty or forty. The gene for the autosomal recessive form of Stargardt's disease was found on the short arm of chromosome 1 and is called the ABCR or ABCA4 gene. The specific gene has been localized to 1p22.1. This gene produces an ATP-binding transport protein; with the mutated gene, the defective protein is unable to perform its transport function and get rid of waste in the cells. This protein is expressed in the inner rod segments, and the defect leads to degeneration of these cells in the retina and vision loss.

However, only 60 percent of people with Star gardt's, or fundus flavimaculatus, have a mutation in the ABCA4 gene. Further research has shown that this locus is involved in the development of age related macular degeneration, autosomal recessive retinitis pigmentosa, and autosomal recessive rod cone dystrophy. It is thought that these diseases are part of a continuum. As with all autosomal recessive disorders, a person must inherit both copies of the gene in each cell from both parents. Children of two carriers have a 25% chance of being affected, a 50% chance of being an asymptomatic carrier, and a 25% chance of being unaffected and not a carrier.

In the more rare autosomal dominant Stargardt's disease, the defect has been mapped to chromosome 6q14.1 and is associated with the mutation located on the ELOVL4 gene. This gene codes for a membrane bound protein that is involved in long-chain fatty acid biosynthesis. Other retinal diseases have been traced back to chromosome 6, such as recessive retinitis pigmentosa, Leber congenital amaurosis, and North Carolina macular dystrophy. Children born to individuals with the ELOVL4 mutation have a 50% chance of inheriting the condition.

SYMPTOMS

The main symptom is bilateral decreased central vision starting in childhood and young adulthood. This vision loss manifests itself as bilateral central scotomas. Color vision is also impacted, but it usually is not noticeable until the later stages of the disease. People with Stargardt's disease generally do not have any decrease in peripheral vision but may have problems with night vision.

SCREENING AND DIAGNOSIS

For people whose parents or genetically related siblings have a diagnosed retinal disease, there should be a genetic screening test done to rule out Stargardt's disease or one of the other related conditions. For many patients, however, this may not be an option, and the disease may be misdiagnosed in the early stages because of lack of changes in the retina. As the disease progresses, there may be yellowish "pisciform" flecks at the level of the retinal pigment epithelium at the posterior pole; a bull's-eye type pattern of retinal degeneration may also become evident later in the disease. Areas of regional geographic atrophy also give the macula what is known as a "beaten bronze" appearance.

Diagnostic tests that may be used to diagnose Stargardt's disease include fluoroscein angiography(FA), fundus autofluorescence (FAF), optical coherence tomography (OCT), and electrooculography. In Stargardt's disease, the FA shows what is known as a dark or silent choroid, irregular hyperfluorescent spots, and the bull's-eye pattern of retinal degeneration. The electrooculography test tends to be subnormal. Visual field tests will be obtained to create a map of the visual field along with visual acuity tests. Genetic testing can confirm the diagnosis.

TREATMENT AND THERAPY

At this time, there is no known treatment for Stargardt's disease. Because of the role of ABCA4 in the processing of vitamin A, some researchers feel that excess vitamin A might make the disease worse. Wearing sunglasses to protect the eyes is often recommended. Gene therapy treatment shows promising results and orphan status in Europe. Other drugs are being tested to prevent the toxic buildup in the macula from the inability to process vitamin A. Clinical trials are underway.

PREVENTION AND OUTCOMES

Genetic screening in couples where one person is known to have the disease or where family members are known to have the disease may help determine if any future children are at risk of developing the disease. It is thought that bright lights and ultra violet rays may accelerate the progression of Star gardt's disease, so it is suggested that people with Stargardt's disease should avoid bright lights and wear UV-blocking sunglasses as much as possible. Early onset, on or before age 10, is associated with the most severe form.

An important factor in improving outcomes in people with Stargardt's disease is to learn about available low vision services and aids that can help a person live a full and functional life.

Dominique Walton Brooks, M.D., M.B.A.; updated by
Deanna M. Neff, M.P.H.

FURTHER READING

Fujinami K, Zernant J, Chana R K, et al. "Clinical and molecular characteristics of childhood-onset Stargardt disease". *Ophthalmology.* 2015;122: 326–334.

Hartnett, Mary Elizabeth, et al. "Pediatric Retina: Medical and Surgical Approaches". Illustrated ed. Philadelphia: Lippincott Williams & Wilkins, 2004. This book looks at pediatric retinal diseases.

Ho, Allen C., et al. *Retina: Color Atlas and Synopsis of Clinical Ophthalmology.* Illustrated ed. New York: McGraw-Hill Professional, 2003. A combination of illustrated atlas and reference book that is easy to understand.

Regillo, Carl D., Gary C. Brown, and Harry W.

Flynn. *Vitreoretinal Disease: The Essentials.* Illustrated ed. New York: Thieme Medical, 1999. This book makes it easier to understand recent ophthalmologic advances.

Lambertus S., van Huet R. A. C., Bax N. M., et al. "Early-onset Stargardt disease: phenotypic and genotypic characteristics. Ophthalmology". 2015; 122: 335–344.

Gene expression pattern of the ABCA4 gene. Genomics Institute of the Novartis Research Foundation, via Wikimedia Commons

figure created by me in chemdraw and illustrator. Roadnottaken at the English language Wikipedia, via Wikimedia Commons

Song H., Rossi E. A., Latchney L., et al. "Cone and rod loss in Stargardt disease revealed by adaptive optics scanning light ophthalmoscopy". *JAMA Ophthal.* 2015; 133: 1198–1203.

Yanoff, Myron, Jay S. Duker, and James J. Augsburger. *Ophthalmology.* 3d ed. New York: Elsevier Health Sciences, 2009. Updated edition of reference book that offers information about almost every ophthalmic condition.

WEB SITES OF INTEREST

American Macular Degeneration Foundation
http://www.macular.org/

Genetic and Rare Diseases Information Center
https://rarediseases.info.nih.gov/diseases

Genetics Home Reference
https://ghr.nlm.nih.gov/condition

Lighthouse International
http://www.lighthouse.org/medical/eye-disorders/
    stargardts-disease/

Macular Degeneration Foundation
http://www.eyesight.org

Macular Degeneration Support
http://www.mdsupport.org/librar y/stargrdt.html

See also: Aniridia; Best disease; Choroideremia; Color blindness; Corneal dystrophies; Glaucoma; Gyrate atrophy of the choroid and retina; Macular degeneration; Norrie syndrome; Progressive external ophthalmoplegia; Retinitis pigmentosa; Retino blastoma.

Sterilization laws

CATEGORY: Human genetics and social issues

SIGNIFICANCE: Forced sterilization for eugenic reasons became legal throughout much of the United States and many parts of the world during the first half of the twentieth century. Though sterilization is an ineffective mechanism for changing the genetic makeup of a population, various sterilization laws remain in effect in many countries throughout the world.

KEY TERMS

negative eugenics: the effort to improve the human species by discouraging or eliminating reproduction among those deemed to be socially or physically unfit

positive eugenics: the effort to encourage more prolific breeding among "gifted" individuals

sterilization: an operation to make reproduction impossible; in tubal ligation, doctors sever the fallopian tubes so that a woman cannot conceive a child

THE EUGENICS MOVEMENT AND STERILIZATION LAWS

The founder of the eugenics movement is considered to be Sir Francis Galton (1822–1911), who carried out extensive genetic studies of human traits. He thought that the human race would be improved by encouraging humans with desirable traits (such as intelligence, good character, and musical ability) to have more children than those people with less desirable traits (positive eugenics). With the development of Mendelian genetics shortly after the beginning of the twentieth century, research on improving the genetic quality of plants and animals was in full swing. Success with plants and domestic animals made it inevitable that interest would develop in applying those principles to the improvement of human beings. As some human traits became known to be under the control of single genes, some geneticists began to claim that all sorts of traits (including many behavioral traits and even social characteristics and preferences) were under the control of a single gene, with little regard for the possible impact of environmental factors.

The Eugenics Record Office at Cold Spring Harbor, New York, was set up by Charles Davenport to gather and collate information on human traits. The eugenics movement became a powerful political force that led to the creation and implementation of laws restricting immigration and regulating reproduction. Some geneticists and politicians reasoned that since mental retardation and other "undesirable" behavioral and physical traits were affected by genes, society had an obligation and a moral right to restrict the reproduction of individuals with "bad genes" (negative genetics).

Exhibit depicting the status compulsory sterilization legislation in the United States in 1921. public domain via wikimedia commons

The couple is in front of a map of Germany, surrounded by the flags of nations which had enacted (to the left) or were considering (bottom and to the right) similar legislation. public domain via wikimedia commons

The state of Indiana passed the first compulsory sterilization law in 1907, which permitted the involuntary sterilization of inmates in state institutions. Inmates included not only "imbeciles," "idiots," and others with varying degrees of intellectual disability (described as "feeble-mindedness") but also people who were committed for behavioral problems such as criminality, swearing, promiscuity, and slovenliness. By 1911, similar laws had been passed in six states, and by the end of the 1920s, twenty-four states had similar sterilization laws. Ultimately, thirty-three states enacted sterilization laws.

The US Supreme Court, in its 1927 *Buck v. Bell* decision, supported the eugenic principle that states could use involuntary sterilization to eliminate genetic defects from the population. The vote of the court was eight to one. The court's reasoning went as follows:

"We have seen more than once that the public welfare may call upon the best citizens for their lives. It would be strange if it could not call upon those who already sap the strength of the state for these lesser sacrifices, often not felt to be such by those concerned, in order to prevent our being swamped with incompetence. It is better for all the world, if instead of waiting to execute degenerate offspring for crime, or to let them starve for their imbecility, society can prevent those who are manifestly unfit from continuing their kind. The principle that sustains compulsory vaccination is broad enough to cover cutting the Fallopian tubes".

Ironically, the sterilization laws of the United States and Canada served as models for the eugenics movement in Nazi Germany in its program to ensure so-called racial purity and superiority.

IMPACT AND APPLICATIONS

Two problems associated with eugenics are the subjective nature of deciding which traits are desirable and determining who should decide. These concerns aside, the question of whether there is a sound scientific basis for the desire to manipulate the human gene pool remains. Does the sterilization of individuals who are intellectually disabled or who have some other mental or physical impairment improve the human genetic composition? Involuntary sterilization of affected individuals would quickly reduce the incidence of dominant genetic traits. Individuals who were homozygous for recessive traits would also be eliminated. However, most harmful recessive genes are carried by individuals who appear normal and, therefore, would not be "obvious" for sterilization purposes. These "normal" people would continue to pass on the "bad" gene to the next generation, and a certain number of affected people would again be born. It would take an extraordinary number of generations to significantly reduce the frequency of harmful genes.

The impact sterilization laws had on the US population by 1960 was far-reaching, as some sixty thousand people were sterilized. In 1978, the federal government passed legislation requiring full, informed consent and a waiting period of more than a month before a publicly funded sterilization may be performed. Other countries also had laws that allowed forced sterilizations, with many programs continuing into the 1970s. The province of Alberta, Canada, sterilized three thousand people before its law was repealed. Another sixty thousand were sterilized in Sweden. The story of sterilization and "euthanasia" in Germany needs no retelling. According to Paul Samakow, legal advice contributor to the *Washington Times*, China and India continued to perform forced sterilizations, sometimes en masse, in the 2010s for reasons of population control. As the United Nations and World Health Organization stated in their inter-agency statement *Eliminating Forced, Coercive and Otherwise Involuntary Sterilization* (2014), involuntary and/or coercive sterilizations of specific populations, such as those with disabilities and those belonging to ethnic, racial, or sexual minority groups, continues around the world. With the ability to decipher the human genome and implement improved genetic testing procedures, a danger exists that new institutionalized programs of eugenics might once again emerge.

Donald J. Nash, Ph.D.

Further Reading

Campbell, Annily. *Childfree and Sterilized: Women's Decisions and Medical Responses.* New York: Cassell, 1999. Print.

42 e-CFR 441 Subpart F—Sterilizations. *Electronic Code of Federal Regulations.* GPO, 4 Aug. 2014. Web. 6 Aug. 2014.

Cussins, Jessica. "Involuntary Sterilization Then and Now." *Psychology Today.* Sussex, 5 Sept. 2013. Web. 6 Aug. 2014.

Gallagher, Nancy L. *Breeding Better Vermonters: The Eugenics Program in the Green Mountain State.* Hanover: UP of New England, 2000. Print.

Human Rights Watch. "Sterilization of Women and Girls with Disabilities: A Briefing Paper." *HRW. org.* Human Rights Watch, 10 Nov. 2011. Web. 6 Aug. 2014.

Kevles, Daniel J. *In the Name of Eugenics: Genetics and the Uses of Human Heredity.* 1995. Cambridge: Harvard UP, 2004. Print.

Lombardo, Paul A. *Three Generations, No Imbeciles: Eugenics, the Supreme Court, and* Buck v. Bell. Baltimore: Johns Hopkins UP, 2010. Print.

Mason, J. K. "Unsuccessful Sterilization." *The Troubled Pregnancy: Legal Wrongs and Rights in Reproduction.* New York: Cambridge UP, 2007. Print.

Meyers, David W. *The Human Body and the Law: A Medico-Legal Study.* New Brunswick: Aldine Transaction, 2006. Print.

Office of the High Commissioner for Human Rights, UN Human Rights Office, UN Women, the Joint UN Programme on HIV and AIDS (UNAIDS), the United Nations Development Programme (UNDP), the United Nations Population Fund (UNFPA), the United Nations Children's Fund (UNICEF), and the World Health Organization (WHO). *Eliminating Forced, Coercive and Otherwise Involuntary Sterilization.* Geneva: Dept. of Reproductive Health and Research, World Health Organization, 2014. PDF file.

Samakow, Paul. "Forced Sterilization of Mentally Incompetent Man Legal in Britain." *Washington Times Communities.* Washington Times, 2013. Web. 6 Aug. 2014.

See also: Criminality; Eugenics; Eugenics: Nazi Germany; Hardy-Weinberg law; Miscegenation and antimiscegenation laws; Race.

Steroid hormones

Category: Developmental genetics; Molecular genetics

Significance: Steroid hormones—hormones containing a steroid ring derived from cholesterol—are important for many processes that control sex determination, reproduction, behavior, and metabolism. Mutations in the genes that produce or regulate the action of specific steroid hormones may lead to infertility, sterility, sex determination, osteoporosis, autoimmune diseases, heart abnormalities, and breast, uterine, and prostate cancer.

Key terms

anabolic steroids: drugs derived from androgens and used to enhance performance in sports

androgens: steroid hormones that cause masculinization

estrogens: steroid hormones that produce female characteristics

glucocorticoids: steroid hormones that respond to stress and maintain sugar, salt, and body fluid levels

hormones: chemical messengers produced by endocrine glands and secreted into the blood

mineralocorticoids: a group of steroid hormones important for maintenance of salt and water balance

progestins: steroid hormones important for pregnancy and breast development *testosterone:* the principal androgen, produced by the testes and responsible for male secondary sexual characteristics

STEROID HORMONE CHARACTERISTICS AND FUNCTION

Steroid hormones represent a group of hormones that all contain a characteristic "steroid" ring structure. This steroid ring is derived from cholesterol, and cholesterol is the starting material for the production of different steroid hormones. Steroid hormones, like other types of hormones, are secreted by endocrine glands into the bloodstream and travel throughout the body before having an effect. All steroid hormones, although specific for the regulation of certain genes, function in a similar manner. Because steroid hormones are derived from cholesterol, they have the unique ability to diffuse through a cell's outer plasma membrane. Inside the cell, the steroid hormone binds to its specific receptor in the cytoplasm. Upon binding, the newly formed hormone-receptor complex relocates to the nucleus. In the nucleus, the hormone-receptor complex binds to the DNA in the promoter region of certain genes at specific nucleotide sequences termed hormone-responsive elements. The binding of the hormone-receptor complex to hormone-responsive elements causes the increased production of transcription and protein production in most cases. In some instances, binding to a specific hormone-responsive element will stop the production of proteins that are usually made in the absence of the hormone.

Chemical structure of 11-ketotestosterone By Boghog2 (Own work), via Wikimedia Commons

Estetrol By Gabethenerd (Own work), via Wikimedia Commons

There are two types (sex steroid and adrenal steroid) and five classes of steroid hormones. The sex steroid hormones include the androgens, estrogens, and progestins and are produced by the male testes (androgens) and female ovaries. Adrenal steroid hormones include glucocorticoids and mineralocorticoids and are produced by the adrenal glands.

SEX STEROID HORMONES

Sex steroid hormone genes are responsible for determining the sex and development of males and females. Androgens are a group of steroid hormones that cause masculinization. The principal androgen is testosterone, which is produced by the testes and is responsible for male secondary sexual characteristics (growth of facial and pubic hair, deepening of voice, sperm production). Estrogens are sex steroid hormones produced in the ovaries and cause femininization. In addition, estrogens control calcium content in the bones, modulate other hormones produced in the ovary, modify sexual behavior, regulate secondary sex characteristics (menstrual periods, breast development, growth of pubic hair), and are essential for pregnancy to occur. The most potent estrogen is 17-beta estradiol. Progestins, including progesterone, are also sex steroid hormones. Progesterone is important for proper breast development and normal and healthy pregnancies; it functions in the mother to alter endometrial cells so the embryo can implant. The loss of progesterone at the end of a pregnancy aids in the beginning of uterine contractions.

Anabolic steroids are drugs derived from the male steroid hormone testosterone and were developed in the late 1930s to treat hypogonadism in men, a condition that results in insufficient testosterone production by the testes. During this same period, scientists discovered that anabolic steroids also increased the muscle mass in animals. These findings led to the use of anabolic steroids by bodybuilders, weightlifters, and other athletes to increase muscle mass and enhance performance. Anabolic steroid use can seriously affect the long-term health of an individual and in women results in masculinization.

Adrenal Steroid Hormones

Adrenal steroid hormones are secreted from the adrenal cortex and are important for many bodily functions, including response to stress and maintenance of blood sugar levels, fluid balance, and electrolytes. The glucocorticoids represent one class of adrenal steroid hormone. The most important, cortisol, performs critically important functions; it helps to maintain blood pressure and can decrease the response of the body's immune system. Cortisol can also elevate blood sugar levels and helps to control the amount of water in the body. Elevated cortisol helps the body respond to stress. The glucocorticoids cortisone and hydrocortisone are used as anti-inflammatory drugs to control itching, swelling, pain, and other inflammatory reactions. Prednisone and prednisolone, also members of the glucocorticoid class of hormones, are the broadest anti-inflammatory and immunosuppressive medications available.

The second class of adrenal steroid hormones is the mineralocorticoids, including aldosterone, which helps maintain salt and water balance and increases blood pressure. Aldosterone is crucial for retaining sodium in the kidney, salivary glands, sweat glands, and colon.

Genetic Defects Affecting Sex Steroid Hormones

Defects in the genes involved in the production of sex steroid hormones can have serious consequences. Mutations in the androgen receptor, the receptor for testosterone, result in androgen insensitivity syndrome. In this syndrome, the individual has the genes of a male (XY) but develops, behaves, and appears female. Other gene defects in androgen biosynthesis often result in sterility. Genetic defects in estrogen receptors or estradiol biosynthesis lead to infertility. Reduced levels of estradiol have also been linked to bone loss (osteoporosis) and infertility, whereas excessive levels are associated with an increased risk of breast and uterine cancer. Similarly, genetic mutations in the progesterone production pathway or the progesterone receptor are associated with infertility. In addition, bone loss is one of the most serious results of progesterone deficiency, made worse by inappropriate diet and lack of exercise.

Genetic Defects Affecting Adrenal Steroid Hormones

Genetic abnormalities in adrenal steroid hormone biosynthesis are known to cause hypertension in some cases of congenital adrenal hyperplasia (CAH). In people with this condition, hypertension usually accompanies a characteristic phenotype with abnormal sexual differentiation. CAH is a family of autosomal recessive disorders of adrenal steroidogenesis. Each disorder has a specific pattern of hormonal abnormalities resulting from a deficiency of one of the enzymes necessary for cortisol synthesis. The most common form of CAH is 21-hydroxylase deficiency; however, in all forms, cortisol production is impaired, which results in an increase in adrenocorticotropin and the overproduction of androgen steroids.

There are two major forms of 21-hydroxylase deficiency. Classic CAH deficiency results in masculinized girls who are born with genital ambiguity and may possess both female and male genitalia. Nonclassic 21-hydroxylase deficiency does not produce ambiguous genitalia in female infants but may result in premature puberty, short stature, menstrual irregularities or lack of a menstrual cycle, and infertility. Familial glucocorticoid deficiency (FGD) is an extremely rare, genetic autosomal recessive condition in which a part of the adrenal glands is destroyed. These changes result in very low levels of cortisol. Although this disease is easily treatable if recognized, when left untreated it is often fatal or can lead to severe mental disability.

The genetic basis of four forms of severe hypertension transmitted on an autosomal basis has also been determined. All of these conditions are characterized by salt-sensitive increases in blood pressure, indicating an increased mineralocorticoid effect. The four disorders—aldosteronism, mineralocorticoid excess syndrome, activating mutation of the mineralocorticoid receptor, and Liddle syndrome—are a consequence of either abnormal biosynthesis, abnormal metabolism, or abnormal action of steroid hormones and the development of hypertension. Adrenal insufficiency is known as Addison's disease and causes death within two weeks unless treated. Classical Addison's disease results from a loss of both cortisol and aldosterone secretion as a result of the near total or total destruction of both adrenal glands.

Thomas L. Brown, Ph.D.

FURTHER READING

Burnstein, Kerry L., ed. *Steroid Hormones and Cell Cycle Regulation*. Boston: Kluwer Academic, 2002. Print.

Ethier, Stephen P., ed. *Endocrine Oncology*. Humana, 2000. Print.

Freedman, Leonard P., and M. Karin, eds. *Molecular Biology of Steroid and Nuclear Hormone Receptors*. Boston: Birkhauser, 1999. Print.

Jameson, J. Larry, ed. *Harrison's Endocrinology*. New York: McGraw, 2006. Print.

Khan, Sohaib A., and George M. Stancel, eds. *Protooncogenes and Growth Factors in Steroid Hormone Induced Growth and Differentiation*. Boca Raton: CRC, 1994. Print.

Moudgil, V. K., ed. *Steroid Hormone Receptors: Basic and Clinical Aspects*. Boston: Birkhauser, 1994. Print.

National Institutes of Health. *Steroid Abuse and Addiction*. NIH 00-3721. Bethesda: Author, 2000. Print.

New, Maria I., et al. *Genetic Steroid Disorders*. Philadelphia: Academic: 2013. Print.

Newton, David E. *Steroids and Doping in Sports: A Reference Handbook*. Santa Barbara: ABC-CLIO, 2014.

Salway, Jack G. "Steroid Hormones: Aldosterone, Cortisol, Androgens, and Oestrogens." *Medical Biochemistry at a Glance*. 3rd ed. Chichester: Wiley, 2012. Print.

Strauss, Jerome F., III, and Robert L. Barbieri, eds. *Yen and Jaffe's Reproductive Endocrinology: Physiology, Pathophysiology, and Clinical Management*. 7th ed. Philadelphia: Saunders/Elsevier, 2014. Digital file.

Tilly, J., J. F. Strauss III, and M. Tenniswood, eds. *Cell Death in Reproductive Physiology*. New York: Springer, 1997. Print.

Wynn, Ralph M., and W. Jollie, eds. *Biology of the Uterus*. 2nd rev. ed. Boston: Kluwer Academic, 1989. Print.

Zorea, Aharon W. *Steroids*. Santa Barbara: Greenwood, 2014. Print.

See also: Aggression; Allergies; Androgen insensitivity syndrome; Autoimmune disorders; Behavior; Cancer; Gender identity; Heart disease; Hermaphrodites; Human genetics; Metafemales; Pseudohermaphrodites; X chromosome inactivation; XYY syndrome.

Sulfite oxidase deficiency

CATEGORY: Diseases and syndromes

ALSO KNOWN AS: Isolated sulfite oxidase deficiency; sulphite oxidase deficiency

DEFINITION

Sulfite oxidase deficiency is a rare deficiency disease in which there is a defect in the enzyme sulfite oxidase, which metabolizes sulfur amino acids. Isolated sulfite oxidase deficiency is characterized by severe neurological abnormalities, seizures, intellectual disability, physical malformations, and dislocation of ocular lenses and is often fatal in infancy.

RISK FACTORS

Inheritance of sulfite oxidase deficiency is autosomal recessive. Individuals who are heterozygous for this condition have no symptoms. Individuals with this disorder belong to both genders and to various ethnic groups. There is a 25 percent risk of sulfite oxidase deficiency occurring in future children of parents who already have a child with this disorder.

Structural drawing of the sulfite oxidase reaction. public domain via wikimedia commons

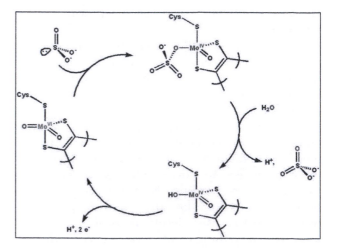

Structural drawing of the proposed mechanism of sulfite oxidase public domain via wikimedia commons

Etiology and Genetics

Sulfite oxidase catalyzes the final reaction in oxidative degradation of sulfur amino acids. Defects in enzyme activity result in sulfite oxidase deficiency. Two conditions that affect enzyme activity include mutations in the enzyme itself and a genetic defect that results in absence of a required molybdenum cofactor.

Normally, the amino acids methionine and cysteine are metabolized to sulfite followed by oxidation to sulfite through the activity of the enzyme sulfite oxidase in a step that requires a molybdenum cofactor. Deficiency of either the enzyme or the cofactor results in similar disease symptoms. A defect in the pathway results in buildup of sulfite, which increases activity of alternate metabolic pathways for sulfite degradation. This results in formation of metabolites, S-sulfocysteine and thiosulfate, which can be used as diagnostic indicators of sulfite oxidase deficiency. The metabolite S-sulfocysteine probably substitutes for cysteine in connective tissues. This substitution weakens the zonule, a tissue in the lens that is normally rich in cysteine, and results in characteristic dislocated lenses associated with this disorder. The pathogenesis of brain damage associated with sulfite oxidase deficiency is not known but is likely related to toxic sulfite accumulation in the brain. As reported by *Orphanet* (January 2012), isolated sulfite oxidase deficiency cases are more rare than those associated with deficiency of the molybdenum cofactor. Individuals with isolated sulfite oxidase deficiency lack sulfite oxidase activity, but are normal with respect to molybdenum cofactor.

Inheritance of isolated sulfite oxidase deficiency is autosomal recessive. Mutations in the gene that codes for sulfite oxidase, *SUOX*, and in genes SUOX that code for molybdenum cofactor components (*MOCS1* or *MOCS2* have been described, although no mutation is clearly predominant. Some mutations in the sulfite oxidase gene have been characterized at the molecular level, with deletions, insertions, and both nonsense and missense mutations identified.

Symptoms

In isolated sulfite oxidase deficiency, severe convulsions begin soon after birth. Individuals with this disorder generally show symptoms such as seizures, neurological disorders, intellectual disability, and physical malformations as newborns. Other symptoms include hypotonia and myclonus. Choreiform movements and symptoms similar to cerebral palsy may be present in individuals with milder forms. Brain pathology in affected individuals shows brain degradation, severe encephalopathy, marked neuronal loss, and white matter demyelination.

Screening and Diagnosis

Although the frequency of sulfite oxidase deficiency is unknown, this disorder is likely underdiagnosed. The condition is rare, with only about fifty cases reported worldwide. A predominance of reported cases in Europe and the United States most likely reflects increased recognition in these areas. Sulfite oxidase deficiency has traditionally been identified in patients during the neonatal period, although an increasing number of diagnoses with later onset have been reported. Elevated urinary sulfite is one indicator used to diagnose sulfite oxidase deficiency; it can be measured using commercially available dipsticks. Enzyme activity in fibroblasts and cofactor levels in liver biopsies are used for confirmation. Sophisticated laboratory techniques can identify characteristic metabolites, S-sulfocysteine and thiosulfate, present in urine or plasma of patients with this disorder. Cranial CT scans or magnetic resonance imaging (MRI) may show characteristic brain abnormalities such as cerebral atrophy, decreased white matter density, neuronal loss, or cerebral edema. Sulfite oxidase activity in chorionic villi or DNA analysis in families known to carry a mutation in the sulfite oxidase gene have been used in prenatal diagnosis.

Treatment and Therapy

There are no effective medical treatments known for sulfite oxidase deficiency, particularly for patients diagnosed in infancy. Treatment for this disorder is supportive. Although diets restricted in cysteine and methionine have been tried and resulted in biochemical improvements, clinical gains were not substantial. Various drug treatments have also been tried, with limited success. High-dose thiamine has been used to replace thiamine destroyed by sulfite. Compounds such as cysteamine and penicillamine have been used to chelate excess sulfite, with some biochemical effects but few or no clinical effects. Some success in controlling seizures has been achieved with the antiepileptic drug vigabatrin.

PREVENTION AND OUTCOMES

Sulfite oxidase deficiency is almost always associated with severe brain damage and death in early childhood, and is generally fatal in infancy. Survival beyond two years is often associated with development of dislocation of the ocular lens and profound intellectual disability. Some cases of individuals with later presentation of sulfite oxidase deficiency symptoms have more favorable outcomes.

FURTHER READING

Bosley, Thomas, et al. "Neurologic Injury in Isolated Sulfite Oxidase Deficiency." *Neurology* 82.10 (2014): P4. Print.

Clarke, Joe T. R. *A Clinical Guide to Inherited Metabolic Diseases.* Cambridge: Cambridge UP, 2002. Print.

"Encephalopathy Due to Sulfite Oxidase Deficiency." *Orphanet.* Orphanet, Jan. 2012. Web. 8 Aug. 2014.

Fernandes, John, Jean-Marie Saudubray, Geroges Van Den Berghe, and John H. Walter. *Inborn Metabolic Diseases.* 4th ed. Berlin: Springer, 2006. Print.

Hoffmann, Georg F., J. Zshocke and W. L. Nyhan. *Inherited Metabolic Diseases: A Clinical Approach.* Berlin: Springer, 2010. Print.

Milunksy, Aubrey. *Genetic Disorders and the Fetus.* Baltimore: Johns Hopkins UP, 2004. Print.

See also: Alkaptonuria; Andersen's disease; Diabetes; Diabetes insipidus; Fabry disease; Forbes disease; Galactokinase deficiency; Galactosemia; Gaucher disease; Glucose galactose malabsorption; Glucose-6-phosphate dehydrogenase deficiency; Glycogen storage diseases; Gm1-gangliosidosis; Hemochromatosis; Hereditary diseases; Hereditary xanthinuria; Hers disease; Homocystinuria; Hunter disease; Hurler syndrome; Inborn errors of metabolism; Jansky-Bielschowsky disease; Kearns-Sayre syndrome; Krabbé disease; Lactose intolerance; Leigh syndrome; Lesch-Nyhan syndrome; McArdle's disease; Maple syrup urine disease; Menkes syndrome; Metachromatic leukodystrophy; Niemann-Pick disease; Ornithine transcarbamylase deficiency; Orotic aciduria; Phenylketonuria (PKU); Pompe disease; Tarui's disease; Tay-Sachs disease.

Synthetic antibodies

CATEGORY: Immunogenetics

SIGNIFICANCE: Synthetic antibodies are artificially produced replacements for natural human antibodies. They are used to treat a variety of illnesses and promise to continue to be an important part of medical technology in the future.

KEY TERMS

antibody: a protein molecule that binds to a substance in order to remove, destroy, or deactivate it
antigen: the substance to which an antibody binds
B cells: white blood cells that produce antibodies
monoclonal antibodies: identical antibodies produced by identical B cells

THE DEVELOPMENT OF ANTIBODY THERAPY

Natural antibodies are protein molecules produced by white blood cells known as B cells in response to the presence of foreign substances. A specific antibody binds to a specific substance, known as an antigen, in a way that renders it harmless or allows it to be removed from the body or destroyed. A person will produce antibodies naturally upon exposure to harmless versions of an antigen, a process known as active immunization. Active immunization was the

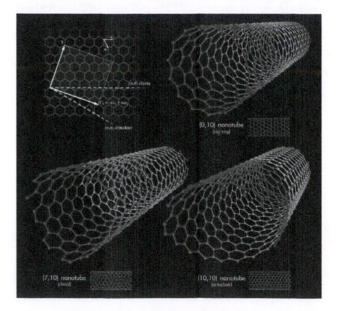

A diagram showing the types of carbon nanotubes. By User Mstroeck on en.wikipedia, via Wikimedia Commons

first form of antibody therapy to be developed and is used to prevent diseases such as measles and polio.

The oldest method of producing therapeutic antibodies outside the human body is known as passive immunization. This process involves exposing an animal to an antigen so that it develops antibodies to it. The antibodies are separated from the animal's blood and administered to a patient. Passive immunization is used to treat diseases such as rabies and diphtheria. A disadvantage of antibodies derived from animal blood is the possibility that the patient may develop an allergic reaction. Because the animal's antibodies are foreign substances, the patient's own antibodies may treat them as antigens, leading to fever, rash, itching, joint pain, swollen tissues, and other symptoms. Antibodies derived from human blood are much less likely to cause allergic reactions than antibodies from the blood of other animals. This led researchers to seek a way to develop synthetic human antibodies.

A major breakthrough in the search for synthetic antibodies was made in 1975 by Cesar Milstein and Georges Köhler. They developed a technique that allowed them to produce a specific antibody outside the body of a living animal. This method involved exposing an animal to an antigen, causing it to produce antibodies. Instead of obtaining the antibodies from the animal's blood, they obtained B cells from the animal's spleen. These cells are then combined with abnormal B cells known as myeloma cells. Unlike normal B cells, myeloma cells can reproduce identical copies of themselves an unlimited number of times. The normal B cells and the myeloma cells fuse to form cells known as hybridoma cells. Hybridoma cells are able to reproduce an unlimited number of times and are able to produce the same antibodies as the B cells. Those hybridoma cells that produce the desired antibody are separated from the others and allowed to reproduce. The antibodies produced this way are known as monoclonal antibodies.

Because human B cells do not normally form stable hybridoma cells with myeloma cells, B cells from mice have been used. Because mouse antibodies are not identical to human antibodies, they may be treated as antigens by the patient's own antibodies, leading to allergic reactions. During the 1980s and 1990s, researchers began to develop methods of producing synthetic antibodies that were similar or identical to human antibodies. An antibody consists of a variable region, which binds to the antigen, and a constant region. The risk of allergic reactions can be reduced by combining variable regions derived from mouse hybridoma cells with constant regions from human cells. The risk can be further reduced by identifying the exact sites on the mouse variable region that are necessary for binding and integrating these sites into human variable regions. This method produces synthetic antibodies that are very similar to human antibodies.

Other methods exist to produce synthetic antibodies that are identical to human antibodies. A species of virus known as the Epstein-Barr virus can be used to change human B cells in such a way that they will fuse with myeloma cells to form stable hybridoma cells that produce human antibodies. Another method involves using genetic engineering to produce mice with B cells that produce human antibodies rather than mouse antibodies. One of the most promising techniques has been the creation of libraries of synthetic human antibodies. This process is done by using the polymerase chain reaction (PCR) to produce multiple copies of the genetic material within B cells. This genetic material contains the information that results in the production of proteins that come together to form antibodies. By causing these proteins to be produced and allowing them to combine at random, researchers are able to produce millions of different antibodies. The antibodies are then tested to detect those that bind to selected antigens.

IMPACT AND APPLICATIONS

Some synthetic antibodies are used to help prevent the rejection of transplanted organs. An antibody that binds to the heart drug digoxin can be used to treat overdoses of that drug. Antibodies attached to radioactive isotopes are used in certain diagnostic procedures. Synthetic antibodies have also been used in patients undergoing a heart procedure known as a percutaneous transluminal coronary angioplasty (PTCA). The use of a particular synthetic antibody has been shown to reduce the risk of having one of the blood vessels that supply blood to the heart shut down during or after a PTCA. Researchers also hope to develop synthetic antibodies to treat acquired immunodeficiency syndrome (AIDS) and septic shock, a syndrome caused by toxic substances released by certain bacteria.

The most active area of research involving synthetic antibodies in the 1990s was in the treatment of cancer. On November 26, 1997, the US Food and Drug Administration approved a synthetic antibody for use in non-Hodgkin's lymphoma, non-Hodgkins a cancer synthetic antibodies of the white blood cells. It was the first synthetic antibody approved for use in cancer therapy.

Antibodies are important for immune system protection against pathogens. They are also important tools in biological research, as with the use of antibodies to help determine the structure of cellular proteins. There may be a role for synthetic antibodies in determining the structure of RNA as well. RNA is genetic material that works with DNA. DNA is the master genetic code, but the role of RNA is a crucial one. More information on RNA structure may unveil more information on RNA function.

New approaches to therapeutic synthetic antibodies are in development. One approach involves the production of symphobodies. Symphobodies are made up of several different synthetic antibodies attacking a variety of antigens on the same target. These targets can be tumor or cancer cells or whole organisms such as viruses. Multiple synthetic antibody attacks on the same pathogen could result in more effective treatment.

Rose Secrest; M.D,
Richard P. Capriccioso, M.D.

FURTHER READING

Coghlan, Andy. "A Second Chance for Antibodies." *New Scientist* 129 (1991). Print.

Doerr, Allison. "RNA Antibodies: Upping the Ante." *Nature Methods* 5.3 (2008): 220. Print.

Inbar, Noa Harel, and Itai Benhar. "Selection of Antibodies from Synthetic Antibody Libraries." *Archives of Biochemistry and Biophysics* 526.2, Sp. Iss. SI (n.d.): 87–98. *Biological Abstracts*. Web. 4 Sept. 2014.

Kontermann, Roland, and Stefan Dübel, eds. *Antibody Engineering*. New York: Springer, 2001. Print.

Mayforth, Ruth D. *Designing Antibodies*. San Diego: Academic, 1993. Print.

Miersch, S., and S. S. Sidhu. "Synthetic Antibodies: Concepts, Potential and Practical Considerations." *Methods* 57.4 (2012): 486-498. *Biological Abstracts*. Web. 4 Sept. 2014.

"The Next Generation of Antibody Therapeutics?" *Pharmaceutical & Diagnostic Innovation* 4.11 (2006): 13–14. Print.

Weber, Marcel, et al. "A Highly Functional Synthetic Phage Display Library Containing over Forty Billion Human Antibody Clones." *Plos ONE* 9.6 (2014): 1–9. *Academic Search Complete*. Web. 4 Sept. 2014.

See also: Allergies; Anthrax; Antibodies; Autoimmune disorders; Biopharmaceuticals; Blotting: Southern, Northern, and Western; Burkitt's lymphoma; Cancer; Central dogma of molecular biology; Cloning; Diabetes; Genetic engineering: Historical development; Genetic engineering: Industrial applications; Hybridomas and monoclonal antibodies; Immunogenetics; Molecular genetics; Multiple alleles; Oncogenes; Organ transplants and HLA genes; Prion diseases: Kuru and Creutzfeldt-Jakob syndrome; Transgenic organisms.

Synthetic genes

CATEGORY: Genetic engineering and biotechnology

SIGNIFICANCE: Synthetic genes have been shown to function in biological organisms. Scientists hope that it will prove possible to restore normal function in diseased humans, animals, and plants by replacing defective natural genes with appropriately modified synthetic genes.

KEY TERMS

restriction enzyme: an enzyme that cleaves, or cuts, DNA at specific sites with sequences recognized by the enzyme; also called restriction endonucleases

reverse transcription: the synthesis of DNA from RNA

A BRIEF HISTORY

In 1871, Swiss physician Johann Friedrich Miescher reported that the chief constituent of the cell nucleus was nucleoprotein, or nuclein. Later it was established that the nuclei of bacteria contained little or no protein, so the hereditary material was named nucleic acid. At the end of the nineteenth century, German biochemist Albrecht Kossel identified the four nitrogenous bases: the purines adenine (A) and guanine (G) and the pyrimidines cytosine (C) and uracil (U).

In the 1920s, Phoebus A. Levene and others indicated the existence of two kinds of nucleic acid: ribonucleic acid (RNA) and deoxyribonucleic acid (DNA); the latter contains thymine (T) instead of uracil.

Har Gobind Khorana (1922 – 2011) See page for author, via Wikimedia Commons

The chemical identity of genes began to unfold in 1928, when Frederick Griffith discovered the phenomenon of genetic transformation. Oswald Avery, Colin MacLeod, and Maclyn McCarty (in 1944) and Alfred Hershey and Martha Chase (in 1952) demonstrated that DNA was the hereditary material. Following the elucidation of the structure of DNA in 1953 by James Watson and Francis Crick, pioneering efforts by several scientists led to the eventual synthesis of a gene. The successful enzymatic synthesis of DNA in vitro (in the test tube) in 1956, by Arthur Kornberg and colleagues, and that of RNA by Marianne Grunberg-Manago and Severo Ochoa, also contributed to the development of synthetic genes. In 1961, Marshall Nirenberg and Heinrich Matthaei synthesized polyphenylalanine chains using a synthetic messenger RNA (mRNA).

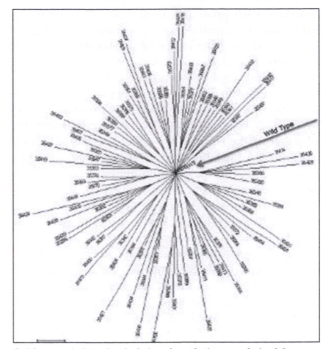

Infologs are independently designed synthetic genes derived from one or a few genes where substitutions are systematically incorporated to maximize information. By Laurawgenesyn (Own work), via Wikimedia Commons

In 1965, Robert W. Holley and colleagues determined the complete sequence of alanine transfer RNA (tRNA) isolated from yeast. The interpretation of the genetic code by several groups of scientists throughout the 1960s was also clearly important.

In 1970, Har Gobind Khorana, along with twelve associates, synthesized the first gene: the gene for an alanine tRNA in yeast. There were no automatic DNA synthesizers available then. In 1976, Khorana's group synthesized the tyrosine suppressor tRNA gene of *Escherichia coli* (*E. coli*). The *lac* operator gene (twenty-one nucleotides long) was also synthesized, introduced into *E. coli*, and demonstrated to be functional. It took ten years to synthesize the first gene; by the mid-1990s, gene machines could synthesize a gene in hours.

GENE SYNTHESIS

Protein engineering is possible by making targeted changes in a DNA sequence to produce a different product (protein) polypeptide with different properties, such as stress tolerance. The process of targeting a specific change in the nucleotide sequence (site-directed mutagenesis) allows the correlation of gene structure with protein function. Rapid sequencing with modern capillary DNA sequencers facilitates determination of the order of nucleotides that make up a gene in a matter of hours.

Once the sequence of a gene is known, it can be synthesized from nucleotides using gene machines. A gene machine is simply a chemical synthesizer made up of tubes, valves, and pumps that bonds nucleotides together in the right order under the direction of a computer. An intelligent person with a minimum of training can produce synthetic genes. A gene may be isolated from an organism using restriction enzymes (any of the several enzymes found in bacteria that serve to chop up the DNA of invading viruses), or it may be made on a gene machine. For example, the chymosin gene (an enzyme used in cheese making) in calves can be synthesized from its known nucleotide sequence instead of isolating it from calf DNA using restriction enzymes. Alternatively, chymosin mRNA can be obtained from calf stomach cells, which can be transformed into DNA through reverse transcription.

New or modified genes may be manufactured to obtain a desired product. Gene synthesis, coupled with automated rapid sequencing and protein analysis, has yielded remarkable dividends in medicine and agriculture. Genetic engineers are designing new proteins from scratch to learn more about protein function and architecture. With synthetic genes, the process of mutagenesis can be explored in greater depth. It is possible to produce various alterations at will in the nucleotide sequence of a gene and observe their effects on protein function. Such studies carry the potential to unravel many biochemical and genetic pathways that could be the key to a better understanding of health and disease.

Manjit S. Kang, Ph.D.

FURTHER READING

Aldridge, Susan. *The Thread of Life: The Story of Genes and Genetic Engineering*. New York: Cambridge UP, 1996. Print.

Carlson, Robert. *Biology Is Technology: The Promise, Peril, and New Business of Engineering Life*. Cambridge: Harvard UP, 2010. Print.

Gibson, Daniel G., et al. "Complete Chemical Synthesis, Assembly, and Cloning of a *Mycoplasma genitalium* Genome." *Science* 319.5867 (29 Feb. 2008): 1215–20. Print.

Greber, David, and Martin Fussenegger. "Synthetic Gene Networks." *Systems Biology and Synthetic Biology*. Ed. Pengcheng Fu and Sven Panke. Hoboken: Wiley, 2009. Print.

Henry, Robert J. *Practical Applications of Plant Molecular Biology*. New York: Chapman, 1997. Print.

Liljeruhm, Josefine, Erik Gullberg, and Anthony C. Forster. *Synthetic Biology: A Lab Manual*. Hackensack: World Scientific, 2014. Print.

Pollack, Andrew. "How Do You Like Your Genes? Biofabs Take Orders." *New York Times*. New York Times, 12 Sept. 2007. Web. 29 Aug. 2014. Print.

Richardson, Sarah M., et al. "GeneDesign: Rapid, Automated Design of Multikilobase Synthetic Genes." *Genome Research* 16.4 (2006): 13. Print.

Specter, Michael. "A Life of Its Own: Where Will Synthetic Biology Lead Us?" *New Yorker* 28 Sept. 2009): 56–65. Print.

Venter, J. Craig. *Life at the Speed of Light: From the Double Helix to the Dawn of Digital Life*. New York: Viking, 2013. Print.

Weber, Wilfried, and Martin Fussenegger. *Synthetic Gene Networks: Methods and Protocols*. New York: Humana, 2012. Print.

See also: Biopharmaceuticals; Cell culture: Plant cells; Cloning; Cloning vectors; DNA sequencing technology; Gene therapy; Genetic engineering; Protein synthesis; Restriction enzymes; Reverse transcriptase; Synthetic antibodies.

T

Tangier disease

CATEGORY: Diseases and syndromes

ALSO KNOWN AS: A-alphalipoprotein neuropathy; alpha high-density lipoprotein deficiency disease; analphalipoproteinemia; cholesterol thesaurismosis; familial high-density lipoprotein deficiency disease; familial hypoalphalipoproteinemia; HDL lipoprotein deficiency disease; lipoprotein deficiency disease, HDL, familial; Tangier disease neuropathy; Tangier hereditary neuropathy

DEFINITION

Tangier disease is a rare, inherited disease that severely reduces blood concentrations of high density lipoprotein (HDL). Cells lack the ability to export fats and cholesterol, and cholesterol accumulates inside cells, causing premature cardiovascular disease and other systemic pathologies.

RISK FACTORS

Because Tangier disease is inherited, it runs in families. A person cannot contract Tangier disease unless both biological parents have at least one mutant copy of the ABCA1 gene. This disease is quite rare, with less than one hundred cases known worldwide, but is it found in many different countries and occurs equally in men and women. It may be underdiagnosed however.

ETIOLOGY AND GENETICS

Mutations in the ABCA1 gene cause Tangier disease, and this disorder is inherited as an autosomal recessive trait. ABCA1 is located on the long arm of chromosome 9 in band 31.1.

To inherit Tangier disease, both parents must carry at least one mutant copy of the ABCA1 gene. Each sibling born to parents who both carry one mutant copy of the ABCA1 gene has a 25 percent chance of contracting Tangier disease.

The ABCA1 gene provides the instructions for the synthesis of a protein called the ATP-binding cassette

Double superhelix model of high density lipoprotein" ACE model showing standardised variance coefficients for a twin study.

Cholesterol By Sbrools (Own work) [GFDL (http://www.gnu.org/copyleft/fdl.html), CC-BY-SA-3.0 (http://creativecommons.org/licenses/by-sa/3.0/) or CC-BY-SA-2.5-2.0-1.0 (http://creativecommons.org/licenses/by-sa/2.5-2.0-1.0)], via Wikimedia Commons

transporter A1. This protein is inserted into cell membranes. The cell membrane delimits the interior of the cell from its exterior, and is composed of phosphate-containing lipids. To function properly, biological membranes must maintain a particular level of fluidity. Animal cells maintain the fluidity of their membranes by interspersing cholesterol molecules between the membrane lipid molecules.

Cholesterol, however, is too bulky a molecule to move across cell membranes without a transport protein. The ATP-binding cassette transporter A1 protein serves as a cholesterol transporter, and it exports lipid and cholesterol molecules from cells.

Since human cells make their own cholesterol and use dietary cholesterol, they must dispose of excess cholesterol. A process called reverse cholesterol transport moves excess cholesterol from the peripheral tissues to the liver where it is converted into bile salts, secreted into the gastrointestinal tract, disposed of in feces. The ATP-binding cassette transporter A1 mediates reverse cholesterol transport.

Reverse cholesterol transport begins when the liver secretes a protein called apoA1 into the blood. ApoA1 binds to blood lipids and forms a nascent discoidal high-density lipoprotein (ndHDL). Cells use the ATP-binding cassette transporter A1 to export lipids and cholesterol into the extracellular spaces and ndHDLs absorb these molecules and use an enzyme called lecithin cholesterol acyltransferase (LCAT) to convert cholesterol into cholesterol esters. This enlarges the ndHDLs and transforms them into spherical, mature HDL particles, which are called HDL-C particles. HDL-C particles are taken up by the liver, and their cholesterol esters are converted into bile salts that are excreted into the small intestine for disposal.

Mutations in the ABCA1 gene that inactivate the ATP-binding cassette transporter A1 protein prevent cells from ridding themselves of excess cholesterol. Without the increased levels of cholesterol near the surfaces of cells, ApoA1 protein molecules never make HDL-C particles and are, instead, rap idly degraded. HDL levels in the blood are extremely low, and cholesterol builds up in cells throughout the body, inflaming tissue, altering cell function, eventually killing cells.

SYMPTOMS

The tonsils are greatly enlarged and have an orange or yellow color. Cholesterol buildup in nerves causes nervous system abnormalities (neuropathy). The large blood vessels show premature buildup of lipids and cholesterol within the inner lining of the vessel wall (atherosclerosis). Mild hypertriglyceridemia is common. Complications include an enlarged spleen (splenomegaly) and liver (hepatomegaly), clouding of the cornea of the eyes, early-onset cardiovascular disease, and type 2 diabetes.

SCREENING AND DIAGNOSIS

Cholesterol deposits in the cornea of the eyes, tonsils, or rectal tissues are diagnostic, especially if combined with unexplained enlargement of the spleen or liver and neurological disturbances. Bio chemically, patients show hypoalphalipoproteinemia, or unusually low blood HDL-C levels (less than 5 mg/dL). Genetic testing to detect mutations in the ABCA1 gene is available.

TREATMENT AND THERAPY

Presently, there is no cure for Tangier disease. Treatment regimes vary, but organs with excessive cholesterol deposits, like the tonsils and spleen, are usually removed. Overall healthy lifestyle and low fat diet are recommended. Treatment of arteriosclerosis requires angioplasty, and coronary artery disease is treated with bypass surgery. Prevention includes reduction of risk factors such as smoking, high blood pressure, diabetes, obesity, high triglycerides and homocysteine. Medications typically show no efficacy, however fibrates can be used to lower triglycerides. Specialized lipid centers and specialist consultation may provide advanced management of the disease.

PREVENTION AND OUTCOMES

The prognosis for Tangier disease is, in most cases, rather good. If patients develop heart disease, then they might have a decreased life span, but this depends on the severity of their disease and the quality of medical care they that receive.

Michael A. Buratovich, Ph.D.; updated by Deanna M. Neff, M.P.H.

FURTHER READING

Andres, Lisa Marie. "Tangier Disease." In Gale Encyclopedia of Genetic Disorders, edited by Stacey L. Blachford. Farmington Hills, Mich.: Thomson Gale, 2005. A focused and easily understood summary of Tangier disease from a genetic and clinical perspective.

Maxfield, Frederick R., and Ira Tabas. "Role of Cholesterol and Lipid Organization in Disease." Nature 438, no. 7068 (2005): 612–621. A technical but very well organized review of cholesterol trafficking and the role of genetic variation in the onset of cardiovascular diseases.

Oram, John. "Tangier Disease and ABCA1." Biochimica et Biophysica Acta 1529 (2000): 321–330. A somewhat technical, biochemical discussion of the link between Tangier disease and the transport protein encoded by the ABCA1 gene. It nicely reviews the research on Tangier disease and other cholesterol-induced pathologies.

Ramasamy I. "Update on the molecular biology of dyslipidemias." Clin chim acta. 2016;454:143–85.

Tietjen I, Hovingh GK, Singaraja R, et al. "Increased self-reported risk of coronary artery disease in Caucasians with extremely low HDL cholesterol due to mutations in ABCA1, APOA1, and LCAT." Biochim biophys acta. 2011.

WEB SITES OF INTEREST

Children Living with Inherited Metabolic Diseases (CLIMB)
http://www.climb.org.uk

Genetics Home Reference: Tangier Disease
http://ghr.nlm.nih.gov/condition=tangierdisease

Medline Plus: HDL Test
http://www.nlm.nih.gov/medlineplus/ency/article/003496.htm

National Organization for Rare Disorders: TangierDisease
http://www.rarediseases.org/search/rdbdetail_abstract.html?disname=Tangier%20Disease

OMIM® Online Mendelian Inheritance in Man
http://www.omim.org/about

Orphanet Journal of Rare Diseases
https://ojrd.biomedcentral.com/

See also: Atherosclerosis; Barlow's syndrome; Cardiomyopathy; Heart disease; Holt-Oram syndrome; Long QT syndrome.

Tarui's disease

CATEGORY: Diseases and syndromes

ALSO KNOWN AS: Glycogenosis type VII; muscle phosphofructokinase deficiency

DEFINITION

Tarui's disease is both a glycogen storage disease and a glycolytic disorder. In glycogen storage diseases, ATP production in muscle tissue is impaired and excessive glycogen amounts are stored in muscles and other tissues. Glycolytic disorders feature a defect in one or more steps in glycogen metabolism. Tarui's disease is caused by an inherited defect in the gene coding for phosphofructokinase (PFK), an enzyme that catalyzes the rate-limiting step in glycolysis.

RISK FACTORS

The main risk factor for Tarui's disease is having a family member who has the disorder. The disease is especially prevalent among Ashkenazi Jewish individuals, with disease onset usually occurring in childhood.

ETIOLOGY AND GENETICS

Tarui's disease is a glycogen storage disease in which the conversion of glycogen to glucose is impaired, resulting in the accumulation of glycogen in tissues. The defective glycogen metabolism is caused by a deficiency in PFK, which catalyzes the rate-limiting conversion of fructose-6-phosphate and fructose-1-phosphate to fructose-1,6-diphosphate. PFK occurs in three forms in humans, the muscle (PFK-M), liver (PFK-L), and platelet (PFK-P) isozymes. PFK-M is the most common form in skeletal muscle, heart, and brain and the only PFK isozyme that metabolizes glucose in muscle. Red blood cells, however, use both PFK-M and PFK-L.

Tarui's disease is inherited as an autosomal recessive trait, meaning that an affected individual will receive one copy of the mutated gene from each parent. J. B. Sherman and colleagues found that the mutation occurs in two major forms in Ashkenazi Tarui's disease patients, as a splicing mutation and as a deletion mutation. The splicing mutation, delta5,

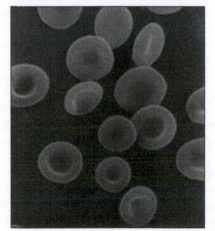

red blood cells, (erythrocytes) public domain via wikimedia commons

Glycolysis diagram. Tekks at en.wikipedia, from Wikimedia Commons

is a G to A point mutation at the 5'-splice donor site of intron 5 of the PFK muscle subunit (PFKM) gene, resulting in the complete deletion of exon 5 from the PFKM mRNA transcript. The delta5 mutation was detected in eleven out of eighteen (60 percent) mutated genes in nine Ashkenazi families affected by the disease. The deletion mutation, which involves deletion of a single base in exon 22, was observed in six out of seven (86 percent) mutated genes in the nine Ashkenazi families. Together, these two mutations accounted for 94 percent of the total mutated genes detected in the members of these families. In contrast, the delta5 gene was detected in only one out of 250 normal Ashkenazi individuals. Mutations in other exons and in an intron between exon 10 and exon 11 have also been associated with the Tarui's disease phenotype.

These pathogenic PFKM mutations cause the muscle symptoms of Tarui's disease, including muscle weakness and exercise intolerance. Because PFK-M is used by red blood cells to metabolize glucose, these mutations can also cause red blood cell impairment in the form of reticulocytosis and hemolysis. Currently, patients with symptoms of Tarui's disease may be genetically tested by a sequencing polymerase chain reaction (PCR) assay on DNA extracted from muscle tissue. Healthcare practitioners will usually offer patients the option of genetic counseling if they are considering genetic testing, especially because there is no specific treatment for Tarui's disease.

SYMPTOMS

Tarui's disease symptoms include muscle weakness, cramps, and exercise intolerance, referring to the excessive fatigue experienced in response to exercise. Some patients experience hemolysis with jaundice or severe renal impairment. This results in muscle necrosis and myoglobinuria, in which myoglobin is released from muscle cells and excreted in the urine, which appears rust-colored. In some cases, myoglobin accumulates in the kidney tubules, causing severe renal insufficiency. The phosphofructokinase defect also affects red blood cells, thus some patients have hemolysis with hyperbilirubinemia or jaundice.

SCREENING AND DIAGNOSIS

Physical examination often does not reveal abnormalities. Taking a patient's history, including response to exercise and family medical history, and lab testing are the most useful tools for diagnosing this disease. If risk factors are identified, laboratory testing is performed. Frequently, a creatine kinase assay is performed on a blood specimen and a myoglobinuria assay is conducted on a urine specimen. Elevated creatine kinase and positive myoglobinuria, especially after exercise, are warning signs of Tarui's disease. Another common assay determines the presence of the PFK enzyme by immunohistochemistry, which involves the binding of PFK-specific antibodies to PFK, if present in the specimen. The absence of PFK implies Tarui's disease. The ischemic forearm test is also frequently performed as a Tarui's disease screening test. In this assay, the patient grasps an object once or twice per second for two to three minutes while a blood pressure cuff is inflated on his or her upper arm. After the patient relaxes his or her grip, creatinine kinase, ammonia, and lactate levels are assayed at five-, ten-, and twenty-minute intervals. A positive ischemic forearm test, suggesting Tarui's disease, is the lack of lactate elevation as ammonia levels rise. Healthy subjects are expected to demonstrate increases in both lactate and ammonia levels. If one or more of these laboratory tests are positive, a muscle biopsy is required for a definitive diagnosis. When the muscle sample is examined under a microscope, the presence of subcarcolemmal vacuoles, abnormal polysaccharide deposits in muscle fibers, or abnormal red blood cells are positive findings for Tarui's disease.

TREATMENT AND THERAPY

Currently, there is no treatment for Tarui's disease, although diet modifications, rest, and exercise avoidance have been shown to be effective for decreasing clinical symptoms. Oral intake of glucose or fructose may also improve exercise tolerance.

PREVENTION AND OUTCOMES

Tarui's disease symptoms can be avoided by minimizing strenuous exercise and by observing a low-carbohydrate, high-protein diet, especially for less severe cases where disease onset occurs later in childhood or in adulthood.

Ing-Wei Khor, Ph.D.

FURTHER READING

Cheng, Liang, et al. *Molecular Genetic Pathology*. 2d ed. New York: Springer, 2013. Print.

Fletcher, H. L., and G. I. Hickey. *Genetics*. New York: Garland Science, 2013. Print.

Gray, R. G. F., et al. "Inborn Errors of Metabolism as a Cause of Neurological Disease in Adults: An Approach to Investigation." *Journal of Neurology, Neurosurgery & Psychiatry* 69 (2000): 5–12. Print.

Raben, N., et al. "Various Classes of Mutations in Patients with Phosphofructokinase Deficiency (Tarui's Disease)." *Muscle & Nerve* 3 (1995): S35–S38. Print.

Sherman, J. B., et al. "Common Mutations in the Phosphofructokinase-M Gene in Ashkenazi Jewish Patients with Glycogenesis vII—and Their Population Frequency." *The American Journal of Human Genetics* 55 (1994): 305–13. Print.

Vasconcelos, O., et al. "Nonsense Mutation in the Phosphofructokinase Muscle Subunit Gene Associated with Retention of Intron 10 in One of the Isolated Transcripts in Ashkenazi Jewish Patients with Tarui Disease." *The Proceedings of the National Academy of Sciences* 92 (1995): 10322–326.

Wiggins, Jennifer, and Anna Middleton. *Getting the Message Across: Communication with Diverse Populations in Clinical Genetics*. Oxford: Oxford UP, 2013. Print.

See also: Andersen's disease; Forbes disease; Galactokinase deficiency; Galactosemia; Gaucher disease; Glucose galactose malabsorption; Glucose-6-phosphate dehydrogenase deficiency; Glycogen storage diseases; Hereditary diseases; Hers disease; Inborn errors of metabolism; McArdle's disease; Pompe disease.

Tay-Sachs disease

CATEGORY: Diseases and syndromes

ALSO KNOWN AS: Hexosaminidase A deficiency; GM2 Gangliosidosis; TSD

DEFINITION

Tay-Sachs disease (TSD) is a lethal disease inherited as an autosomal recessive disorder. With TSD, nerve cells in the brain and spinal cord are destroyed. Affected children are normal at birth, and symptoms are usually noticed by six months of age, after which they progressively worsen; the child usually dies at or before four years of age. There is no cure for this severe disorder of the nervous system, but an understanding of the genetic nature of the disorder has led to effective population screening, prenatal diagnosis, and genetic counseling.

RISK FACTORS

One of the interesting features of TSD, as is true of some other genetic disorders, is its variation across ethnic groups. While people of any ethnic descent can be TSD carriers, there is a greatly increased risk among people of Ashkenazi Jewish or Eastern European descent. Approximately 1 in 27 Ashkenazi Jews is a TSD carrier, compared to perhaps 1 in 250 for the rest of the world's population (including Sephardic Jews). Other groups with a higher incidence of TSD include French Canadians who live near the St. Lawrence River, Old Order Amish community in Pennsylvania, and members of the Cajun community of Louisiana.

ETIOLOGY AND GENETICS

Tay-Sachs disease (TSD) is named after Warren Tay, an English ophthalmologist, and Bernard Sachs, an American neurologist, who first described the disorder. TSD is one of the lysosomal storage disorders, as are Hurler syndrome, Hunter syndrome, Gaucher disease, and Fabry disease. Lysosomes are organelles found in the cytoplasm of cells and contain many enzymes that digest the cell's food and waste. TSD is caused by the lack of the enzyme beta-hexosaminidase A (Hex A), which facilitates the breakdown of fatty substances called GM2 gangliosides in the brain and spinal cord. This mutation occurs in the HEXA gene located at 15q23, responsible for instructing the Hex A protein. When Hex A is sufficiently lacking, as in TSD, gangliosides accumulate in the body and eventually lead to the destruction of the nervous system. In type 1, onset occurs in infancy between three and six months of age. The juvenile form, type 2, begins between the ages of two and six years old. The adult form may begin as early as age 10, and is the most slowly progressing. Other sub-variants of the disease have been identified.

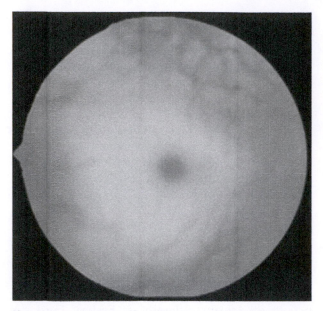

Cherry red spot as seen in Tay Sachs disease. The center of the fovea appears bright red because it is surrounded by a milky halo. By Jonathan Trobe, M.D., via Wikimedia Commons

Structure of the HEXA protein. Based on PyMOL rendering of PDB 2gjx. By Emw (Own work), via Wikimedia Commons

All forms of TSD are inherited as autosomal recessive disorders. Individuals with only one copy of the defective gene will not manifest the disease, while individuals with two copies of the gene will be afflicted with the disease. Couples in which only one partner carries the defective gene have no risk of having a baby with TSD, while couples in which both partners have the gene have a 25 percent risk of having a baby with TSD.

SYMPTOMS
Children with type 1 TSD appear normal at birth and up to six months of age. During this time,

they may show an exaggerated startle response to sound. Shortly after six months, more obvious symptoms appear. The child may show poor head control and an involuntary back-and-forth movement of the eyes. Also distinctive of TSD is a "cherry red spot" on the retina of the eye, first described by Tay, that usually appears after one year of age as atrophy of the optic nerve head occurs. The symptoms are progressive, and the child loses all the motor and mental skills developed to that point. Convulsions, increased motor tone, and blindness develop as the disease progresses. The buildup of storage material in the brain causes the head to enlarge, and brain weight may be 50 percent greater than normal at the time of death. There is no cure for TSD, and death usually occurs between two and four years of age, with the most common cause of death being pneumonia.

There are several forms of Tay-Sachs disease in addition to the classical type 1, or infant, form already described. There is a juvenile form in which similar symptoms appear between two and six years of age, with death occurring around age fifteen. A chronic or adult form of TSD has symptoms beginning around adolescence that are far milder than those of the infant and juvenile forms. Late-onset Tay-Sachs disease (LOTS) is a rare form in which there is some residual Hex A activity so that symptoms appear later in life and the disease progresses much more slowly.

SCREENING AND DIAGNOSIS
Screening and educational programs among at risk groups (in particular, the Ashkenazi Jews) have been very effective. Couples with advance knowledge of their carrier status can receive genetic counseling so that they understand their risk of having a child affected with TSD.

Diagnosis of TSD often occurs when a "cherry red" spot is noted during an eye exam. Blood testing will reveal decreased hexosaminidase A activity. The parents' blood may be tested to determine their carrier status.

TREATMENT AND THERAPY
Unfortunately, there is no treatment available for TSD. Researchers continue to work towards some form of gene therapy or enzyme replacement therapy

that could slow or halt the relentless progression of TSD in an affected baby.

Therapy is aimed at providing comfort for the affected child and support for the family. The child may be made more comfortable by helping to clear accumulated mucus from the lungs via chest physiotherapy, thus improving breathing and decreasing the risk of infection. A nasogastric tube or percutaneous esophago-gastrostomy tube may be required for feeding, in order to avoid aspiration of liquids or foods into the lungs. Antiseizure medications may be necessary, and physical therapy may be provided in order to prevent joint stiffness and/or muscle contractures. Nutrition supplementation, treatments to prevent constipation, and adequate hydration are provided.

Prevention and Outcomes

Although much has been learned about the genetics of the Tay-Sachs gene and the protein deficiency that causes the disease, there is still no cure. Nevertheless, TSD provides an excellent example of how the medical community can assist a susceptible population in confronting an incurable genetic disease. The effective screening of populations at risk for TSD and prenatal detection of fetuses with TSD have served to dramatically reduce the overall incidence of this terrible disease.

Individuals who want to determine whether they carry the defective gene can undergo a blood plasma assay that identifies differences in Hex A activity. If one or both parents are not TSD carriers, then they will not be at risk of having an affected child. However, if both couples are carriers, then they have a 25 percent risk of bearing a child with TSD. Once a woman is pregnant, prenatal diagnosis (chorionic villus sampling at ten to twelve weeks of pregnancy, or amniocentesis at approximately fifteen to twenty weeks of pregnancy) can be used to ascertain whether the fetus has Tay-Sachs disease, allowing the couple to receive counseling regarding therapeutic pregnancy termination.

Donald J. Nash, Ph.D.; updated by Rosalyn Carson-De-Witt, M.D. and Deanna M. Neff, M.P.H.

Further Reading

Bach G., J. Tomczak, N. Risch, and J. Ekstein. "Tay Sachs Screening in the Jewish Ashkenazi Population: DNA Testing Is the Preferred Procedure." "American Journal of Medical Genetics" 99 (February 15, 2001). Argues for using DNA testing as the most cost-effective and efficient way to screen for TSD. Bembi, B. "Substrate Reduction Therapy in the In fantile Form of Tay-Sachs." "Neurology" 66 (January 24, 2006). The researchers explored the use of miglustat to treat TSD; neurological deterioration was not arrested, although the drug concentrated in the cerebrospinal fluid (CSF) and did decrease the risk of macrocephaly.

Desnick, Robert J., and Michael M. Kaback, eds. "Tay Sachs Disease." San Diego: Academic, 2001. Detailed analysis of Tay-Sachs. Illustrations, bibliography, index.

Hall P, Minnich S, Teigen C, Raymond K. "Diagnosing Lysosomal Storage Disorders: The GM2 Gangliosidoses." "Curr Protoc Hum Genet." 2014;83:17.16.1–8.

Leavitt, J. A. "The 'Cherry Red' Spot." "Pediatric Neurology" 37 (July 1, 2007). Discusses the clinical appearance and etiology of this pathognomonic finding. National Tay-Sachs and Allied Diseases Association. "A Genetics Primer for Understanding Tay-Sachs and the Allied Diseases." Brookline, Mass.: Author, 1995. An introductory over view of Tay-Sachs disease.

Parker, James N., and Philip M. Parker, eds. "The Official Parent's Sourcebook on Tay-Sachs Disease: A Revised and Updated Directory for the Internet Age." San Diego: Icon Press, 2002. Topics include the essentials on Tay-Sachs disease, parents' rights, and insurance. Shapiro, B. E. "Late-Onset Tay-Sachs Disease: Adverse Effects of Medications and Implications for Treatment." "Neurology" 67 (September 12, 2006). The authors studied the use of about 350 different medications in individuals with late-onset Tay-Sachs disease, to identify which medications are relatively safe, and which may actually worsen the clinical picture.

Rose E, Schreiber-Agus N, Bajaj K, Klugman S, Goldwaser T. "Challenges of Pre and Post-Test Counseling for Orthodox Jewish Individuals in the Premarital Phase." "J Genet Couns." 2016 Feb;25(1):18–24.

Zallen, Doris Teichler. "Does It Run in the Family? A Consumer's Guide to DNA Testing for Genetic Disorders." New Brunswick, N.J.: Rutgers University Press, 1997. Covers the applications and social implications of testing for genetic disorders. Bibliography, index.

WEB SITES OF INTEREST

Cure Tay Sachs Foundation
http://www.curetay-sachs.org/
Dolan DNA Learning Center: Your Genes Your Health
http://www.ygyh.org
Sponsored by the Cold Spring Harbor Laboratory, this site, a component of the DNA Interactive Web site, offers information on more than a dozen inherited diseases and syndromes, including Tay Sachs disease.
National Human Genome Research Institute
http://www.genome.gov/10001220
Provides a vast amount of information regarding advances made in the study of genetics as related to human disease.
National Institute of Neurologic Disorders and Stroke
http://www.ninds.nih.gov/disorders/taysachs/tay-sachs.htm
A division of the National Institutes of Health, this Web site provides information on a variety of neurological disorders, including Tay-Sachs disease.
National Tay-Sachs and Allied Diseases Association
https://www.ntsad.org/
OMIM® Online Mendelian Inheritance in Man
http://www.omim.org/about

See also: Fabry disease; Gaucher disease; Genetic counseling; Genetic screening; Genetic testing; Genetic testing: Ethical and economic issues; Hereditary diseases; Hunter disease; Hurler syndrome; In vitro fertilization and embryo transfer; Inborn errors of metabolism; Prenatal diagnosis.

T-cell immunodeficiency syndrome

CATEGORY: Diseases and syndromes

DEFINITION

T-cell immunodeficiency syndrome refers to the group of immunodeficiencies that increase susceptibility to infection as a result on an immune system with deficient, absent, or defective T cells. This immunodeficiency can be expressed as a primary (con genital) or a secondary (acquired) disorder.

Primary T-cell immunodeficiency results from autosomal or X-linked genetic defects.

RISK FACTORS

Secondary T-cell immunodeficiency is the most common and develops as a result of chronic infection, malnutrition, systemic disease, malignancy, or drug therapy. Although primary T-cell immunodeficiency is less common than secondary forms, they are rare genetic disorders and generally develop in infancy or early childhood accompanied by recur rent unusual infections.

ETIOLOGY AND GENETICS

Considering that T cells (a type of white blood cells) are the dominant type of lymphocytes in circulating blood, it is very likely that a significant T cell deficiency usually may cause a decrease in the number of blood lymphocytes. Several genetic abnormalities may prevent T cells from identifying and destroying foreign or abnormal cells circulating in the body. An impaired T-cell immunity dam ages the immune system's ability to protect the body against bacterial, viral, fungal, or cancer cell at tacks. The two general reasons contributing to the development of T-cell immunodeficiency syndrome are either autosomal or X-linked gene disorders resulting from mutations or deletions. These hereditary genetic disorders give rise to partial or absolute defects in T-cell function resulting in a defective immune system at birth or early in life. The most common forms of T-cell immunodeficiency disorders are severe combined immune deficiency (SCID), X-linked lymphoproliferative syndrome, X-linked hyper-IgM immunodeficiency, hyper-IgE syndrome, DiGeorge syndrome, ataxia telangectasia, Nijmegen breakage syndrome, Wiskott-Aldrich syndrome (WAS), and T-cell immunodeficiency, recurrent infections, and autoimmunity with or without cardiac malformations (TIIAC). Severe combined immune deficiency (SCID or bubble boy syndrome) is the most serious immunodeficiency disorder. A mutation in the IL2RG gene of the X chromosome, responsible for making a protein that helps immune cells grow and mature, most commonly causes SCID. This results in low levels of antibodies (immunoglobulins) and no T cells. The severity of this deficiency results in the development of more serious infections with infants not growing or developing normally. Untreated children frequently

Scanning electron micrograph of a human T lymphocyte (also called a T cell) from the immune system of a healthy donor. Credit: NIAID By NIAID/NIH (NIAID Flickr's photostream), via Wikimedia Commons

From left to right: erythrocyte, thrombocyte, leukocyte By Electron Microscopy Facility at The National Cancer Institute at Frederick (NCI-Frederick) ([1]), via Wikimedia Commons

die before the age of one. The X-linked disorder affects males more than females. Males only have one X chromosome and therefore the mutation is enough to cause the disease, whereas females would need to inherit the same mutation in both X chromosomes. Omenn syndrome is an example of an autosomal recessive form of severe combined immunodeficiency

(SCID). In this case both parents pass on the mutation typically to the RAG1 or RAG2 genes.

In DiGeorge syndrome, a deletion of chromosome 22 (at 22q11.2) results in a thymus gland absent or underdeveloped at birth. The fetus has heart, face, thymus, and parathyroid gland abnormalities, leading to a mild to moderate T-cell deficiency. The X-linked lymphoproliferative (XLP) syndrome (Duncan disease) is caused by mutations in the SH2D1A (Type 1) and XIAP (Type 2) genes. It results in defective T cells and natural killer (NK) cells and is characterized by extreme sensitivity to Epstein-Barr (mononucleosis) virus infection, resulting in liver failure, immunodeficiency, and malignant lymphoma.

Hyper-IgM syndrome is an antibody deficiency known by normal or elevated IgM levels and decreased levels or absence of other serum antibodies. It is caused by a mutation in the CD40LG gene of the X chromosome and leads into susceptibility to bacterial infections. The gene makes CD40 ligand protein necessary to make antibodies.

Hyper-IgE syndrome (Buckley or Job syndrome) is caused by a mutation in the STAT3 gene of chromosome 17, which results in high levels of IgE and normal levels of the other antibody classes. These patients suffer from chronic eczema, recurrent lung infections, weak bones, coarse facial features, and pus abscesses.

The mutation in the ATM gene of chromosome 11, results in ataxia telangiectasia (AT). AT is characterized by dilated capillaries, higher susceptibility to infections, body movement in coordination, and malignancy predisposition.

A mutation in the NBN gene located on chromosome 8 (at position 8q21.3) is responsible for the Nijmegen (Berlin) breakage syndrome, which is characterized by microcephaly, sinopulmonary infections, immunodeficiency, and high risk for lymphoma cancer. People with Nijmegen breakage syndrome have abnormally low levels of immunoglobulin G (IgG), immunoglobulin A (IgA), and T cells. Because Wiskott-Aldrich syndrome is caused by mutation in the WAS gene on the X chromosome at Xp11.23, immunodeficiencies are characterized by thrombocytopenia, eczema, and recurrent respiratory infections. There is abnormal antibody production and defective T-cell function, affecting boys only. There is a higher incidence of developing cancers such as lymphoma and leukemia.

Mutations in STK4 on chromosome 20 has been identified as responsible for T-cell immunodeficiency, recurrent infections, and autoimmunity with or without cardiac malformations (TIIAC). TIIAC is a primary T-cell immunodeficiency syndrome causing recurrent infections, warts, and abscesses, autoimmune diseases, and cardiac malformations, including atrial septal defect.

SYMPTOMS

A history of recurrent unusual infections might suggest T-cell immunodeficiency syndrome. Frequently, respiratory infections arise first and reappear, becoming severe and persistent and leading to complications. Generally, the earliest the symptoms in life arise in children, the more severe will be the T-cell immunodeficiency syndrome. Other different ailments may contrast or change based on the infections' severity and length. Chronic diarrhea may cause infants or young children not to grow or develop (failure to thrive) due to weight loss.

Type 1 diabetes, hypoadrenalism, hypothyroidism, glomerulonephritis, and autoimmune enteropathy often develop in children with immune disorders at a very early age.

SCREENING AND DIAGNOSIS

Doctors suspecting a primary T-cell immunodeficiency will run a battery of tests to identify the specific genetic abnormality, immunoglobulin levels, white blood microscopic irregularities, skin tests, number of circulating B and T cells, and proper B and T cell function. Upon physical examination, rashes, weight loss, chronic cough, hair loss, and/or enlarged spleen or liver may suggest a particular disorder to doctors based on disease-specific clinical manifestations. An early onset of recurring or unusual infections is a key determinant in identifying the type of immunodeficiency disorder. Adverse prognosis follows a delayed diagnosis. The particular form of infection will also help healthcare professionals pinpoint the T-cell immunodeficiency variant.

TREATMENT AND THERAPY

Symptoms suggest the type of genetic disorder, and treatment strategies are tailored to meet specific immunodeficiencies needs. Many patients will require prompt aggressive treatment. General guide lines for these patients include: periodic IV immunoglobulin replacement therapy, practicing

excellent personal hygiene, avoiding undercooked food, drinking boiled water, routine non-live vaccines, and avoiding contact with infected people. SCID patients are kept in protected environments, preventing exposure to pathogens and are treated with antibiotics, antivirals, and anti bodies. Bone marrow stem cell transplantation from an unaffected sibling matching the same tissue type is the only effective treatment for SCID and WAS. Thymus transplantation for DiGeorge syndrome patients can cure the immunodeficiency, and corrective heart surgery is done for severe heart conditions. Chemotherapy for malignancy may need to be tailored to lower doses and longer therapies due to DNA instability.

Gene therapy is being studied for many of these diseases, particularly SCID and WAS.

PREVENTION AND OUTCOMES

Prevention and outcome strategies depend on the type of T-cell immunodeficiency disorder diagnosed and time of diagnosis. Some T-cell immunodeficiency syndromes shorten life span while others can be managed throughout life. When the disorder does not impair antibody production, vaccination is recommended only with killed viral and bacterial vaccines since live vaccines might cause disease in immunodeficient patients. There is no effective form of prevention; therefore, genetic testing and counseling should be provided to people with family history previously identified for these types of hereditary immunodeficiencies. Early diagnosis is critical in improving patient outcome since many children die young if untreated. The role of alert healthcare professionals to recognize T-cell immunodeficiency clinical findings can play an essential part confirming rapid accurate diagnosis, ultimately resulting in improved patient outcome.

Ana Maria Rodriguez-Rojas, M.S.; updated by Deanna M. Neff, M.P.H.

FURTHER READING

Bonilla, F. A., et al. "Practice Parameter for the Diagnosis and Management of Primary Immunodeficiency." "Annals of Allergy, Asthma & Immunology" 94, no. 5 Suppl 1 (May, 2005): S1-63.

Boztug, K., et al. "Multiple Independent Second Site Mutations in Two Siblings with Somatic Mosaicism for Wiskott-Aldrich Syndrome." "Clinical Genetics" 74 (2008): 68–74.

Conley, Mary Ellen. "Antibody Deficiencies." In "The Metabolic and Molecular Bases of Inherited Disease", edited by Charles Scriver et al. 8th ed. New York: McGraw-Hill, 2001.

Cooper, Megan A., Thomas L. Pommering, and Katalin Koranyi. "Primary Immunodeficiencies." "American Family Physician" 68 (2003): 2001–2008, 2011.

Edgar, J. D. "T Cell Immunodeficiency." "Journal of Clinical Pathology" 61 (2008): 988–993.

Pachlopnik Schmid J, Güngör T, Seger R. "Modern management of primary T-cell immunodeficiencies." "Pediatr Allergy Immunol." 2014;25 (4):300–13.

Kingsmore, S. F., et al. "Identification of Diagnostic Biomarkers for Infection in Premature Neonates." "Molecular & Cellular Proteomics" 7, no. 10 (October, 2008): 1863–1875.

WEB SITES OF INTEREST

Genetics Home Reference

https://ghr.nlm.nih.gov/condition

Immune System Poster

http://www.info4pi.org/aboutPI/pdf/ ImmuneSystemPoster.pdf

Immunodeficiency Disorders

http://www.nlm.nih.gov/medlineplus/ency/ article/000818.htm

Jeffrey Modell Foundation: Primary Immunodeficiency FAQs

http://www.info4pi.org/aboutPI/index. cfm?section=aboutPI&content=faq&C-FID=32813331&CFTOKEN=3862055

National Institute of Child Health and Human Development (NICHD): Primary Immunodeficiency

http://www.nichd.nih.gov/publications/pubs/ primary_immuno.cfm#WhatisPrimaryImmuno deficiency

Nemours Foundation: Immune System

http://kidshealth.org/parent/general/body_ basics/immune.html

OMIM® Online Mendelian Inheritance in Man

http://www.omim.org/about

Warning Signs of Primary Immunodeficiency

http://www.aafp.org/afp/20031115/2011ph.html

See also: Ataxia telangectasia; DiGeorge syndrome; Immunodeficiency with hyper-IgM; Severe combined immune deficiency; Wiskott-Aldrich syndrome.

Telomeres

CATEGORY: Cellular biology

SIGNIFICANCE: Telomeres, the ends of the arms of chromosomes of eukaryotes, become shorter as organisms age. They are thought to act biologically to slow chromosome shortening, which can lead to cell death caused by the loss of genes and may be related to aging and diseases such as cancer. Telomeric DNA may also be involved in chromosome movement and localization in the nucleus, as well as transcriptional regulation of genes near the telomeres.

KEY TERMS

eukaryote: a unicellular or multicellular organism with cells that contain a membrane-bound nucleus, multiple chromosomes, and membrane-bound organelles

prokaryote: a unicellular organism with a single chromosome and lacking a nucleus or any other membrane-bound organelles

EUKARYOTIC CHROMOSOMES AND TELOMERES

The DNA of bacteria and other related simple organisms (prokaryotes) consists of one double-stranded DNA molecule. Structurally and functionally, the prokaryotic chromosome contains one copy of most genes as well as DNA regions that control expression of these genes. Prokaryotic gene expression depends primarily upon a cell's moment-to-moment needs. An entire prokaryotic chromosome, its genome, usually encodes about one thousand genes.

The genomes of eukaryotes are much more complex and may include 100,000 or more genes. The number of chromosomes in different types of eukaryotes can range from just a few to several hundred. Each of these huge DNA molecules is linear rather than the circular molecule seen in prokaryotes. In addition, many individual segments of eukaryotic DNA exist in multiple copies. For example, about 10 percent of the DNA of a eukaryote consists of "very highly repetitive segments" (VRS's), units that are less than ten deoxyribonucleotides long that are repeated up to several million times per cell. DNA segments that are several hundred deoxyribonucleotide units long represent about 20 to 25 percent of the DNA. They are repeated one thousand times or more per cell. The rest of the eukaryote DNA (from 65 to 70 percent of the total) consists of larger segments repeated once or a few times, the genes, and the DNA regions that control the expression of the genes.

Much of the repetitive DNA, called satellite DNA, does not seem to be involved in coding for proteins or RNAs involved in making proteins. Telomeres are part of this DNA and consist of pieces of DNA that are several thousand deoxyribonucleotide units long, found at both chromosome ends. They are believed to act to stabilize the ends of chromosomes and protect them from exonuclease enzymes that degrade DNA from the ends. Researchers have concluded this for two reasons. First, the enzymes that make two chromosomes every time a cell reproduces are unable to operate at the chromosome ends. Hence, the repeated reproduction of a eukaryote cell and its DNA will lead to the creation of shorter and shorter chromosomes, a process that can cause cell death when essential genes are lost. Second, as organisms age, the telomeres of their cells become shorter and shorter.

TELOMERASE ENZYMES

When chromosomes are replicated in preparation for cell division, the internal segments are replicated by a complex process involving the enzymes primase and DNA polymerase. Primase lays down a small segment of RNA on the template strand of DNA, and DNA polymerase uses the primer to start replication. Making the end of a linear chromosome is a problem, however, because primers cannot consistently be produced at the very ends of the chromosomes. Consequently, with each cell division a small portion of the ends of newly replicated chromosomes is single-stranded and is trimmed off by exonucleases. This problem is solved by enzymes known as telomerases, which add telomeres to eukaryote chromosomes. Each telomerase contains a nucleic acid subunit, known as human telomerase RNA component (hTERC), which is about 150 ribonucleotides long. This length is equivalent to 1.5 copies of the appropriate repeat in the DNA telomere to be made.

The catalytic subunit of telomerase is called the human telomerase reverse transcriptase enzyme (hTERT). hTERT uses this piece of RNA as a template to make the desired DNA strand of the telomere. At the telomere, these two telomerase subunits

are present along with other telomere-associated proteins and telomere-binding proteins, which affect the localization and activity of telomerase. The exact mechanism by which the DNA strand is made is not yet confirmed; however, it is thought that telomerase uses its RNA sequence (AACCCC) to bind to the target complementary DNA sequence (TTGGGG) at the end of the parent DNA strand. The polymerase activity and RNA template allows for the addition of nucleotides to the telomere. After six new nucleotides have been added (TTGGGG), the telomerase unit moves down the DNA parent strand and continues adding nucleotides. How the telomerase in any given species identifies the correct length of telomere repeat for a specific chromosome is not clearly understood, although it may be regulated by various telomere-associated proteins. After the addition of telomeric DNA sequences, the parent DNA strand will be longer than the complementary daughter DNA strand. This so-called "end-replication problem" is hypothesized to be solved by the enzyme primase, which uses the extended telomere to create a primer on the daughter DNA strand that DNA polymerase can then extend to fill in the gap.

A picture depicting a telomere forming a loop. public domain via wikimedia commons

Telomerase activity can be lost in certain strains of simple eukaryotes, such as protozoa. When this happens to a given cell line, each cell division leads to the additional shortening of its telomeres. This procedure continues for a fixed number of cell divisions; it then ends with the death of the telomerase-deficient cell line in a process known as replicative senescence.

A related observation has been made in humans. It has been shown that when human fibroblasts are grown in tissue culture, telomere length is longest

Telomere Length in Clones

Dolly the sheep, the first mammal to be cloned from adult cells, was born on July 5, 1996. While Dolly ushered in a new era of mammalian cloning, her tenure as the cloning community's lovable mascot was, quite literally, short-lived. Dolly was euthanized on February 14, 2003, after being diagnosed with a progressive lung disease; she had already been suffering from debilitating arthritis. While Dolly's health problems could have resulted from "natural causes," both ailments are more characteristic of much older sheep. Sheep normally live to an age of about twelve, Dolly was only half that.

Dolly's early demise was actually foreshadowed in 1999, when the group which cloned her reported that Dolly's telomeres were shorter than expected for a sheep of her age. Dolly's telomeres were about the length one would expect if her cells had been six years old on the day she was born (Dolly was cloned from a six-year-old ewe). Since telomere length acts as a "molecular clock" that determines the age of a cell, researchers had hoped that this clock would somehow be "reset" upon transfer of an adult nucleus to a host ovum.

While clearly not the case for Dolly, this resetting of telomere length has been demonstrated in cloned cows. In 2000, Robert Lanza and colleagues reported that cloned cows had longer-than-normal telomeres. Will these "super cows" be able to live appreciably longer than normal cows? Only time will tell, since cows have a normal life span of about twenty years. What accounts for the difference between Dolly and these cloned cows? Subsequent research has shown that the type of cell used in the cloning process may be an important factor. In 2002, Norikazu Miyashita and colleagues reported that cows cloned from mammary gland cells (like Dolly) had shorter-than-normal telomeres, clones obtained from skin fibroblasts (connective tissue precursors, those used by Lanza) had longer-than-normal telomeres, and clones obtained from muscle cells showed no significant differences in telomere length.

The telomere length of clones may also be species-specific. Teruhiko Wakayama and colleagues cloned mice sequentially for six generations but saw no difference in telomere length in any of the clones produced. Mice, however, are known to have extremely long telomeres to begin with; also, unlike the somatic cells of cows or sheep, many of the somatic cells of mice are known to express the telomerase enzyme.

More research is necessary to understand exactly why certain animal clones are produced with shortened telomeres and others are not. Currently, our lack of knowledge on the subject remains one of the more compelling reasons not to attempt to clone a human at this time. A human clone produced with unusually short telomeres may, like Dolly, meet with an untimely death. In fact, patients with a human genetic disease called Hutchinson-Gilford progeria have skin fibroblasts with greatly reduced telomere lengths; persons affected with this disease live to an average age of about thirteen years.

James S. Godde, Ph.D.

when cells are obtained from young individuals. They are shorter in cells taken from the middle-aged, and very short in cells taken from the aged. Similar observations have been made with the fibroblasts from other higher eukaryotes as well as with other human cell types. In contrast, the process of telomere shortening does not happen when germ-cell lines—which in the whole organism produce sperm and ova—are grown in tissue culture. This suggests a basis for differences in longevity of the germ cells and the somatic cells that make up other human tissues.

Impact and Applications

The discovery and study of telomeres and telomerases produced new insights into DNA synthesis, the number of times a cell can reproduce, and the aging process. The circular DNA of bacteria (which are prokaryotes) allows them to undergo many more cycles of reproduction than the somatic cells of the eukaryotes. The linear eukaryote chromosome may have evolved because such DNA molecules were too large to survive as circular molecules given their rigidity and fragility. In addition, the observation of telomere shortening in simple and complex eukaryotes raises the fascinating possibility that the life spans of organisms may be related to the conservation of telomeres associated with the replication of these structures by telomerases.

The role of telomere length in longevity is uncertain, but apparently significant. Cells grown in cell multiplying at greater rates rather than stagnating or dying, will give researchers a greater number of cells to study, especially in the context of disease treatment. The scientists used a modified messenger RNA that contains the coding sequence for the active component of telomerase in the lengthening process.

Sanford S. Singer, Ph.D.;
updated by Elizabeth A. Manning, Ph.D.

FURTHER READING

Blackburn, Elizabeth H. "Telomeres, Telomerase, and Cancer." *Scientific American* February 1996. Print.

Blackburn, Elizabeth H., and Carol W. Greider, eds. *Telomeres.* Cold Spring Harbor: Cold Spring Harbor Laboratory, 1995. Print.

Chan, S. R. W. L., and E. H. Blackburn. "Telomeres and Telomerase." *Philosophical Transactions of the Royal Society B: Biological Sciences* 359 (2004): 109–21. Print.

Conger, Krista. "Telomere Extension Turns Back Aging Clock in Cultured Human Cells, Study Finds." *Stanford Medicine.* Stanford Medicine, 22 Jan. 2015. Web. 21 Jan. 2016.

De Lange, Titia, Roger R. Reddel, and Virginia A. Zakia, eds. *Abstracts of Papers Presented at the 2013 Meeting on Telomeres and Telomerase.* Cold Spring Harbor: Cold Spring Harbor Laboratory, 2013. Print.

Double, John A., and Michael J. Thompson, eds. *Telomeres and Telomerase: Methods and Protocols.* Totowa: Humana, 2002. Print.

Jain, K. K. *Applications of Biotechnology in Oncology.* New York: Humana, 2014. Print.

Kipling, David, ed. *The Telomere.* New York: Oxford UP, 1995. Print.

Krupp, Guido, and Reza Parwaresch, eds. *Telomerases, Telomeres, and Cancer.* New York: Kluwer Academic/Plenum, 2003. Print.

Lewis, Ricki. "Telomere Tales." *Bioscience* 48.12 (1998). Print.

Phatak, P., and A. M. Burger. "Telomerase and Its Potential for Therapeutic Intervention." *British Journal of Pharmacology* 152.7 (2007): 1003011. Print.

Trusina, Ala. "Stress Induced Telomere Shortening: Longer Life with Less Mutations?" *BMC Systems Biology* 8.1 (2014): 1–17. Print.

See also: Aging; Animal cloning; Chromosome mutation; Chromosome structure; Cloning vectors; DNA replication; Molecular genetics; Reverse transcriptase.

Thalassemia

CATEGORY: Diseases and syndromes
ALSO KNOWN AS: Mediterranean anemia; Cooley's anemia; thalassemia major; thalassemia minor; Alpha/beta thalassemia

DEFINITION

Thalassemia is an inherited disorder. It leads to the decreased production and increased destruction of red blood cells. Hemoglobin in the red blood cells carry oxygen for all organs in the body. The loss of red blood cells results in low hemoglobin. This leads to anemia. The decreased oxygen will impair the ability to maintain normal functions.

Hemoglobin is made of two separate amino acid chains. They are alpha and beta. Thalassemias are categorized by the specific chain and number of genes affected.

In alpha thalassemia, the alpha chain is affected. Silent carrier thalassemia affects one gene; thalassemia trait affects two genes; Hemoglobin H disease affects three genes; alpha hydrops fetalis, the most severe form, affects four genes and results in fetal or newborn death.

In beta thalassemia, the beta chain is affected. Thalassemia minor involves one abnormal gene; thalassemia major (Cooley's anemia) involves two abnormal genes.

RISK FACTORS

Risk factors that increase an individual's chance of thalassemia include the geographic location of his or her ancestors. Individuals with ancestors from southeast Asia (highest risk), Mediterranean countries, North Africa, the Middle East, India, Central Asia and southern China are at risk for alpha thalassemias; individuals of southeast Asian, Chinese, and Filipino ancestry are at risk for alpha hydrops fetalis; those with ancestors from Africa, Mediterranean countries, the Middle East, India, Central Asia, and southeast Asia are at risk for beta thalassemias. A family history of the disorder is another risk factor.

ETIOLOGY AND GENETICS

Mutations in the HBB gene, located on the short arm of chromosome 11 at position 11p15.5, are the cause of beta thalassemia. This gene encodes

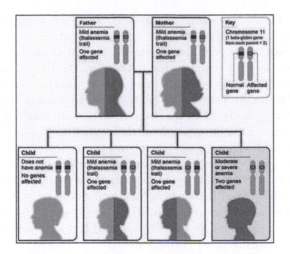

The picture shows one example of how beta thalassemia is inherited. The beta globin gene is located on chromosome 11. A child inherits two beta globin genes (one from each parent). In this example, each parent has one altered beta globin gene. Each child has a 25 percent chance of inheriting two normal genes (no anemia), a 50 percent chance of inheriting one altered gene and one normal gene (beta thalassemia trait), or a 25 percent chance of inheriting two altered genes (beta thalassemia major). By National Heart Lung and Blood Institute (NIH) (National Heart Lung and Blood Institute (NIH)), via Wikimedia Commons

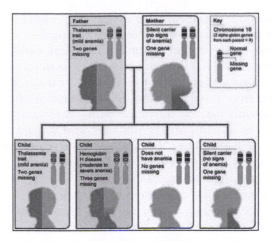

The picture shows one example of how alpha thalassemia is inherited. The alpha globin genes are located on chromosome 16. A child inherits four alpha globin genes (two from each parent). In this example, the father is missing two alpha globin genes and the mother is missing one alpha globin gene. Each child has a 25 percent chance of inheriting two missing genes and two normal genes (thalassemia trait), three missing genes and one normal gene (hemoglobin H disease), four normal genes (no anemia), or one missing gene and three normal genes (silent carrier). By National Heart Lung and Blood Institute (NIH) (National Heart Lung and Blood Institute (NIH)), via Wikimedia Commons

the beta-globin polypeptide, which is one of the major components of hemoglobin. Some mutations completely inactivate the gene and stop the production of beta-globin (β0 thalassemia), while others result in only a decreased amount of beta-globin in red blood cells (β+ thalassemia). In either case, insufficient amounts of hemoglobin are formed, and anemia and other growth problems associated with beta thalassemia result. The inheritance pattern for this disease is usually autosomal recessive, meaning that both copies of the gene must be deficient in order for the individual to be afflicted. Typically, an affected child is born to two unaffected parents, both of whom are carriers of the recessive mutant allele. The probable outcomes for children whose parents are both carriers are 75 percent unaffected and 25 percent affected.

The inheritance of alpha thalassemia is more complex, since two genes are involved. About 35 mutations have been identified. The HBA1 and HBA2 genes are virtually identical copies of each other, and they are found in adjacent positions on the short arm of chromosome 16 at position 16p13.3. Each encodes an alpha-globin polypeptide, one of the four subunits of a mature hemoglobin molecule. Alpha thalassemia results when one or more copies of these genes are deleted from the genome. Since each individual has two copies of each gene, there are four functional genes that encode alpha-globin in healthy individuals. Different degrees or severities of alpha thalassemia are recognized when one, two, three, or all four copies of the gene are missing. If both parents are missing at least one copy of either HBA1 or HBA2, their children could inherit anywhere from zero to four alpha-globin genes and present clinically with anywhere from the most severe form of alpha thalassemia to no thalassemia at all. The precise risk in each particular case depends entirely on the number and orientation of the missing genes in each parent.

Symptoms

Symptoms most often begin within three to six months of birth. Symptoms may include anemia, which may be mild, moderate, or severe; jaundice; an enlarged spleen; fatigue (tiredness); listlessness; and reduced appetite. Another symptom may be enlarged and fragile bones, including thickening and roughening of facial bones, bones that break easily, and teeth that do not line up properly. Growth problems, increased susceptibility to infection, and skin that is paler than usual may also be symptoms. Additional symptoms may be hormone problems, such as delayed or absent puberty, diabetes, and thyroid problems. Heart failure, shortness of breath, liver problems, and gallstones may be other symptoms.

Alpha thalassemia usually causes milder forms of the disease with varying degrees of anemia.

Beta thalassemia can be asymptomatic or be a mild form of disease. The mild form is known as thalassemia intermedia. This form rarely needs extensive medical care.

Beta thalassemia major (Cooley's anemia) has symptoms within the first two years of a child's life. Children are pale and listless. They often have poor appetites. They grow slowly and often develop jaundice (yellowing of skin). It is a serious disease. It requires regular blood transfusions and extensive medical care.

Without treatment, the spleen, liver, and heart soon become very enlarged. Bones become thin and brittle. Abnormal deposits of iron in body can lead to organ failure. This is called secondary hemochromatosis. It most often affects the heart, liver, and pancreas. Heart failure and infection are the leading causes of death among children with untreated thalassemia major.

SCREENING AND DIAGNOSIS
The doctor will ask about a patient's symptoms and medical history. A physical exam will be done. Blood tests may include a complete blood count, which is a count of the different types of blood cells; a blood smear; hemoglobin electrophoresis; quantitative hemoglobin analysis; and iron levels.

Genetic testing is available for HBB, HBA1, and HBA2. Screening tests are available for possible carriers, and prenatal testing is available if the familial mutation is known.

TREATMENT AND THERAPY
Folic acid supplementation is recommended to help the body make healthy blood cells. Treatment may also include blood transfusions. These are done to replace abnormal red blood cells with healthy new ones.

Iron chelation therapy is another form of treatment. Excess iron can accumulate in the body after repeated blood transfusions. Too much iron can damage the heart, liver, and other vital organs. A drug called deferoxamine (Desferal) can be given to bind to excess iron in the body. It is then carried out through the urine. This drug is given through the skin or by vein using a small infusion pump. Deferasirox (Exjade) was approved in 2013 for chronic iron overload caused by non–transfusion-dependent thalassemia. It can be given as a drink or mixed with water or juice. Another drug, deferiprone was approved by the FDA in 2011. They may be used alone or in combination.

Splenectomy is a surgical procedure done to re move the spleen. It may help reduce the number of blood transfusions that are needed.

In a bone marrow transplant, healthy stem cells from a donor's bone marrow are injected into a patient's vein. The new cells travel through the blood stream to the bone cavities; there they can produce new blood cells, including red blood cells. This is usually only done in severe cases. A compatible sib ling donor is required.

Keeping vaccines up to date and avoiding infection is prudent for those with thalassemia.

PREVENTION AND OUTCOMES
This disease is inherited. Blood tests and family genetic studies will show if an individual is a carrier. A genetic counselor can discuss the risks of passing on the disease. The counselor can also provide information on testing. Outcomes for those with the disease depend on the type and severity of the condition. Many people live normal lifespan with proper medical management. In severe cases, early death, often from heart failure, is a possibility.

Jenna Hollenstein, M.S., RD; reviewed by Igor Puzanov, M.D. "Etiology and Genetics" by Jeffrey A. Knight, Ph.D.; updated by Deanna M. Neff, M.P.H.

FURTHER READING
EBSCO Publishing. "Health Librar y: Thalassemia." Ipswich, Mass.: Author, 2009. Available through http://www.ebscohost.com.

Perrine SP, Pace BS, Faller DV. "Targeted fetal hemoglobin induction for treatment of beta hemoglobinopathies." "Hematol Oncol Clin North Am." 2014;28(2):233-48.

Piel FB, Weatherall DJ. "The a-thalassemias." " N Engl J Med." 2014;371(20):1908-16.

Rivella S. "β-thalassemias: paradigmatic diseases for scientific discoveries and development of innovative therapies." "Haematologica." 2015;100 (4):418-30.

Steinberg, Martin H., et al., eds. "Disorders of Hemoglobin: Genetics, Pathophysiology, and Clinical Management." New York: Cambridge University Press, 2001.

Weatherall, D. J., and J. B. Clegg. "The Thalassaemia Syndromes." 4th ed. Malden, Mass.: Blackwell Science, 2001.

Web Sites of Interest

Canadian Hemophiliac Society
http://www.hemophilia.ca/en
Centers for Disease Control and Prevention
http://www.cdc.gov
Genetic and Rare Diseases Information Center
https://rarediseases.info.nih.gov/diseases
Genetics Home Reference
http://ghr.nlm.nih.gov
National Heart, Lung, and Blood Institute
http://www.nhlbi.nih.gov
Northern California Comprehensive Thalassemia Center
http://www.thalassemia.com
The Thalassemia Foundation of Canada
http://www.thalassemia.ca

See also: ABO blood group system; Fanconi anemia; Hereditary diseases; Sickle-cell disease.

Thalidomide and other teratogens

CATEGORY: Diseases and syndromes

SIGNIFICANCE: Teratogenesis is the development of defects in the embryo or fetus caused by exposure to chemicals, radiation, or other environmental conditions. Thalidomide, a sedative whose ingestion by pregnant women led to the birth of abnormal babies in the late 1950s and early 1960s, is one of the more publicized examples of a chemical teratogen.

Key terms

congenital defect: a defect or disorder that occurs during prenatal development

peromelia: the congenital absence or malformation of the extremities caused by abnormal development of the limb bud from about the fourth to the eighth week after conception; the ingestion of thalidomide by pregnant women can cause this disorder in fetuses

Teratogenesis and Its Causes

Teratogenesis is the development of structural or functional abnormalities in an embryo or fetus due to the presence of a toxic chemical or other environmental factor. The term is derived from the Greek words *teras* (monster) and *genesis* (birth). The phenomenon is usually attributed to exposure of the mother to some causative agent during the early stages of pregnancy. These may include chemicals, excessive radiation exposure, viral infections, or drugs. Drugs that are taken by the father may be teratogenic only if they damage the chromosomes of a spermatozoan that then joins with the egg to form a zygote.

For many centuries, the impression that malformed babies were conceived as a result of the intercourse between humans and devils or animals dominated society. Seventeenth century English physiologist William Harvey attributed teratogenesis to embryonic development. In the nineteenth century, the French brothers Étienne and Isidore Geoffroy Saint-Hilaire outlined a systematic study on the science of teratology. In the United States, the importance of teratogens was first widely covered during the 1940s, when scientists discovered that pregnant women who were affected by German measles (rubella) often gave birth to babies that had one or more birth defects. In the 1940s and 1950s, the consumption of diethylstilbestrol (DES) before the ninth week of gestation to prevent miscarriage was found to produce cancer in the developing fetus. Animal studies have also shown that defective offspring result from the use of hallucinogens such as lysergic acid diethylamide (LSD).

Left: S isomer. Right: R isomer public domain via wikimedia commons

A broader definition of teratogenesis may include other minor birth defects that are more likely to be genetically linked, such as clubfoot, cleft lip, and cleft palate. These defects can often be treated in a much more effective way than those caused by toxic substances. Clubfoot, for example, which can be detected by the unusual twisted position of one or both feet, may be treated with surgery and physical therapy within the first month after birth. Brachydactyly (short digits) in rabbits has been linked to a recessive gene that causes a local breakdown of the circulation in the developing bud of the embryo, which is followed by necrosis (tissue death) and healing. In more extreme cases of agenesis, such as limb absence, a fold of amnion (embryonic membrane) was found to cause strangulation of the limb. Agenesis has been

Structure of afimoxifene By Boghog at en.wikipedia (Own work), via Wikimedia Commons

observed with organs such as kidneys, bladders, testicles, ovaries, thyroids, and lungs. Other genetic teratogenic malformations include anencephaly (absence of brain at birth), microcephaly (small-size head), hydrocephaly (large-size head caused by accumulation of large amounts of fluids), spina bifida (failure of the spine to close over the spinal cord), cleft palate (lack of fusion in the ventral laminae), and hermaphrodism (presence of both male and female sexual organs).

THALIDOMIDE AND ITS IMPACT

Thalidomide resembles glutethimide in its sedative action. Laboratory studies of the late 1950s and early 1960s had shown thalidomide to be a safe sedative for pregnant women. As early as 1958, the West German government made the medicine available without prescription. Other Western European countries followed, with the medicine available only upon physician's prescription. It took several years for the human population to provide the evidence that laboratory animals could not. German physician Widukind Lenz established the role of thalidomide in a series of congenital defects. He proved that administration of the drug during the first twelve weeks of the mother's pregnancy led to the development of phocomelia, a condition characterized by peromelia (the congenital absence or malformation of the extremities caused by the abnormal formation and development of the limb bud from about the fourth to the eighth week after conception), absence or malformation of the external ear, fusion defects of the eye, and absence of the normal openings of the gastrointestinal system of the body.

The United States escaped the thalidomide tragedy to a great extent because of the efforts of Frances O. Kelsey, MD, of the US Food and Drug Administration (FDA). She had serious doubts about the drug's safety and was instrumental in banning the approval of thalidomide for marketing in the United States. Other scientists such as Helen Brooke Taussig, a pioneer of pediatric cardiology and one of the physicians who outlined the surgery on babies with the Fallot (blue baby) syndrome, played a key role in preventing the approval of thalidomide by the FDA. It is estimated that about seven thousand births were affected by the ingestion of thalidomide.

The thalidomide incident made all scientists more skeptical about the final approval of any type of medicine, especially those likely to be used during pregnancy. The trend intensified the fight against any chemicals that might affect the fetus during the first trimester, when it is particularly vulnerable to teratogens. Alcohol and tobacco drew many headlines in the media in the 1990s. Both have been shown to create congenital problems in mental development and learning abilities. At the same time, regulation of new FDA-approved medicine became much stricter, and efforts to study the long-term effects of various pharmaceuticals increased. Surprisingly, thalidomide itself has been used successfully in leprosy cases and, in conjunction with cyclosporine, to treat cases of the immune reaction that appears in many bone-marrow transplant patients. There is also a movement to use thalidomide in the treatment of acquired immunodeficiency syndrome (AIDS).

In addition to drugs, many other agents can affect fetal development. Essentially, any factor with the potential to cause DNA mutations has a high probability of being teratogenic. Consequently, early in pregnancy, women are advised to limit their exposure to a variety of potential teratogens, such as excess radiation, toxic chemicals, tobacco, alcohol, and other drugs. Prevention might even include work reassignment to limit or eliminate the woman's normal exposure to teratogens. Unfortunately, teratogenesis can occur early in the pregnancy, before the woman is even aware that she is pregnant. Prevention by avoidance is therefore essential.

Soraya Ghayourmanesh, Ph.D.;
updated by Bryan Ness, Ph.D.

FURTHER READING

Ferretti, Patrizia, et al., eds. *Embryos, Genes, and Birth Defects.* 2d ed. Hoboken: Wiley, 2006. Print.

Giavini, Erminio, and Elena Menegola. "Biomarkers of Teratogensis: Suggestions from Animal Studies." *Reproductive Toxicology* 34.2 (2012): 180–85. Print.

Holmes, L. B. "Teratogen-Induced Limb Defects." *American Journal of Medical Genetics* 112.3 (2002): 297–303. Print.

McCredie, Janet. *Beyond Thalidomide: Birth Defects Explained.* London: Royal Society of Medicine, 2007. Print.

Moore, Keith L., T. V. N. Persaud, and Mark H. Torchia. *Before We Are Born: Essentials of Embryology and Birth Defects.* 8th ed. Philadelphia: Elsevier, 2013. Print.

Schardein, James L. *Chemically Induced Birth Defects.* 3d ed. New York: Dekker, 2000. Print.

Stephens, Trent D., and Rock Brynner. *Dark Remedy: The Impact of Thalidomide and Its Revival as a Vital Medicine.* Cambridge, Mass.: Perseus, 2001. Print.

Vajda, Frank J. E., et al. "Teratogenesis in Repeated Pregnancies in Antiepileptic Drug-Treated Women." *Epilepsia* 54.1 (2013): 181–86. Print.

See also: Congenital defects; Prenatal diagnosis.

Totipotency

CATEGORY: Cellular biology

SIGNIFICANCE: Totipotency is the ability of a living cell to express all of its genes to regenerate a whole new individual. Totipotent cells from plants have been used in tissue-culture techniques to produce improved plant materials that are pathogen-free and disease-resistant. Totipotent cells from animals are now being used to clone mammals, although ethical questions remain over whether cloning a human should be done.

KEY TERMS

multipotent cell: a stem cell capable of forming multiple differentiated tissues

parthenogenesis: asexual reproduction from a single egg without fertilization by sperm

pluripotent cell: a stem cell that forms all types of differentiated tissues

unipotent cell: a stem cell that forms only one differentiated tissue

EGG AND SPERM CELLS

In plants and animals, a whole organism is sexually reproduced from a zygote, a product of fusion between egg and sperm. Zygotes are totipotent. A zygote in the seed of a plant or in the uterus of a mammal divides by mitosis and has the potential to produce more cells, called embryonic cells, before developing into an adult individual. During embryonic cell division, the cells begin to differentiate. Once differentiated, these specialized cells still

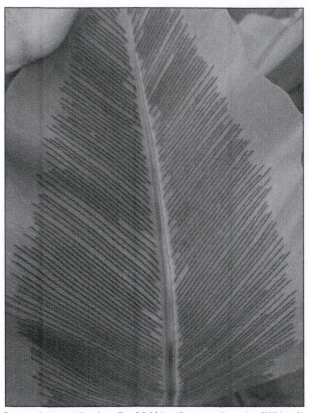

Spores for reproduction By Mokkie (Own work), via Wikimedia Commons

zygote public domain via wikimedia commons

possess all the genetic materials inherited from the zygote. Differentiated cells express or use some of their genes (not all) to produce their own specific proteins. For example, epidermal cells in human beings produce fibrous proteins called keratin to protect the skin, and red blood cells produce hemoglobin to help transport oxygen. Due to the differences in gene expression, differentiated cells have their own distinct structures and functions, and some differentiated cells are totipotent.

A whole organism can be asexually reproduced from a single egg without the sperm by a process called parthenogenesis. This occurs naturally in some insects, snakes, lizards, and amphibians, as well as in some plants. In this type of reproduction, the haploid chromosomes within an unfertilized egg duplicate, and the embryo develops as if the egg had been fertilized. The pseudo-fertilized eggs are totipotent and generate all female individuals. The females can reproduce under favorable environmental conditions without waiting for a mate. Like in vitro fertilization, parthenogenesis is used as a technique to create an embryo in the laboratory. Chromosomal duplication is induced in the egg cell to reproduce female individuals.

It may become possible to produce males through a process called androgenesis. In the laboratory, the haploid chromosomes from one sperm may be induced to duplicate. As in animal cloning, the duplicated chromosomes, which are diploid, can be implanted into an enucleated egg cell (a cell from which the nucleus has been removed). Although androgenesis holds some promise, so far it has not produced normal embryos.

CELL DIFFERENTIATION

Cell differentiation is a process whereby genetically identical cells become different or specialized for their specific functions. During differentiation, enzymes and other polypeptides, including other large molecules, are synthesized. Ribosomes and other cell structures are assembled. Differentiated cells express only some of their genes to make enzymes and other proteins.

Tissue differentiation is usually triggered by mitosis, followed by cytokinesis. Then differentiation occurs in the daughter cells. Often the two daughter cells have different structures and functions, but both retain the same genes. For example, the epidermal cell mitotically divides to produce one large and one small cell on the root surface; the large one maintains the role of epidermal cell as a root covering, whereas the small one becomes the root hair.

TOTIPOTENT CELLS IN PLANT-TISSUE CULTURE

Cuttings of plants and tissue-culture techniques have proven that many plant cells are totipotent. Tissue culture, however, helps to identify what specific type of cell is totipotent, because the technique uses a very small piece of known tissue. For example, if pith tissues from tobacco (*Nicotiana tobaccum*), soybean (*Glycine max*), and other dicot stems are cut off and cultured aseptically on an agar medium with proper nutrients and hormones, a clump of unspecialized and loosely arranged cells, called a callus, is formed. Each cell from the callus begins to divide and differentiate, forming a multicellular embryoid. One test tube can accommodate thousands of cells, and each embryoid has the potential to become a complete plantlet. Plantlets can be transplanted into the soil to develop into adult plants.

The phloem tissues from the roots of carrots (*Daucus* species) also exhibit totipotency. Cells in pollen grains of tobacco are totipotent, and they produce haploid plants. Using meristem tissues of shoot and root tips, the cells regenerate new plants that are free of viruses, bacteria, and fungi. Pathogen elimination is possible because vascular tissues (xylem and phloem), in which viruses move, do not reach the root or shoot apex. The protoplasts (cells without cell walls) from mesophyll cells of the leaf regenerate new plants.

PLANT HORMONES

Totipotency of plant cells is enhanced by the presence of hormones, such as auxins and cytokinins, in the culture media. Addition of auxins influences the expression of genes and causes physiological and morphological changes in plants. Addition of cytokinins promotes cell division, cytokinesis, and organ formation. If these are present in the proper ratio, callus from many plant species can be made to develop into an entire new plant. If the cytokinin-to-auxin ratio is high, cells in the callus divide and give rise to the development of buds, stems, and leaves. If the cytokinin-to-auxin ratio is low, root formation is favored. Totipotency of some plant cells is promoted by the addition of coconut water to the culture media—an indication that coconut water has the right proportion of cytokinin and auxin to regenerate an entire plant.

IMPORTANCE OF TOTIPOTENCY IN PLANTS

Clonal propagation of plants using tissue culturing is used commercially to mass-produce numerous ornamentals, vegetables, and forest trees. A major use of pathogen-free plants is for the storage of germ plasm and for transport of plant materials into different countries. It is also posssible to generate plants with desirable traits, such as resistance to herbicides and environmental stressors or tolerance of soil salinity, soil acidity, and heavy-metal toxicity. It is easier to select resistant or tolerant plants from a thousand cells than from a thousand plants.

SOMATIC CELLS IN ANIMAL CLONING

Animals are more difficult to reproduce asexually than plants are. Somatic cells of animals become totipotent when used as donor cells in cloning. The first animal successfully cloned was a frog, *Xenopus laevis*. This cloning involved the use of a nucleus from the intestinal epithelial cells of a tadpole and an egg cell from a mature frog. In the laboratory, the nucleus from the egg cell was removed (enucleated) by micropipette. The tadpole's nucleus (the donor cell) was inserted into the enucleated frog's egg cell. The nuclei-injected egg cell underwent a series of embryonic developmental stages, including the blastula stage, developing into tadpoles that later died before becoming adults.

Cloning of Dolly the sheep (*Ovis* species) used the mammary cell of a six-year-old ewe as the donor cell. It was injected into the enucleated sheep's egg cell. Cloning a mammal requires a surrogate mother. The blastula stage of the embryo was developed in vitro and was implanted into a surrogate mother. After five months, a lamb was born. The lamb was genetically identical to the sheep from which the mammary cell was taken. Cloning is now done by scientists to produce other animals, including cattle, pigs, monkeys, cats, and dogs. Cloning a human seems possible, but there are many ethical and moral questions about whether it should or should not be done.

STEM CELLS IN ANIMAL CLONING

Stem cells exhibit totipotency because they can generate new types of tissues. Some sources of stem cells are the blastocyst (the immature embryo), the fetus, the placenta, bone marrow, blood, skeletal muscle, and brain. Because there is no proof yet whether a single embryonic stem cell has the ability to regenerate into a complete individual, stem cells are generally only partially totipotent. A unipotent stem cell can form only one differentiated tissue. A multipotent stem cell can form multiple differentiated tissues. For example, stem cells from blood can form platelets, white blood cells, or red blood cells. The stem cells from skeletal muscle can form smooth muscle, cardiac muscle, bone, or cartilage. A pluripotent stem cell from embryo, brain, or bone marrow has the ability to develop all types of differentiated tissues of the body. For example, brain stem cells can be turned into all tissue types, including brain, muscles, blood cells, and nerves.

Domingo M. Jariel, Ph.D.

FURTHER READING

Bhojwani, S. S., and Prem Kumar Dantu. *Plant Tissue Culture: An Introductory Text.* New Delhi: Springer, 2013. Print.

Condic, Maureen L. "Totipotency: What It Is and What It Is Not." *Stem Cells & Development* 23.8 (2014): 796–812. Print.

Galan, Amparo, et al. "Defining the Genomic Signature of Totipotency and Pluripotency During Early Human Development." *PLoS ONE* 8.4 (2013): 1–12. Print.

Gibbs, Melissa. "Plant Cell Totipotency." *A Practical Guide to Developmental Biology.* New York: Oxford UP, 2003. Print.

Lanza, Robert, et al., eds. *Essentials of Stem Cell Biology.* 2d ed. San Diego: Academic Press, 2009. Print.

Prentice, David A. *Stem Cells and Cloning.* New York: Cummings, 2003. Print.

Russell, Peter J. *Genetics.* San Francisco: Cummings, 2002. Print.

Smith, Roberta H. *Plant Tissue Culture Techniques and Experiments.* New York: Academic Press, 2000. Print.

Stillman, Bruce, et al. *Control and Regulation of Stem Cells.* Woodbury: Cold Spring Harbor Laboratory, 2008. Print.

See also: Cell culture: Plant cells; Stem cells.

Tourette syndrome

CATEGORY: Diseases and syndromes
ALSO KNOWN AS: Tourette's syndrome

DEFINITION

Tourette syndrome is a chronic, neurological disorder that is a member of a larger group of primary tic disorders. It is characterized by motor and vocal tics. Both motor and vocal tics must be present, though not necessarily at the same time. Tics must be present for more than one year, and its onset must be prior to age eighteen. Tics are rapid, in voluntary movements or sounds that occur repeatedly.

RISK FACTORS

Patients should tell their doctors if they have any of the risk factors, which include a family history of Tourette syndrome, other tic disorders, or obsessive-compulsive disorder. Males are three to four times more likely to be affected. Another risk factor is strep infection (may be a risk in some children) as some researchers believe an abnormal immune response to strep may be a factor.

There are many secondary causes of tics, including hereditary disorders, carbon monoxide poisoning, traumatic brain injury, cerebral infections, medications, and illegal drugs.

ETIOLOGY AND GENETICS

The causes of Tourette syndrome are complex and poorly understood, but it is likely that both genetic and environmental factors are involved. A clear inheritance pattern has not been established. The characteristic tics expressed by individuals with Tourette syndrome probably result from changes in levels or activities of any of several different neurotransmitters, chemicals produced in the brain that help produce and control voluntary motion.

The only specific gene reported to be associated with a small number of cases of Tourette syndrome is the SLITRK1 gene, found on the long arm of chromosome 13 at position 13q31.1. The normal protein product of this gene is a member of a family of proteins that or chestrate the growth and development of neurons. Specifically, the SLITRK1 protein may be important for the development of the long extensions of nerve cells, called dendrites and axons, which facilitate chemical communication between cells. It is unclear, however, how mutations in this gene might lead to the behavioral features characteristic of the syndrome and if other genes play a role. The majority of people with Tourette syndrome do not have mutations in the SLITRK1 gene, so it is clear that a variety of genetic and environmental factors must be involved as opposed to changes in this one single gene. While some cases of the syndrome do appear to cluster in families, there are also many examples of isolated diagnoses in which there is no previous family history. Researchers continue to study twins, siblings, and families to identify other genes or factors. A sibling study has identified DLGAP3 as a possible candidate gene for Tourette syndrome as it may play a role in the organization of synapses and neuronal cell signaling.

SYMPTOMS

Symptoms range from mild to severe, but most cases are mild and begin during ages three to nine. They can occur suddenly, and the length of time they last can vary. Tics may temporarily decrease with concentration or distraction. During times of stress, they may occur more often.

Tics are divided into motor and vocal, and then subdivided into simple and complex. Common examples of motor tics include simple tics, such as eye blinking, facial grimacing, head jerking, and arm or leg thrusting; and complex tics, such as jumping, smelling, touching things or other people, and twirling around. Common examples of vocal tics include simple tics, such as throat clearing, coughing, sniffing, grunting, yelping, and barking; and complex tics, such as saying words or phrases that do not make sense in a given situation and saying obscene or socially unacceptable words (called coprolalia).

Collage representing groups affected by Tourette syndrome By Content Providers(s): CDC/National Center on Birth Defects and Developmental DisabilitiesXyzzy n at en.wikipedia, from Wikimedia Commons

Portrait of Georges Gilles de la Tourette (1857–1904) By Georges_ Gilles_de_la_Tourette.jpg: Unknown, the plate was photographed by an E. Pirou who might be Eugène Pirou (1841–1909). derivative work: Mikhail Ryazanov, via Wikimedia Commons

Many people with Tourette syndrome also have one or more of the following problems: obsessions, compulsions, and ritualistic behaviors; attention deficit disorder, with or without hyperactivity (ADD or ADHD); learning disabilities; difficulties with impulse control; and sleep disorders.

While tics may occur throughout life, older teens may find that symptoms improve. In less than 10 to 40 percent of cases, people have remission from symptoms.

SCREENING AND DIAGNOSIS

The doctor will ask about a patient's symptoms and medical history and will perform a physical exam. Tourette syndrome is diagnosed by observing the symptoms and reviewing when they began and how they progressed. There are no blood or neurological tests to diagnose Tourette syndrome. Some doctors may order a magnetic resonance imaging (MRI) scan, a computed tomography (CT) scan, an electroencephalogram (EEG), or blood tests to rule out other disorders.

TREATMENT AND THERAPY

Most people with Tourette syndrome do not need medical treatment. If patients have a tic that disrupts daily activities, there are treatments. The most common is neuroleptic medication. No single treatment is helpful for all people with Tourette syndrome.

Treatment may not completely eliminate symptoms and come with side effects.

Several medications can help control tics, including clonidine (Catapres), pimozide (Orap), risperidone (Risperdal), and haloperidol (Haldol), as well as newer antipsychotic medications, such as aripiperazole (Abilify) and ziprasidone (Geodon). Obsessive-compulsive symptoms may be treated with fluoxetine (Prozac), clomipramine (Anafranil), sertraline (Zoloft), or other similar medications. Symptoms of ADHD may be treated with stimulants, such as methylphenidate (Ritalin), pemoline (Cylert), or dextroamphetamine sulfate (Dexedrine), the sympatholytic drug guanfacine (Estulic), or tricyclic antidepressants.

Other forms of treatment include behavior therapy, which can help people with Tourette syndrome learn to substitute their tics with alternative movements or sounds that are more acceptable. Cognitive behavioral therapy can help reduce obsessive-compulsive symptoms. Relaxation, biofeedback, and exercise can reduce the stress that often makes symptoms worse.

Psychotherapy can help people with Tourette syndrome and their families cope with the disorder. In tic disorders associated with pediatric autoimmune neuropsychiatric disorders associated with streptococcal (PANDAS), intravenous immunoglobulin therapy has been used with some success in a small number of patients, but this therapy is still considered experimental.

For severe tic symptoms that interfere with daily functioning, deep brain stimulation to target areas of the brain that control movement may help, but more research is necessary to evaluate its effectiveness.

PREVENTION AND OUTCOMES

There is currently no known way to prevent Tourette syndrome. In some people symptoms improve during the late teens or early 20's, while for others it is chronic and lifelong. The condition does not alter life expectancy.

Laurie Rosenblum, M.P.H.;
reviewed by Rimas Lukas, M.D.
"Etiology and Genetics" by Jeffrey A. Knight, Ph.D.;
updated by Deanna M. Neff, M.P.H.

FURTHER READING

Bruun, Ruth Dowling, and Bertel Bruun. "*A Mind of Its Own: Tourette's Syndrome—A Story and a Guide.*" New York: Oxford University Press, 1994.

Crane J, Fagerness J, Osiecki L, et al. "Family-based" genetic association study of DLGAP3 in Tourette Syndrome. "Am J Med Genet B Neuropsychiatr Genet." 2011;156(1):108-14.

EBSCO Publishing. "DynaMed: Tourette Syndrome." Ipswich, Mass.: Author, 2009. Available through http://www.ebscohost.com/dynamed.

"Health Librar y: Tourette Syndrome." Ipswich, Mass.: Author, 2009. Available through http://www.ebscohost.com.

Mell, L. K., R. L. Davis, and D. Owens. "Association Between Streptococcal Infection and Obsessive-Compulsive Disorder, Tourette's Syndrome, and Tic Disorder." *Pediatrics* 116, no. 1 (July, 2005): 56-60.

Menkes, John H., and Har vey B. Sarnat, eds. "*Child Neurology.*" 6th ed. Philadelphia: Lippincott Williams & Wilkins, 2000.

Samuels, Martin A., and Steven K. Feske, eds. "Office Practice of Neurology." 2d ed. Philadelphia: Churchill Livingstone, 2003.

Tamara P. "Tourette syndrome and other tic disorders of childhood." "Handb Clin Neurol." 2013. 112:853-6.

WEB SITES OF INTEREST

About Kids Health
http://www.aboutkidshealth.ca
Genetics Home Reference
http://ghr.nlm.nih.gov
National Institute of Neurological Disorders and Stroke: NINDS Tourette Syndrome Information Page
http://www.ninds.nih.gov/disorders/tourette/tourette.htm
OMIM® Online Mendelian Inheritance in Man
http://www.omim.org/about
Orphanet Journal of Rare Diseases
https://ojrd.biomedcentral.com/
Tourette Syndrome Association
http://www.tsa-usa.org
Tourette Syndrome Foundation of Canada
http://www.tourette.ca

See also: Attention deficit hyperactivity disorder (ADHD); Autism; Bipolar affective disorder; Dyslexia; Fragile X syndrome; Schizophrenia.

Transgenic organisms

CATEGORY: Genetic engineering and biotechnology

SIGNIFICANCE: Implanting genes from one organism into the genome of another enables scientists to study basic genetic mechanisms and inherited diseases and to create plants and animals with traits that are beneficial to humans.

KEY TERMS

genome: the complete genetic material carried by an individual

plasmid: a circular piece of bacterial DNA that is often used as a vector

transformation: integration of foreign DNA into a cell

transgene: the foreign gene incorporated into a cell's DNA during transformation

vector: a carrier molecule that introduces foreign genetic materials into a cell

ENGINEERING ORGANISMS

Domestication and selective breeding of animals and plants began before recorded history. In fact, historians propose, the shaping of organisms to fit human needs contributed to the rise of settled complex cultures. Until late in the twentieth century, farmers and scientists could breed novel strains only from closely related species or subspecies because the DNA had to be compatible in order to produce offspring that in turn were fertile.

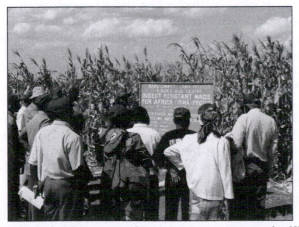

In an effort to reduce corn stem-borer infestations, corporate and public researchers partner to develop local Bt (Bacillus thuringiensis) corn varieties suitable for Kenya. By Dave Hoisington/CIMMYT, via Wikimedia Commons

Transgenic mouse hippocamus By National Institutes of Health (NIH) (National Institutes of Health (NIH)), via Wikimedia Commons

In the late 1970s and early 1980s, molecular biologists learned how to surpass the limitations of selective breeding. They invented procedures for combining the DNA of species as distantly related as microbes, plants, and animals. These organisms carrying the novel heritable genetic material derived from different species using recombinant molecular biology techniques are termed as transgenic or genetically modified organisms (GMO). Genetic engineering makes it possible to design novel organisms for genetic and biochemical research and for medical, agricultural, and ecological innovations. However, commercial use of transgenic organisms created worldwide controversy because of their potential threat to human health and the environment.

Transgenesis seeks to produce an entirely modified organism by incorporating the transgene into all the cells of the mature organism and changing the genome. This is done by transforming not only the somatic (body) cells of the host organism but also the germ cells, so that when the organism reproduces, the transgene will pass to the next generation. Transgenes can block the function of a host gene, replace the host gene with one that codes for a variant protein, or introduce additional proteins.

TRANSGENIC ANIMALS

In recent years the use of transgenic organisms has become widespread and a large variety of animals and plants has been successfully engineered. Some examples of transgenic mammals include mice, rabbits, pigs, sheep, and cows. Birds such as chickens as well as fishes like salmon and trout, and even amphibians like frogs and toads have been made transgenic. Among invertebrates, transgenic fruit flies (*Drosophila melanogaster*) and nematodes (*Caenorhabditis elegans*) have become indispensable for research.

The first transgenic mice were created by Rudolf Jaenisch in 1974, showing that SV40 viral DNA had integrated into mouse genome. In 1982, Richard Palmiter and Ralph Brinster created "supermice" that grew much larger than ordinary mice because these had received the rat growth hormone gene. Most of these transformations were generated by microinjection of DNA directly into cells. Later, scientists were able to deliver foreign genes into hosts by several other methods: incorporating them into retroviruses and then infecting target cells; electroinfusion, whereby an electric current passed the foreign DNA through the relatively flimsy animal cell wall; and biolistics, a means of mechanically shooting a DNA bullet into cells. Two methods, developed at first for mice, are particularly successful in creating genetically modified animals. The first entails injecting transformed embryonic stem cells into a blastocyst (an early spherical form of an embryo). In the second, the DNA is inserted into the pronucleus of a freshly fertilized egg. The blastocyst or egg is then implanted into a foster mother for gestation.

Initially, the modified transgenic animals were intended for scientific research studies. After disabling a specific gene, scientists could study its effect on the structure, metabolic processes, and health of the mature animal. By 2003, thousands of genes had been tested. Studies on mice transformed with human DNA enabled scientists to identify genes associated with breast and prostate cancers, cystic fibrosis, Alzheimer's disease, and severe combined immunodeficiency disorder (SCID). In 2001, the first transgenic primate, a rhesus monkey, expressing the green fluorescent protein was created. It took quite a few years before the first transgenic primate model for the human disorder Huntington's disease, was generated in rhesus macaque in 2008. However, both these animals were unable to give birth to offspring carrying the transgene. In 2009, scientists in the laboratory of Tatsuji Nomura created transgenic marmosets that are the first transgenic primates that

were able to pass the foreign gene to their offspring, potentially supplying a research model genetically much more similar to humans than mice.

Beginning in the late 1990s, transgenic animals were developed for production of proteins that can be used in pharmaceutical drugs to treat human disease. Accordingly, they have become known as "pharm animals." This new technology is known as biopharming and has a potential for producing large quantities of pharmaceutical products and vaccines at much lower costs. A number of companies are developing bioproducts using transgenic domestic lifestock. They include blood clotting factors, malarial antigens for vaccine against malaria, and spider silk protein for fiber development. One example of a transgenic animal is lactating transgenic mice producing tissue plasminogen activator in their milk. Similarly, transgenic sheep supply blood coagulation factor IX and alpha1-antitrypsin, transgenic pigs produce human hemoglobin, and transgenic cows make human lactoferrin. Scientists have also developed transgenic pigs that may supply tissue and organs for transplantation into humans without tissue rejection.

TRANSGENIC PLANTS

Plant cells present greater difficulties for transformation because their cell walls are sturdier than animal cell walls. Microinjection and biolistics are possible, but tricky and slow. A breakthrough for plant transgenesis came in 1983, when three separate teams of scientists used plasmids as vectors (carrier molecules) to infect plants with foreign DNA. The achievement came about because of research into plant tumors caused by crown gall disease. The pathogen, the soil bacterium, *Agrobacterium tumefaciens*, caused the disease by ferrying bits of its own DNA into the genome of plants via plasmids, circular bits of extranuclear DNA. Scientists found that they could take the same plasmid, cut out bits of its DNA with enzymes and insert transgenes, and then use the altered plasmids as vectors to transform plants. Subsequently, scientists discovered that liposomes can be vectors. A liposome is a tiny ball of lipids that binds readily to a cell wall, opens a passage, and delivers any DNA that has been put inside it.

A great variety of transgenic plants have been designed for agriculture to produce genetically modified (GM) foods. The first to be marketed was a strain of tomato that ripened slowly so that it gained flavor by staying longer on the vine and remained ripe longer on supermarket shelves. However this Flavr Savr tomato was not a commercial success. Other crops have been made resistant to herbicides so that weeds can be easily killed without harming the food plants. Corn, cotton, soybeans, potatoes, and papayas received a gene from the bacterium *Bacillus thuringiensis* (*Bt*) that enables them to make a caterpillar-killing toxin; these are frequently referred to as *Bt* crops. Herbicide resistant (HT) soybeans were cultivated in 94 percent of the total US soybean acreage in 2014, according to the US Department of Agriculture. Other transgenic crops such as pest-resistant (*Bt*) cotton was grown in 84 percent of cotton acreage while *Bt* corn was grown in 80 percent of the total corn acreage. Despite the expanding acreage, the diversity of crop types and traits in commercial production is tightly regulated by government agencies.

Like transgenic animals, some transgenic crops promise to deliver pharmaceuticals at lower costs and more conveniently than factory-made drugs. In 2000, scientists reported invention of rice and wheat strains that produce anticancer antibodies. Golden rice, a transgenic strain that contains vitamin A, was developed to ward off blindness from vitamin A deficiency, which is a problem in countries that subsist largely on rice. Another strain has elevated iron levels to combat anemia. Also in a bid to reduce the health risk from smoking, a tobacco company developed a strain free of nicotine. In recent years, maize, potato, soybean, and tomato have been used to produce vaccines for both humans and animals against pneumonic and bubonic plague. A vaccine for hepatitis B has been developed in transgenic potatoes that raises an immunological response in humans. Also edible rice-based vaccine targeted to allergic diseases such as asthma, seasonal allergies, and atopic dermatitis has been developed.

THE DEBATE OVER TRANSGENESIS

Transgenic organisms offer great benefits to humankind: deeper understanding of the genetic component in disease and aids in diagnosis; new, cheaper, more easily produced drugs; and crops that could help alleviate the growing hunger in the world. Yet during the 1990s protests against transgenesis began that are as contentious as any since the controversy over the pesticide DDT during the 1960s.

Some opponents object to the very fact that organisms are modified strictly for human benefit. They find such manipulations of life's essential code blasphemous and arrogant, or at the very least unethical and reckless. Furthermore, animal rights groups regard the production of transgenic pharm and research animals as cruel and in violation of the natural rights of other species.

The greater portion of opponents, however, are concerned with specific dangers that transgenic organism may pose. Many consumers, most noticeably those in Europe, worry that GM foods contain hidden health risks. After transgenes were found to escape from crops and become part of wild plants, environmentalists proposed that there could be unforeseen and harmful ecological consequences, especially in the destruction of natural species and reduction of biodiversity.

Even those who welcome the creation of transgenic animals and plants are concerned about the legal and social effects. Principally, because biotechnology corporations can patent transgenic organisms, they potentially have great influence on agribusiness, perhaps to the detriment of small farmers and consumers.

Therefore, as with the development of any new technology, it is critical to conduct extensive studies and peer reviewed research for harnessing the power of genetic engineering. The close scrutiny and appropriate policies would allow the human society to reap its immense benefits without compromising biodiversity or creating environmental imbalance.

Roger Smith, Ph.D.;
updated by Poonam Bhandari, Ph.D.

FURTHER READING

Brown, Kathryn, Karen Hopkin, and Sasha Nemecek. "GM Foods: Are They Safe?" *Scientific American* 284.4 (2001): 52–57. Print.

Fernandez-Cornejo, Jorge. "Recent Trends in GE Adoption." *USDA.gov.* US Dept. of Agriculture, 14 July 2014. Web. 21 Aug. 2014.

Houdebine, Louis-Marie. "Production of Pharmaceutical Proteins by Transgenic Animals." *Comparative Immunology, Microbiology, and Infectious Diseases* 32 (2009): 107–21. Print.

Lurquin, Paul F. *The Green Phoenix: A History of Genetically Modified Plants.* New York: Columbia UP, 2001. Print.

MacKellar, C., and David Albert Jones. *Chimera's Children: Ethical, Philosophical, and Religious Perspectives on Human-Nonhuman Experimentation.* London: Continuum, 2012. Print.

Nicholl, Desmond S. T. *An Introduction to Genetic Engineering.* 2d ed. New York: Cambridge UP, 2002. Print.

Piguet, Pascale, and Philippe Poindron. *Genetically Modified Organism and Genetic Engineering in Research and Therapy.* New York: Krager, 2012. Print.

Rehbinder, E., et al. *Pharming: Promises and Risks of Biopharmaceuticals Derived from Genetically Modified Plants and Animals.* Berlin: Springer-Verlag, 2009. Print.

Velander, William, et al. "Transgenic Livestock as Drug Factories." *Scientific American* 276 (Jan. 1997). Print.

Winston, Mark L. *Travels in the Genetically Modified Zone.* Cambridge: Harvard UP, 2002. Print.

See also: Antibodies; Biopesticides; Biopharmaceuticals; Genetic engineering; Genetic engineering: Agricultural applications; Genetic engineering: Medical applications; Genetic engineering: Risks; Genetic engineering: Social and ethical issues; Genetically modified foods; Genomics; Human growth hormone; Hybridization and introgression; Knockout genetics and knockout mice; Lateral gene transfer; Model organism: *Drosophila melanogaster*; Model organism: *Mus musculus*; Model organism: *Xenopus laevis*; Molecular genetics; Viroids and virusoids.

Transposable elements

CATEGORY: Bacterial genetics; Molecular genetics

SIGNIFICANCE: Transposable elements are discrete DNA sequences that have evolved the means to move (transpose) within the chromosomes. Transposition results in mutation and potentially large-scale genome rearrangements. Transposable elements contribute to the problem of multiple antibiotic resistance by mobilizing the genes of pathogenic bacteria for antibiotic resistance.

KEY TERMS

composite transposon: a transposable element that contains genes other than those required for transposition

resistance plasmid (R plasmid): a small, circular DNA molecule that replicates independently of the bacterial host chromosome and encodes a gene for antibiotic resistance

selfish DNA: a DNA sequence that has no apparent purpose for the host and that spreads by forming additional copies of itself within the genome

transposase: an enzyme encoded by a transposable element that initiates transposition by cutting specifically at the ends of the element and randomly at the site of insertion

JUMPING GENES

Transposable elements are DNA sequences that are capable of moving from one chromosomal location to another in the same cell. In some senses, transposable elements have been likened to intracellular viruses. The first genetic evidence for transposable elements was described by Barbara McClintock in the 1940s. She was studying the genetics of the pigmentation of maize (corn) kernels and realized that the patterns of inheritance were not following Mendelian laws. Furthermore, she surmised that insertion and excision of genetic material were responsible for the genetic patterns she observed. McClintock was recognized for this pioneering work with a Nobel Prize in Physiology or Medicine in 1983. It was not until the 1960s that the jumping genes that McClintock postulated were isolated and characterized. The first transposable elements to be well characterized were found in the bacteria *Escherichia coli* but have subsequently been found in the cells of many bacteria, plants, and animals.

McClintock giving her Nobel Lecture at Karolinska Institute in Stockholm during the week of the Nobel Prize ceremony. See page for author, via Wikimedia Commons

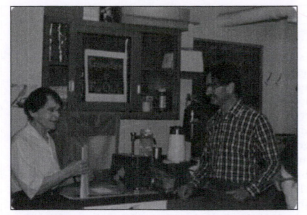

Barbara McClintock with George P. Redei at the Stadler Genetics Symposium, University of Missouri-Columbia. Courtesy of the Barbara McClintock Papers, American Philosophical Society. See page for author, via Wikimedia Commons

Transposable elements are discrete DNA sequences that encode a transposase, an enzyme that catalyzes transposition. Transposition refers to the movement within a genome. The borders of the transposable element are defined by specific DNA sequences; often the sequences at either end of the transposable element are inverted repeats of one another. The transposase enzyme cuts the DNA sequences at the ends of the transposable element to initiate transposition and cuts the DNA at the insertion site. The site for insertion of the transposable element is not specific. Therefore, transposition results in random insertion into chromosomes and often results in mutation and genome rearrangement. In many organisms, transposition accounts for a significant fraction of all mutation. Although the details of the mechanism may vary, there are two basic mechanisms of transposition: conservative and replicative. In conservative transposition, the transposable element is excised from its original site and inserted at another. In replicative transposition, a copy of the transposable element is made and is inserted in a new location. The original transposable element remains at its initial site.

A subset of the replicative transposable elements includes the retrotransposons. These elements transpose through an RNA intermediate. Interestingly, their DNA sequence and organization are similar to those of retroviruses. It is likely that either retroviruses evolved from retrotransposons by gaining the genes to produce the proteins for a viral coat or retrotransposons evolved from retroviruses that lost the genes for a viral coat. This is one of the reasons that transposons are likened to viruses. Viruses can be thought of as transposons that gained the genes for a protein coat and thus the ability to leave one cell and infect others; conversely, transposons can be thought of as intracellular viruses.

GENETIC CHANGE AND SELFISH DNA

Transposition is a significant cause of mutation for many organisms. When McClintock studied the genetic patterns of maize kernel pigmentation, she saw the results of insertion and excision of transposable elements into and out of the pigment genes. Subsequently, it has been well established that mutations in many organisms are the result of insertion of transposable elements into and around genes. Transposition sometimes results in deletion mutations as well. Occasionally the transposase will cut at one end of the transposable element but skip the other end, cutting the DNA further downstream. This can result in a deletion of the DNA between the end of the transposable element and the cut site.

In addition to these direct results, it is believed that transposable elements may be responsible for large-scale rearrangements of chromosomes. Genetic recombination, the exchange of genetic information resulting in new combinations of DNA sequences, depends upon DNA sequence homology. Normally, recombination does not occur between nonhomologous chromosomes or between two parts of the same chromosome. However, transposition can create small regions of homology (the transposable element itself) spread throughout the chromosomes. Recombination occurring between homologous transposable elements can create deletions, inversions, and other large-scale rearrangements of chromosomes.

Scientists often take advantage of transposable elements to construct mutant organisms for study. The random nature of insertion ensures that many different genes can be mutated, the relatively large insertion makes it likely that there will be a complete loss of gene function, and the site of insertion is easy to locate to identify the mutated region.

Biologists often think of natural selection as working at the level of the organism. DNA sequences that confer a selective advantage to the organism are increased in number as a result of the increased reproductive success of the organisms that possess

Barbara McClintock

Though best known for her research on mobile genetic elements (for which she won the first unshared Nobel Prize in Physiology or Medicine awarded to a woman), Barbara McClintock's contributions to the field of genetics were many. McClintock's career in genetics spanned the development of the field itself. While an undergraduate at Cornell University (from which she earned her bachelor of science degree in 1923), she was invited to participate in a graduate course in genetics, then a fledgling discipline. She continued at Cornell as a graduate student (earning her Ph.D. in 1927), combining her interests in the microscopic internal structure of the cell (cytology) with the transmission of heritable traits (genetics).

McClintock's keen observational skills and her holistic approach to science allowed her to make significant advancements. It had only recently been established that the chromosomes (visible under the microscope) were the carriers of Gregor Mendel's "factors," or genes.

McClintock used information gleaned from characteristics of the corn plant, Zea mays (maize), in conjunction with changes in its chromosomes to elucidate many aspects of genetic control. Her first major contribution was the identification and naming of the maize chromosomes. Shortly after, using cytological markers on the chromosomes, McClintock and graduate student Harriet Creighton demonstrated the correlation between patterns of inheritance and chromosomal crossover—the exchange of material between chromosomes. Breeding experiments focusing on "linkage groups" allowed McClintock to associate each of corn's ten chromosomes with the genes they carry.

At that point, Lewis Stadler, who was studying the mutagenic effects of X rays, sent some irradiated corn to McClintock. McClintock demonstrated that the resultant broken chromosomes can fuse into a ring, and she then hypothesized the existence of the telomere, a protective stabilizing structure at the end of the chromosome. At the University of Missouri, McClintock observed the ability of such broken chromosomes to go through a series of breakages and fusions (the breakagefusion-bridge cycle) and identified concomitant chromosomal inversions and deletions. She ultimately discovered that certain genes could transfer from cell to cell and between chromosomes, thereby influencing the color patterns in the leaves and kernels of corn.

In 1941, McClintock moved to Cold Spring Harbor, New York, where she would remain. Doing much of her work before the discovery of the double helical structure of DNA, she rejected the simplistic one-way flow from DNA to RNA to protein outlined in the central dogma of molecular biology, seeking instead an explanation for the spatial and temporal variation in gene expression needed to link genetics to developmental and evolutionary change. Her own work showed that both the location and direction of genetic material, as well as the presence of other "controlling elements," had important effects on the expression of the gene. In addition to this better-known work, McClintock identified the chromosomes of the bread mold *Neurospora* and described its meiotic cycle. She also headed a study aimed at conserving indigenous corn varieties in the Americas. In recognition of her place as one of the most distinguished scientists of the twentieth century, *The Barbara McClintock Papers* are available through the National Library of Medicine through its "Profiles in Science" Web site. Barbara McClintock (© The Nobel Foundation)

Lee Anne Martínez, Ph.D.

those sequences. It has been said that organisms are simply DNA's means of producing more DNA. In 1980, however, W. Ford Doolittle, Carmen Sapienza, Leslie Orgel, and Francis Crick elaborated on another kind of selection that occurs among DNA sequences within a cell. In this selection, DNA sequences are competing with each other to be replicated. DNA sequences that spread by forming additional copies of themselves will increase relative to other DNA sequences. There is selection for discrete DNA sequences to evolve the means to propagate themselves. One of the key points is that this selection does not work at the level of the organism's phenotype. There may be no advantage for the organism to have these DNA sequences. In fact, it may be that there is a slight disadvantage to having many of these DNA sequences. For this reason, DNA sequences that are selected because of their tendency to make additional copies of themselves are referred to as "selfish" DNA. Transposable elements are often cited as examples of selfish DNA.

COMPOSITE TRANSPOSONS AND ANTIBIOTIC RESISTANCE

Some transposable elements have genes unrelated to the transposition process located between the inverted, repeat DNA sequences that define the ends of the element. These are referred to as composite transposons. Very frequently, bacterial composite transposons contain a gene that encodes resistance to antibiotics. The consequence is that the antibiotic resistance gene is mobilized. It will jump along with the rest of the transposable element to new DNA sites. Composite transposons may be generated when two of the same type of transposable elements end up near each other and flanking an antibiotic resistance gene. If mutations occurred to change the sequences at the "inside ends" of the transposable elements, the transposase would then only recognize and cut at the two "outside end" sequences to cause everything in between to be part of a new composite transposon.

Resistance to antibiotics is a growing public health problem that threatens to undo much of the progress that the antibiotic revolution made against infectious disease. Transposition of composite transposons is part of the problem. Transposition can occur between any two sites within the same cell, including between the chromosome and plasmid DNA. Plasmids are small, circular DNA molecules that replicate independently of the bacterial host chromosome. Resistance plasmids (R plasmids) are created when composite transposons carrying an antibiotic resistance gene insert into a plasmid. What makes this particularly serious is that some plasmids encode fertility factors (genes that promote the transfer of the plasmid from one bacterium to another). This provides a mechanism for rapid and widespread antibiotic resistance whenever antibiotics are used. The great selective pressure exerted by antibiotic use results in the spread of R plasmids throughout the bacterial population. This, in turn, increases the opportunities for composite transposon insertion into R plasmids to create multiple drug-resistant R plasmids. The first report of multiple antibiotic resistance caused by R plasmids was in Japan in 1957 when strains of *Shigella dysenteriae*, which causes dysentery, became resistant to four common antibiotics all at once. Some R plasmids encode resistance for up to eight different antibiotics, which often makes treatment of bacterial infection difficult. Furthermore, some plasmids are able to cause genetic transfer between bacterial species, limiting the usefulness of many antibiotics.

Craig S. Laufer, Ph.D.

FURTHER READING

Boyd, Gregory A. *Transposable Elements.* New York: Springer, 2012. Print.

Bushman, Frederic. *Lateral DNA Transfer: Mechanisms and Consequences.* Cold Spring Harbor: Cold Spring Harbor Laboratory, 2002. Print.

Capy, Pierre, et al. *Dynamics and Evolution of Transposable Elements.* New York: Chapman, 1998. Print.

Galun, Esra. *Transposable Elements: A Guide to the Perplexed and the Novice, with Appendices on RNAi, Chromatin Remodeling, and Gene Tagging.* Boston: Kluwer Academic, 2003. Print.

Kazazian, Haig H. Jr. *Mobile DNA: Finding Treasure in Junk.* Upper Saddle River: FT, 2011. Print.

Keller, Evelyn Fox. *A Feeling for the Organism: The Life and Work of Barbara McClintock.* 10th anniversary ed. New York: Freeman, 1993. Print.

McClintock, Barbara. *The Discovery and Characterization of Transposable Elements: The Collected Papers of Barbara McClintock.* New York: Garland, 1987. Print.

McDonald, John F., ed. *Transposable Elements and Genome Evolution.* London: Kluwer Academic, 2000. Print.

Peterson, Thomas. *Plant Transposable Elements: Methods and Protocols.* New York: Humana, 2013. Print.

See also: Antisense RNA; Archaea; Bacterial resistance and super bacteria; Immunogenetics; Lateral gene transfer; Model organism: *Escherichia coli*; Molecular genetics; Mutation and mutagenesis; Plasmids; Repetitive DNA.

Triple X

ALSO KNOWN AS: Multiple X syndrome; metafemale

SIGNIFICANCE: Genetic defects are quite common in humans. The frequency of females born with XXX chromosomes, called triple X or multiple X syndrome, generally occurs in about one in one thousand but may be less in some populations. Although most such females have normal

Drosophila repleta, lateral

Different types of sex determination depending on chromosomes.

appearance and sexual reproduction, this abnormality needs to be better understood so that the affected individuals' lives are bettered medically and socially.

KEY TERMS

autosomes: all chromosomes other than sex chromosomes in a cell nucleus

Barr body: named after its discoverer, Murray L. Barr, a dark-stained sex chromatin body in nuclei of females, which represents the inactivated X chromosome; the number of Barr bodies in any cell is generally one less than the number of X chromosomes

Lyon hypothesis: proposed by Mary Lyon in 1962, a hypothesis that during development one of the two X chromosomes in normal mammalian females is inactivated at random; the inactivated X chromosome is a Barr body

meiosis: the process by which gametes (sperm and eggs) are produced in sexually reproducing organisms

nondisjunction: the failure of homologous chromosomes to disjoin during meiosis I, or the failure of sister chromatids to separate and migrate to opposite poles during meiosis II

sex chromosomes: the homologous pair of chromosomes that determines the sex of an individual; in humans, XX is female and XY is male; XX females produce one kind of gamete, X (homogametic sex), and XY males produce two kinds of gametes, X and Y (heterogametic sex)

HISTORY AND SYMPTOMS

Bridges, Calvin discovered nondisjunction of sex chromosomes in the fruit fly, *Drosophila melanogaster.* In 1925, he proposed the genic or sex balance theory, which defined the relationship between sex chromosomes and autosomes (A) for sex determination. According to this theory, the following ratios of sex chromosomes and numbers of sets of autosomes determine what sex phenotype will emerge in humans. For example, XX + 2 sets of autosomes (2X:2A, ratio = 1.0) = normal female; XY + 2 sets of autosomes (1X:2A, ratio = 0.5) = normal male; and XXX + 2 sets of autosomes (3X:2A, ratio = 1.5) = metafemale, or superfemale.

TYPES OF SEX DETERMINATION

The term "metafemale" was first applied to the XXX (triple X) condition by Curt Stern around 1959. The US National Library of Medicine stated in 2014 that the frequency of the triple X phenotype in the general human population was approximately one in one thousand newborn girls. The XXX females are characterized by the presence of two Barr bodies in their cells. They have a total of 47 chromosomes instead of the normal complement of 46.

Affected individuals have variable fertility, ranging from normal to sterile. They may be phenotypically normal but are often slightly taller than average, with longer legs. These individuals may have widely spaced nipples and a webbed neck. Studies have shown that most affected individuals lead a normal sexual life and have normal children. In some cases, menstruation may begin at an older age, menstrual cycles may be irregular or temporarily interrupted, and menopause may begin earlier compared to normal XX women. Abnormal kidney development and seizures may occur in as many as 10 percent of those with triple X syndrome, as reported by the US National Library of Medicine.

GENETIC CAUSE

The basic causes of XXX females are best explained through meiosis, the cell division that halves the number of chromosomes in gametes, and nondisjunction. From a single human cell (46 chromosomes) designated for sexual reproduction, meiosis produces four cells, each with 23 chromosomes. Thus, normal human eggs carry one-half ($22A + 1X = 23$) of the total number of chromosomes ($44A + 2X = 46$). Occasionally, a mistake occurs during meiosis, called nondisjunction. Nondisjunction during meiosis I or meiosis II can produce eggs with 2X chromosomes ($22A + 2X = 24$). Usually the nondisjunction that gives rise to XXX females occurs in the female parent during meiosis I.

Fertilization of an egg carrying two X chromosomes by an X-bearing ($22A + 1X = 23$) sperm results in an individual with $44A + 3X = 47$ chromosomes, or triple X. The extra X chromosome is not usually transmitted to the children. Thus, affected individuals can have normal children. Triplo-X, trisomy X, and 47 XXX are also the names given to the triple

X phenotype. This genetic condition has also been referred to as extra X aneuploidy, multiple X syndrome, or metafemale.

The intelligence quotient (IQ) of affected individuals is usually low normal to normal. In some studies, IQ was found to be lower by 30 points than that of their normal siblings; only a few had an IQ lower than 70. Language learning in XXX children is usually delayed. Emotional maturation may also be delayed. These delays in development are preventable by providing increased psychological, social, and motor stimulation both at home and at school. Tutoring is often needed at some time during development.

The 47 XXX condition can put some affected individuals at risk for speech disorders, learning disabilities, and neuromotor deficits, which ultimately could lead to decreased psychosocial adaptation, especially during adolescence. One study found young females with 47 XXX to be less well adapted in both their teen and adult years; they described their lives as more stressful. On average, they experienced more work, social, and relationship problems than their siblings. Affected individuals may encounter behavioral problems, including mild depression, conduct disorder, immature behavior, and socializing problems. Good parenting and a supportive home may assure a better social and behavioral development.

FURTHER READING

Bender, B., et al. "Psychological Competence of Unselected Young Adults with Sex Chromosome Abnormalities." *American Journal of Medical Genetics* 88.2 (1999): 200–206. Print.

Jones, Kenneth Lyons, Marilyn Crandall Jones, and Miguel del Campo Casanelles. "XXX and XXXX Syndromes." *Smith's Recognizable Patterns of Human Malformation.* 7th ed. Philadelphia: Elsevier Saunders, 2013. Print.

Migeon, Barbara R. *Females Are Mosaics: X Inactivation and Sex Differences in Disease.* 2nd ed. New York: Oxford UP, 2014. Print.

Redei, G. P. *Genetics Manual.* River Edge: World Scientific, 1998. Print.

Rovet, J., et al. "Intelligence and Achievement in Children with Extra X Aneuploidy." *American Journal of Medical Genetics* 60.5 (1995): 356–63. Print.

"Triple X Syndome." *Genetics Home Reference.* US National Library of Medicine, June 2014. Web. 1 Aug. 2014.

Walsh, Beth. "Chromosomal Abnormalities." *Health Library.* EBSCO, May 2014. Web. 1 Aug. 2014.

Derived from: "Metafemales." *Genetics & Inherited Conditions.* Salem Press. 2010.

Tuberous sclerosis

CATEGORY: Diseases and syndromes
ALSO KNOWN AS: Tuberous sclerosis complex (TSC)

DEFINITION

Tuberous sclerosis (TS) is a rare autosomal dominant genetic disease whose name comes from *tuber* (Latin for "swelling") and *skleros* (Greek for "hard"). The condition results from mutations in one of two genes, *TSC1* (coding for hamartin) or *TSC2* (coding for tuberin). TS is a multi-organ disease and is characterized by tumor-like benign lesions called hamartomas in a variety of organs such as the brain, skin, eyes, heart, lungs, and kidneys.

RISK FACTORS

The mutation occurs spontaneously in people with no family history for unknown reasons (in two-thirds of cases) or may be inherited as an autosomal dominant trait (familial; one-third of cases). The estimated prevalence of TS is 1 in 6,000 people. It affects males and females equally, and there is 50 percent chance that the defective gene will be passed on to their offspring. There are no identified risk factors.

ETIOLOGY AND GENETICS

Mutations that render the *TSC1* and *TSC2* genes inactive may be missense, nonsense, deletions, or insertions. Studies have demonstrated that mutations in *TSC2* are about five times more common than mutations in *TSC1* in the sporadic TS population, but occur equally in familial cases at about fifty percent for each gene. There is no clearly identified "hotspot" (preferred site) for mutations; more than four hundred fifty different mutations are known in the *TSC1* gene and approximately thirteen hundred different mutations in the *TSC2* gene. Any particular

Adenoma sebaceum. Multiple wart-like, waxy lumps consisting of angiomatous and fibrous tissue associated with tuberous sclerosis. By M. Sand, D. Sand, C. Thrandorf, V. Paech, P. Altmeyer, F. G. Bechara, via Wikimedia Commons

Cerebral tuberous sclerosis showing sclerotic, hypertrophic circumvolutions Désiré-Magloire Bourneville, via Wikimedia Commons

mutation accounts for around 1 percent of the disease in the affected population. The TSC genes are located on two different chromosomes with TSC1 on chrommosome 9 (9q34) and TSC2 on chromosome 16 (16p13.3). TSC1 encodes the protein hamartin, while TSC2 encodes the protein tuberin.

The harmartin and tuberin proteins have been shown to form heterodimers that play a role in cell division and the production of tumor-suppressor proteins. The proteins are found all over the body. One particular downstream protcin cascade is affected by the pathogenesis of the disease; the pathway of the mammalian target of rapamycin (mTOR). mTOR detects signals of nutrient avail ability, hypoxia, or growth factor stimulation and is part of many cell processes, such as cell-cycle progression, transcription and translation control, and nutrient uptake. Tuberin and hamartin form an intracellular complex that reduces mTOR stimulation.

In families with more than one child with TS complex, no extended family history, and no clinical features of the TS complex, germline mosaicism is the likely explanation. Germ-line mosaicism is when the individual's eggs or sperm may carry the mutation, even though it is absent from the somatic cells. The carrier of germ-line mosaicism may be asymptomatic or may present with various symptoms of the disease.

Symptoms

The symptoms of tuberous sclerosis vary from person to person. The most common presentation is seizures in infancy or early childhood, particularly infantile spasms. Delayed development and skin lesions usually appear shortly after birth but may remain very discrete in children. Other manifestations include kidney and lung disease, skin abnormalities, and vision problems. Skin abnormalities are common marked by light-colored skin, raised and thickened skin, and growths under the nails. Some affected individuals have normal intelligence and no seizures. Others have severe retardation, serious tumors, or difficult-to-control seizures.

Screening and Diagnosis

Diagnosis of TS is usually based on clinical and radiological findings; however, no single feature of TS is diagnostic. Therefore, an evaluation including all clinical features is necessary. The clinical mani festations of TS appear at distinct developmental points. For example, cortical tubers and cardiac rhabdomyomas form during embryogenesis and are typical in infancy. Skin lesions are detected at all ages in more than 90 percent of patients. Hypo pigmented macules (formerly known as ash-leaf spots) are generally detected in infancy or early childhood, whereas the so-called shagreen patch is identified with increasing frequency after the age of five. Ungual fibromas typically appear after puberty and may develop in adulthood.

Genetic testing for either of the two genes that cause this disease (*TSC1* or *TSC2*) is available. Carrier and prenatal testing are available for those with known familial TSC1 or TSC2 mutation.

Treatment and Therapy

There is no specific treatment for TS. Because the disease can differ from person to person, treatment is based on the symptoms. Finding the right anticonvulsant medications to control seizures is often difficult. De pending on the severity of the mental retardation, the child may need special education. Those with renal disease often require antihypertensive medication. Preventative antiepileptic medication has been shown to reduce later seizure activity.

Small growths on the face may be removed by laser treatment, but tend to come back, making repeat treatments necessary. Rhabdomyomas commonly disappear after puberty, so surgery is usually not necessary.

A multidisciplinary team approach is useful to address the many organ systems that may be affected.

Prevention and Outcomes

Molecular genetic testing of the *TSC1* and *TSC2* genes is complicated by the large size of the two genes and the large number of disease-causing mutations. Genetic counseling for families with one affected child should include a small (1 to 2 percent) possibility of recurrence, even for parents without evidence of TS after a thorough diagnostic evaluation.

Prognosis for people with TS can range depending on the severity of symptoms. Individuals with mild forms do not have a shortened life expectancy, while individuals with more severe forms may have serious disabilities. Currently, there is no cure for TS. However, with appropriate medical care (such as lung transplant or surgical removal of tumors) most individuals with the disorder can look for ward to a normal life expectancy.

Maria Mavris, Ph.D.;
updated by Deanna M. Neff, M.P.H.

FURTHER READING

Crino, P. B., K. L. Nathanson, and E. P. Henske. "The Tuberous Sclerosis Complex." *New England Journal of Medicine* 355 (2006):" 1345-1356. Print.

Curatolo, P., R. Bombardieri, and S. Jozwiak. "Tuberous Sclerosis." *Lancet* 372 (2008): 657–668. Print.

Mayer K, Fonatsch C, Wimmer K, van den Ouweland AM, Maat-Kievit AJ. "Clinical utility gene card for: Tuberous sclerosis complex (TSC1, TSC2)." "Eur J Hum Genet." 2013.

Yu Z, Zhang X, Guo H, et al. "A novel TSC2 mutation in a Chinese family with tuberous sclerosis complex." "J Genet." 2014;93(1):169-72.

WEB SITES OF INTEREST

European Organisation for Rare Diseases (EURORDIS)
http://www.eurordis.org
Genetic and Rare Diseases Information Center
https://rarediseases.info.nih.gov/diseases
Genetics Home Reference
https://ghr.nlm.nih.gov/condition
National Organization for Rare Diseases (NORD)
http://www.rarediseases.org
Orphanet: The Portal for Rare Diseases and Orphan Drugs
http://www.orphanet.org
Tuberous Sclerosis Alliance
http://www.tsalliance.org/

See also: Albinism; Chediak-Higashi syndrome; Epidermolytic hyperkeratosis; Hermansky-Pudlak syndrome; Ichthyosis; Melanoma; Palmoplantar keratoderma.

Tumor-suppressor genes

CATEGORY: Molecular genetics

SIGNIFICANCE: Molecular analysis of tumor-suppressor genes has provided important information on mechanisms of cell cycle regulation and patterns of growth control in normal dividing cells and cancer cells. Tumor-suppressor genes represent cell cycle control genes that inhibit cell division and initiate cell death (apoptosis) processes in abnormal cells. Tumor-suppressor genes cause cancer when they are inactivated (turned off), unlike oncogenes which cause cancer when they are activated (turned on). Tumor-suppressor genes can be inherited as well as acquired, unlike oncogenes, which are typically acquired by mutation or improper expression of normal genes (proto-oncogenes). Mutations in tumor-suppressor genes have been identified in many types of human cancer and play a critical role in the genetic destabilization (e.g., through DNA rearrangement) and loss of growth control characteristic of malignancy.

KEY TERMS

cell cycle: a highly regulated series of events critical to the initiation and control of cell division processes

oncogenes: mutated or improperly expressed genes known to cause cancer; the normal form of an oncogene is called a proto-oncogene, which is usually involved in regulating the cell cycle; however, activating or "turning on" the proto-oncogene (through mutation or improper expression) results in cancer

p53 gene: a tumor-suppressor gene implicated in many types of cancer

Rb gene: a tumor-suppressor gene, when inactivated, is associated with several cancers including the formation of a rare and lethal eye tumor (retinoblastoma) in infants

DISCOVERY OF TUMOR-SUPPRESSOR GENES

The existence of genes playing critical roles in cell cycle regulation by inhibiting cell division was predicted by several lines of evidence. In vitro studies involving the fusion of normal and cancer cell lines were observed to result in suppression of the malignant phenotype, suggesting normal cells contained inhibitors with the ability to reprogram the abnormal growth behavior of the cancer cell lines. In addition, back in 1971, studies by Alfred Knudsen on inherited and noninherited forms of retinoblastoma, a childhood cancer associated with tumor formation in the eye, suggested the inactivation of recessive genes as a consequence of mutation, resulted in the loss of function of inhibitory gene products critical to cell division control. With the advent of molecular methods of genetic analysis, the gene whose inactivation is responsible for retinoblastoma was identified and designated *Rb*.

Structure of the RB1 protein. Based on PyMOL rendering of PDB 1ad6. By Emw (Own work), via Wikimedia Commons

Cartoon representation of a complex between DNA and the protein p53 (described in Cho et al. Science 265 pp. 346, 1994 [1]*)* By Thomas Splettstoesser, via Wikimedia Commons

Additional tumor-suppressor genes were identified by studies of DNA tumor viruses whose cancer-causing properties were found to result, in part, from the ability of specific viral gene products to inactivate host cell inhibitory gene products involved in cell cycle regulation. By inactivating these host cell proteins, the tumor virus removes the constraints on viral and cellular proliferation. The most important cellular gene product to be identified in this way is the p53 protein, named after its molecular weight. Genetic studies of human malignancies have implicated mutations in the *p53* gene in up to 75 percent of tumors of diverse tissue origin, including an inherited disorder called Li-Fraumeni syndrome, which is associated with a higher risk for developing sarcomas, brain tumors, adrenal gland cancers, and leukemias. In addition, studies of other rare inherited malignancies have led to the identification of about thirty recessive tumor-suppressor genes whose inactivation contributes to oncogenic or cancer-causing cell proliferation. The accompanying table provides examples of the chromosomal locations for several tumor-suppressor genes. Included in the list are the *BRCA1* and *BRCA2* genes in breast cancer, the *NF1* gene in neurofibromatosis, the *p16* gene in melanoma, and the *APC* gene in colorectal carcinoma. Each of these genes has also been implicated in nonhereditary cancers. Three types of tumor-suppressor genes are generally recognized: genes controlling cell division, DNA repair, and cell death.

The Properties of Tumor-Suppressor Genes

Molecular analyses of the genetic and biochemical properties of tumor-suppressor genes have suggested some of these gene products play critical but distinct roles in regulating processes involved in cellular division and proliferation. The *Rb* gene product represents a prototype tumor-suppressor gene of this type. The *Rb* gene product normally blocks progression of the cell cycle and cell division by binding to transcription factors in its active form. In order for cell division to occur in response to growth factor stimulation, elements of the signal cascade inactivate *Rb*-mediated inhibition by a mechanism involving the addition of phosphate to the molecule, a reaction called phosphorylation. In cancer, loss of *Rb* function results as a consequence of mutation which removes the brakes on this form of normal inhibitory control; the cell division machinery proceeds without appropriate initiation by growth factors or other stimuli.

Like the *Rb* tumor-suppressor gene, most tumor-suppressor genes become active due to a loss of heterozygosity (LOH). Since chromosomes (and the genes residing within the chromosomes) are paired, a mutation in one gene of the pair is called heterozygosity. For *Rb*, a single gene mutation (the heterozygous condition for the trait encoded by the gene pair) is inherited as a recessive condition where no cancer results (since the infant has one normal gene and one mutated *Rb* gene). During development however, a random mutation can occur in the normal *Rb* gene. As soon as the second *Rb* gene mutates in a single cell, cancer can begin.

Tumor-suppressor genes are also found among the genes specifically involved in DNA repair. Whenever a cell divides the DNA must be duplicated, and errors in the duplication process must be repaired in order for the new cell to function properly. The protein products of DNA repair gene errors in duplicated DNA by proofreading the DNA sequence; however, if the DNA repair genes are mutated, errors will slip by and these mutations can create proteins which may activate oncogenes, or the mutations may create abnormal, mutated tumor-suppressor genes. For example, when DNA repair genes fail to repair DNA errors, some endometrial cancers and hereditary nonpolyposis colon cancer (HNPCC) can result (about 5 percent of all colon cancers).

If the cell's DNA is damaged beyond repair by the DNA repair proteins, then the *p53* tumor-suppressor gene is among the family of genes responsible for destroying the cell by causing cell death (also called "cell suicide" or "programmed cell death" or "apoptosis"). The *p53* tumor-suppressor gene product is a DNA-binding protein with the ability to regulate the expression of other genes in response to genetic damage or other abnormal events occurring during cell cycle progression. In response to p53 activation, the cell will normally arrest the process of cell division (by indirectly blocking Rb inactivation). This cell cycle arrest may allow time for the cell machinery to repair genetic damage before proceeding further along the cell cycle; alternatively, if the damage is too great, the *p53* gene product may initiate a process

of apoptosis. The loss of *p53* activity in the cell as a consequence of mutation results in genetic destabilization and the failure of cell death mechanisms to eliminate damaged cells from the body; both events appear to be critical to late-stage oncogenic mechanisms. Mutations of the *p53* gene may be inherited (as in the Li-Fraumeni syndrome, LFS); however, mutations in *p53* are also routinely found in many sporadic (noninherited) cancers (including lung, colon, breast, and other cancer types).

IMPACT AND APPLICATIONS

The discovery of tumor-suppressor genes has revealed the existence of inhibitory mechanisms critical to the regulation of cellular proliferation. Mutations that destroy the functional activities of these gene products cause the loss of growth control characteristic of cancer cells. Taken together, research on the patterns of oncogene activation and the loss of tumor-suppressor gene function in many types of human malignancy suggest a general model of oncogenesis. Molecular analyses of many tumors show multiple genetic alterations involving both oncogenes and tumor-suppressor genes, suggesting that oncogenesis (development of cancer) requires unregulated stimulation of cellular proliferation pathways along with a loss of inhibitory activities that operate at cell cycle checkpoints.

Some tumor-suppressor gene mutations are inherited and, in rare cases, testing for these gene mutations (which have been found often enough in the general population, like *BRCA 1* and *BRCA 2*) may be helpful to determine which people are at higher risk for certain cancers. Genetic testing for families at risk requires careful screening and counseling and might allow surgical intervention, lifestyle changes, or more frequent cancer screening steps to minimize the individual's familial cancer risk.

Genetic tests for oncogenes and tumor-suppressor genes have become commonplace in cancer diagnosis and treatment. Some genetic tests have been shown to help diagnose the type of cancer, guide cancer treatment, predict survival for patients with cancer, and sometimes to produce novel therapies for cancer patients.

With respect to clinical applications, restoration of *p53* tumor-suppressor gene function by gene therapy appears to result in tumor regression in some experimental systems; however, much more work needs to be done in this area to achieve clinical relevance. More important, research on the mechanism of action of standard chemotherapeutic drugs suggests that cytotoxicity may be caused by p53-induced cell death; the absence of functional p53 in many tumors may account for their resistance to chemotherapy. Promising research is investigating new ways to elicit cell death in tumor cells lacking functional *p53* gene product in response to chemotherapy. The clinical significance of activating these p53-independent cell death mechanisms may be extraordinary.

Sarah Crawford Martinelli, Ph.D.;
updated by Joy Frestedt, Ph.D., RAC, CCTI

FURTHER READING

DeCaprio, J. A. "How the Rb Tumor-Suppressor Structure and Function Was Revealed by the Study of Adenovirus and SV40." *Virology* 384.2 (2009): 274–84. Print.

Ehrlich, Melanie, ed. *DNA Alterations in Cancer: Genetic and Epigenetic Changes*. Natick: Eaton, 2000. Print.

Fearon, Eric, and Bert Vogelstein. "Tumor Suppressor Gene Defects in Human Cancer." *Cancer Medicine*. Ed. Robert C. Bast, Jr., et al. 5th ed. Atlanta: American Cancer Society, 2000. Print.

Fisher, David E., ed. *Tumor Suppressor Genes in Human Cancer*. Totowa: Humana, 2001. Print.

Gunduz, Mehmet, and Esra Gunduz. *Tumor Suppressor Genes: Functions, Regulation and Health Effects*. New York: Nova Biomedical, 2013. Print.

Habib, Nagy A. *Cancer Gene Therapy: Past Achievements and Future Challenges*. New York: Kluwer Academic/Plenum, 2000. Print.

Iglehart, J. Dirk, and Daniel P. Silver. "Synthetic Lethality: A New Direction in Cancer-Drug Development." *New England Journal of Medicine* 361.2 (2009): 189–91. Print.

Lattime, Edmund C., and Stanton L. Gerson, eds. *Gene Therapy of Cancer: Translational Approaches from Preclinical Studies to Clinical Implementation*. 3rd ed. San Diego: Academic, 2014. Print.

Maruta, Hiroshi, ed. *Tumor-Suppressing Viruses, Genes, and Drugs: Innovative Cancer Therapy Approaches*. San Diego: Academic, 2002. Print.

Nguyen, Susan D. *Tumor Suppressors*. New York: Nova Science, 2011. Print.

Oliff, Alan, et al. "New Molecular Targets for Cancer Therapy." *Scientific American* 275 (September, 1996). Print.

Ruddon, Raymond. *Cancer Biology*. 3rd ed. New York: Oxford UP, 1995. Print.

See also: Aging; Breast cancer; Cancer; Cell cycle; Cell division; DNA repair; Human genetics; Human Genome Project; Model organism: Mus musculus; Oncogenes; RB1 gene; RhoGD12 gene.

Turner syndrome and genetics

CATEGORY: Diseases and syndromes

DEFINITION

Turner syndrome is caused by a chromosomal abnormality and is one of the most common genetic problems in women, affecting 1 out of every 2,500 women born, according to the National Institutes of Health. Henry H. Turner, an eminent clinical endocrinologist, is credited with first describing Turner syndrome. In 1938, he published an article describing seven patients, ranging in age from fifteen to twenty-three years, who exhibited short stature, a lack of sexual development, arms that turned out slightly at the elbows, webbing of the neck, and low posterior hairline. He did not know what caused this condition.

In 1959, C. E. Ford discovered that a chromosomal abnormality involving the sex chromosomes caused Turner syndrome. He found that most girls with Turner syndrome did not have all or part of one of their X chromosomes and argued that this missing genetic material accounted for the physical findings associated with the condition.

RISK FACTORS

Only females are at risk for Turner syndrome. The loss or alteration of the X chromosome that characterizes the disorder is not inherited but takes place spontaneously. For this reason, parents who have one child with Turner syndrome will most likely not have another child with this disorder.

Girl with Turner syndrome before and immediately after her operation for neck-webbing By Johannes Nielsen (http://www.aaa. dk/TURNER/ENGELSK/TURN_ORI.HTM#baby), via Wikimedia Commons

Puffiness of feet as a sign of Turner syndrome See page for author, via Wikimedia Commons

ETIOLOGY AND GENETICS

Turner syndrome begins at conception. The disorder results from an error during meiosis in the production of one of the parents' sex cells, although the exact cause remains unknown.

SYMPTOMS

Shortness is the most common characteristic of Turner syndrome. The incidence of short stature among women with Turner syndrome is virtually 100 percent. Women who have this condition are, on average, 4 feet 8 inches (1.4 meters) tall. The cause of the failure to grow is unclear. However, growth-promoting therapy with growth hormones has become standard. Most women with the syndrome also experience ovarian failure. Since the ovaries normally produce estrogen, women with Turner syndrome lack this essential hormone. This deficit results in infertility and incomplete sexual development. Cardiovascular disorders are the single source of increased mortality in women with this condition. High blood pressure is common.

Other physical features often associated with Turner syndrome include puffy hands and feet at birth, a webbed neck, prominent ears, a small jaw, short fingers, a low hairline at the back of the neck, and soft fingernails that turn up at the ends. Some women with Turner syndrome have a tendency to become overweight. Many women will exhibit only a few of these distinctive features, and some may not show any of them. This condition does not affect general intelligence. However, another possible symptom is poor spatial perception abilities. For example, women with this condition may have difficulty driving, recognizing subtle social clues, and solving nonverbal mathematics problems; they may also suffer from clumsiness and attention deficit disorder.

SCREENING AND DIAGNOSIS

Girls suspected of having Turner syndrome, usually because of their short stature, often undergo chromosomal analysis. A simple blood test and laboratory analysis called a karyotype are done to document the existence of an abnormality.

Additional tests to diagnose Turner syndrome include measuring blood hormone levels, an echocardiogram (the use of ultrasound to measure heart defects), ultrasound examinations of reproductive organs and kidneys, and a pelvic exam. Pregnant women can receive chromosome analysis to determine whether their children will have the disorder.

Treatments and Therapy

No treatment is available to correct the chromosome abnormality that causes this condition. However, injections of human growth hormone can restore most of the growth deficit. Unless they undergo hormone replacement therapy, girls with Turner syndrome will not menstruate or develop breasts and pubic hair. In addition to estrogen replacement therapy, women with Turner syndrome are often advised to take calcium and exercise regularly. Although infertility cannot be altered, pregnancy may be made possible through in vitro fertilization and embryo transfer. Individuals with Turner syndrome can be healthy, happy, and productive members of society.

Nevertheless, because of its relative rarity, a woman with Turner syndrome may never meet another individual with this condition and may suffer from self-consciousness, embarrassment, and poor self-esteem. The attitudes of parents, siblings, and relatives are important in helping develop a strong sense of identity and self-worth. The Turner Syndrome Society of the United States is a key source of information and support groups.

Prevention and Outcomes

Although there is no treatment to cure the chromosomal abnormality, advances in chromosomal analysis have proved helpful in the diagnosis and management of Turner syndrome. In addition, new developments in hormonal therapy for short stature and ovarian failure, combined with advances in vitro fertilization, have significantly improved the potential for growth, sexual development, and fertility for afflicted individuals.

Fred Buchstein, M.A.

Further Reading

Albertsson-Wikland, Kerstin, and Michael B. Ranke, eds. *Turner Syndrome in a Life Span Perspective: Research and Clinical Aspects.* New York: Elsevier, 1995. Print.

Broman, Sarah H., and Jordan Grafman, eds. *Atypical Cognitive Deficits in Developmental Disorders: Implications for Brain Function.* Hillsdale: Lawrence Erlbaum, 1994. Print.

Goldstein, Sam, and Cecil R. Reynolds. *Handbook of Neurodevelopmental and Genetic Disorders in Children.* New York: Guilford, 2011. Print.

Gould, Harley N., et al. "High Levels of Education and Employment Among Women with Turner Syndrome." *Journ. of Women's Health* 22.3 (2013): 230–35. Print.

Powell, M. Paige, and Kimberly R. Snapp. "Turner Syndrome." *Handbook of Neurodevelopmental and Genetic Disorders in Adults.* Ed. Sam Goldstein and Cecil R. Reynolds. New York: Guilford, 2005. Print.

Power, Theresa, et al. "The Forensic Implications of Turner's Syndrome." *Journ. of Forensic Sciences* 59.3 (2014): 671–75. Print.

Rieser, Patricia A., and Marsha Davenport. *Turner Syndrome: A Guide for Families.* Houston: Turner Syndrome Society, 1992. Print.

Rosenfeld, Ron G. *Turner Syndrome: A Guide for Physicians.* 2d ed. Houston: Turner Syndrome Society, 1992. Print.

Saenger, Paul. "Turner Syndrome." *Pediatric Endocrinology.* Ed. Mark A. Sperling. Rev. 3d ed. Philadelphia: Saunders/Elsevier, 2008. Print.

Saenger, Paul, and Anna-Maria Pasquino, eds. *Optimizing Health Care for Turner Patients in the Twenty-first Century.* New York: Elsevier, 2000. Print.

Sybert, Virginia P. "Turner Syndrome." *Management of Genetic Syndromes.* Ed. Suzanne B. Cassidy and Judith E. Allanson. 2d ed. Hoboken: Wiley-Liss, 2005. Print.

See also: Amniocentesis; Chorionic villus sampling; Dwarfism; Hereditary diseases; Infertility; Klinefelter syndrome; Mutation and mutagenesis; Nondisjunction and aneuploidy; X chromosome inactivation; XY Y syndrome.

Twin studies

Category: Techniques and methodologies

Significance: Studies of twins are widely considered to be the best way to determine the relative contributions of genetic and environmental factors to the development of human physical and psychological characteristics.

Key terms

dizygotic: developed from two separate zygotes; fraternal twins are dizygotic because they develop from two separate fertilized ova (eggs) *monozygotic:* developed from a single zygote; identical twins are monozygotic because they develop from a single fertilized ovum that splits in two

zygosity: the degree to which two individuals are genetically similar

zygote: a cell formed from the union of a sperm and an ovum

THE ORIGIN OF TWIN STUDIES

Sir Francis Galton, an early pioneer in the science of genetics and a founder of the theory of eugenics, conducted some of the earliest systematic studies of human twins in the 1870s. Galton recognized the difficulty of identifying the extent to which human traits are biologically inherited and the extent to which traits are produced by diet, upbringing, education, and other environmental influences. Borrowing a phrase from William Shakespeare, Galton called this the "nature vs. nurture" problem. Galton reasoned that he could attempt to find an answer to this problem by comparing similarities among people who obviously shared a great deal of biological inheritance, with similarities among people sharing less biological inheritance. Twins offered the clearest example of people who shared common biological backgrounds.

Galton contacted all of the twins he knew and asked them to supply him with the names of other twins. He obtained information on ninety-four sets of twins. Of these, thirty-five sets were very similar, people who would now be called identical twins. These thirty-five pairs reported that people often had difficulty telling them apart. Using questionnaires and interviews, Galton compared the thirty-five identical pairs with the other twins.

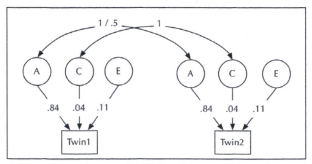

ACE model showing standardised variance coefficients for a twin study. By Tim bates (Own work), via Wikimedia Commons

Twin Study MZ discordant positive_example By Tim bates (Own work), via Wikimedia Commons

He found that the identical twins were much more similar to one another in habits, interests, and personalities, as well as in appearance. They were even much more alike in physical health and susceptibility to illness. The one area in which all individuals seemed to differ markedly was in handwriting.

MODERN TWIN STUDIES

Since Galton's time, researchers have discovered how biological inheritance occurs, and this has made possible an understanding of why twins are similar. It has also enabled researchers to make more sophisticated use of twins in studies that address various aspects of the nature vs. nurture problem. Parents pass their physical traits to their children by means of genes in chromosomes. Each chromosome carries two genes (called alleles) for every hereditary trait. One allele comes from the father and one comes from the mother. Any set of full brothers and sisters will share many of the same alleles, since all of their genes come from the same parents. However, brothers and sisters usually also differ substantially; each zygote (ovum, or egg, fertilized by a sperm cell) will combine alleles from the father and the mother in a unique manner, so different zygotes will develop into unique individuals. Even when two fertilized eggs are present at the same time, as in the case of dizygotic or fraternal twins, the two will have different combinations of genes from the mother and the father.

Identical twins are an exception to the rule of unique combinations of genes. Identical twins develop from a single zygote, a cell created by one union of egg and sperm. Therefore, monozygotic twins (from one zygote) will normally have the same genetic makeup. Differences between genetic twins, researchers argue, must therefore be produced by environmental factors following birth.

The ideal way to conduct twin studies is to compare monozygotic twins who have been reared apart from each other in vastly different types of families or environments. This is rarely possible, however, because the number of twins separated at birth and adopted is relatively small. For this reason, researchers in most twin studies use fraternal twins as a comparison group, since the major difference between monozygotic and dizygotic twins is that the former are genetically identical. Statistical similarities among monozygotic twins that are not found among dizygotic twins are therefore believed to be caused by genetic inheritance.

Researchers use several types of data on twins to estimate the extent to which human characteristics are the consequence of genetics. One of the main sources for twin studies is the Minnesota Twin Registry. In the 1990s, this registry consisted of about 10,500 twins in Minnesota. They were found in Minnesota birth records from the years 1936 through 1955, and they were located and recruited by mail between 1985 and 1990. A second major source of twin studies is the Virginia Twin Registry. This is a register of twins constructed from a systematic review of public birth records in the Commonwealth of Virginia. A few other states also maintain records of twins. Some other organizations, such as the American Association of Retired Persons (AARP), keep records of twins who volunteer to participate and make these records available to researchers.

Zygosity, or degree of genetic similarity between twins, is usually measured by survey questions about physical similarity and by how often other people mistake one twin for the other. In some cases, zygosity may be determined more rigorously through analysis of DNA samples. The emerging field of epigenetics has also found that the epigenomes of twins can display the differences caused by environmental factors after birth. For example, a study from the university of Utah's Genetic Science Learning Center found that fifty-year-old twins have significantly more variation in epigenetic tags than do three-year-old twins. This understanding can help reveal the influence of both genetics and the environment on various characteristics and conditions.

PROBLEMS WITH TWIN STUDIES

Although twin studies are one of the best available means for studying genetic influences in human beings, there are a number of problems with this approach. Although twin studies assume that monozygotic twins are biologically identical, some critics have claimed that there are reasons to question this assumption. Even though these twins tend to show greater uniformity than other people, developmental differences may emerge even in the womb after the splitting of the zygote.

Twins who show a great physical similarity may also be subject to environmental similarities so that traits believed to be caused by genetics may, in fact, be a result of upbringing. Some parents, for example, dress twins in matching clothing. Even when twins grow up in separate homes without being in contact with each other, their appearances and mannerisms may evoke the same kinds of responses from others. Physical attractiveness, height, and other characteristics often affect how individuals are treated by others so that the biologically based resemblances of twins can lead to common experiences. The discovery of the influence of epigenetics on twins further suggests that the nature-nurture relationship is extremely complicated and may be oversimplified by relying on a traditional understanding of twin studies.

Finally, critics of twin studies point out that twins constitute a special group of people and that it may be difficult to apply findings from twin studies to the population at large. Some studies have indicated that intelligence quotient (IQ) scores of twins, on average, are about five points below IQ scores in the general population, and twins may differ from the general population in other respects. It is conceivable that genetics plays a more prominent role in twins than in most other people.

IMPACT AND APPLICATIONS

Twin studies have provided evidence that a substantial amount of human character and behavior may be genetically determined. In 1976, psychologists John C. Loehlin and Robert C. Nichols published their analyses of the backgrounds and performances of 850 sets of twins who took the 1962 National Merit Scholarship test. Results showed that identical twins showed greater similarities than fraternal twins in abilities, personalities, opinions, and ambitions. A careful examination of backgrounds indicated that these similarities could not be explained by the similar treatment received by identical twins during upbringing.

Later twin studies continued to provide evidence that genes shape many areas of human life. Monozygotic twins tend to resemble each other in probabilities of developing mental illnesses, such as schizophrenia and depression, suggesting that these psychological problems are partly genetic in origin. A 1996 study published in the *Journal of Personality and Social Psychology* used a sample from the Minnesota Twin Registry to establish that identical twins are similar in probabilities of divorce. A 1997 study in the *American Journal of Psychiatry* indicated that there is even a great resemblance between twins in intensity of religious faith. Twin studies have offered evidence that homosexual or heterosexual orientation may be partly a genetic matter, although researcher Scott L. Hershberger has found that the genetic inheritance of sexual orientation may be greater among women than among men. Similar studies have suggested that there may be some genetic influence in the development of transgender identities.

Twin studies have been particularly insightful regarding the genetic or environmental origin of various diseases and disorders. For example, evidence from research on identical and fraternal twins suggests that there is a strong genetic influence on conditions such as reading disability, autism, and Alzheimer's disease. In comparison, Crohn's disease, strokes, and rheumatoid arthritis are much more dependent on environmental factors. These studies allow researchers to potentially identify triggers and

risk factors for diseases as well as their mechanisms of action, aiding the development of preventative measures and treatments.

FURTHER READING

Asbury, Kathryn, and Robert Plomin. *G is for Genes: The Impact of Genetics on Education and Achievement.* Hoboken: Wiley, 2014. Print.

Fletcher, H. L., and G. I. Hickey. *Genetics.* New York: Garland Science, 2013. Print.

Hershberger, Scott L. "A Twin Registry Study of Male and Female Sexual Orientation." *Journal of Sex Research* 34, no. 2 (1997). Print.

Joseph, Jay. *The Gene Illusion: Genetic Research in Psychiatry and Psychology Under the Microscope.* New York: Algora, 2004. Print.

Kendler, Kenneth S., and Carol A. Prescott. *Genes, Environment, and Psychopathology: Understanding the Causes of Psychiatric and Substance Use Disorders.* New York: Guilford, 2006. Print.

"Insights from Identical Twins." *Learn.Genetics.* University of Utah Health Sciences, 2016. Web. 27 Jan. 2016.

Loehlin, John C., and Robert C. Nichols. *Heredity, Environment, and Personality: A Study of 850 Sets of Twins.* Austin: U of Texas P, 1976. Print.

Piontelli, Alessandra. *Twins: From Fetus to Child.* New York: Routledge, 2002. Print.

Spector, Tim D. *Identically Different: Why You Can Change Your Genes.* London: Phoenix, 2013. Print.

Spector, Tim D., Harold Snieder, and Alex J. MacGregor, eds. *Advances in Twin and Sib-Pair Analysis.* New York: Oxford UP, 2000. Print.

Steen, R. Grant. *DNA and Destiny: Nurture and Nature in Human Behavior.* New York: Plenum, 1996. Print.

"Twin Studies." *Genetics and Social Science.* NCHPEG, 2016. Web. 27 Jan. 2016.

TwinStudies.org. International Society for Twin Studies, 2016. Web. 27 Jan. 2016.

Wright, Lawrence. *Twins: And What They Tell Us About Who We Are.* New York: John Wiley and Sons, 1997. Print.

See also: Aging; Animal cloning; Behavior; Cloning: Ethical isdsues; Diabetes; DNA fingerprinting; Gender identity; Genetic testing; Genetics in television and films; Heredity and environment; Homosexuality; Intelligence; Prenatal diagnosis; Quantitative inheritance.

Tyrosinemia type I

CATEGORY: Diseases and syndromes

ALSO KNOWN AS: Hepatorenal tyrosinemia; fumary-
lacetoacetase deficiency

DEFINITION

Tyrosinemia type I is a hereditary disorder affecting
primarily the liver and kidneys. It is caused by mutations in the *FAH* gene that lead to an inability to
fully break down the amino acid tyrosine. It can lead
to liver failure, liver cancer, rickets, pain crises, and
death if untreated.

RISK FACTORS

Tyrosinemia type I is an autosomal recessive disorder
and affects males and females equally. Parents who are
carriers of a mutation in the *FAH* gene have a 25 percent risk of having an affected child. Overall, the disorder has a prevalence of 1 in 100,000 live births but is
more common in the Saguenay Lac St-Jean region of
Quebec, Canada, where the prevalence is 1 in 1,846,
according to the US National Institutes of Health.

ETIOLOGY AND GENETICS

Amino acids are the building blocks of protein. The
amino acid tyrosine is broken down via several steps
to form fumarate and acetoacetate, which are then
sent through other metabolic pathways to create
energy. Fumarylacetoacetate hydrolase (FAH) is the
last enzyme in this pathway and is defective in tyrosinemia type I. FAH deficiency leads to the accumulation of fumarylacetoacetate (FAA), which is converted to succinylacetoacetate and succinylacetone.
The accumulated FAA is predicted to cause cellular
damage and premature cell death in the liver and
kidneys. Succinylacetone inhibits two enzymes: par-
ahydroxyphenylpyruvic acid dioxygenase (*p*-HPPD)
which increases plasma tyrosine concentration, and
PBG synthase, which leads to reduced heme synthesis
and increased delta-aminolevulinic acid which can
induce neurologic pain episodes.

The FAH enzyme is encoded by the *FAH* gene,
located on the long arm of chromosome 15. More specifically, *FAH* is located at 15q25.1. The *FAH* gene consists of fourteen exons and is primarily expressed in
the liver and kidney, but it can be found at low levels in
all tissues. There are several mutations found more frequently in specific populations due to founder effects

L-tyrosine-skeletal public domain via wikimedia commons

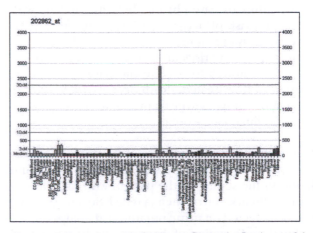

Gene expression pattern of the FAH gene. Genomics Institute of the
Novartis Research Foundation, via Wikimedia Commons

or genetic drift. The p.P261L mutation accounts for
virtually 100 percent of alleles in affected individuals
of Ashkenazi Jewish descent. The common French
Canadian mutation is c.1062+5GA (IVS 12+5 GA).
There are common mutations in Finland, Turkey,
Pakistan, Northern Europe, Southern Europe, and
individuals of Scandinavian descent. Reported mutations are missense, nonsense, and splice-site mutations, and small deletions have been reported but no
large multi-exon deletions that cannot be picked up
by standard DNA sequencing methodology.

In the childhood-onset chronic form, the liver nodules show a high incidence of allele reversion-that is, the mutant allele self-corrects to the normal allele, yielding a normal genotype and normal expression of the FAH enzyme in those cells. Milder expression of symptoms can be correlated to the amount of allelic reversion; the corrected cells modify the phenotype. Gene reversion may explain the variability of symptoms within the same family.

SYMPTOMS
Infants presenting earlier than six months of age have severe liver dysfunction. Symptoms include markedly reduced ability to clot, ascites, jaundice, and gastrointestinal bleeding. Untreated affected infants can die from liver failure within weeks of first symptoms. Children presenting at older than six months can have chronic liver dysfunction with significant risk of hepatocellular carcinoma (HCC) and renal dysfunction causing rickets. Episodes of neurologic pain crises are not uncommon and can be severe enough to require mechanical breathing assistance. If untreated, death occurs typically before the age of ten from liver failure, neurologic crisis, or hepatocellular carcinoma.

SCREENING AND DIAGNOSIS
The presence of succinylacetone in the urine and blood in the setting of the patient with liver disease is the hallmark of tyrosinemia type I. Succinylacetone can be detected on urine organic acid analysis.

Final confirmation of diagnosis can be performed by DNA sequencing of the *FAH* gene. Measuring FAH enzyme activity in cultured skin fibroblasts will also provide confirmation.

Tyrosinemia type I has been added to state newborn screening programs. Measuring succinylacetone from the newborn blood spot by tandem mass spectroscopy is a more sensitive indicator of tyrosinemia type I than measuring tyrosine.

TREATMENT AND THERAPY
Treatment consists of medication and dietary restriction. Orfadin (nitisinone) formerly known as NTBC, prevents FAA and succinylacetone formation, but elevates blood tyrosine levels. A low tyrosine diet is required to keep levels in a safe range. Liver transplantation was once the only treatment, but it is used much less frequently now, given the effectiveness of nitisinone and the significant risks associated with liver transplant. Patients should be monitored with regular lab tests for liver and kidney function, plasma amino acids, succinylacetone, blood nitisinone levels, and yearly liver imaging for risk of HCC.

PREVENTION AND OUTCOMES
Response to nitisinone has markedly increased life spans, reduced the incidence of HCC, and dramatically lowered the need for liver transplant. Patients who have had transplants may still require nitisinone to prevent ongoing renal damage from FAA and succinylacetone that is still being produced in kidney cells.

FURTHER READING
Barnby, Elizabeth. "Tyrosinemia Type 1: An Overview of Nursing Care." *Pediatric Nursing* 40.2 (2014): 61–90. Print.

Nussbaum, Robert L., Roderick R. McInnes, and Huntington F. Willard. *Thompson and Thompson Genetics in Medicine*. 7th ed. New York: Saunders, 2007. Print.

Nyhna, William L., Bruce A. Barshop, and Pinar T. Ozand. *Atlas of Inherited Metabolic Disorders*. London: Hodder Edu., 2011. Print.

Suchy, Frederick J., Ronald J. Sokol, and William F. Balistreri. *Liver Disease in Children*. Philadelphia: Lippincott, 2001. Print.

van Dyk, E., and P. J. Gene Pretorius. "Impaired DNA Repair and Genomic Stability in Hereditary Tyrosinemia Type 1." *Gene* 495.1 (2012): 56–61. Print.

See also: Alkaptonuria; Andersen's disease; Diabetes; Diabetes insipidus; Fabry disease; Forbes disease; Galactokinase deficiency; Galactosemia; Gaucher disease; Glucose galactose malabsorption; Glucose-6-phosphate dehydrogenase deficiency; Glycogen storage diseases; Gm1-gangliosidosis; Hemochromatosis; Hereditary diseases; Hereditary xanthinuria; Hers disease; Homocystinuria; Hunter disease; Hurler syndrome; Inborn errors of metabolism; Jansky-Bielschowsky disease; Kearns-Sayre syndrome; Krabbé disease; Lactose intolerance; Leigh syndrome; Lesch-Nyhan syndrome; McArdle's disease; Maple syrup urine disease; Menkes syndrome; Metachromatic leukodystrophy; Niemann-Pick disease; Ornithine transcarbamylase deficiency; Orotic aciduria; Phenylketonuria (PKU); Pompe disease; Sulfite oxidase deficiency; Tarui's disease; Tay-Sachs disease.

U

Usher syndrome

CATEGORY: Diseases and syndromes

ALSO KNOWN AS: Deafness-retinitis pigmentosa syndrome; Dystrophia retinae pigmentosa-dysostosis syndrome; Graefe-Usher syndrome; Hallgren syndrome; Usher's syndrome

DEFINITION

Usher syndrome is a rare inherited disorder that involves loss of both hearing and sight. Hearing loss is usually present at birth or soon thereafter. It is due to an impaired ability of the auditory nerves to transmit sensory input to the brain. It is called sensorineural hearing loss.

The vision loss, called retinitis pigmentosa (RP), begins later in childhood, usually after age ten. It slowly gets worse over time. During the teen years, loss of vision is characterized by night blindness and loss of peripheral vision. RP is a deterioration of the retina. The retina is a layer of light-sensitive tissue that lines the back of the eye. It converts visual images into nerve impulses in the brain that allow people to see.

Three types of Usher syndrome have been identified: types I, II, and III. The age of onset and severity of symptoms distinguish the different types.

Approximately 4 out of 100,000 infants born in the United States have Usher syndrome. Usher syndrome accounts for 3 to 6 percent of all deaf children, 3 to 6 percent of all hard-of-hearing children, and half of all blind-deaf adults.

RISK FACTORS

The only known risk factor for Usher syndrome is having parents with the disorder and/or parents who carry the genes for the disorder. If both parents carry the abnormal gene, their child has a 25 per cent chance of inheriting both of these abnormal genes and therefore developing Usher syndrome.

Mutations for type I and type III have been identified in the Ashkenazi Jewish population.

ETIOLOGY AND GENETICS

Nearly 20 genes have now been identified that are associated with Usher syndrome. All these genes specify proteins that function in the development maintenance of specialized sensory cells in the inner ear and light-sensing cells in the retina (rods and cones). While the exact functions of some of these proteins in the processes of hearing and vision may be poorly understood, the effect of mutations in the associated genes is most often observed as the gradual loss of rods and cones in the retina and of hair cells in the inner ear.

Type I Usher syndrome can result from mutations in any of the following genes: MYO7A (located on chromosome 11 at position 11q13.5), USH1C (at position 11p15.1), CDH23 (at position 10q21-q22), USH1H (at position 15q22-q23), USH1G (at position 17q24-q25), PCHD15 (at position 10q21-q22), SANS, or USH1G, (at position 17q25.1), CIB2 (at position 15q25.1), USH1K (at position 10p11.21-q21.1). Mutations resulting in Usher syndrome type II occur in the following genes: USH2A (at position 1q41), ADGRV1 (at position 5q14.3), WHRN (at position 9q32-q34), and GPR98 (at position 5q14) and PDZD7 (at position 10q24.31). The gene known as USH3A, also called CLRN1, (at position 3q21-q25) and HARS (at position 5q31.3) are the only genes so far identified in which mutations lead to type III Usher syndrome.

All forms of Usher syndrome are inherited in an autosomal recessive fashion, which means that both copies of the particular gene must be deficient in order for the individual to be afflicted. Typically, an affected child is born to two unaffected parents, both of whom are carriers of the recessive mutant allele. The probable outcomes for children whose

Scottish ophthalmologist Charles Usher (2 March 1865 – 3 March 1942) By Unknown photographer (The Usher Family of Scotland), via Wikimedia Commons

parents are both carriers are 75 percent unaffected and 25 per cent affected. If one parent has Usher syndrome and the other is a carrier of the same type, there is a 50 percent probability that each child will be affected.

SYMPTOMS

The main symptoms of Usher syndrome are hearing and vision loss. Some people also have balance problems due to inner ear problems.

RP begins in the early teenage years as night blindness and leads to blindness by mid-adulthood. The progression of RP limits a person's ability to see in dim light or in the dark (night blindness). It also causes a person to lose peripheral (side) vision slowly over time. Eventually, any vision left is only in a small tunnel-shaped area. Almost everyone with RP becomes legally blind. There is no known way of predicting when or how quickly a person will lose vision.

Symptoms of type I Usher syndrome include being deaf at birth and receiving little or no benefit from hearing aids, having severe balance problems, being slow to sit without support, and rarely learning to walk before the age of eighteen months. RP begins by age ten with difficulty seeing at night, and it quickly progresses to blindness.

Symptoms of type II Usher syndrome include being born with moderate to severe hearing loss, benefitting from hearing aids, and not having balance problems. RP begins in the teenage years.

Symptoms of type III include being born with normal hearing that gets worse in the teenage years and leads to deafness by mid to late adulthood and being born with near-normal balance. Vision loss develops around adolescence. Individuals may develop some balance issues.

SCREENING AND DIAGNOSIS

The doctor will ask about symptoms and medical history and will perform a physical exam. Hearing loss is determined with standard hearing tests. Balance problems can be detected with a test called electronystagmography (ENG). In this test, the doctor flushes the ears with warm and then cool water. This causes nystagmus, which is rapid eye movements that can help the doctor detect a balance disorder.

An eye doctor will perform an eye exam, which will likely include a visual field test to check side vision, a test to check for ability to adapt to seeing in the dark, and a test to check sensitivity to color and contrast.

If any problems are found on these tests, an electroretinography (ERG) is done. This test confirms a diagnosis of RP. It measures the electricity given off by the nerves in the retina. The test is done while wearing special contact lenses and looking at a flashing light.

Genetic testing is feasible for some of the genes responsible for Usher syndrome.

TREATMENT AND THERAPY

There is no cure for Usher syndrome. The best treatment is to identify the disorder as early as possible and begin educational programs and other services right away. This helps reduce the communication and learning problems that can result from hearing and vision loss.

The specific programs and services depend on the severity of the hearing, vision, and balance problems and the person's age and abilities. Options include hearing aids; assistive listening devices; cochlear implant, in which a small device is surgically put under the skin behind the ear to give deaf people some ability to hear; adjustment and career

Fundus of patient with retinitis pigmentosa By Christian Hamel (Retinitis pigmentosa by Christian Hamel), via Wikimedia Commons

counseling; training to help with balance and movement; low-vision services; communications training; and skills in living independently. Vitamin A palmitate is used to treat vision loss in people with type II.

PREVENTION AND OUTCOMES

Currently, there is no known way to prevent Usher syndrome. With treatment, education, and training programs, children and adults can live full and happy lives.

Laurie Rosenblum, M.P.H.; reviewed by Kari Kassir, M.D. "Etiology and Genetics" by Jeffrey A. Knight, Ph.D.; updated by Deanna M. Neff, M.P.H.

FURTHER *Reading*

Bernardis I, Chiesi L, Tenedini E, et al. *Unravelling the Complexity of Inherited Retinal Dystrophies Molecular Testing: Added Value of Targeted Next-Generation Sequencing.* Biomed Res Int. 2016:6341870.

Bonnet C, El-Amraoui A. Usher syndrome (sensorineural deafness and retinitis pigmentosa): *pathogenesis, molecular diagnosis and therapeutic approaches.* Curr Opin Neurol. 2012; 25(1):42–49.

EBSCO Publishing. Health Librar y: *Usher Syndrome. Ipswich, Mass.: Author, 2009.* Available through http://www.ebscohost.com.

Sutton, Amy L. Eye Care Sourcebook: *Basic Consumer Health Information About Eye Care and Eye Disorders.* Detroit: Omnigraphics, 2008.

Williams, David. *"Retinal Degeneration in Usher Syndrome." In Retinal Degenerations: Biology, Diag nostics, and Therapeutics, edited by Joyce Tombran Tink and Colin J. Barnstable. Totowa, N.J.:* Hu mana Press, 2007.

WEB *Sites of Interest*
Boys Town National Research Hospital
http://www.boystownhospital.org/home.asp

Canadian National Institute for the Blind
http://www.cnib.ca/en/Default.aspx

Genetics Home Reference
http://ghr.nlm.nih.gov

National Eye Institute
http://www.nei.nih.gov

National Institute on Deafness and Other Communication Disorders: Usher Syndrome
http://www.nidcd.nih.gov/health/hearing/usher.asp

OMIM® Online Mendelian Inheritance in Man
http://www.omim.org/about

Orphanet Journal of Rare Diseases
https://ojrd.biomedcentral.com/
Usher Syndrome Coalition
http://www.usher-syndrome.org/

See also: Aniridia; Best disease; Choroideremia; Color blindness; Corneal dystrophies; Deafness; Glaucoma; Gyrate atrophy of the choroid and retina; Macular degeneration; Norrie syndrome; Pendred syndrome; Progressive external ophthalmoplegia; Retinitis pigmentosa; Retinoblastoma; Stargardt's disease.

V

Vanishing white matter disease

CATEGORY: Diseases and syndromes

ALSO KNOWN AS: Myelinosis centralis difusa; child hood ataxia with central nervous system hypo my elination (CACH); Cree leukoencephalopathy; leukoencephalopathy with vanishing white matter; VWM

DEFINITION

Vanishing white matter (VWM) disease is a rare, progressive, panethnic autosomal recessive disorder that affects the central nervous system predominantly in children, but also in young adults. Approximately150 cases have been reported thus far. The disease leads to a deterioration of the white matter (leuko dystrophy) and though it is quite rare, it is the most common disease affecting white matter. The fatty myelin sheath that insulates nerve fibers, giving white matter its color, is affected.

RISK FACTORS

Family history is an important risk factor.

ETIOLOGY AND GENETICS

The disease in about 90% of cases is caused by mutations in one of the five genes coding for the eukaryotic initiation factor 2B (eIF2B): EIF2B1, EIF2B2, EIF2B3, EIF2B4, and EIF2B5, located on chromosomes 12q24.3, 14q24, 1p34.20, 2p23.3, and 3q27, respectively. The genes encode the five subunits of EIF2B complex protein, which regulate translation initiation and ultimately protein synthesis in the cell. A defective EIF2B leads to an impaired cellular ability to regulate protein synthesis under normal conditions, as well as in response to physical, chemical, and oxidative stress. This might explain the exacerbation of clinical symptoms under stress conditions as the loss of EIF2B function makes it difficult for cells to deal with changing conditions and stress.

White matter is particularly susceptible to the defect. Additional genes not yet identified may explain the small percentage of cases without mutation in one of these five genes.

To date, more than eighty mutations have been identified, including punctiform mutations (the majority), deletions, and insertions. The process of identification of the first two genes involved in VWM, EIF2B5 and EIF2B2, was facilitated by two founder effects in the Dutch population. At present, it appears that gene EIF2B5 contains most mutations (65per cent), frequently R113H. Interestingly, brain glial cells (astrocytes and oligodendrocytes) are particularly susceptible to EIF2B5 mutations. Neuropathologic examination reveals a unique and selective disruption of the glial cells, with spared neurons. White matter rarefaction, cavitating lesions, and increased numbers of "foamy" oligodendrocytes are observed. Studies show that, in astrocytes, EIF2B5 alterations lead to cellular maturation defects, but the basis of their selective vulnerability is still poorly understood. Other frequent changes are present on genes EIF2B4 (17 percent) and EIF2B2 (15 percent), followed by EIF2B3 (7 percent) and EIF2B1 (4 percent). A report on Chinese patients identified several novel mutations, including missense, and estimated the frequency of EIF2B3 alterations to be 20 percent, but the full spectrum of mutations among all populations is still unclear. Of note, many mutations, regardless of type, involve highly conserved amino acids. Half of the amino acids involved are conserved in human, rat, and mouse and a quarter are conserved starting with insects. A correlation between genotype and the severity of the phenotype is difficult to establish. However, an association between the mildest phenotype, with onset after five years of age, and mutations in nonconserved amino acids (R113H and E213G) was suggested. In addition, a severe phenotype with mutations in highly conserved amino acids (R195H and V309L) was reported.

The pattern of inheritance is autosomal recessive, signifying that both copies of the gene in each cell display the mutation. Patients are homozygotes or compound heterozygotes for mutations that are on the same gene. The parents of a patient each carry a copy of the affected gene without showing any signs of disease.

SYMPTOMS

Frequently reported clinical characteristics include spasticity, cerebellar ataxia, optic atrophy (in constant), ovarian insufficiency, and seizures. The first signs may occur antenatally, in infancy, early childhood, late childhood or adulthood. The severity of clinical presentation is highly variable. Mental abilities are relatively preserved. The progression is slow, with exacerbations (triggered by injuries, febrile illness, even fright) leading to partial recovery or coma and death. Lengthy periods of relative stability and even mild improvements are possible. Age of onset is correlated with the severity of the condition with early onset the most severe presentation.

diffusion MRI Tractography in the brain white matter. By Xavier Gigandet et. al., via Wikimedia Commons

SCREENING AND DIAGNOSIS

The initial diagnosis relies on clinical symptoms and magnetic resonance imaging (MRI) findings. Imaging reveals diffuse abnormal signal of the cerebral white matter and cystic degeneration (cavitation). The diagnosis also involves detection of EIF2B mutations via sequence analysis or mutation scanning. Carrier testing is available for family members once mutation has been identified in a proband. Routine studies of cerebrospinal fluid (CSF), blood, and urine are unremarkable. The lymphoblasts of these patients show a decreased intrinsic activity of the eIF2B factor. A marked reduction in the amount of asialo-transferrin in CSF is a recently described biochemical abnormality that can become a clinical diagnostic biomarker.

TREATMENT AND THERAPY

At present, there is no cure for this disease. Treatment is symptomatic. Antibiotics and vaccines should be used rigorously. In children with frequent upper respiratory infections, daily low-dose antibiotics can be considered. Corticosteroids are sometimes useful in the acute phase. Minimizing "cellular stress" is important. Affected individuals should avoid psychological stressors, trauma (contact sports), and high body temperature.

Regulation of eIF2 By Hannes Röst (Own work), via Wikimedia Commons

PREVENTION AND OUTCOMES

Genetic counseling, prenatal testing, and testing of family members can be pursued by individuals with relevant family history. Prognosis appears to correlate with the time of onset, with early forms being more severe (for example, Creeleukoencephalopathy, a fatal infantile form). The phenotype varies widely, from early demise in antenatal onset to slowly progressive disease in the adult form. Most patients survive for a few years after diagnosis.

Mihaela Avramut, M.D., Ph.D.; updated by Deanna M. Neff, M.P.H.

Further Reading

Donkelaar, Hans J., Martin Lammens, and Akira Hori. "Clinical Neuroembriology: Development and Developmental Disorders of the Human Central Nervous System." New York: Springer, 2006. Introduction to developmental disorders, in the context of neurogenetics and neuropathology advances.

Lynch DS, Rodrigues Brandão de Paiva A, Zhang WJ. "Clinical and genetic characterization of leukoencephalopathies in adults. Brain." 2017.

Nussbaum, Robert L., Roderick R. McInnes, and Huntington F. Willard. "Thompson and Thompson Genetics in Medicine." 7th ed. New York: Saunders,2007. A classic medical school textbook.

Raini G, Sharet R, Herrero M, et al. "Mutant eIF2B leads to impaired mitochondrial oxidative phosphorylation in vanishing white matter disease. J Neurochem." 2017

Rosenberg, Roger N., et al., eds. "The Molecular and Genetic Basis of Neurologic and Psychiatric Disease." 4th ed. Philadelphia: Lippincott Williams and Wilkins, 2007. Comprehensive review of molecular, genetic, and genomic features, with fresh in sights into pathogenesis.

Web Sites of Interest

National Ataxia Foundation
http://www.ataxia.org

National Library of Medicine, Genetics Home Reference: Leukoencephalopathy with Vanishing White Matter
http://ghr.nlm.nih.gov/condition=*leukoencephalopathywithvanishingwhitematter*

NINDS Leukodystrophy Information Page
http://www.ninds.nih.gov/disorders/ leukodystrophy/leukodystrophy.htm

United Leukodystrophy Foundation
http://www.ulf.org/index.html

See also: Adrenoleukodystrophy; Alexander disease; Alzheimer's disease; Amyotrophic lateral sclerosis; Arnold-Chiari syndrome; Ataxia telangiectasia; Canavan disease; Cerebrotendinous xanthomatosis; Charcot-Marie-Tooth syndrome; Chediak-Higashi syndrome; Dandy-Walker syndrome; Deafness; Epilepsy; Essential tremor; Friedreich ataxia; Hunting ton's disease; Jansky-Bielschowsky disease; Joubert syndrome; Kennedy disease; Krabbé disease; Leigh syndrome; Leukodystrophy; Limb girdle muscular dystrophy; Maple syrup urine disease; Metachromatic leukodystrophy; Myoclonic epilepsy associated with ragged red fibers (MERRF); Narcolepsy; Nemaline myopathy; Neural tube defects; Neurofibromatosis; Parkinson disease; Pelizaeus-Merzbacher disease; Pendred syndrome; Periodic paralysis syndrome; Prion diseases: Kuru and Creutzfeldt-Jakob syndrome; Refsum disease; Sandhoff disease; San filippo syndrome; Spinal muscular atrophy; Spino cerebellar ataxia.

Viral genetics

Category: Viral genetics

Significance: The composition and structures of virus genomes are more varied than any identified in the entire bacterial, botanical, or animal kingdoms. Unlike the genomes of all other cells, which are composed of DNA, virus genomes may contain their genetic information encoded in either DNA or RNA. Viruses cannot replicate on their own but must instead use the reproductive machinery of host cells to reproduce themselves.

Key terms

capsid: the protective protein coating of a virus particle

ribosome: a cytoplasmic organelle that serves as the site for amino acid incorporation during the synthesis of protein

virions: mature infectious virus particles

What Is a Virus?

Viruses are submicroscopic, obligate intracellular parasites. This definition differentiates viruses from all other groups of living organisms. There exists more biological diversity within viruses than in all other known life-forms combined. This is the result of viruses successfully parasitizing all known groups of living organisms. Viruses have evolved in parallel with other species by capturing and using genes from infected host cells for functions that they require to produce their progeny, to enhance their escape from their host's cells and immune system, and to survive the intracellular and extracellular environment. At the molecular level, the composition and structures of virus genomes are more varied than any others identified in the entire bacterial, botanical, or animal kingdoms. Unlike the genomes of all other cells composed of DNA, virus genomes may contain their genetic information encoded in either DNA or RNA. The nucleic acid comprising a virus genome may be single-stranded or double-stranded and may occur in a linear, circular, or segmented configuration.

THE NEED FOR A HOST

It must be understood that virus particles themselves do not grow or undergo division. Virus particles are produced from the assembling of pre-formed components, whereas other agents actually grow from an increase in the integrated sum of their components and reproduce by division. The reason is that viruses lack the genetic information that encodes the apparatus necessary for the generation of metabolic energy or for protein synthesis (ribosomes). The most critical interaction between a virus and a host cell is the need of the virus for the host's cellular apparatus for nucleic acid and for the synthesis of proteins. No known virus has the biochemical or genetic potential to generate the energy necessary for producing all biological processes. Viruses depend totally on a host cell for this function.

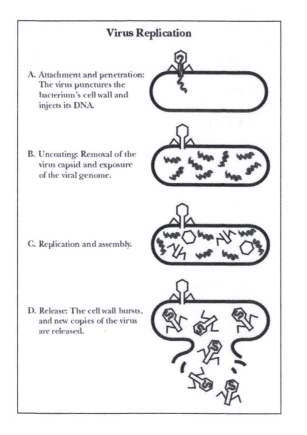

Virus Replication

A. Attachment and penetration: The virus punctures the bacterium's cell wall and injects its DNA.

B. Uncoating: Removal of the virus capsid and exposure of the viral genome.

C. Replication and assembly.

D. Release: The cell wall bursts, and new copies of the virus are released.

Viruses are therefore not living in the traditional sense, but they nevertheless function as living things; they do replicate their own genes. Inside a host cell, viruses are "alive," whereas outside the host they are merely a complex assemblage of metabolically inert chemicals—basically a protein shell. Therefore, while viruses have no inner metabolism and cannot reproduce on their own, they carry with them the means necessary to get into other cells and then use those cells' own reproductive machinery to make copies of themselves. Viruses thrive at the host cells' expense.

REPLICATION

The sole goal of a virus is to replicate its genetic information. The type of host cell infected by a virus has a direct effect on the process of replication. For viruses of prokaryotes (bacteria, primarily), reproduction reflects the physical simplicity of the host cell. For viruses with eukaryotic host cells (plants and animals), reproduction is more complex. The coding capacity of the genome forces the virus to choose a reproductive strategy. The strategy might involve near-total reliance on the host cell, resulting in a compact genome encoded for only a few essential proteins (+), or could involve a large, complex virus genome encoded with nearly all the information necessary for replication, relying on the host cell only for energy and ribosomes. Those viruses with an RNA genome plus messenger RNAs (mRNAs) have no need to enter the nucleus of their host cell, although during replication many often do. DNA genome viruses mostly replicate in the host cell's nucleus, where host DNA is replicated and the biochemical apparatus required for this process is located. Some DNA viruses (poxviruses) have evolved to contain the biochemical capacity to replicate in their host's cytoplasm, with a minimal need for the host cell's other functions.

Virus replication involves several stages carried out by all types of viruses, including the onset of infection, replication, and release of mature virions from an infected host cell. The stages can be defined in eight basic steps: attachment, penetration, uncoating, replication, gene expression, assembly, maturation, and release.

The first stage, attachment, occurs when a virus interacts with a host cell and attaches itself—binds with a virus-attachment protein (antireceptor)—to a cellular receptor molecule in the cell membrane. The receptor may be a protein or a carbohydrate residue.

Some complex viruses, such as herpes viruses, use more than one receptor and therefore have alternate routes of cellular invasion.

Shortly after attachment the target cell is penetrated. Cell penetration is usually an energy-dependent process, and the cell must be metabolically active for penetration to occur. The virus bound to the cellular receptor molecule is translocated across the cell membrane by the receptor and is engulfed by the cell's cytoplasm.

Uncoating occurs after penetration and results in the complete or partial removal of the virus capsid and the exposure of the virus genome as a nucleoprotein complex. This protein complex can be a simple RNA genome or can be highly complex, as in the case of a retrovirus containing a diploid RNA genome responsible for converting a virus RNA genome into a DNA provirus.

How a virus replicates and the resulting expression of its genes depends on the nature of its genetic materials. Control of gene expression is a vital element of virus replication. Viruses use the biochemical apparatus of their infected host cells to express their genetic information as proteins and do this by using the appropriate biochemical language recognized by the host cell. Viruses include double-stranded DNA viruses such as papoviruses, poxviruses, and herpesviruses; single-stranded sense DNA viruses such as parvoviruses; double-stranded RNA reoviruses; single-stranded sense RNA viruses such as flaviviruses, togaviruses, and claiciviruses; single-stranded antisense RNA such as filoviruses and bunyaviruses; single-stranded sense RNA with DNA intermediate retroviruses; and double-stranded DNA with RNA intermediate-like hepadnaviruses.

During assembly, the basic structure of the virus particle is formed. Virus proteins anchor themselves to the cellular membrane, and, as virus proteins and genome molecules reach a critical concentration, assembly begins. The result is that a genome is stuffed into a completed protein shell. The process of maturation prepares the virus particle for infecting subsequent cells and usually involves the cleavage of proteins to form matured products or conformational structural changes.

For most viruses, release is a simple matter of breaking open the infected cell and exiting. The breakage normally occurs through a physical interaction of proteins against the inner surface of the host cell membrane. A virus may also exit a cell by budding. Budding involves the creation of a lipoprotein envelope around the virion prior to the virion's being extruded out through the cell membrane.

Randall L. Milstein, Ph.D.

Further Reading

Becker, Yechiel, and Gholamreza Darai, eds. *Molecular Evolution of Viruses: Past and Present.* Boston: Kluwer Academic, 2000. Print.

Dimmock, N. J., A. J. Easton, and K. N. Leppard. *Introduction to Modern Virology.* 6th ed. Malden: Blackwell, 2007. Print.

Domingo, Esteban, Colin R. Parrish, and John J. Holland, eds. *Origin and Evolution of Viruses.* 2nd ed. Boston: Elsevier/Academic, 2008. Print.

Holland, J. J., ed. *Current Topics in Microbiology and Immunology: Genetic Diversity of RNA Viruses.* New York: Springer, 1992. Print.

Poehlmann, Stefan, and Graham Simmons. *Viral Entry into Host Cells.* New York: Springer, 2013. Print.

Shors, Teri. *Understanding Viruses.* 2nd ed. Sudbury: Jones, 2013. Print.

Tibayrenc, Michel. *Genetics and Evolution of Infectious Disease.* Boston: Elsevier, 2011. Print.

Yang, Decheng, ed. *RNA Viruses: Host Gene Responses to Infections.* Hackensack: World Scientific, 2009. Print.

Zimmer, Carl. *Parasite Rex: Inside the Bizarre World of Nature's Most Dangerous Creatures.* New York: Free, 2000. Print.

See also: DNA structure and function; Gene regulation: Viruses; Genetic engineering; Hybridomas and monoclonal antibodies; Oncogenes; Organ transplants and HLA genes; RNA structure and function; Viroids and virusoids.

Viroids and virusoids

Category: Viral genetics

Significance: Viroids are naked strands of RNA, 270 to 380 nucleotides long, that are circular and do not code for any proteins. However, some viroids are catalytic RNAs (ribozymes), able to cleave and ligate themselves. In spite of their simplicity, they are able to cause disease in susceptible plants, many of them economically important. Virusoids are similar to viroids, except that they require a helper virus to infect a plant and reproduce.

Putative secondary structure of the PSTV (potato spindle tuber viroid)
   Black: secondary structure of the viroid   Red: GAAAC sequence common to all viroids   Yellow: central conservative sequence   Blue: nucleotide numbers By Author: Jakub Friedl (user kyknos) (Source file with layers (gimp xcf file):), via Wikimedia Commons

KEY TERMS

RNA polymerase: an enzyme that catalyzes the joining of ribonucleotides to make RNA using DNA or another RNA strand as a template

RNase: an enzyme that catalyzes the cutting of an RNA molecule

GENERAL CHARACTERISTICS OF VIROIDS AND VIRUSOIDS

Viroids, and some virusoids, are circular, single-stranded RNA molecules, which normally appear as rods but when denatured by heating appear as closed circles. The rod-shaped structure is formed by extensive base pairing within the RNA molecule, and the secondary structure is divided into five structural domains. One domain is called the pathogenicity (P) domain, because differences among variant strains of the same species of viroid seem to correlate with differences in pathogenicity.

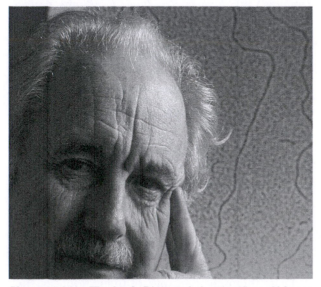

Plant pathologist Theodor O. Diener took the scientific world by surprise in 1971 when he discovered the viroid, a plant pathogen 80 times smaller than a virus. public domain via wikimedia commons

Virusoids may also comprise linear RNA or, rarely, double-stranded circular RNA.

The difference between viroids and virusoids is in their mode of transmission. Viroids have no protective covering of any kind and are no more than the RNA that makes up their genetic material. They depend on breaks in a plant's epidermis or can travel with pollen or ovules to gain entry. Virusoids, also known as satellite RNAs, are packaged in the protein coat of other plant viruses, referred to as helpers, and are therefore dependent on the other virus.

Viroids are typically divided into two groups based on the nature of their RNA molecule. Group A is the smallest group, and their RNA has the ability to self-cleave. These include the avocado sunblotch and peach latent mosaic viroids. Group B contains all the other viroids, and their RNA is not capable of self-cleavage. Species in group B include the potato spindle tuber, coconut cadang, tomato plant macho, and citrus bent leaf viroids.

Virusoids are less well studied than viroids and, although more diverse, are most similar to group B viroids in that they cannot self-cleave. Examples include the tomato black ring virus viroid, the peanut stunt virus viroid, and the tobacco ringspot virus viroid. Because so little is known about virusoids, the remainder of this article will focus on viroids.

VIROID PATHOGENESIS

If infected leaves are homogenized in a blender and passed through an "ultrafilter" fine enough to exclude bacteria, the infection is easily transmitted to another plant by painting some of the filtrate on a leaf. Even billionfold dilutions of the filtrate retain the ability to cause infection, suggesting that it is being replicated. RNase destroys infectivity, suggesting that the genetic material (RNA) is exposed to the medium, unlike viruses, which have a protective protein coat. When isolated from other cell components, an absorbance spectrum shows that viroids are pure nucleic acid, lacking a protein coat.

Although viroids are structurally simple and do not code for any proteins, they still cause disease. Although the molecular mechanisms of viroid pathogenesis are unknown, it is clear that the pathogenesis domain (P domain) is primarily responsible.

Changes in the sequence of nucleotides in the P domain have been correlated with pathogenicity. Some research suggests that the pathogenicity of a viroid strain is related to the resistance of the P domain to heat denaturation, with stability of this region being inversely related to severity. However, some evidence suggests that this may not be entirely true. In a series of nucleotide substitutions introduced by researchers into the P region of an intermediate strain (that is, intermediate in pathogenicity) of potato spindle tuber viroid (PSTVd), four showed viroid infectivity and pathogenicity that were the same as those of a previously reported severe strain of PSTVd. Altogether, eight different mutant strains were analyzed, and resistance to denaturation and PSTVd pathogenicity were not correlated in all cases.

Research is under way to understand how viroids move from cell to cell and traverse the cytoplasm to the nucleus, where many viroids replicate. There is evidence that a possible interaction might involve viroid RNA activating an RNA-activated protein kinase in response to a nucleotide sequence similar to that of the normal RNA activator. Protein kinases are integral to intracellular signaling pathways that control many aspects of cell metabolism. Once researchers understand the signals that viroids use to get around, it may be possible to devise treatments against them. A better understanding of the process may also shed light on normal biochemical communication pathways in plant cells.

Viroid Replication

Viroids replicate by a rolling circle mechanism, a method also used by some viruses. The original strand is referred to as the "(+) strand," and complementary copies of it are called "(−) strands." Type A and B viroids replicate slightly differently. In type A viroids, the circular (+) strand is replicated by RNA-dependent RNA polymerase to form several linear copies of the RNA (−) strand connected end to end. Site-specific self-cleavage produces individual (−) strands later circularized by a host RNA ligase. Each (−) strand is finally copied by the RNA polymerase to make several linear copies of (+) strand RNA.

Cleavage of this last strand makes individual RNA (+) strands, which are then circularized. Self-cleavage in viroids represents one of the cases in which RNA acts as an enzyme. The RNA forms a "hammerhead" structure that enzymatically cleaves the longer RNAs at just the right sites.

Replication of type B viroids is apparently mediated by normal host DNA-dependent RNA polymerase, which mistakes the viroid RNA for DNA. The overall process is similar to what happens with type A viroids, except that the (−) strand is not cleaved but instead is copied directly, yielding a (+) strand that is cleaved by host RNase to form individual copies that are ligated to become circular.

Economic Impact of Viroids

Genetically engineered plants in the future might make proteins that would essentially confer immunity by preventing viroids from entering the nucleus. With no access to the nucleus, a viroid would be incapable of replicating, effectively preventing the damage normally associated with viroid infection. Currently, no such transgenic plants exist, and viroids can reduce agricultural productivity if outbreaks are not checked quickly. The typical treatment is simply to destroy the affected plants, as there is no cure.

Although predominantly negative, viroids may have some potentially positive benefits. They have already been used in unique ways to study plant genetics, and they may provide insights into how plant proteins and nucleic acids move in and out of cell nuclei. It may also be possible to harness the benefits of viroid infection for certain agricultural applications, such as dwarfing citrus trees. Considerably more will need to be learned about viroids before they can be adequately controlled or used for human benefit.

Bryan Ness, Ph.D.

Further Reading

Dalakouras, Athanasios, Elena Dadami, and Michael Wassenegger. "Viroid-Induced DNA Methylation in Plants." *Biomolecular Concepts* 4.6 (2013): 557–65. Print.

Diener, T. O., R. A. Owens, and R. W. Hammond. "Viroids, the Smallest and Simplest Agents of Infectious Disease: How Do They Make Plants Sick?" *Intervirology* 35.1–4 (1993): 186–95. Print.

Duran-Vila, Núria, et al. "Structure and Evolution of Viroids." *Origin and Evolution of Viruses.* Ed. Esteban Domingo, Colin R. Parrish, and John J. Holland. 2nd ed. Boston: Elsevier/Academic, 2008. Print.

Gómez, Gustavo, and Vicente Pallás. "Viroids: A Light in the Darkness of the lnc RNA-Directed Regulatory Networks in Plants." *New Phytologist* 198.1 (2013): 10–15. Print.

Hadidi, Ahmed, et al., eds. *Viroids.* Enfield: Science, 2003. Print.

Hammond, R. W. "Analysis of the Virulence Modulating Region of Potato Spindle Tuber Viroid (PSTVd) by Site-Directed Mutagenesis." *Virology* 187.2 (1992): 654–62. Print.

Owens, R. A., W. Chen, Y. Hu, and Y-H. Hsu. "Suppression of Potato Spindle Tuber Viroid Replication and Symptom Expression by Mutations, Which Stabilize the Pathogenicity Domain." *Virology* 208.2 (1995): 554–64. Print.

Shors, Teri. "What About Prions and Viroids?" and "Plant Viruses." *Understanding Viruses.* 2nd ed. Sudbury: Jones, 2013. Print.

Wassenegger, M., et al. "RNA-Directed *De Novo* Methylation of Genomic Sequences in Plants." *Cell* 76.3 (1994): 567–76. Print.

See also: DNA structure and function; Gene regulation: Viruses; Genetic engineering; Hybridomas and monoclonal antibodies; Oncogenes; Organ transplants and HLA genes; RNA structure and function; Viral genetics.

Von Gierke disease

CATEGORY: Developmental genetics
ALSO KNOWN AS: Glycogen storage disease type I; von Gierke's disease

DEFINITION

Von Gierke disease is a rare inherited glycogen storage disease. It is characterized by the inability to break down glycogen into glucose because of the absence of the enzyme glucose-6-phosphatase (G6P). There are two types of von Gierke disease, Ia and Ib. Type Ia is caused by lack of G6P, and type Ib is caused by the lack of G6P translocase, the main transporter substance for G6P.

RISK FACTORS

Von Gierke disease is an autosomal recessive trait that requires that both parents pass on the mutations. In September 2013, Deeksha Bali reported eighty percent of cases are type Ia, and 20 percent are type Ib. The incidence is about one case per 100,000 births. Type Ia is more common in Ashkenazi Jewish populations, where the incidence is 1 case per 20,000 births.

Glucose-6-phosphate   Zephyris at the English language Wikipedia, from Wikimedia Commons

Glycogen bonds By Boumphreyfr (Own work), via Wikimedia Commons

Etiology and Genetics

Normally, the body stores excess sugar as glycogen in the liver and kidneys. As the glucose is needed for energy and to support body functions, it is freed from the glycogen by a process that requires the enzyme G6P. A similar process converts proteins and fats to glucose. Without G6P, blood glucose levels are unstable, and the body develops large stores of glycogen. The drop in blood glucose levels several hours after meals or at night causes severe hypoglycemia, which can be fatal. Chronic hypoglycemia causes other problems of metabolism. Levels of lactic acid, triglycerides, and uric acid are elevated.

Von Gierke type Ia is caused by mutations on chromosome 17 at 17q21. As reported by Roseline Froissart et al, more than eighty-five mutations had been identified as of May 2011. Mutations tend to vary according to country of origin. The more common mutations are *R83C, Q347X, 459insTA,* and *R83H.* These mutations stop production of G6P. According to Deeksha Bali et al, there have been no strong genotype-phenotype correlations identified for Von Gierke disease.

Von Gierke type Ib is caused by the absence of translocator1 gene (*G6PT1*) located on chromosome 11 at 11q23. Some of the mutations are due to splicing bases from one exon to another. Froissart reports more than eighty mutations have been identified. The more common mutations are *1211delCT, G339C,* and *W188Rv.*

Symptoms

Symptoms of von Gierke disease develop right after birth and can be fatal if not treated. The infant can demonstrate symptoms of irritability, tremors, cyanosis, seizures, apnea, and coma. Usually, the disease is diagnosed at this time. If not, the child exhibits lethargy, difficult arousal from overnight sleep, overwhelming hunger, poor growth, increase in abdominal girth, easy bruising, and puffy cheeks as a result of fat deposits.

Older patients have poor tolerance of fasting, severe hepatomegaly, growth retardation, osteoporosis, gout, and enlarged kidneys. With type Ib, there are frequent infections.

Screening and Diagnosis

Due to its rarity, von Gierke disease is not screened for unless there is a family history. The diagnosis includes the presenting symptoms. Blood tests of glucose, lactic acid, triglycerides, and uric acid are performed four hours after eating. Typically, the blood glucose is quite low, while lactic acid, triglycerides, and uric acid are elevated. For type Ib, a complete blood count with white cell differential is performed to evaluate for decreased neutrophils. Ultrasounds of the liver and kidneys demonstrate organ enlargement.

The liver is biopsied and examined for G6P activity and deposits of glycogen. Growth and development is behind schedule. Genetic testing is performed for the chromosomal changes that occur with von Gierke disease.

Treatment and Therapy

Von Gierke disease is treated by a diet that is high in starches and glucose. According to guidelines from the *European Study on Glycogen Storage Disease,* as reported by Rake et al, this diet should be 60 to 70 percent carbohydrate, 10 to 15 percent protein, and the remainder from fat. Galactose, fructose, sucrose, and lactose should be avoided, since these sugars require G6P to be converted to glucose. Carbohydrates, such as glucose or corn starch, are provided during the night. This is done using a gastric tube with continuous infusion of glucose or starch, or by night feedings with uncooked corn starch.

Elevated uric acid levels are treated with the drug allopurinal, which interferes with its production. During childhood, episodes of metabolic acidosis can occur during minor illnesses or vomiting. They are treated with intravenous fluids in order to restore glucose levels. If all else fails, a liver transplant can be performed to treat von Gierke disease.

Prevention and Outcomes

There is no way to prevent von Gierke disease unless there is a family history of the condition. In this case, genetic testing is performed.

There is no cure for the disease. Patients should be taught to observe for hypoglycemia and how to treat it. Long-term complications of von Gierke disease include seizures, kidney failure, hepatic tumors, kidney stones, and brain damage. Type Ib can also lead to inflammatory bowel disease, frequent lung and skin infections, secondary diabetes mellitus, and acute myelogenous leukemia.

Christine M. Carroll, R.N., B.S.N., M.B.A.

FURTHER READING

"Type I Glycogen Storage Disease." *Association for Glycogen Storage Disease.* Assoc. for Glycogen Storage Disease, 10 Aug. 2014. Web. 11 Aug. 2014.

Bali, Deeksha S., Yuan-Tsong Chen and Jennifer L Goldstein. "Glycogen Storage Disease Type I." *GeneReviews.* Ed. Roberta A. Pagon et al. Seattle: U of Washington, Seattle, 1993–2014. *NCBI Bookshelf.* Natl. Center for Biotechnology Information, 19 Sept. 2013. Web. 11 Aug. 2014.

Froissart, Roseline, et al. "Glucose-6-Phosphatase Deficiency." *Orphanet Journal of Rare Diseases* 6.27 (2011): n. pag. Web 18 Aug. 2014.

Haldeman-Englert, Chad. "Von Gierke Disease." *MedlinePlus.* US Natl. Lib. of Medicine, 7 May 2013. Web. 11 Aug. 2014.

Nussbaum, Robert, Roderick R. McInnes, and Huntington F. Willard. *Thompson and Thompson Genetics in Medicine.* 7th ed. Philadelphia: Saunders, 2007. Print.

Pritchard, Dorian J., and Bruce R. Korf. *Medical Genetics at a Glance.* 3rd ed. Hoboken: Wiley-Blackwell, 2013. Print.

Rake, JP, et al. "Guidelines for Management of Glycogen Storage Disease Type I - European Study on Glycogen Storage Disease Type I (ESGSD I)." *European Journal of Pediatrics.* 161 (2011): S112-S119. PDF File.

See also: Andersen's disease; Forbes disease; Galactokinase deficiency; Galactosemia; Gaucher disease; Glucose galactose malabsorption; Glucose-6-phosphate dehydrogenase deficiency; Glycogen storage diseases; Hereditary diseases; Hers disease; Inborn errors of metabolism; McArdle's disease; Pompe disease; Tarui's disease.

Von Hippel-Lindau syndrome

CATEGORY: Diseases and syndromes
ALSO KNOWN AS: Von Hippel-Lindau disease; VHL

DEFINITION

Von Hippel-Lindau (VHL) syndrome is a rare genetic disorder (affecting approximately 1 in 36,000 people) in which some blood vessels grow in an abnormal way and cause tumors in parts of the body that are rich in blood vessels.

RISK FACTORS

The only known risk factor for VHL is having family members with this syndrome.

ETIOLOGY AND GENETICS

A single gene, *VHL*, located on the short arm of chromosome 3 at position 3p25.3, is known to be associated with Von Hippel-Lindau syndrome. There are actually two different proteins specified by this gene, depending on how the coding portions of the messenger ribonucleic acid (RNA) are spliced together. These proteins normally move back and forth in cells between the nucleus and the cytoplasm, and they form complexes with several other proteins in a pathway that targets yet other proteins to be degraded when they are no longer needed. One such protein that is often targeted for degradation is the hypoxia-inducible factor (HIF), which acts to control cell division and the formation of new blood vessels. When mutations in the *VHL* gene result in missing or

These lesions may be a part of von Hippel-Lindau syndrome By Nephron (Own work), via Wikimedia Commons

CT in patient with VHL syndrome through the petrous ridge demonstrates bone erosion at the site of the endolymphatic sac tumor, typical of the locally aggressive behavior of this tumor (curved arrow). public domain via wikimedia commons

altered VHL proteins, an excess of HIF may develop. This can lead to uncontrolled cell division with superfluous blood vessels, resulting in the characteristic tumors and cysts seen in patients with VHL.

The inheritance of VHL follows a classic autosomal dominant pattern, meaning that a single copy of the mutation is sufficient to cause full expression of the syndrome. An affected individual has a 50 percent chance of transmitting the mutation to each of his or her children. In about 20 percent of cases, however, the disease results from a spontaneous new mutation, so in these instances affected individuals will have unaffected parents. Curiously, it has been shown that at the molecular level within cells, both copies of the *VHL* gene must be mutated in order to initiate the formation of tumors and cysts. One of these mutations is the inherited one that is present in all cells, while the second occurs randomly during normal cell growth in tissues, such as the kidney, brain, or retina. It is this acquired second mutation that triggers tumor or cyst formation in the affected tissue.

Symptoms

There is wide variation in the age at which VHL begins, the organs where problems occur, and the types and severity of symptoms. These differences occur even among members of the same family.

Although there is no consistent set of symptoms, the most common ones are vision problems (retinal angiomatosis), headaches, signs of elevated intracranial pressure, and trouble walking (cerebellar hemangioblastoma). Less common findings include pheochromocytoma, a tumor of the adrenal gland that leads to many problems, including very high or spiking blood pressure; and tumors and/or cysts in the spinal cord, lungs, liver, pancreas, and epididymis (part of the scrotum). Renal cell carcinoma is the most common cause of death.

Few people with VHL have all these problems. Full-blown symptoms usually occur in adulthood, but they can begin in childhood.

Screening and Diagnosis

The doctor will ask about a patient's symptoms and medical history and will perform a physical exam. A blood test that analyzes DNA may be done to determine if the patient has the VHL gene. Not all families with VHL have an identifiable VHL mutation. If members of the patient's family are positive for the gene and the patient is not, the patient does not need any further testing.

However, if other family members have been diagnosed with VHL despite a negative genetic test, or if the patient tests positive for the VHL gene, the patient needs to have regular medical exams and tests to uncover early signs. Even in the absence of symptoms, screening should begin in childhood and continue periodically throughout life.

Screening for VHL complications includes a physical exam with special attention to the patient's eyes and nervous system. Tests may include a magnetic resonance imaging (MRI) scan, a test that uses powerful magnets and radio waves to generate images of the inside of the body; a computed tomography (CT) scan, a type of X ray that uses a computer to generate images of the inside of the body; ultrasound, a test that uses high-pitched sound waves to examine the inside of the body; angiography, X rays taken after a dye is injected into the arteries allowing their interior to be seen; and a twenty-four-hour urine test for elevated levels of hormones. Depending on the test results, the doctor will tell the patient what symptoms to watch for and if the patient needs treatment.

If the patient has any VHL symptoms, he or she should consider being tested for the gene. This is advised even if the patient has no known family history of the disease. The patient could be the first person in his or her family to have VHL, or he or she could be the first one to have it properly diagnosed since many people are not aware they have it.

Treatment and Therapy

There is no known cure for VHL. Treatment depends on a patient's specific symptoms, test results, and general health. Retinal angiomas may be treated with photocoagulation or cryocoagulation. When treatment is needed (for example, for cerebellar lesions), it usually involves surgery to remove tumors. However, tumors are usually removed only if they are cancerous or causing other problems, such as preventing an organ from working properly. If tumors are not removed, they must be watched carefully for further growth.

Prevention and Outcomes

There is no known way to prevent the VHL gene from causing its many manifestations. Therefore, genetic counseling is advised for families with known VHL or who test positive for the gene.

Individuals who have a family history of the disease or know they have the gene can reduce their risks of serious health problems by having regular screening tests to detect VHL complications early, watching carefully for any suspicious symptoms, and getting treatment as soon as symptoms occur. Individuals can also take steps to reduce their risk of the cancers associated with VHL, such as eating a diet high in fruits and vegetables, not smoking, and limiting their consumption of alcohol.

Laurie Rosenblum, M.P.H.;
reviewed by Rosalyn Carson-DeWitt, M.D.
"Etiology and Genetics" by Jeffrey A. Knight, Ph.D.

FURTHER READING

Choyke, P. L., et al. "Von Hippel-Lindau Disease: Genetic, Clinical, and Imaging Features." *Radiology* 194.3 (March, 1995): 629–42. Print.

Kleigman, Robert M., et al., eds. *Nelson Textbook of Pediatrics*. 18th ed. Philadelphia: Elsevier, 2007. Print.

Mahon, Suzanne M., and Laura Waldman. "Von Hippel-Lindau Syndrome: Implications for Nursing Care." *Oncology Nursing Forum* 39.6 (2012): 533–36. Print.

Murray, Michael F., et al. *Clinical Genomics: Practical Applications in Adult Patient Care*. New York: McGraw-Hill Education/Medical, 2014. Print.

O'Brien, F. J., et al. "Manifestations of Von Hippel-Lindau Syndrome: A Retrospective National Review." *QJM: An Intl. Journ. of Medicine* 107.4 (2014): 291–96. Print.

Schmike, R. Neil, and Debra L. Collins. "Von Hippel-Lindau Syndrome." *Management of Genetic Syndromes*. Ed. Suzanne B. Cassidy and Judith E. Allanson. Hoboken: Wiley-Liss, 2005. Print.

See also: Atherosclerosis; Barlow's syndrome; Cardiomyopathy; Heart disease; Holt-Oram syndrome; Long QT syndrome; Wolff-Parkinson-White syndrome.

Von Willebrand disease and genetics

CATEGORY: Diseases and syndromes
ALSO KNOWN AS: vWD

DEFINITION

Von Willebrand disease (vWD) is an inherited blood disorder. It decreases the blood's ability to clot. As a result, bleeding lasts longer than usual.

Von Willebrand disease is the most common hereditary bleeding disorder, affecting about 1 percent of the population. It affects both sexes approximately equally. There are no racial or ethnic associations with this disorder.

RISK FACTORS

The only risk factor for vWD is having family members with this disease.

ETIOLOGY AND GENETICS

Von Willebrand disease is caused by mutations in a gene called *VWF*, which is found on the short arm of chromosome 12 at position 12p13.3. This gene encodes a protein known as the von Willebrand factor (vWF), which plays an important role in the formation of blood clots. It is the von Willebrand factor that causes platelets to aggregate together and to help plug the holes in damaged blood vessel walls, a critical first step in clot formation. Some mutations in the gene cause a reduced amount of von Willebrand factor to be produced, and these result in the mildest (type 1) form of the disease. Type 2 disease usually results from different mutations that do not reduce the amount of protein but instead compromise the ability of the protein to perform its normal function. In the severest form (type 3), mutations typically result in an abnormally short protein that is completely nonfunctional.

All cases of type 1 vWD and a minority of type 2 cases are inherited in an autosomal dominant fashion, meaning that a single copy of the mutation is sufficient to cause full expression. An affected individual

PBB Protein VWF image By ProteinBoxBot at en.wikipedia, from Wikimedia Commons

has a 50 percent chance of transmitting the mutation to each of his or her children. Some of these cases, however, result from a spontaneous new mutation, so in these instances, affected individuals will have unaffected parents. All cases of type 3 disease and most instances of type 2 disease are inherited in an autosomal recessive manner, which means that both copies of the gene must be deficient in order for the individual to be afflicted. Typically, an affected child is born to two unaffected parents, both of whom are carriers of the recessive mutant allele. The probable outcomes for children whose parents are both carriers are 75 percent unaffected and 25 percent affected.

SYMPTOMS

Many people with the vWD gene have very mild symptoms or none at all. When symptoms do occur, the severity varies from person to person. Many people only notice symptoms after taking aspirin or similar medications that interfere with clotting. Symptoms usually begin in childhood and fluctuate throughout life.

Common symptoms include easy bruising, frequent or prolonged nosebleeds, prolonged bleeding from the gums and minor cuts, heavy or prolonged bleeding during menstrual periods, and bleeding in the digestive system. Another symptom is prolonged bleeding after injury, childbirth, surgery, or invasive dental procedures.

SCREENING AND DIAGNOSIS

The doctor will ask about a patient's symptoms and medical history and will perform a physical exam. Blood tests may be done to check for bleeding time, which in vWD will be prolonged, particularly after the administration of aspirin. Blood tests can also check for the factor VIII antigen. This indirectly measures levels of vWF in the blood; in vWD, it will be reduced. Ristocetin cofactor activity can also be checked by a blood test. This shows how well a patient's vWF works; in vWD, it will be decreased. In addition, a blood test can check the von Willebrand factor multimer. This examines the different structural types of vWF in the blood; in vWD, it will be reduced.

TREATMENT AND THERAPY

Many people with vWD do not need treatment. For patients who do, their treatment will depend on the type and severity of their vWD. In many cases, treatment is only necessary for patients who are having a surgical or dental procedure that is likely to cause bleeding.

Treatment may include desmopressin. This medicine usually controls bleeding in mild cases of type I vWD by raising the level of vWF in the blood. It can be taken as a nasal spray (Stimate) or an injection (DDAVP). Intravenous infusions control a patient's bleeding. These infusions are concentrates that contain factor VIII and the von Willebrand factor. Birth control pills may be used to control heavy menstrual periods in women with type 1 vWD. Antifibrinolytic medicine (often Amicar) can be used for bleeding in the nose or mouth. It helps keep a clot that has already formed from being dissolved.

PREVENTION AND OUTCOMES

There are no guidelines for preventing vWD. Genetic counseling can be helpful to review a detailed family history and discuss risks and tests available for von Willebrand disease.

Laurie Rosenblum, M.P.H.;
reviewed by Rosalyn Carson-DeWitt, M.D.
"Etiology and Genetics" by Jeffrey A. Knight, Ph.D.

FURTHER READING

Antovic, Jovan P., and Margareta Blombäck. *Essential Guide to Blood Coagulation*. 2d ed. Chichester: Wiley, 2013. Print.

Greer, John P. *Wintrobe's Clinical Hematology*. Philadelphia: Kluwer, 2014. Print.

Hoffman, Ronald, et al. *Hematology: Basic Principles and Practice*. 6th ed. Philadelphia: Elsevier, 2013.

Kouides, Peter A. "Von Willebrand Disease." *Inherited Bleeding Disorders in Women*. Ed. Christine A. Lee, Rezan A. Kadir, and Kouides. Hoboken: Wiley, 2009. Print.

Longe, Jacqueline L., and the Gale Group. *The Gale Encyclopedia of Medicine*. 3d ed. Detroit: Gale, 2006. Print.

Strozewski, Susan M. "Von Willebrand's Disease." *American Journal of Nursing* 100.2 (Feb. 2000): 24AA–24BB, 24DD. Print.

See also: ABO blood types; Chronic myeloid leukemia; Fanconi anemia; Hemophilia; Hereditary spherocytosis; Infantile agranulocytosis; Myelodysplastic syndromes; Paroxysmal nocturnal hemoglobinuria; Porphyria; Rh incompatibility and isoimmunization; Sickle-cell disease.

W

Waardenburg syndrome

CATEGORY: Diseases and syndromes

ALSO KNOWN AS: Waardenburg type I (WSI); type II (WSII); type III (WSIII, Klein-Waardenburg syndrome); type IV (WSIV, Shah-Waardenburg syndrome, Waardenburg-Hirschsprung disease)

DEFINITION

Waardenburg syndrome (WS) is a genetic disorder first described in 1951 by Petrus Johannes Waardenburg. Since the original publication, at least four types (I–IV) have been described. All forms are classified as hereditary auditory-pigmentary syndromes characterized by congenital sensorineural hearing loss, patchy depigmentation, and defects of neural-crest-derived tissues. WS is caused by mutations in many genes, including *EDN3*, *EDNRB*, *MITF*, *PAX3*, *SNAI2*, and *SOX10*.

RISK FACTORS

Individuals without a family history presumably have de novo (sporadic) mutations. Advanced paternal age is a risk factor for sporadic mutations including those that cause WS. The new mutation rate is estimated at 0.4 per 100,000. Both sexes and people of all races are affected equally, with an overall prevalence of 1 in 32,400–42,000.

Patient with Waardenburg-Klein syndrome. See page for author, via Wikimedia Commons
Patient with Waardenburg-Klein syndrome (one of two identical twins described by van der Hoeve)) See page for author, via Wikimedia Commons

ETIOLOGY AND GENETICS

WS is a genetically heterogeneous group of conditions. Approximately 96 percent of individuals who meet the diagnostic criteria for WSI have a detectable mutation (90 percent) or a whole or partial gene deletion (6 percent) of the *PAX3* gene located on chromosome 2q35. *PAX3* mutations have also been found in individuals with WSIII. Mutations in the microphthalmia-associated transcription factor (*MITF*) gene, located on chromosome 3p14.1-p12.3, are found in approximately 15 percent of individuals with WSII. Additional subtypes of WSII have been linked to other loci including 1p, 8p23, 8q11 (*SNAI2*), and 22q13 (*SOX10*). WSIV is associated with mutations in the endothelin-B-receptor gene (*EDNRP*) on chromosome 13q22, the endothelin-3 gene (*EDN3*) on 20q13.2-q13.3, and the *SOX 10* gene on 22q13.

WS is inherited in both an autosomal dominant (AD) and autosomal recessive (AR) manner. AD refers to a type of condition that can be inherited by a single parent. A person who is heterozygous (one working gene and one nonworking gene) is affected with the condition. The recurrence risk for the offspring of individuals who are affected is 50 percent. AR refers to a type of condition that has to be inherited by both parents. A person who is heterozygous is referred to as a carrier and is unaffected. When two carriers of the same nonworking gene have children, they have a 25-percent chance of having a child homozygous (with two nonworking genes) and thus, of having a child affected with the condition. WS types I, II, and in some cases IV (when *SOX10*) are AD. When WSIII occurs in families it is AD; however, it is usually sporadic. There have also been cases reported of individuals with WSIII who are homozygous for *PAX3* mutations. WS type IV (when *EDNRP* and *EDN3*) is AR.

The genes that cause WS are important in the regulation of melanocyte development. Melanocytes produce melanin, which contributes to the pigmentation of skin, hair, and eye color and is important for the proper function of the cochlea. Mutations in any of these genes may result in hearing loss and changes in pigmentation. Genes responsible for WSIV (*SOX10, EDN3,* or *EDNRB*) are involved in the development of nerve cells in the large intestine, leading to problems related to Hirschsprung's disease. All forms of WS show marked interfamilial and intrafamilial variability, indicating that modifier genes probably play a role in the expression of the disease.

SYMPTOMS

Major features of WS include sensorineural hearing loss, a white forelock or premature graying of the hair, different colored eyes (one blue and one brown), and patchy skin dipigmentation. WSI is associated with dystopia canthorum, a condition in which the inner corners of the eyes are spaced farther apart than normal. WSII appears similar to WSI without dystopia canthorum. The principal feature of WSIII is musculoskeletal anomalies of the upper limbs, including hypoplasia (underdevelopment), contractures, and syndactyly (fused fingers). WSIV includes features of type II combined with Hirschsprung's disease.

SCREENING AND DIAGNOSIS

The Waardenburg Consortium has proposed clinical diagnostic criteria. Molecular genetic testing may be available to confirm the diagnosis, clarify risks for family members, and provide prenatal diagnosis. Testing is offered clinically for all types. Population screening for WS is not available.

TREATMENT AND THERAPY

There is no cure for WS. Treatment depends on manifestations as appropriate. Often the most significant complication is hearing loss; benefits are gained from early detection and treatment with hearing aids or cochlear implants. Individuals may also require orthopedic interventions or treatment for Hirschsprung's disease. For optimal care, patients should see a variety of specialists, including a clinical geneticist, genetic counselor, otolaryngologist, audiologist, speech-language pathologist, and possibly an ophthalmologist, dermatologist, craniofacial surgeon, and gastrointestinal specialist.

PREVENTION AND OUTCOMES

Prenatal or preimplantation genetic diagnoses are available if the cause is known. Women at risk of having a child with WSI are recommended to take folic acid supplementation. Most individuals with WS have normal intelligence and live long, productive lives.

Amber M. Mathiesen, M.S.

FURTHER READING

Bansal, Yuvika, et al. "Waardenburg Syndrome: A Case Report." *Contact Lens and Anterior Eye* 36.1 (2013): 49–51. Print.

Farrer, L. A., et al. "Waardenburg Syndrome (WS) Type I Is Caused by Defects at Multiple Loci, One of Which Is Near ALPP on Chromosome 2: First Report of the WS Consortium." *American Journal of Human Genetics* 50 (1992): 902–13. Print.

Garg, Uma, and Ritesh Surana. "Waardenburg Syndrome 2." *Indian Journal of Otology* 18.4 (2012): 220–22. Print.

Kontorinis, Georgios, et al. "Inner Ear Anatomy in Waardenburg Syndrome: Radiological Assessment and Comparison with Normative Data." *International Journal of Pediatric Otorhinolaryngology* 78.8 (2014): 1320–26. Print.

Newton, V. E. "Clinical Features of the Waardenburg Syndromes." *Advances in Oto-Rhino-Laryngology* 61 (2002): 201–8. Print.

See also: Albinism; Chediak-Higashi syndrome; Epidermolytic hyperkeratosis; Hermansky-Pudlak syndrome; Hirschsprung's disease; Ichthyosis; Melanoma; Palmoplantar keratoderma.

Waldenström macroglobulinemia (WM)

CATEGORY: Diseases and syndromes
ALSO KNOWN AS: Lymphoplasmacytic lymphoma

DEFINITION

Waldenström macroglobulinemia (WM) is a rare and indolent form of non-Hodgkin's lymphoma and is one of the malignant monoclonal gammopathies. In WM, lymphoplasmacytic cells that are in the process of maturing from B cells into plasma cells multiply abnormally and produce large amounts of monoclonal immunoglobulin M antibody (IgM). High levels of IgM create hyperviscosity of the serum, and lymphoplasmacytic cells infiltrate into the bone marrow, spleen, and lymph nodes.

Spontaneous splenic rupture in Waldenstrom's macroglobulinemia
By Michail Charakidis, David Joseph Russell, via Wikimedia Commons

Lymphocyte
B cell

B cell. By BruceBlaus (Own work), via Wikimedia Commons

RISK FACTORS

The most significant risk factor for WM is age. Median age at diagnosis is sixty-three. Men are at greater risk than women, and white men are at higher risk than African Americans. People who have monoclonal gammopathy of undetermined significance (MGUS) have a higher risk of developing non-Hodgkin's lymphoma and WM within twenty years. Having a first-degree relative with WM may also increase the risk.

ETIOLOGY AND GENETICS

The cause of WM remains unknown, although mutations in gene *MYD88* have been observed in over 90 percent of patients. There is some evidence that IgM in some patients with WM may have specificity for the same myelin-associated glycoprotein that has been associated with demyelinating diseases such as multiple sclerosis. This may explain why some patients with WM develop peripheral neuropathy before the onset of neoplastic disease. Speculation exists that this immunologic response may be triggered by viral infection. Hepatitis C, hepatitis G, and human herpes virus 8 have been suspected in the etiology of WM, but the data are not strong enough for these viruses to be considered causative at this time.

Evidence of a genetic etiology for WM comes from reports of family history. In one study approximately 20 percent of people with WM were found to have a first-degree relative with WM or a similar B cell-associated disease. Various other studies have documented immunoglobulin abnormalities in first-degree relatives of people diagnosed with WM, including monoclonal gammopathy, polyclonal gammopathy, and decreased levels of immunoglobulins. In a recent report published in *Clinical Cancer Research*, a follow-up study of twenty-two first-degree relatives of patients with WM found that IgM macroglobulinemia seems to be a phenotypic marker of WM in some families and carries a high risk of progression to WM. The frequency of IgM macroglobulinemia was found to be greater than thirty times what would normally be expected in a general population. Of five relatives who initially had IgM monoclonal gammopathy, after a median time period of seventeen years, all had persisted or progressed and three had gone on to develop WM.

Several types of chromosomal abnormalities have been observed in patients with WM. Deletions of chromosome 6q, including 6q21-22, have been reported in about 75 percent of patients with WM. Prognostic indications of these findings is uncertain, and there is not enough evidence to link WM with any consistent chromosomal or genetic change.

SYMPTOMS

Signs and symptoms of WM are caused by secretion of IgM, which causes hyperviscosity and vascular complications because of the physical, chemical, and immunologic properties of the IgM paraprotein, and by direct infiltration of neoplastic lymphoplasmacytic cells into bone marrow, spleen, and lymph nodes.

The onset of WM may be gradual and nonspecific, and many asymptomatic patients are diagnosed by routine blood work abnormalities. The most common presenting symptoms are weakness, severe fatigue, anorexia, peripheral neuropathy, weight loss, fever, and Raynaud's phenomenon. Common symptoms due to hyperviscosity may include abnormal bleeding from the nose, gums, or gastrointestinal tract, headache, blurred vision, dizziness, or hearing loss.

Common signs of WM found on physical examination include enlargement of the spleen and liver as well as generalized lymphadenopathy. Examination of the skin may reveal signs of increased bleeding tendency such as bruising or purpura. Ophthalmoscopic evaluation may reveal dilation of retinal veins, which is characteristic of hyperviscosity.

Infiltration of the central nervous system can cause Bing-Neel syndrome, which is characterized by lethargy, stupor, confusion, memory loss, and motor abnormalities. The neuropathy of WM is typically distal, sensorimotor, symmetrical, and slowly progressive. The constellation of polyneuropathy, organomegaly, endocrinopathy, M protein, and skin changes is known as POEMS syndrome and can be seen in patients with WM.

The signs and symptoms of WM are most similar to multiple myeloma (MM). WM can be differentiated from MM by enlargement of the spleen and liver, which is common in WM but rare in MM. Lytic bone lesions and renal disease that are commonly seen in MM are rarely seem in WM.

SCREENING AND DIAGNOSIS

WM is a rare condition with about 1,500 cases diagnosed each year in the United States, accounting for about 2 percent of hematologic malignancies. Diagnosis is based on finding evidence of a monoclonal spike on serum electrophoresis. Immunoelectrophoresis and immunofixation studies can help identify the spike as M component. About 80 percent of patients will present with a normocytic normochromic anemia. Thrombocytopenia and leukopenia are also common.

Malignant lymphocytes are usually present in peripheral blood. About 10 percent of macroglobulins in WM are cryoglobulins, but unlike the mixed cryoglobulins seen in rheumatoid arthritis or other autoimmune diseases, the cryoglobulins seen in WM are purely composed of IgM. Like the mixed cryoglobulins, the cryoglobulins of WM may cause Raynaud's phenomenon or other vascular symptoms precipitated by cold.

Bone marrow aspiration and biopsy are needed to confirm the diagnosis of WM. Bone marrow examination will show lymphoplasmacytic and small lymphocyte infiltration. Infiltration may be described on histology as diffuse, nodular, or packed. Nodular infiltration has the best prognosis and packed infiltration has the poorest prognosis.

Urinary immunoglobulins are usually light chain kappa type. Proteinuria is found in 40 percent of patients but exceeds 1 gram per day in only 3 percent of patients. Imaging studies including chest radiographs, computed tomography (CT), and magnetic resonance imaging (MRI) may be done to rule out infiltrates and organomegaly. Mental status symptoms should be evaluated by obtaining cerebrospinal fluid to rule out the presence of IgM.

TREATMENT AND THERAPY

Although there is no cure for WM, treatment can be effective and there are many treatment options available. Treatment for symptomatic hyperviscosity is considered to be a medical emergency and should be instituted promptly. The treatment of choice is plasmapheresis since 80 percent of IgM is confined in the intravascular space. Treatment of macroglobulinemia is by alkylating agents, nucleoside analogues, monoclonal antibodies, or combination therapy. The alkylating agent chlorambucil has been used for more than forty years. The response rate is about 60 percent when chlorambucil is used with or without prednisone. In patients who are resistant to alkylating agents, the purine nucleosides fludarabine or cladribine are often effective. The monoclonal antibody rituximab produces response rates of 20 to 50 percent. Combination therapies have reached response rates of 75 percent in some studies.

Other therapies that have been effective for WM include thalidomide, autologous blood cell transplantation, and interferon alpha. Autologous transplantation is reserved for younger patients who have not responded to other treatment. Interferon alpha given for six months has shown a response rate of 50 percent for a duration of more than two years. In cases where other treatments are not effective, splenectomy is occasionally performed because it removes a major reservoir of IgM.

PREVENTION AND OUTCOMES

There is no way to prevent WM. Some patients meet the diagnostic criteria for WM but remain asymptomatic. These patients are considered to have smoldering or indolent disease and can be followed carefully without treatment for many years. Complications of WM include renal disease, amyloidosis, cardiac failure, infections, and increased risk for lymphomas, myelodysplasia, and leukemia.

Median survival for all patients with WM is 78 months. About 80 percent of patients respond to some type of chemotherapy, and their median survival rate exceeds three years. In patients whose macroglobulin level can be reduced by 75 percent, median survival increases to 7.7 years. Incidence of WM rises sharply with age. Half of all patients with WM are diagnosed after the age of sixty-three. Older age, male sex, general symptoms, and cytopenia are associated with a worse prognosis.

Chris Iliades, M.D.

FURTHER READING

Cashen, Amanda F., and Brian Van Tine, eds. *The Washington Manual Hematology and Oncology Subspecialty Consult.* 3rd ed. Philadelphia: Kluwer/Lippincott, 2012. Print.

Fauci, Anthony S., et al. *Harrison's Principles of Internal Medicine.* 18th ed. New York: McGraw, 2012. Print.

"Macroglobulinemia of Waldenstrom." *MedlinePlus.* Natl. Lib. of Medicine, 30 Apr. 2012. Web. 2 Sept. 2014.

See also: Burkitt's lymphoma; Cancer; Chronic myeloid leukemia; Multiple endocrine neoplasias; Mutagenesis and cancer; Mutation and mutagenesis; Oncogenes; Tumor-suppressor genes.

Walker-Warburg Syndrome

CATEGORY: Diseases and syndromes

ALSO KNOWN AS: POMT1-Related hydrocephalus, agyria and retinal dysplasia; Hard syndrome; Hard +/- E syndrome; Warburg syndrome; Chemke syndrome; Pagon syndrome; Cerebroocular dysgenesis; Cerebroocular dysplasia muscular dystrophy syndrome; COD-MD syndrome

DEFINITION

Walker-Warburg Syndrome is a genetic disorder that causes profound muscle, brain, and eye abnormalities at birth. It is the most severe form of one of several related phenotypes that affect glycosylation including Fukuyama Congenital Muscular Dystrophy and Muscle-eye-brain disease. The specific group of disorders is known as dystroglycanopathies. The larger group of disorders is known as congenital muscular dystrophies (CMD). Survival is limited.

RISK FACTORS

The disease affects about 1 in 60,500 newborns worldwide. Consanguineous families are at highest risk. Carrier prevalence is about 1 in 120 in the Ashkenazi Jewish population.

ETIOLOGY AND GENETICS

At least 13 genes are responsible for Walker-Warburg Syndrome. Phenotypes are sometimes classified as Muscular Dystrophy-Dystroglycanopathy (MDDGA) 1-13. The most common gene mutations are those in POMT1 (located at 9q34.13), POMT2 (14q24.3), ISPD (located at 7p21.2), FKTN (located at 9q31.2), FKRP (located at 19q13.32), and LARGE1 (located at 22q12.3), affecting half of individuals. These and other genes are responsible for proteins to support glycosylation. This process allows the -dystroglycan protein to attach the stable framework in each cell (cytoskeleton) to extracellular proteins and other molecules. It stabilizes and protects muscle fibers and directs the migration of nerve cells during fetal development. Disruption of the glycosylation process through the various mutations damages muscle and brain tissue profoundly as the cells die and malfunction. It is unclear how the effects on glycosylation impact the eyes and other parts of the body.

The disease is inherited in an autosomal recessive manner. Both parents must be carriers and pass on a mutated gene. In this case, each offspring has a 25 percent chance of inheriting the disease, a 50 percent chance of becoming a carrier, and a 25 percent chance of being unaffected.

SIGNS AND SYMPTOMS

The most consistent feature of the disease is the smooth surface of the brain (lissencephaly). Signs and symptoms are typically present at birth and include hypotonia (with poor suck and swallow) and muscle atrophy ("floppy baby"), and serious brain malformations such as lissencephaly, hydrocephalus, and cerebellar malformations. Affected infants also have eye abnormalities, and other abnormalities, such as cleft lip/palate and contractures. Some infants have seizures. Intellectual disability and developmental delay are commonly seen. Eye abnormalities can vary significantly and may include small eyes (microphthalmia), optic nerve hypoplasia, malformations of the space behind the cornea and in front of the iris, defects of the retina, cataracts, a cleft or loss of tissue of the retina or iris (colobomas), abnormally large and protruding eyes (buphthalmos), or glaucoma. These malformations can cause partial or complete loss of vision.

SCREENING AND DIAGNOSIS

Brain defects can be seen in prenatal ultrasound. The conditions are diagnosed on the basis of clinical features and autopsy findings such as: congenital hydrocephalus, bilateral microphthalmos, severe developmental retardation, and several brain malformations. The findings can overlap with other muscular dystrophies, making myopathy a key distinguishing feature.

Prenatal, carrier, and genetic testing are available to confirm the presence of Walker-Warburg mutation.

TREATMENT AND THERAPY

There are no targeted treatments or cures for the disease. Treatment may include reducing occasional seizures with anticonvulsants and correction of hydrocephalus through surgical shunting. Supportive care may include physical therapy to treat contractures and feeding support.

PREVENTION AND OUTCOMES

In its most severe form, infant survival is limited to approximately nine months. Most children with Walker-Warburg do not live past three years of age.

Amber M. Mathiesen, M.S.

FURTHER READING

Abumansour IS, Al Sulmi E, Chodirker BN, Hunt JC. "Prenatal diagnosis of Walker–Warburg syndrome using single nucleotide polymorphism array: A clinical experience from three related palestinian families with congenital hydrocephalus." *AJP Rep.* 2015; 5(2): e116–e120.

Genetics Home Reference. "Walker-Warburg Syndrome." Available from https://ghr.nlm.nih.gov/condition/walker-warburg-syndrome#genes. Accessed July 27, 2017.

National Organization for Rare Disorders. "Walker Warburg Syndrome." Available from https://rarediseases.org/rare-diseases/walker-warburg-syndrome/. Accessed July 27, 2017.

Sparks SE, Quijano-Roy S, Harper A, et al. "Congenital Muscular Dystrophy Overview." 2001 Jan 22 [Updated 2012 Aug 23]. In: Pagon RA, Adam MP, Ardinger HH, et al., editors. GeneReviews® [Internet]. Seattle (WA): University of Washington, Seattle; 1993–2017. Available from: https://www.ncbi.nlm.nih.gov/books/NBK1291/.

Vitaliti G, Pavone P, Romano C, Barbagallo M, Vecchio M, Ledda C, Lubrano R, Falsaperla R. "Congenital muscular dystrophy and epilepsy: A prospective case series of pediatric patients. J Biol Regul Homeost Agents." 2016;30(4):1217–1221.

WEB SITES OF INTEREST

Cure CMD - Congenital Muscular Dystrophy
http://curecmd.org/
Muscular Dystrophy Association (MDA)
http://www.mdausa.org/
Muscular Dystrophy Family Foundation
http://www.mdff.org
OMIM® - Online Mendelian Inheritance in Man
http://www.omim.org/about

Deanna M. Neff, M.P.H.

See also: Aniridia; Best disease; Brachydactyly; Choroideremia; Color blindness; Corneal dystrophies; Glaucoma; Gyrate atrophy of the choroid and retina; Macular degeneration; Norrie syndrome; Progressive external ophthalmoplegia; Retinitis pigmentosa; Retinoblastoma; Stargardt's disease.

Weill-Marchesani syndrome

CATEGORY: Diseases and syndromes
ALSO KNOWN AS: WMS; WM syndrome; spherophakia-brachymorphia syndrome; congenital mesodermal dysmorphology

DEFINITION

Weill-Marchesani syndrome (WMS) is a genetic disorder first reported by George Weill in 1932 and subsequentially delineated by Oswald Marchesan in 1939. WMS is classified as a disorder of connective tissue, which binds together, supports, and strengthens muscles, joints, organs, and skin. Short stature, brachydactyly, joint stiffness, and characteristic eye anomalies including microspherophakia, ectopia of the lens, severe myopia, and glaucoma are all characteristic of WMS. Both autosomal recessive and dominant modes of inheritance have been described. Although not all causes are known, mutations in both *ADAMTS10* and *FBN1* genes have been found.

RISK FACTORS

The offspring of consanguineous relationships are at a higher risk for autosomal recessive conditions.

Many people reported with autosomal recessive WMS were members of consanguineous families. The majority of individuals with the autosomal dominant form have a family history. If no family history is found, it is likely a result of a de novo (sporadic) mutation. There are no other reported factors associated with an increased risk for having a child with WMS. The prevalence has been estimated at 1 in 100,000 people.

ETIOLOGY AND GENETICS

The etiology of WMS syndrome depends on the mode of inheritance. WMS is inherited in both an autosomal dominant (AD) and autosomal recessive (AR) manner. AD refers to a type of condition that can be inherited by a single parent. A person who is heterozygous (one working gene and one nonworking gene) is affected with the condition. The recurrence risk for the offspring of individuals who are affected is 50 percent. AR refers to a type of condition that has to be inherited by both parents. In an AR condition, a person who is heterozygous is referred to as a carrier and is unaffected. When two carriers of the same nonworking gene have children, they have a 25 percent chance of having a child who is homozygous (with two nonworking genes) and thus affected with the condition. The AR mode of inheritance seems to be more frequent then the AD form.

Homozygous mutations within the *ADAMTS10* gene located on chromosome locus 19p13.3-p13.2 are responsible for the AR form. The *ADAMTS10* gene codes for a protein product belonging to the ADAMTS family of proteins, which are involved in the extracellular matrix. The protein is expressed in the skin, fetal chondrocytes (a cartilage cell), and in the fetal and adult heart. Mutations in the *ADAMTS10* gene are associated with impairment of support, adhesion, movement, and regulation of cells.

Heterozygous mutations within the *FBN1* gene located on chromosome locus 15q21.1 have been found in a large Lebanese family where mode of inheritance is AD. The significance of this finding remains unclear in the etiology of WMS. *FBN1* codes for the protein fibrillin-1, involved in making fibers that help strengthen and allow for flexibility of the connective tissues. Mutations lead to a nonfunctional protein product, leaving the connective tissue compromised.

SYMPTOMS

Despite the genetically heterogeneous nature of WMS, there is clinical homogeneity between all forms. The major features of WMS involve ocular (eye) problems including microspherophakia (small lens) in 84 percent, ectopia (abnormal placement) of the lens in 73 percent, severe myopia (nearsightedness) in 94 percent, glaucoma in 80 percent, and cataracts in 23 percent. Usually myopia is the first finding, while glaucoma is the most serious and may lead to blindness. Other features include brachydactyly (short fingers) in 98 percent, joint stiffness in 62 percent, and short stature in 98 percent with an average adult height of 130 to 157 centimeters (cm) for females and 142 to 169 cm for males. Cardiac anomalies are seen in 24 percent of patients, including pulmonary stenosis, mitral valve insufficiency, aortic valve stenosis, ductus ateriosus, and ventricular septal defects. Intelligence is usually normal.

SCREENING AND DIAGNOSIS

The diagnosis of WMS is made clinically; however, no diagnostic criteria have been proposed. Molecular genetic testing may be available to confirm the diagnosis, clarify risks for family members, and allow for prenatal diagnosis. Currently testing is offered clinically for *ADAMTS10*. The detection rate is unknown, however, and many people with a clinical diagnosis have no mutation found. Carrier and prenatal testing require prior identification of the disease-causing mutation. Population screening for WMS is not available.

TREATMENT AND THERAPY

There is no cure for WMS. Treatment depends on manifestations as appropriate. Often the most significant complication is the optical manifestations of this condition and cardiac abnormalities when seen. For optimal care, patients should see a variety of specialists, including a clinical geneticist, genetic counselor, ophthalmologist, physical therapist, and cardiologist.

PREVENTION AND OUTCOMES

Prenatal or preimplantation genetic diagnosis is available if the cause is known. Benefits are gained from early detection and treatment of ocular manifestations. The use of ophthalmic miotics and mydriatics should be avoided, as they can induce pupillary block. Although mild intellectual deficits have been reported, most individuals have normal intelligence and live long and productive lives.

Amber M. Mathiesen, M.S.

FURTHER READING
"Weill-Marchesani Syndrome." *Gene Reviews.* NCBI, 14 Feb. 2013. Web. 2 Sept. 2014.
"Weill-Marchesani Syndrome." *Genetics Home Reference.* Nat'l. Lib. of Medecine, Oct. 2008. Web. 2 Sept. 2014.
Dagoneau, N., et al. "*ADAMTS10* Mutations in Autosomal Recessive Weill-Marchesani Syndrome." *American Journal of Human Genetics* 75.5 (2005): 801–6. Print.
Faivre, L., et al. "Clinical Homogeneity and Genetic Heterogeneity in Weill-Marchesani Syndrome." *American Journal of Medical Genetics Part C* 123 (2003): 204–7. Print.

See also: Aniridia; Best disease; Brachydactyly; Choroideremia; Color blindness; Corneal dystrophies; Glaucoma; Gyrate atrophy of the choroid and retina; Macular degeneration; Norrie syndrome; Progressive external ophthalmoplegia; Retinitis pigmentosa; Retinoblastoma; Stargardt's disease.

Werner syndrome

CATEGORY: Diseases and syndromes
ALSO KNOWN AS: Progeroid syndrome; adult progeria; adult premature aging syndrome; Werner's syndrome; WS

DEFINITION

Werner syndrome (WS), named after the German scientist who first described it, Otto Werner, is a rare, hereditary disorder characterized by premature aging. Patients typically have thin arms and legs, a thick torso, and a characteristic facial appearance described as "bird-like."

RISK FACTORS

The Werner syndrome (*WRN*) gene is transmitted as an autosomal recessive trait. The risk for Werner syndrome is related to the level of consanguinity (close relation) in a population.

In the United States, Werner syndrome occurs in approximately 1 in 200,000 births. However, it is more common in the Japanese population (approximately 1 in 20,000 to 1 in 40,000; based on the frequencies of detectable heterozygous mutations). This is likely the result of a founder mutation in the Japanese population.

ETIOLOGY AND GENETICS

The *WRN* gene is located on chromosome 8 (cytogenetic location: 8p12-p11.2) and codes for a DNA helicase belonging to the RecQ family. This DNA helicase normally plays an important role in cell division, maintenance, and repair of DNA, and the regulation of telomeres. DNA helicases are critical for preserving genome integrity. The molecular role of the *WRN* gene in Werner syndrome is not yet known. Mutations in the *WRN* gene (also called *RECQL2* or *REQ3*) lead to the production of an abnormally short, nonfunctional Werner protein. This mutated form of *WRN* cannot interact with DNA, probably because of defective transport of the WRN protein to the nucleus. It is thought that cells with the mutated form of *WRN* may divide more slowly or stop dividing earlier than normal, thus causing growth problems. Additionally, without a functional WRN protein, DNA damage may accumulate that could prevent normal cell functions and cause the health problems seen in Werner syndrome. The genome of Werner syndrome cells is highly unstable, with large, spontaneous DNA deletions. Telomere length dynamics are abnormal—that is, as cells divide, telomeres shorten more rapidly than normal. The unstable genome of Werner syndrome cells may play a key role in the pathogenesis of Werner syndrome.

So far, fifty distinct mutations have been discovered since the *WRN* gene was first cloned in 1996. All these mutations result in the elimination of the nuclear localization signal, thus impeding any functional interactions in the nucleus.

SYMPTOMS

The age of onset of Werner syndrome is variable, but patients develop normally until they reach puberty. One of the first signs of Werner syndrome is the lack of a growth spurt in the early teen years, which results in short stature. After puberty, patients begin to age rapidly, and by age forty, they appear several decades older than they are.

Gene expression pattern of the WRN gene. Genomics Institute of the Novartis Research Foundation, via Wikimedia Commons

Werner syndrome ATP-dependent helicase WRN By English: Jawahar Swaminathan and MSD staff at the European Bioinformatics Institute Deutsch: Jawahar Swaminathan und MSD Mitarbeiter am Europäischen Institut für Bioinformatik Plattdüütsch: Jawahar Swaminathan un de Lüüd von MSD an dat Europääsche Inst

The cardinal signs and symptoms (onset after age ten years) of Werner syndrome include cataracts in both eyes; characteristic skin patterns (tight skin, atrophic skin, pigmentary alterations, ulceration, hyperkeratosis, regional subcutaneous atrophy); characteristic birdlike faces (nasal bridge appears pinched and subcutaneous tissue is diminished); short stature; premature graying and/or thinning of scalp hair; and parental consanguinity (third cousin or closer) or affected sibling.

Additional signs and symptoms include type II diabetes mellitus; hypogonadism (secondary sexual underdevelopment, diminished fertility, testicular or ovarian atrophy); osteoporosis; osteosclerosis of distal phalanges of fingers and/or toes; soft-tissue calcification; premature atherosclerosis (history of myocardial infarction); neoplasms; abnormal voice (high-pitched, squeaky, or hoarse); and flat feet.

SCREENING AND DIAGNOSIS

In families in which the disease-causing mutations have been identified in an affected family member, prenatal screening (genetic testing) is available and family members may be tested. Diagnosis is based on the presence of the cardinal signs and symptoms of Werner syndrome.

TREATMENT AND THERAPY

There is no cure for Werner syndrome. Therapy is based on the treatment of symptoms: aggressive treatment of skin ulcers with standard therapies; control of type II diabetes mellitus; cholesterol-lowering drugs if the lipid profile is abnormal; surgical treatment of ocular cataracts; treatment of malignancies in a standard fashion (except that radiation therapy is not used, as it may do more harm than good to those with Werner syndrome). Current clinical trials are studying the treatment of symptoms. Preliminary laboratory findings suggest restoring normal WRN function in cells from a patient with Werner syndrome may correct the molecular defects.

PREVENTION AND OUTCOMES

Early diagnosis is useful so that screening for cancer and associated diseases such as diabetes can then be performed on a regular basis. Genetic counseling for patients and their family is advised.

Patients usually live to their late forties or early fifties, the most common cause of death being cancer or atherosclerosis.

Anita P. Kuan, Ph.D.

FURTHER READING

Ariyoshi, Kentaro, et al. "Introduction of a Normal Human Chromosome 8 Corrects Abnormal Phenotypes of Werner Syndrome Cells Immortalized by Expressing an hTERT Gene." *Journal of Radiation Research* 50.3 (2009): 253–59.

Chen, Lishan, and Junko Oshima. "Werner Syndrome." *Journal of Biomedicine and Biotechnology* 2.2 (2002): 46–54.

Coppedè, Fabio. "The Epidemiology of Premature Aging and Associated Comorbidities." *Clinical Interventions in Aging* 8 (2013): 1023–32.

Goto, Makoto, Robert W. Miller, and Nihon Gan Gakkai. *From Premature Gray Hair to Helicase-Werner Syndrome: Implications for Aging and Cancer.* Tokyo: Japan Scientific Societies, 2001.

Muftuoglu, Meltem, et al. "The Clinical Characteristics of Werner Syndrome: Molecular and Biochemical Diagnosis." *Human Genetics* 124.4 (2008): 369–77.

Parker, Philip M. *Werner Syndrome: A Bibliography and Dictionary for Physicians, Patients, and Genome Researchers.* San Diego: Icon Group International, 2007.

See also: Aging; Congenital defects; Diabetes; Hereditary diseases.

WHIM Syndrome

CATEGORY: Diseases and syndromes
ALSO KNOWN AS: Warts, Hypogammaglobulinemia, Infections, and Myelokathexis; WHIMS

DEFINITION

WHIM syndrome, Warts, Hypogamma-globulinemia, Infections, and Myelokathexix, is a genetic immunodeficiency disorder in which the development and maturation of immune cells are affected. Onset occurs during infancy or early childhood. Recurring bacterial infections and widespread warts, due to severe human papillomavirus (HPV) infection, are the main features. Mutations in the CXCR4 gene are responsible for the condition.

RISK FACTORS

Males and females are affected equally. The condition is extremely rare. Frequency is estimated at 0.2 cases per million live births.

ETIOLOGY AND GENETICS

The syndrome is caused by at least nine mutations in the CXCR4 (chemokine receptor) gene located on the long (q) arm of chromosome 2 at position 22.1. CXCR4 encodes for a receptor protein found in the outer membrane of white blood, brain, and spinal cord cells. The protein stimulates a signaling pathway inside the cell after attaching to its ligand, SDF-1, and regulates cell proliferation, differentiation, and migration, otherwise known as cell "trafficking." In WHIM syndrome the mutation is a gain-of-function mutation; the protein becomes overactive and cannot be removed from the cell after signaling, causing immunological dysfunctions and retention of neutrophils, a type of white blood cell, in the bone marrow

(myelokathexix). The molecular pathways that lead to all of WHIM syndrome symptoms, such as B cell levels and HPV susceptibility, are not well understood.

A few individuals have the disease without the CXCR4 mutation, and therefore, other genes may be responsible.

The syndrome is inherited in an autosomal dominant manner. Either the father or mother pass on the condition. Each offspring has a 50 percent chance of inheriting the condition.

SIGNS AND SYMPTOMS

Symptoms vary significantly from mild to severe and life-threatening. Features include chronic HPV and bacterial sinopulmonary infections, low immunoglobulin levels, peripheral neutropenia from bone marrow hypercellularity, and neutrophil abnormalities. Infection profile is varied but limited to some degree and may include recurring middle ear infection; skin infections such as cellulitis, folliculitis, impetigo; pneumonia; sinusitis; septic arthritis; tooth and gum infections; urinary tract infections and meningitis. Repeated infections may lead to other complications such as respiratory failure, heart failure, or hearing loss. Susceptibility to HPV infection leads to widespread warts and an increased risk for oral and genital cancers.

Migration and maturation dysfunction can lead to low levels of several types of white blood cells and antibodies. Neutropenic, B-lymphocyte, T cells, natural killer cells, and other immune cells may be affected.

SCREENING AND DIAGNOSIS

The rarity of the disorder make diagnosis a challenge. Diagnosis is made based on clinical features, patient history, and specialized genetic tests. Blood tests to assess immune cell activity and bone marrow biopsy to reveal myelokathexis are also performed. Genetic testing can confirm the diagnosis. Genetic counseling can help family members understand the syndrome and future risk.

Examination of the bone marrow can distinguish WHIM syndrome from similar conditions such as severe chronic neutropenia, Kostmann syndrome, Barth syndrome, cyclic neutropenia, X-linked congenital neutropenia, and Shwachman-Diamond syndrome.

TREATMENT AND THERAPY

Treatment may include medicines that replace antibodies (intravenous immunoglobulin) or increase the number of neutrophils, mainly granulocyte colony-stimulating factor (G-CSF). Prompt treatment of infections is essential. HPV lesions are surgically removed.

Regular vaccinations and prophylactic antibiotics can lower the risk of infections. Regular monitoring of skin and wart manifestations is also performed.

Researchers continue to study medications that inhibit the hyper function of CXCR4 and assess bone marrow transplant as a potential to cure some aspects of the disease. A new drug called plerixafor, which blocks the activity of CXCR4, may hold promise for affected individuals.

PREVENTION AND OUTCOMES

Early diagnosis, surveillance, and prompt infection treatment are essential to preventing and managing infections and complications. Recurring infections can lead to early mortality.

Deanna M. Neff, M.P.H.

FURTHER READING

Dotta L, Tassone L, Badolato R. "Clinical and genetic features of Warts, Hypogammaglobulinemia, Infections and Myelokathexis (WHIM) syndrome." *Curr Mol Med.* 2011;11(4):317–25.

National Organization for Rare Disorders. "WHIM Syndrome." Available from https://rarediseases.org/rare-diseases/whim-syndrome/. Accessed July 28, 2017.

Online Inheritance of Man. "WHIM Syndrome; WHIMS." 2016. Available from https://www.omim.org/entry/193670?search=whim%20syndrome&highlight=syndromic%20whim%20syndrome.

Ustwani O, Kurzrock R, and Wetzler M. "Genetics on a WHIM." *British Journal of Haematology.* 2014;164: 15–23.

WEB SITES OF INTEREST

Canadian Immunodeficiencies Patient Organization (CIPO)
http://cipo.ca
Genetic and Rare Diseases Information Center
https://rarediseases.info.nih.gov/diseases
Immune Deficiency Foundation
http://www.primaryimmune.org/
Jeffrey Modell Foundation/National Primary Immunodeficiency Resource Center

http://www.info4pi.org/
National Primary Immunodeficiency Resource Center
http://www.info4pi.org
United States Immunodeficiency Network (USIDNET)
http://www.usidnet.org

Williams syndrome

CATEGORY: Diseases and syndromes
ALSO KNOWN AS: Williams-Beuren syndrome; WBS; WS; Elfin Facies syndrome

DEFINITION

Williams syndrome (WS) is a rare developmental disorder that affects many parts of the body. The condition is characterized by a distinctive cheerful facial appearance, unique behavioral and cognitive traits, mild to moderate intellectual disabilities, and cardiovascular problems. Williams syndrome is due to a deletion of several genes on chromosome 7.

RISK FACTORS

There are no known risk factors. According to the Williams Syndrome Association in 2016, the incidence of Williams syndrome is estimated to be approximately 1 in 10,000 people. The disease almost always occurs sporadically. In the few reported examples of familial transmission, the deletion acts as an autosomal dominant mutation. Williams syndrome affects males and females equally.

ETIOLOGY AND GENETICS

Williams syndrome is caused by a loss of DNA from band 7q11.23 of chromosome 7. Therefore while the normal number of chromosomes is maintained, approximately twenty-five genes are lost because of the deletion. This region is referred to as the Williams-Bueren syndrome critical region (WBSCR). The deletion of the WBSCR in chromosome 7 is believed to be the result of unequal crossover events during meiosis. This region is flanked by low copy repeats that increase the likelihood of nonallelic homologous recombination. The deletion arises with equal frequency on the maternally or the paternally inherited chromosome 7. The size of the deletion can vary from 1.5 to 1.8 Mb pairs of DNA. Amongst the deleted genes is the elastin

Williams Syndrome is an unusual genetic condition characterized by inadequate mental development, an atypical appearance of the face, problems of the circulatory system including the heart and blood vessels, and discrepancies in the level of blood calcium. By Poornima P, Patil P, Subbareddy. .

(*ELN*) gene. Loss of this gene is associated with the connective tissue abnormalities, cardiovascular disease (specifically supravalvular aortic stenosis), and facial dysmorphology found in people with this disease. Additionally, scientists believe that the deletion of the *NCF1* gene on chromosome 7 reduces the risk of a person with Williams syndrome developing hypertension.

Other genes contained in this region include *LIMK1* (lim kinase 1), *GTF2IRD1* (part of the TFII-1 transcription family), and *GTF2I* (general transcription factor II, I). Their deletion may be responsible for the characteristic difficulties with visual-spatial tasks. Evidence also exists that the loss of the *CLIP2* gene, among others, may contribute to the learning disabilities and other cognitive difficulties seen in Williams syndrome.

Most cases of Williams syndrome occur as random events during the formation of reproductive cells in a parent of an affected individual. These cases occur in people with no history of the disorder in their family. Williams syndrome is an autosomal dominant mutation. Williams syndrome should be distinguished from other syndromes that include developmental delay, short stature, distinctive facies, and congenital heart disease, such as Noonan syndrome (deletion in chromosome 22q11) and Smith-Magenis syndrome (deletion in chromosome 17p11.2).

Symptoms

The onset of symptoms usually occurs just after birth or during infancy and begins with physical characteristics, irritability, colic, and feeding problems. Almost all cases of Williams syndrome have typical facial features that can be recognized even at birth. Williams patients usually have problems with spatial-visual tasks but have strong abilities in the area of music and spoken language. They often have outgoing and engaging personalities. Children often have delays in walking and speaking; however, the latter improves with age. Motor difficulties persist at all ages. Symptoms progress to abdominal pain in adolescents, diabetes, high blood pressure, heart failure (specifically supravalvular aortic stenosis, SVAS, and supravalvular pulmonary stenosis, SVPS), and hearing loss in adults.

Elastin arteriopathy is present in about 75 percent of Williams individuals, with the most common being SVAS. In most cases, morbidity is due to this aortic narrowing, which can lead to elevated left heart pressure, cardiac hypertrophy, and eventually cardiac failure.

Screening and Diagnosis

The clinical manifestations include a distinct facial appearance, which can be observed early after birth. Other characteristics such as cardiovascular anomalies and hypocalcemia, can be detected via electroencephalogram and routine blood examinations. The deletion in chromosome 7 is not detected through standard karyotyping but rather through fluorescence in situ hybridization (FISH). Testing is routinely performed on peripheral blood leukocytes. FISH testing and karyotype are performed in cytogenetics laboratories.

Prenatal testing is clinically available but is rarely used because most cases occur in a single family member only and no prenatal indicators exist for low-risk pregnancies.

Treatment and Therapy

There is currently no cure for Williams syndrome. Williams syndrome is a complex multisystem medical condition that requires the attention of multiple health care professionals. Initial care often centers on failure to thrive, hypocalcemia, or repair of the cardiac lesion. Physical therapy is helpful to patients with joint stiffness. Developmental and speech

Human Chromosom 7 public domain via wikimedia commons

therapy can also help affected children; for example, verbal strengths can help make up for other weaknesses. Other treatments are based on a patient's symptoms.

PREVENTION AND OUTCOMES

There is no known way to prevent the genetic problem that causes Williams syndrome. Prenatal testing is available for couples with a family history of Williams syndrome who wish to conceive. According to the National Institutes of Health's National Library of Medicine in 2016, about 75 percent of those with Williams syndrome have some intellectual disability. Most patients will not live as long as normal, due to complications. Most patients require full-time caregivers and often live in supervised group homes.

Maria Mavris, Ph.D.

FURTHER READING

"What Is Williams Syndrome?" *Williams Syndrome Association*. Williams Syndrome Assn., n.d. Web. 27 Jan. 2016.

"Williams Syndrome." *Genetics Home Reference*. Natl. Library of Medicine, Natl. Inst. of Health, 18 Jan. 2016. Web. 22 Jan. 2016.

"Williams Syndrome." *MedlinePlus*. Natl. Library of Medicine, Natl. Inst. of Health, 13 Jan. 2016. Web. 22 Jan. 2016.

Bayes, M., et al. "Mutational Mechanisms of Williams-Beuren Syndrome Deletions." *American Journal of Human Genetics* 73 (2003): 131–51. Print.

Cassidy, Suzanne B., and Judith E. Allanson. *Management of Genetic Syndromes*. 3rd ed. Hoboken: Wiley, 2010. Print.

Farran, Emily K., and Annette Karmiloff-Smith. *Neurodevelopmental Disorders Across the Lifespan: A Neuroconstructivist Approach*. Oxford: Oxford UP, 2012. Print.

Martens, Marilee. "Developmental and Cognitive Troubles in Williams Syndrome." *Pediatric Neurology*. Ed. Olivier Dulac, Maryse Lassonde, and Harvey B. Sarnat. Edinburgh: Elsevier, 2013. 291–93. Print.

Morris, C. A., et al. "Natural History of Williams Syndrome: Physical Characteristics." *Journal of Pediatrics* 113 (1988): 318–26. Print.

Morris, C., H. Lenhoff, and P. Wang. *Williams-Beuren Syndrome: Research, Evaluation, and Treatment*. Baltimore: Johns Hopkins UP, 2006. Print.

See also: Apert syndrome; Brachydactyly; Carpenter syndrome; Cleft lip and palate; Congenital defects; Cornelia de Lange syndrome; Cri du chat syndrome; Crouzon syndrome; Down syndrome; Edwards syndrome; Ellis-van Creveld syndrome; Holt-Oram syndrome; Ivemark syndrome; Meacham syndrome; Opitz-Frias syndrome; Patau syndrome; Polydactyly; Robert syndrome; Rubinstein-Taybi syndrome; Werner syndrome.

Wilms' tumor

CATEGORY: Diseases and syndromes

ALSO KNOWN AS: Nephroblastoma; kidney tumor

DEFINITION

Wilms tumor is a type of kidney cancer that predominantly affects children. It is the most common renal tumor of childhood. It usually occurs in the first five years of life, especially around ages three and four. In most cases, Wilms tumor affects only one of the two kidneys. The frequency of this tumor is 1 in 200,000-250,000 children.

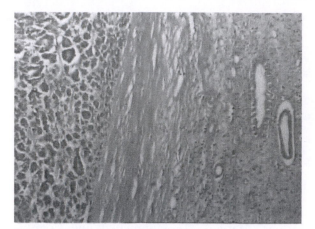

Triphasic pattern showing tubules, solid sheets of cells, and stromal differentiation in a pathological specimen of adult Wilms' tumour. By V Geethamani, V Kusuma, KM Srinivasa Gowda and Monika Lamba Saini., via Wikimedia Commons

Wilms tumor is generally divided into two types based on how it looks under the microscope. Favorable types of Wilms tumor generally have a better outcome and require less aggressive treatment. The unfavorable or anaplastic histology of Wilms tumor is still curable but requires more aggressive chemotherapy and higher doses of radiation therapy. Despite the more aggressive therapies, survival is generally more limited. However, the overall five-year survival rate for Wilms tumor is greater than 90 percent, varying according to the stage of disease at diagnosis, tumor size, histopathologic features (with worse outcomes for diffuse anaplasia), and age.

RISK FACTORS

One likely risk factor for Wilms tumor is having a family member with a Wilms tumor; approximately 1 to 2 percent of patients have one or more relative with a history of Wilms tumor. Certain birth defects also increase the risk of a Wilms tumor. These include WAGR, a syndrome that includes Wilms tumor; aniridia—a completely or partially missing iris (colored part) of the eyes; genitourinary abnormalities, such as defects of the kidneys, urinary tract, penis, scrotum, testicles, clitoris, or ovaries; and mental retardation.

Additional risk factors include Beckwith-Wiedemann syndrome, in which patients have a larger than normal tongue, larger than normal internal organs, and one arm or leg that may be larger than the other; Denys-Drash syndrome, which is the absence of the penis, scrotum, and testicles; Perlman

syndrome, which is characterized by fetal gigantism, renal dysplasia, and multiple congenital abnormalities; and hemihypertrophy, in which one side of the body is larger than the other. Other genetic defects, including defects on chromosome 11, also increase risk. A persistence of nephrogenic rests (embryonic tissue that is retained in the kidney) beyond early childhood is also a risk factor for Wilms tumor. Patients with these abnormalities should be regularly screened for Wilms tumor during childhood.

ETIOLOGY AND GENETICS

The great majority of cases of Wilms tumor are sporadic (nonfamilial), and they are believed to arise as the result of genetic mutations in the kidney tissue either before or shortly after birth. Less than 5 percent of all cases are inherited, and even among these it appears that mutations in any of several different genes may be responsible. About one-third of patients with familial Wilms tumor have mutations in the WT1 gene, located on the short arm of chromosome 11 at position 11p13. The protein encoded by this gene is a regulatory molecule that acts to turn other genes on at appropriate times during the development of kidney and reproductive tissue. Failure to do so as a result of mutations in the WT1 gene may result in the uncontrolled growth of kidney tumors characteristic of the disease.

Other genes known to be associated with genetic predisposition to Wilms tumor include WT2 (at position 11p15.5) and WTX (on the X chromosome). Other genes and chromosomes that may be involved in Wilms tumor include chromosomes 16q and 1p, gene CACNA1E (at position 1q25.3), genes MEOX2

Wilms tumor By The Armed Forces Institute of Pathology, via Wikimedia Commons

and *SOSTDC1* (at position 7p21), *SKCG-1* (at position 11q23.2), *TP53* gene, *FBXW7* gene, and *MYCN* gene. A small percentage of patients with Wilms tumor have identifiable genetic syndromes in which this malignancy is one manifestation of a larger panoply of clinical presentations. These include Denys-Drash syndrome, Beckwith-Wiedemann syndrome, Perlman syndrome, and WAGR syndrome.

The inheritance of familial Wilms tumor follows a classic autosomal dominant pattern, meaning that a single copy of the mutation is sufficient to cause full expression of the disease. An affected individual has a 50 percent chance of transmitting the mutation to each of his or her children. In some cases, however, the disease results from a spontaneous new mutation, so in these instances affected individuals will have unaffected parents. Curiously, it has been shown that at the molecular level within cells, both copies of the *WT1* gene must be mutated in order to initiate the formation of kidney tumors. One of these mutations is the inherited one that is present in all cells, while the second occurs randomly during normal cell growth in kidney tissue. It is this acquired second mutation that triggers tumor formation in the affected tissue.

Symptoms

The first noticeable symptom is usually a large lump or hard mass in the abdomen. Other symptoms may include stomach pain, fever, blood in the urine (hematuria), high blood pressure, loss of appetite, weight loss, nausea, vomiting, and constipation. Erythrocytosis (a condition where there are too many red cells in the blood) may also be a presenting sign that the doctor finds when taking a blood test. This is because Wilms tumor makes a protein that causes increased production of red cells. Wilms tumors may grow larger without causing any pain or other symptoms.

Screening and Diagnosis

The doctor will ask about a child's symptoms and medical history and will perform a physical exam. Blood and urine tests may be done. The child will need one or more tests in order to look for tumors. These tests provide pictures of the kidney, surrounding blood vessels, and other organs to which the cancer may have spread.

These tests include ultrasound, a test that uses sound waves to examine the kidneys. A computed tomography (CT) scan, a type of x-ray that uses a computer to make pictures of the inside of the body, may also be done. In some CT scans, a dye is first injected into a vein. This dye makes structures in the body more visible on an x-ray. Additional tests include a functional magnetic resonance imaging (fMRI) scan, a test that uses magnetic waves to make pictures of the inside of the body; a chest x-ray, a test that uses radiation to look for the spread of cancer to the lungs; a bone scan, in which a small amount of a radioactive material is injected into a vein to highlight any cancer that may have spread to the bones; and a biopsy, the removal of a sample of tissue to test for cancer cells. In Wilms tumor, the biopsy may actually be a major surgical procedure to remove the kidney.

Except for removal of the kidney, these tests are not invasive but require the child to remain still. Sedation may be needed.

Children who have risk factors for Wilms tumor should have a physical exam with a specialist and an ultrasound every three months until age six or seven. This screening should be done even if they do not have symptoms. It can help find tumors while they are small and have not yet spread to other parts of the body.

Treatment and Therapy

Wilms tumor can be cured in most children. The specific treatment depends on if the cancer has spread beyond the kidney to other parts of the body and, if so, how far. The process for determining this, called staging, uses the results of the diagnostic tests. Tumor size, cell type, whether the tumor is favorable or unfavorable, and the child's age and health are also considered in choosing treatment. The National Wilms Tumor Study Group and the Children's Oncology Group recommend nephrectomy (removal of part or all of a kidney), followed by chemotherapy with or without radiation therapy.

Chemotherapy is the use of drugs to kill cancer cells. Chemotherapy can be given in many forms, including pill, injection, and via a catheter placed in a blood vessel. The drugs enter the bloodstream and travel through the body killing mostly cancer cells, but also some healthy cells.

Radiation therapy is the use of radiation to kill cancer cells and shrink tumors. Radiation may be external radiation therapy, in which radiation is directed at the tumor from a source outside the body.

PREVENTION AND OUTCOMES

Currently, there is no known way to prevent the majority of cases of Wilms tumor. Genetic counseling is recommended for pregnancies at risk for inheriting the *WT1* gene or 11p15 genomic alteration, including prenatal testing of the fetus or preimplantation genetic testing for embryos created by in vitro fertilization.

Laurie Rosenblum, M.P.H.;
reviewed by Mohei Abouzied, M.D.
"Etiology and Genetics" by Jeffrey A. Knight, Ph.D.

FURTHER READING

Driskoll, K. M. Isakoff, and F. Ferrer. "Update on Pediatric Genitourinary Oncology." *Current Opinion in Urology* 17.4 (2007): 281–86. Print.

Kalapurakol, John A., and Patrick R. M. Thomas. "Wilms' Tumor." *Perez and Brady's Principles and Practice of Radiation Oncology.* Ed. Edward C. Halperin, Carlos A. Perez, and Luther W. Brady. Philadelphia: Wolters, 2008. Print.

Pritchard, Jones, Kathy, et al. "Omission of Doxorubicin from the Treatment of Stage II–III, Intermediate-Risk Wilms' Tumour (SIOP WT 2001): An Open-Label, Non-Inferiority, Randomised Controlled Trial." *Lancet* 386.999 (2015): 1156–64. PDF file.

See also: Alport syndrome; Bartter syndrome; Cancer; Chemical mutagens; Chromosome mutation; Hereditary leiomyomatosis and renal cell cancer; Hereditary non-VHL clear cell renal cell carcinomas; Hereditary papillary renal cancer; Mutagenesis and cancer; Mutation and mutagenesis; Oncogenes; Polycystic kidney disease; Tumor-suppressor genes.

Wilms' tumor aniridia-genitourinary anomalies-mental retardation (WAGR) syndrome and genetics

CATEGORY: Diseases and syndromes

ALSO KNOWN AS: 11p deletion syndrome; chromosome 11p deletion syndrome; WAGR complex; Wilms' tumor-aniridia-gonadoblastoma-mental retardation syndrome

DEFINITION

WAGR syndrome is a rare genetic condition. Children born with this syndrome often have an unusual group of developmental abnormalities. Generally, they have problems with their eyes, are at risk for developing certain types of cancer, and may be at risk for intellectual disability.

RISK FACTORS

WAGR syndrome usually occurs spontaneously during fetal development. Several genes on chromosome 11 have been linked to this condition. Therefore, individuals who have a deleted portion of chromosome 11 are at risk of developing WAGR syndrome. Wilms' tumor occurs in approximately 8 per 1 million white children in the United States, and the incidence is somewhat higher in black children.

ETIOLOGY AND GENETICS

Several different disorders are associated with WAGR syndrome, each of which make up the acronym WAGR. *Wilms'* tumor is the most common type of pediatric kidney cancer, and children with WAGR syndrome have a 50 percent chance of developing it. *Aniridia* is characterized by a missing iris, the colored part of the eye. *Genitourinary* anomalies include undescended testes, abnormal locations of the opening for urination, and urinary problems in girls. Mental Retardation or intellectual disability may also occur and can vary in severity between individuals. The majority of children with WAGR syndrome experience at least two of these conditions, but they do not always have all the described conditions.

WAGR syndrome occurs when part of chromosome 11 is missing, and therefore it sometimes is referred to as a contiguous gene deletion syndrome. This designation means that WAGR syndrome develops when an individual does not have certain genes located on a specific part of chromosome 11 (11p13). In the majority of cases, this mutation is de novo, meaning that it occurs spontaneously during the early stages of fetal development. In other cases, this dysfunctional chromosome is passed from parent to offspring. This occurs when the chromosomes within a parent undergo a translocation event. Translocation of two chromosomes (one being chromosome 11) can lead to a loss of some of the genes on the chromosome. When such a translocation event occurs and is passed on to a new generation, the offspring may contain normal cells and ones that have the 11p13 deletion, a condition referred to as mosaic WAGR syndrome.

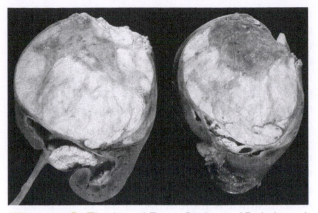

Wilms tumor. By The Armed Forces Institute of Pathology, via Wikimedia Commons

It is not surprising that the severity of WAGR syndrome will depend on how large the chromosomal deletion is (how many and which genes are missing). Individuals with smaller deletions usually have aniridia and Wilms' tumor. Larger deletions are responsible for genitourinary defects and intellectual disability. The deleted region of chromosome 11 contains an ocular development gene called *PAX6*. When absent, this gene causes aniridia. Some studies suggest that the *PAX6* gene may also be responsible for pancreatic and brain deficiencies. The Wilms' tumor-suppressor gene, *WT1*, also is deleted in individuals with WAGR syndrome. Although it is best known for causing Wilms' tumor when it is missing, the *WT1* gene also may be associated with some of the genitourinary manifestations of WAGR syndrome.

SYMPTOMS

Symptoms of WAGR syndrome manifest soon after birth. Aniridia is commonly apparent first in both males and females. In boys, undescended testes also are noticeable soon after the baby is born. The specific symptoms experienced by each person who has WAGR syndrome depend on the combination of

Aniridia By Gardar Rurak at en.wikipedia, from Wikimedia Commons

disorders that are present, since each individual may have varying physical and mental disorders.

SCREENING AND DIAGNOSIS

Aniridia is a rare symptom that manifests almost immediately and may indicate that a patient has WAGR syndrome. To diagnose WAGR syndrome definitively, genetic tests such as karyotyping are performed to analyze the chromosomes and determine whether the chromosome 11p13 deletion is present. Another test that may be employed during the genetic testing is a fluorescence in situ hybridization (FISH) test, which also will evaluate whether the deletion is present.

TREATMENT AND THERAPY

Treatment of children with WAGR syndrome depends on the appearance of Wilms' tumor. The features and the stage of the tumor determine the appropriate management for each individual. Close to 50 percent of Wilms' tumors are diagnosed before reaching stage II, meaning that they are confined to the kidney and can be surgically excised. Approximately 90 percent of children with Wilms' tumor are cured. Depending on how far the cancer has spread, chemotherapy and radiation may also be used.

PREVENTION AND OUTCOMES

WAGR syndrome patients can survive long-term, and early detection of the disorder improves their prognosis. However, lifelong disabilities such as vision loss and intellectual disability may afflict these patients.

Kelly L. McCoy

FURTHER READING

Fischbach, Bernard V., et al. "WAGR Syndrome: A Clinical Review of 54 Cases." *Pediatrics* 116 (2005): 984–88. Print.

Kliegman, Robert M. *Nelson Textbook of Pediatrics.* 19th ed. Philadelphia: Saunders, 2011. Print.

Kumar, Vinay, Abul K. Abbas, and Jon C. Aster. *Robbins and Cotran Pathologic Basis of Disease.* 9th ed. Philadelphia: Saunders Elsevier, 2015. Print.

Rosenblum, Laurie. "Wilms' Tumor." *Health Library.* EBSCO Information Services, 28 May 2014. Web. 2 Sept. 2014.

See also: Alagille syndrome; Attention deficit hyperactivity disorder (ADHD); Autism; Cockayne syndrome; Congenital defects; Dwarfism; Dyslexia; Fragile X syndrome; Hermaphrodism; Smith-Lemli- Opitz syndrome; Werner syndrome; Williams syndrome.

Wilson disease and genetics

CATEGORY: Diseases and syndromes
ALSO KNOWN AS: Wilson's disease

DEFINITION

Wilson disease is a rare, inherited, genetic disorder of copper metabolism.

Copper is a trace mineral that the human body needs in small amounts. Most people get a lot more copper from food than they need. However, most people are also able to excrete the excess copper. People with Wilson disease cannot excrete the excess cop per because of a deficiency in ceruloplasmin, a copper-carrying protein.

As a result, copper begins to build up in the liver right after birth and eventually damages the organ. When the liver can no longer hold the excess cop per, the mineral goes into the bloodstream. It travels to other organs and may damage the brain, central nervous system, kidneys, and eyes. This disease is fatal unless it is treated before serious illness develops.

RISK FACTORS

The only known risk factor for Wilson disease is a family history of the disease. It tends to be most common in eastern Europeans, Sicilians, and southern Italians. It occurs in one out of every thirty thousand people.

ETIOLOGY AND GENETICS

Wilson disease results from mutations in a gene called ATP7B, which is located on the long arm of chromosome 13 at position 13q14.2-q21. This gene belongs to a family of genes called the ATPase super family, and it specifies a protein known as copper transporting ATPase 2. Found mainly in the liver, this protein normally acts to transport copper from the liver to other parts of the body where it is needed in minute quantities as a cofactor for some enzymatic reactions. Additionally, if copper levels in the liver get too high,

this protein can facilitate the transport of excess copper to bile sacs in the liver where it can be eliminated. If concentrations of this protein are drastically reduced or eliminated altogether because of mutations in the ATP7B gene, removal of the excess copper is compromised. Copper may then accumulate in tissues to toxic levels, causing the clinical symptoms characteristic of Wilson disease.

Mutations in a second gene, PRNP (found on chromosome 20 at 20pter-p12), have been found that delay the age of onset of Wilson disease and ameliorate the symptoms somewhat. This gene en codes the prion protein, which is most active in the brain. In addition to its other functions, prion protein may also be involved in the intercellular transport of copper. For those with mutations in ATP78, it appears that having the amino acid methionine instead of valine at position 129 on PRNP is associated with delayed onset of Wilson disease, but further research is necessary.

Dr Samuel Alexander Kinnier Wilson (1878–1937), U.S.-born British neurologist best known for his description of Wilson's disease. Undated portrait by Carl Vandyk of Vandyk studios, London. By Carl Vandyk (1851–1931), via Wikimedia Commons

Wilson disease is inherited in a classic autosomal recessive manner, which means that both copies of the ATP7B gene must be deficient in order for the individual to be afflicted. Typically, an affected child is born to two unaffected parents, both of whom are carriers of the recessive mutant allele. The probable outcomes for children whose parents are both carriers are 75 percent unaffected and 25 percent affected.

SYMPTOMS

Symptoms most commonly appear in people less than forty years of age. In children, the symptoms usually begin to be expressed around four years of age. Chronic liver disease is often a sign in adolescence or early twenties.

Symptoms of excess copper in the liver include jaundice, a swelled abdomen or legs, pain in the abdomen, nausea, weight loss, and vomiting blood. Symptoms of excess copper in the brain include depression, anxiety, mood swings, aggressive or other inappropriate behaviors, difficulty speaking and swallowing, tremors, rigid muscles, and problems with balance and walking. Symptoms of excess copper in the eyes include Kayser-Fleischer rings (rusty or brown-colored ring around the iris).

Some patients develop additional psychiatric symptoms, such as abrupt personality changes, suicidal thoughts, and psychosis. Other signs include menstruation irregularities, infertility, anemia, easy bruising or bleeding, kidney stones, arthritis, and osteoporosis.

With rare exceptions, they are diagnostic of inherited hepatolenticular degeneration—Wilson's disease. By Herbert L. Fred, MD, Hendrik A. van Dijk (http://cnx.org/content/m15007/latest/), via Wikimedia Commons

SCREENING AND DIAGNOSIS

Wilson disease is easy to diagnose when it is suspected. However, because it is relatively rare, common signs, such as psychiatric symptoms or hepatitis, may initially be attributed to other causes. A patient may appear healthy even while his or her liver is getting damaged. Sometimes the liver symptoms are mistaken for infectious hepatitis or mononucleosis. Doctors may not recognize psychiatric symptoms caused by Wilson disease. However, it is very important to get diagnosed and treated early to avoid organ damage and early death.

The doctor will ask about a patient's symptoms and medical history and will perform physical and mental exams. Tests may include blood and urine tests to measure levels of copper and ceruloplasmin (a copper carrying protein); an eye exam to look for brown, ring-shaped color in the cornea (Kayser-Fleischer rings); and a liver biopsy, in which a small sample of liver tissue is removed and tested for excess copper.

When there is a known family history of Wilson disease, early testing may prevent symptoms and organ damage. Genetic testing may be possible if a family member with the diagnosis of Wilson disease has identifiable changes in the gene. Because there are so many gene mutations that result in Wilson disease, there is no single, simple test for everyone.

Nonetheless, recent advances in the understanding of the ATP7B gene have increasingly allowed a diagnosis to be made by direct genetic analysis. This technique is particularly useful when other tests are negative or equivocal. Experts now think that when a condition known as "fatty liver" occurs in people who do not consume large amounts of alcohol (excessive alcohol intake is the most common cause of fatty liver), specific testing for Wilson disease is recommended.

Since diagnosis of this disease can be very difficult, experts have devised a scoring system that combines many of the available tests into a single score that is positive in over 90 percent of people who truly have the disease and negative in nearly 97 percent of people whose symptoms are caused by some other condition. Genetic counseling may be helpful to review risks and discuss appropriate testing and management.

TREATMENT AND THERAPY

The goals of treatment are to remove the excess copper, prevent copper from building up again, and improve all associated symptoms of copper over load. Treatment cannot cure the underlying problem of copper accumulation; therefore, patients must continue treatment throughout their lives.

Medications used to treat Wilson disease include zinc acetate, which blocks the absorption of copper in the intestinal tract; penicillamine (chelates, or binds, with copper, causing its increased urinary excretion); tetrathiomolybdolate (may be better than a similar drug called trientine due to its lower toxic profile); and dimercaprol. Penicillamine is probably the best-studied treatment and is commonly used, especially in severely symptomatic persons, however trientine and ammonium tetrathiomolybdate are considered to be safer alternatives to D-penicillamine. Zinc has gained increasing importance in recent years because it is often effective in long-term maintenance and has fewer side effects than penicillamine. The role of tetrathiomolybdo late has not yet been clearly established and it still considered experimental.

If a patient has severe liver damage, he or she may need a liver transplant. Liver transplantational lows the body to correct its copper metabolism and can at least prevent the disease from worsening. Transplantation also affords an effective treatment for patients who cannot tolerate the sometimes serious side effects of penicillamine.

PREVENTION AND OUTCOMES

Currently, there are no guidelines to prevent Wilson disease. However, when identified early, treatment can prevent the development of symptoms and patients can live a normal lifespan. Untreated, it can lead to severe brain damage, liver failure, and death.

Laurie Rosenblum, M.P.H.; reviewed by Rosalyn Carson-DeWitt, M.D. "Etiology and Genetics" by Jeffrey A. Knight, Ph.D.; updated by Deanna M. Neff, M.P.H.

FURTHER READING

Brewer, G. J., et al. "Treatment of Wilson Disease with Ammonium Tetrathiomolybdate, IV: Comparison of Tetrathiomolybdate and Trientine in a Double-Blind Study of Treatment of the Neurologic Presentation of Wilson Disease." *Archives of Neurology 63*, no. 4 (April, 2006): 521–527.

EBSCO Publishing. "Health Library: Wilson Disease." Ipswich, Mass.: Author, 2009. Available through http://www.ebscohost.com.

Ferenci, P. "Wilson's Disease." "Clinical Gastroenterology and Hepatology" 3, no. 8 (August, 2005): 726–733.

Li WJ, Chen C, You ZF, Yang RM, Wang XP. "Current Drug Managements of Wilson's Disease: From West to East. Curr Neuropharmacol." 2016;14(4):322–5.

Parker, James N. "The Official Patient's Sourcebook on Wilson's Disease." San Diego: Icon Health, 2002. Wakim-Fleming, Jamile, and Kevin D. Mullen. "Wilson's Disease." In "Practical Management of Liver Diseases", edited by Zobair M. Younossi. New York: Cambridge University Press, 2008.

Rodriguez-Castro KI, Hevia-Urrutia FJ, Sturniolo GC. "Wilson's disease: A review of what we have learned. World J Hepatol". 2015; 7 (29):2859–70.

WEB SITES OF INTEREST

American Association for the Study of Liver Diseases
http://www.aasld.org/Pages/Default.aspx

American Liver Foundation
http://www.liverfoundation.org/

Canadian Liver Foundation
http://www.liver.ca/Home.aspx

Genetics Home Reference
http://ghr.nlm.nih.gov

Health Canada
http://www.hc-sc.gc.ca/index-eng.php

Mayo Clinic.com: Wilson's Disease
http://www.mayoclinic.com/health/wilsons-disease/DS00411

Wilson's Disease Association
http://www.wilsonsdisease.org

See also: Alkaptonuria; Andersen's disease; Diabetes; Diabetes insipidus; Fabry disease; Forbes disease; Galactokinase deficiency; Galactosemia; Gaucher disease; Glucose galactose malabsorption; Glucose-6-phosphate dehydrogenase deficiency; Glycogen storage diseases; Gm1-gangliosidosis; Hemochromatosis; Hereditary diseases; Hereditary xanthinuria; Hers disease; Homocystinuria; Hunter disease; Hurler syndrome; Inborn errors of metabolism; Jansky-Bielschowsky disease; Kearns-Sayre syndrome; Krabbé disease; Lactose intolerance; Leigh syndrome; Lesch-Nyhan syndrome; McArdle's disease; Maple syrup urine disease; Menkes syndrome; Metachromatic leukodystrophy; Niemann-Pick disease; Ornithine transcarbamylase deficiency; Orotic aciduria; Phenylketonuria (PKU); Pompe disease; Sulfite oxidase deficiency; Tarui's disease; Tay-Sachs disease; Tyrosinemia, type I; Von Gierke disease.

Wiskott-Aldrich syndrome and genetics

CATEGORY: Diseases and syndromes
ALSO KNOWN AS: Eczema-thrombocytopenia-immunodeficiency syndrome; Aldrich syndrome

DEFINITION

Wiskott-Aldrich syndrome is an inherited disorder in which cells of the blood function improperly. The disease is caused by mutation of the gene encoding for Wiskott-Aldrich syndrome protein (WASP), which controls the shape, attachment, division, and movement of blood cells. Patients with Wiskott-Aldrich syndrome have problems with blood clotting and increased rates of infection, autoimmune disease, and cancers of the immune system.

RISK FACTORS

Wiskott-Aldrich syndrome is caused by a rare, recessive, sex-linked allele. The disease is seen almost exclusively in males. Cases in females are exceedingly rare. The global incidence of Wiskott-Aldrich syndrome is estimated at 1 to 10 in 1,000,000 males. There are no environmental risk factors.

ETIOLOGY AND GENETICS

The *WAS* gene encoding for WASP is found on the X chromosome (Xp11.22-23). Wiskott-Aldrich syndrome is caused by a rare recessive allele that causes disease predominantly in males because they have only one copy of the X chromosome. Although most cases of Wiskott-Aldrich syndrome are inherited from the mother, as many as one-third arise from spontaneous mutation. WASP is expressed predominantly in blood cells where its cellular function is to transmit signals to the cytoskeleton, thereby controlling the shape, attachment, division, and movement of these cells. Expression of nonfunctional WASP results in defects in platelets and cells of the immune system.

Many mutations in WASP have been found to cause Wiskott-Aldrich syndrome, and the severity of disease corresponds to the specific mutation that is present. Some patients with mild mutations may exhibit only low platelet counts, small platelet size, and bleeding, while others with more severe phenotypes may exhibit eczema, infections, autoimmune disease, and/or cancers of the immune system.

A specific activating mutation in the *WAS* gene is associated with a distinct disease, X-linked neutropenia.

SYMPTOMS

All patients with Wiskott-Aldrich syndrome exhibit platelets that are reduced in number and in size. Platelets play important roles in blood clotting, and bruising and bleeding may be present from birth. The spleen, which is responsible for removing damaged platelets, is sometimes enlarged. Eczema is also common in Wiskott-Aldrich patients. Many patients are immunodeficient, and at increased risk for bacterial, viral, and fungal infections due to defects in the activity of T cells and B cells. Patients may also exhibit autoimmune disease that can affect a variety of tissues. Patients are also at a higher risk for leukemia and lymphoma.

SCREENING AND DIAGNOSIS

Because patients with Wiskott-Aldrich syndrome invariably have platelets that are small and reduced in number, careful analysis of platelet number and size can be useful in determining diagnosis. Antibody levels are also abnormal in patients due to improper immune cell function and can be analyzed to aid diagnosis. Levels of IgG are low and levels of IgA and sometimes IgE are elevated. Genetic testing that confirms the presence of a mutation in the *WAS* gene provides the most definitive diagnosis.

TREATMENT AND THERAPY

Treatments vary depending on the severity of the disease. Patients with severe bleeding may require transfusions of red blood cells or platelets. Splenectomy results in increased platelet numbers and reduced bleeding but may make patients more susceptible to infection. Young boys may wear helmets to protect from head injuries that might result in bleeding in the brain. Susceptibility to various infectious agents may be a major problem in Wiskott-Aldrich syndrome patients, and proper antimicrobial therapy is essential. Patients may also benefit from immunoglobulin replacement therapy, in which antibodies from many donors are administered intravenously to provide some protection against infection, raise platelet levels, and reduce auto-immune disease. Patients should not receive live virus vaccines because they may cause infection.

Bone marrow transplantation or cord blood stem cell transplantation is the only cure for Wiskott-Aldrich syndrome. Because this technology has the potential to eliminate disease, a search for a matched donor usually occurs immediately following confirmation of diagnosis. In transplantation, the blood-producing cells of the patient are destroyed and replaced with those from a non-diseased individual. The new cells make normal platelets and immune cells, thereby eliminating symptoms. Although success rates of transplantation are high and improving, not all patients are good candidates for transplantation and significant risks are associated with transplantation.

PREVENTION AND OUTCOMES

There is no means to prevent Wiskott-Aldrich syndrome. One-half of the brothers of patients with Wiskott-Aldrich syndrome also have the disease, and one-half of sisters are unaffected carriers of the disease-causing allele. Genetic counseling should be made available for parents of an affected child. Genetic testing can detect the presence of the disease in the fetus and determine if unaffected females are carriers. Outcome depends on the severity of disease and the response to treatment. Before modern treatment, the life expectancy of Wiskott-Aldrich patients was between two and three years. Today, nearly 90 percent of patients that receive tissue-matched bone marrow from unaffected siblings can be cured. The overall cure rate is lower because patients with infection or cancer may not be good candidates for transplantation.

Kyle J. McQuade, Ph.D.

FURTHER READING

Lewis, Ricki. *Human Genetics.* 11th ed. New York: McGraw, 2015. Print.

Rezaie, Nima, Asghar Aghamohammadi, and Luigi D. Notarangelo. *Primary Immunodeficiency Diseases.* Berlin: Springer, 2008. Print.

"Wiskott-Aldrich Syndrome." *Be the Match.* Nat'l. Marrow Donor Program, 2014. Web. 2 Sept. 2014.

"Wiskott-Aldrich Syndrome." *Genetics Home Reference.* Nat'l. Lib. of Medicine, Feb. 2013. Web. 2 Sept. 2014.

See also: ABO blood types; Agammaglobulinemia; Allergies; Anthrax; Antibodies; Ataxia telangiectasia; Autoimmune disorders; Autoimmune polyglandular syndrome; Chediak-Higashi syndrome; Chronic granulomatous disease; Chronic myeloid leukemia; Fanconi anemia; Hemophilia; Hereditary sphero-cytosis; Hybridomas and monoclonal antibodies; Immunodeficiency with hyper-IgM; Immunogenetics; Infantile agranulocytosis; Myelodysplastic syndromes; Myeloperoxidase deficiency; Paroxysmal nocturnal hemoglobinuria; Porphyria; Purine nucle-oside phosphorylase deficiency; Rh incompatibility and isoimmunization; Severe combined immunodeficiency syndrome (SCID); Sickle-cell disease; Wolf-Hirschhorn syndrome.

Wolff-Parkinson-White syndrome

CATEGORY: Diseases and syndromes

ALSO known as: WPW syndrome; Ventricular familial pre-excitation syndrome; Auriculoventricular accessory pathway syndrome; False bundle branch block syndrome; Anomalous ventricular excitation syndrome; Pre-excitation syndrome

DEFINITION

Wolff-Parkinson-White (WPW) syndrome is a disorder of the heart's electrical activity. People with the syndrome have an extra electrical pathway present at birth. It causes the heart to beat with an irregular rhythm and faster than normal. This is called tachyarrhythmia.

RISK FACTORS

There are no known risk factors for WPW syndrome.

ETIOLOGY AND GENETICS

The etiology of Wolff-Parkinson-White syndrome is complex, involving both genetic and environmental determinants, most of which are not at all well understood. The great majority of cases are sporadic, and these individuals have no apparent family history of the disease. In a small minority of cases, mutations in the PRKAG2 gene, located on the long arm of chromosome 7 at position 7q36.1, have been shown to cause the condition. Roughly six mutations have been found. This gene encodes a protein known as protein kinase, AMP-activated, gamma 2 non-catalytic subunit (AMPK). An important cellular regulatory molecule, AMPK senses and responds to energy demands within the cell by helping to regulate the concentrations of the cell's main energy source, adenosine triphosphate (ATP). AMPK is known to be active during heart development in the fetus, although its exact role in the process is not well understood. Mutations in the PRKAG2 gene may result in either an overactive or underactive AMPK protein, but in either case heart function is compromised.

The familial form of WPW syndrome, caused by mutations in the PRKAG2 gene, is inherited in an autosomal dominant fashion. This means that a single copy of the mutation is sufficient to cause full expression of the syndrome. An affected individual has a 50 percent chance of transmitting the mutation to each of his or her children. Many cases of familial WPW syndrome, however, result from a spontaneous new mutation, so in these instances affected individuals will have unaffected parents.

Given its potentially fatal cardiac effects, the syndrome is currently under extensive study.

SYMPTOMS

Infants may show irritability, feeding problems, or evidence of congestive heart failure. Older children often describe chest pain, palpitations, and have sudden change in activity level and trouble breathing while previously well. Some people with WPW syndrome never have tachyarrhythmia and its associated symptoms. In those who do, symptoms usually begin between ages eleven and fifty. The frequency and severity of the tachyarrhythmia varies from one person to another and may be associated with any or all of these symptoms: palpitations (sensation of a pounding heart beat), chest pain or tightness, dizziness, fainting, and shortness of breath. In rare cases, a person will go into cardiac arrest (the heart stops pumping) and lose consciousness.

Graphic representation of the bundle of Kent in Wolff–Parkinson–White syndrome. By Tom Lück (Own work), via Wikimedia Commons

SCREENING AND DIAGNOSIS

The doctor will ask about a patient's symptoms and medical history and will perform a physical exam. If the patient has a tachyarrhythmia due to WPW syndrome, he or she will have normal or low blood pressure and a heart rate of 150-250 beats per minute. (A normal heart rate is 60-100 beats per minute.) If a patient is not having irregular heart rhythms during the exam, the results of the exam may be normal. In either case, an electrocardiogram (a test that records the heart's activity by measuring electrical currents through the skin) will usually show a "delta wave" that signals an extra electrical pathway.

Other tests may include treadmill testing and monitoring with a Holter monitor for twenty-four to forty-eight hours to check for any episodes of irregular heartbeat and an electrophysiology study, in which a catheter (a thin tube designed to be inserted into a blood vessel) is passed to the interior of the heart, where it takes de tailed measurements of its electrical activity. This study will detect the extra pathway. Genetic testing can be performed on patients and relatives to look for WPW mutations and related

One beat from a rhythm strip in V2 demonstrating characteristic findings in Wolff–Parkinson–White syndrome: Note the characteristic delta wave (above the blue bar), the short PR interval (red bar) of 80 ms, and the long QRS complex (blue bar plus green bar) at 120 ms. By Ksheka at en.wikipedia diseases such as Pompe disease, Ebstein's anomaly, Danon disease, tuberous sclerosis complex, Leber's hereditary optic neuropathy (LHON), as well as diabetes and deafness presenting as subtle features of mitochondrial disease.

TREATMENT AND THERAPY

The goal of treatment is to reduce or eliminate episodes of tachyarrhythmia and associated symptoms. If a patient does not have symptoms, treatment is usually not necessary.

If a patient does need treatment, it may include medication. Antiarrhythmics may be given to coordinate the heart's electrical signals. This can control or prevent episodes of rapid heartbeat. However, the patient must take the medicine carefully because it can sometimes make an abnormal heart rhythm worse.

Radiofrequency ablation is the gold standard procedure in which a catheter delivers energy at a particular radio frequency to the heart. This destroys (ablates) the abnormal electrical pathway. In most cases, ablation is successful and ends the need to take medicine.

Open-heart surgery may be done to destroy the abnormal pathway. However, this procedure is rarely necessary.

Monitoring and treatment of triggers such as coronary heart disease, ischemia, cardiomyopathy, pericarditis, electrolyte disturbances, thyroid disease, and anemia are important. Specialist consultations are often needed.

Defibrillation is done in the case of cardiac arrest, which is rare. Defibrillation gives the heart a brief electric shock. This procedure converts a rapid, irregular heartbeat back into a normal heartbeat.

PREVENTION AND OUTCOMES

There is no known way of preventing WPW syndrome. However, symptoms can be prevented with proper treatment.

Laurie Rosenblum, M.P.H.; reviewed by Michael J. Fucci, D.O. "Etiology and Genetics" by Jeffrey A. Knight, Ph.D.; updated by Deanna M. Neff, M.P.H.

FURTHER READING

Beers, Mark H., et al. "The Merck Manual of Diagnosis and Therapy". 18th ed. Whitehouse Station, N.J.: Merck Research Laboratories, 2006.

Bunch TJ, May HT, Bair TL, et al. "Long-term" natural history of adult Wolff-Parkinson-White syndrome patients treated with and without catheter ablation. "Circ Arrhythm Electrophysiol". 2015.

EBSCO Publishing. "Health Library: Wolff-Parkinson White Syndrome". Ipswich, Mass.: Author, 2009. Available through http://www.ebscohost.com.

Khairy P, Van Hare GF, Balaji S, Berul CI, Cecchin F, Cohen MI, et al. "PACES/HRS Expert Consensus Statement on the Recognition and Management of Arrhythmias in Adult Congenital Heart Disease: developed in partnership between the Pediatric and Congenital Electrophysiology Society (PACES) and the Heart Rhythm Society (HRS)". Endorsed by the governing bodies of PACES, HRS, the American College of Cardiology (ACC), the American Heart Association (AHA), the European Heart Rhythm Association (EHRA), the Canadian Heart Rhythm Society (CHRS), and the International Society for Adult Congenital Heart Disease (ISACHD). Heart Rhythm. 2014;(10):e102-65.

WEB SITES OF INTEREST

American Heart Association
http://www.americanheart.org

Cleveland Clinic: Wolff-Parkinson-White Syndrome (WPW)
http://my.clevelandclinic.org/heart/disorders/electric/wpw.aspx

Genetic Home Reference: Wolff-Parkinson-White Syndrome
http://ghr.nlm.nih.gov/condition=wolffparkinsonwhitesyndrome

MedLine Plus: Wolff-Parkinson-White Syndrome
http://www.nlm.nih.gov/medlineplus/ency/article/000151.htm

National Organization for Rare Diseases.
https://rarediseases.org/rare-diseases/wolff-parkinson-white-syndrome/

SADS Foundation
http://www.sads.org/What-is-SADS/Wolff-Parkinson-White-Syndrome#.WS72-WjyvIU

See also: Atherosclerosis; Barlow's syndrome; Cardiomyopathy; Heart disease; Holt-Oram syndrome; Long QT syndrome.

Wolf-Hirschhorn syndrome

CATEGORY: Diseases and syndromes

ALSO KNOWN AS: 4p-syndrome; monosomy 4p; del(4p); includes Pitt-Rogers-Danks syndrome

DEFINITION

Wolf-Hirschhorn syndrome (WHS) is caused by a partial deletion of the short arm of human chromosome 4. The syndrome is characterized by multiple congenital malformations accompanied by intellectual disability and is estimated to occur in at least 1 out of 50,000 births.

RISK FACTORS

Two-thirds of existing cases of Wolf-Hirschhorn syndrome occur in females. About 75 percent of WHS cases can be linked to a paternal origin, which is likely the result of the preponderance of subtelomeric genetic recombination that is known to occur during meiosis in the male germ line.

Photograph of a neonate with the Wolf-Hirschhorn syndrome. Note the hypospadias and calcaneovalgus deformity of the foot. By see above, via Wikimedia Commons

deletion of short arm of the chromosome 4 in a patient with Wolf-Hirschhorn syndrome By see above, via Wikimedia Commons

ETIOLOGY AND GENETICS

A case report of a child exhibiting symptoms now associated with WHS was first published in 1961 by the laboratory of Kurt Hirschhorn, an Austrian-born American geneticist and pediatrician who also linked this disorder with a deletion on either human chromosome 4 or 5. Three years later, a partial deletion of the short arm of chromosome 5 was demonstrated to be the causal factor of cri du chat syndrome, and the following year WHS was described in detail in simultaneous reports by Hirschhorn's group as well as by German geneticist Ulrich Wolf and colleagues.

As techniques were later developed that allowed for the physical mapping of human chromosomes, scientists sought to delineate the minimal deletion which would define WHS, as well as to characterize the genes that contribute to the disorder. Noting that about 20 percent of WHS cases have deletions restricted to 4p16.3, the terminal 2 percent of the chromosome, a WHS "critical region" was defined that encompassed this area. The subsequent description of rare patients who had submicroscopic deletions was able to reduce this critical region by more than half, an area in which the human genome sequencing project revealed there were at least a dozen genes, including *WHSC1* (Wolf-Hirschhorn syndrome candidate 1), *LETM1* (Leucine zipper-EF-hand containing transmembrane protein 1), and *FGFR3* (Fibroblast growth factor receptor 3).

The most promising research to determine how the WHS critical region contributes to the disorder comes from mouse models in which the corresponding homologous genes have been mutated experimentally. Mice with mutations in *WHSC1* are seen to have growth impairment accompanied by craniofacial deformations and congenital heart defects, while those with mutations in *FGFR3* demonstrate specific skeletal defects. Although no mice-bearing mutations in the *LETM1* homolog have been reported, this gene has been linked with the appearance of seizures by examining patients with atypical patterns of deletion. It is clear that experiments involving mice will play a central role in elucidating the etiology of this syndrome in the future.

SYMPTOMS

WHS can display a wide range of symptoms, but just four are considered to define the core set of minimal diagnostic criteria. The first of these is a facial appearance which has been described as a "Greek warrior helmet." This includes a broad bridge of the nose which continues to the forehead, a prominent space between the eyebrows, an increased distance between the eyes, and high-arched eyebrows. Other facial features include a small head with an undersized jaw, a "carp-shaped" mouth with a short infranasal depression, and low-set ears. The other core symptoms are growth delay, intellectual disability, and seizures (or at least detectable EEG anomalies). In addition to these core characteristics, some patients display a set of symptoms which have been characterized as "midline defects" and which include a cleft lip/palate; specific defects in such organs as the heart, esophagus, and diaphragm; and skeletal malformations such as scoliosis and clubfoot.

SCREENING AND DIAGNOSIS

Initial screening techniques used to detect WHS included basic cytogenetic procedures such as human karyotyping accompanied by staining to detect chromosome banding patterns, but these tended to miss about 40 percent of WHS cases. High-resolution banding techniques or FISH (fluorescence in situ hybridization), using probes which bind to the WHS critical region, are required to detect the smaller deletions which can lead to WHS.

TREATMENT AND THERAPY

The two most consistent treatable medical problems in children with WHS are major feeding difficulties and seizures. The former is usually treated by gastrostomy, creating a surgical opening into the stomach for feeding via a tube, while the latter has often been controlled by the use of antiepileptic drugs. Surgical intervention is also available to treat clubfoot and scoliosis, as well as to repair congenital heart defects.

PREVENTION AND OUTCOMES

There is presently no cure for WHS. Over time, all cases of WHS will be expected to make improvements in communication skills, with about half of the cases learning how to walk, a fifth helping with simple household tasks, and a tenth becoming self-feeders. A tenth of WHS cases will also go on to achieve fecal continence during the day.

James S. Godde, Ph.D.

FURTHER READING

Bailey, Regina. "Wolf-Hirschhorn Syndrome." *Advances in Neonatal Care* 14.5 (2014): 318–21. Print.

Battaglia, Agatino, John C. Carey, and Tracy J. Wright, "Wolf-Hirschhorn (4p-) Syndrome." *Advances in Pediatrics* 48 (2001): 75–113. Print.

Kerzendorfer, C., et al. "Meier-Gorlin Syndrome and Wolf-Hirschhorn Syndrome: Two Developmental Disorders Highlighting the Importance of Efficient DNA Replication for Normal Development and Neurogenesis." *DNA Repair* 12.8 (2013): 637–44. Print.

Nimura, Keisuke, et al. "A Histone H3 Lysine 36 Trimethyltransferase Links Nkx2-5 to Wolf-Hirschhorn Syndrome." *Nature* 9 July 2009: 287–91. Print.

Searle, Claire J., Emma Shearling, and Oliver W. Quarrell. "Wolf-Hirschhorn Syndrome." *Clinical Dysmorphology* 22.4 (2013): 149–51. Print.

Simon, Ruth, and Andrew D. Bergemann. "Mouse Models of Wolf-Hirschhorn Syndrome." *American Journal of Medical Genetics Part C (Seminars in Medical Genetics)* 148C (2008): 275–80. Print.

See also: ABO blood types; Agammaglobulinemia; Allergies; Anthrax; Antibodies; Ataxia telangiectasia; Autoimmune disorders; Autoimmune polyglandular syndrome; Chediak-Higashi syndrome; Chronic granulomatous disease; Chronic myeloid leukemia; Fanconi anemia; Hemophilia; Hereditary spherocytosis; Hybridomas and monoclonal antibodies; Immunodeficiency with hyper-IgM; Immunogenetics; Infantile agranulocytosis; Myelodysplastic syndromes; Myeloperoxidase deficiency; Paroxysmal nocturnal hemoglobinuria; Porphyria; Purine nucleoside phosphorylase deficiency; Rh incompatibility and isoimmunization; Severe combined immunodeficiency syndrome (SCID); Sickle-cell disease; Wiskott-Aldrich syndrome.

Wolman disease

CATEGORY: Diseases and syndromes

ALSO KNOWN AS: Lysosomal acid lipase deficiency; acid lipase deficiency; cholesteryl ester storage disease; familial xanthomatosis; LAL deficiency; LIPA deficiency

DEFINITION

Wolman disease is a rare, autosomal recessive disorder caused by deficiency of the enzyme lysosomal acid lipase (LAL). Insufficiency of this enzyme causes accumulation of cholesteryl esters and triglycerides throughout the body, resulting in multisystem organ damage and death.

RISK FACTORS

Individuals with mutations in both copies of the *LIPA* gene are at risk for either Wolman disease or a milder condition known as cholesteryl ester storage disease (CESD). Full siblings of affected individuals have a 25 percent risk of inheriting the disorder. Males and females are affected with equal frequency. Cases have been reported in a variety of different ethnic groups; given the rarity of the condition, it is difficult to ascertain whether a higher prevalence truly exists among any particular group.

ETIOLOGY AND GENETICS

Located on chromosome 10q23.2q23.3, the *LIPA* gene produces the LAL enzyme, which is involved in the breakdown of cholesteryl esters and triglycerides within the lysosomes of the cell. This process is part of a tightly regulated system allowing the body to use these and other lipids (fats) appropriately, then recycle or dispose of them as needed.

Deficient LAL activity prevents the breakdown of cholesteryl esters and triglycerides; the effects of their subsequent accumulation within the lysosomes disrupt lipid processing throughout the body. The lysosomes become engorged, ultimately destroying the cell and eventually impairing the function of involved organs, such as the liver.

Mutations in the *LIPA* gene and subsequent deficiency of LAL can also result in the comparatively milder CESD phenotype. Whereas the Wolman phenotype is characterized by the tissue storage of both cholesteryl esters and triglycerides, CESD is characterized by cholesteryl ester storage. While Wolman disease is typically diagnosed in infancy and characterized by rapid progression and death, CESD (while quite variable) can remain undiagnosed into adulthood and be compatible with a normal life span.

The factors determining the expression of the Wolman disease phenotype versus the CESD phenotype have not been completely elucidated. Studies of *LIPA* gene mutations indicate the presence of one common mutation involved with CESD not typically seen in individuals with Wolman disease. This mutation (called Δ254-277) affects how the *LIPA* gene is put together (spliced) and read by the body and is believed to result in the production of both normal

Picture of Moshe Wolman By Wolman529 (Own work), via Wikimedia Commons

and unstable LAL enzyme. The production of at least some normal LAL enzyme is thought to play a role in the milder phenotype of CESD.

Mutation type, however, may not be the only factor that determines the clinical expression of this condition, as evidenced by the clinical variability among individuals with the common mutation. It is postulated that environmental risk factors and genetic background may also play a role, though the specific factors remain to be determined.

SYMPTOMS

Wolman disease initially manifests in infancy with excessive vomiting and diarrhea. Affected infants typically have markedly distended abdomens due to enlargement of the liver and spleen (hepatosplenomegaly), in addition to progressive anemia and developmental regression. Calcification of the adrenal glands, a characteristic feature, can be observed on certain imaging studies, such as computed tomography (CT) scan. In contrast, hepatosplenomegaly is often the only physical sign of CESD, though affected individuals are at increased risk for premature atherosclerosis. Adrenal calcifications are rarely noted.

SCREENING AND DIAGNOSIS

Aside from looking for adrenal calcifications on abdominal imaging, there is no screening test that suggests a diagnosis of Wolman disease. Though tissue lipid levels are remarkably high, plasma lipids are typically within normal range in Wolman disease. If suspected based on clinical presentation, both Wolman disease and CESD can be diagnosed by assaying LAL enzyme activity in white blood cells, liver biopsy, or fibroblasts. Further confirmation of the diagnosis can be achieved by sequencing of the *LIPA* gene.

TREATMENT AND THERAPY

The only treatment currently available for infants diagnosed with Wolman disease is hematopoietic stem cell transplantation (HSCT). Donor stem cells with normal LAL activity are transplanted into an affected individual; if successful, the LAL expressed by the donor cells is enough to constitute normal activity within the host. Few reports are available regarding outcomes of HSCT therapy in Wolman disease. These reports indicate that, among those that survive the HSCT process and for whom the procedure is successful (complete donor cell engraftment), the features of Wolman syndrome are largely ameliorated. Widely used for standard hypercholesterolemia therapy, cholesterol-lowering drugs have been used in the treatment of CESD.

PREVENTION AND OUTCOMES

Without treatment with HSCT, affected infants typically die within the first year of life. The life span after successful HSCT treatment is unknown, though ongoing survival into early adolescence has been documented. Though widely variable, individuals with CESD can have a normal life span with symptomatic treatment. There is no effective way to prevent Wolman disease or CESD, though prenatal diagnostic options and genetic counseling should be made available to those individuals with a family history of these conditions.

Erin Rooney Riggs, M.S.

FURTHER READING

Anderson, R., et al. "Lysosomal Acid Lipase Mutations That Determine Phenotype in Wolman Disease and Cholesterol Ester Storage Disease." *Molecular Genetics and Metabolism* 68 (1999): 333–45. Print.

Assman, G., and U. Seedorf. "Acid Lipase Deficiency: Wolman Disease and Cholesteryl Ester Storage Disease." *Metabolic and Molecular Bases of Inherited Disease.* Ed. Charles Scriver et al. 8th ed. New York: McGraw, 2001.

MacSween, Roderick N. M., Alastair D. Burt, Bernard Portmann, and Linda D. Ferrell. *MacSween's Pathology of the Liver.* Edinburgh: Churchill, 2012. Print.

Milunsky, Aubrey, and Jeff M. Milunsky. *Genetic Disorders and the Fetus: Diagnosis, Prevention, and Treatment.* 6th ed. Chichester: Wiley, 2010. Print.

Noggle, Chad A., Raymond S. Dean, and Arthur MacNeill Horton. *The Encyclopedia of Neuropsychological Disorders.* New York: Springer, 2012. Print.

Tolar, J., et al. "Long-Term Metabolic, Endocrine, and Neuropsychological Outcome of Hematopoietic Cell Transplantation for Wolman Disease." *Bone Marrow Transplantation* 43 (2009): 21–27.

See also: Fabry disease; Gaucher disease; Gm1-gangliosidosis; Hereditary diseases; Hunter disease; Hurler syndrome; Inborn errors of metabolism; Jansky-Bielschowsky disease; Krabbé disease; Metachromatic leukodystrophy; Niemann-Pick disease; Pompe disease; Sandhoff disease; Tay-Sachs disease.

X chromosome inactivation

CATEGORY: Developmental genetics

SIGNIFICANCE: Normal females have two X chromosomes, and normal males have one X chromosome. In order to compensate for the potential problem of doubling of gene products in females, one X chromosome is randomly inactivated in each cell.

KEY TERMS

Barr body: a highly condensed and inactivated X chromosome visible in female cells as a darkly staining spot in a prepared microscope slide

dosage compensation: an equalization of gene products that can occur whenever there are more or fewer genes for specific traits than normal

mosaic: an individual possessing cells with more than one type of genetic constitution

sex chromosomes: the X and Y chromosomes; females possess two X chromosomes, while males possess one X and one Y chromosome

THE HISTORY OF X CHROMOSOME INACTIVATION

In 1961 Mary Lyon hypothesized that gene products were found in equal amounts in males and females because one of the X chromosomes in females became inactivated early in development. This hypothesis became known as the Lyon hypothesis, and the process became known as Lyonization, or X chromosome inactivation. Prior to this explanation, it was recognized that females had two X chromosomes and males had only one X chromosome, yet the proteins encoded by genes on the X chromosomes were found in equal amounts in females and males because of dosage compensation.

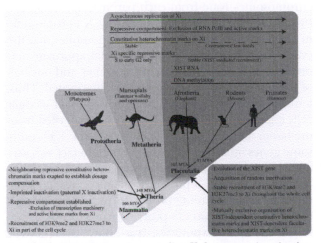

A model for the evolution of mammalian X-chromosome inactivation. Arrows above the phylogeny show epigenetic features underlying X chromosome inactivation (solid arrows indicate stable components of XCI within the clades, whereas dashed lines indicate unstable repressive modification). We propose that in the ancestral therian mammal neighbouring centromeric constitutive heterochromatin histone modifications were exapted to reduce transcription from the paternal X chromosome in females. H3K27me3 and H3K9me2 were also recruited to the Xi in a cell-cycle and/or cell-lineage dependent manner. After the divergence of placental from marsupial mammals, the XIST gene evolved and H3K27me3 and H3K9me2 (along with H4K20me1) were stably recruited into the XCI machinery. In placental mammals the original silencing machinery was restricted, and organised in mutually exclusive domains with the Xi-specific facultative heterochromatin. In marsupials, much of the original silencing machinery that was recruited from constitutive heterochromatin remains in place. By Chaumeil J, Waters PD, Koina E, Gilbert C, Robinson TJ, Graves JA., via Wikimedia Commons

The principles of inheritance dictate that individuals receive half of their chromosomes from their fathers and the other half from their mothers at conception. Therefore, a female possesses two different X

Site of the X chromosome inactivation in mouse. By Helixitta (Own work), via Wikimedia Commons

chromosomes (one from each parent). In addition to hypothesizing the inactivation of one X chromosome in each cell, the Lyon hypothesis also implies that the event occurs randomly. In any individual, approximately one-half of the paternal X chromosomes and one-half of the maternal X chromosomes are inactivated. Thus, females display a mosaic condition since half of their cells express the X chromosome genes inherited from the father and half of their cells express the X chromosome genes inherited from the mother. In fact, this situation can be seen in individuals who inherit an allele for a different form of a protein from each parent: Some cells express one parent's protein form, while other cells express the other parent's protein form.

Prior to Lyon's hypothesis, it was known that a densely staining material could be seen in cells from females that was absent in cells from males. This material was termed a "Barr body," after Murray Barr. Later, it was shown that Barr bodies were synonymous with the inactivated X chromosome. Other observations led scientists to understand that the number of Barr bodies in a cell was always one less than the number of X chromosomes in the cell. For example, one Barr body indicated the presence of two X chromosomes, and two Barr bodies indicated the presence of three X chromosomes.

CLINICAL SIGNIFICANCE

The significance of Barr bodies became apparent with the observation that females lacking one Barr body or possessing more than one Barr body developed an abnormal appearance. Particularly intriguing were females with Turner syndrome. These females possess only one X chromosome per cell, a condition that is not analogous to normal females, who possess only one functional X chromosome per cell as a result of inactivation. The difference in the development of a Turner syndrome female and a normal female lies in the fact that both X chromosomes are active in normal females during the first few days of development. After this period, inactivation occurs

randomly in each cell, as hypothesized by Lyon. In cases in which inactivation is not random, individuals may have a variety of developmental problems. Therefore, there is apparently a critical need for both X chromosomes to be active in females in early development for normal development to occur.

It is equally important that there not be more than two X chromosomes present during this early development. Females possessing three X chromosomes, and therefore two Barr bodies, are sometimes called superfemales or metafemales because of a tendency to be taller than average. These females are also two to ten times more likely to suffer from mild to moderate intellectual disability.

The same phenomenon has been observed in males who possess Barr bodies. Barr bodies are not normally present in males because they have only one X chromosome. The presence of Barr bodies indicates the existence of an extra X chromosome that has become inactive. Just as in females, extra X chromosomes are also expressed in early development, and abnormal amounts of gene products result in abnormal physical characteristics and mental retardation. Males with Klinefelter syndrome have two X chromosomes and a Y chromosome. In cases in which males have more than two X chromosomes, the effects are even more remarkable.

MECHANISM OF X INACTIVATION

While it has been apparent since the 1960s that X inactivation is required for normal female development, the mechanism has been elusive. Only with the development of techniques to study the molecular events of the cell and its chromosomes has progress been made in understanding the process of inactivation. One process involved in turning off a gene (thus "shutting down" the process of transcription) is the alteration of one of the molecules of DNA known as cytosine. When a methyl group is added to the cytosine, the gene cannot produce the RNA necessary to make a protein. It is thought that this methyl group blocks the proteins that normally bind to the DNA, so that transcription cannot occur. When methyl groups are removed from cytosines, the block is removed and transcription begins. This is a common means of regulating transcription of genes. Methylation is significantly higher in the inactivated X chromosome than in the activated X chromosome. As the genes on the chromosome become inactive, the chromosome condenses into the tightly packed mass known as the Barr body. However, the process of methylation alone cannot entirely account for inactivation.

A region on the X chromosome called the X inactivation center (XIC) is considered the control center for X inactivation. In this region is a gene called X inactive specific transcript (non-protein coding), or *XIST*. At the time of its discovery, this gene was the only gene known to be functional in an inactivated chromosome. It produces an RNA that remains inside the nucleus.

Evidence in humans supports the hypothesis that the *XIST* gene is turned on and begins to make its RNA when the egg is fertilized. Studies with mice have shown that RNA is produced, at first, in low levels and from both X chromosomes. It has been shown in mice, but not humans, that prior to inactivation, Xist (lowercased when referring to mouse genes) RNA is localized at the XIC site only, thus suggesting a potential role prior to actual inactivation of the chromosome. At this point, one X chromosome will begin to increase its production of XIST RNA; shortly thereafter, XIST RNA transcription from the other X chromosome ceases. It is not clear how XIST RNA initiates the process of inactivation and condensing of the inactive chromosome, but XIST RNA binds along the entire length of the inactive X chromosome in females. These results suggest that inactivation spreads from the XIC region toward the end of the chromosome and that XIST RNA is required to maintain an inactive state. If a mouse's *Xist* gene is mutated and cannot produce its RNA, inactivation of that X chromosome is blocked. Other studies have suggested that a product from a nonsex chromosome may interact with the XIC region, causing it to remain active. As expected, but not explained, the *XIST* gene is repressed, or expresses XIST RNA at only very low levels, in males with only one X chromosome.

No difference has been detected between maternally and paternally expressed *XIST* genes in humans. This has led scientists to suspect that *XIST* gene RNA may not be responsible for determining which X chromosome becomes inactivated. It is also not clear how the cell knows how many X chromosomes are present. The search for other candidates for these roles is under way. Finally, there are a few genes besides the *XIST* gene that are also active on the inactive X chromosome. How they escape the inactivation process and why this is necessary are also questions that must be resolved.

Linda R. Adkison, Ph.D.

Further Reading

Bainbridge, David. "The Double Life of Women." *The X in Sex: How the X Chromosome Controls Our Lives.* Cambridge: Harvard UP, 2003. Print.

Deng, X., J. B. Berletch, D. K. Nguyen, and C. M. Disteche. "X Chromosome Regulation: Diverse Patterns in Development, Tissues and Disease." *Nature Reviews. Genetics* 15.6 (2014): 367–378. *MEDLINE with Full Text.* Web. 2 Sept. 2014.

Erbe, Richard W. "Single-Active-X Principle." *Scientific American Medicine* 2.9.IV (1995). Print.

Latham, Keith E. "X Chromosome Imprinting and Inactivation in the Early Mammalian Embryo." *Trends in Genetics* 12.4 (1996): 134–138. Print.

McKusick, Victor A., and Ada Hamosh. "*314670 X Inactivation-Specific Transcript; XIST." *OMIM.org.* Johns Hopkins U, 15 Jan. 2014. Web. 2 Sept. 2014.

Migeon, Barbara R. *Females Are Mosaics: X Inactivation and Sex Differences in Disease.* 2d ed. New York: Oxford UP, 2014. Print.

"X in a Cage." *Discover* 15.3 (1994): 14. Print.

See also: Androgen insensitivity syndrome; Fragile X syndrome; Gender identity; Hermaphrodites; Infertility; Klinefelter syndrome; Metafemales; Pseudohermaphrodites; Turner syndrome; XY Y syndrome.

Xenopu laevis

Category: Diseases and syndromes

Significance: *Xenopus laevis*, the African clawed frog, has been used widely in the field of developmental biology. By following the development of this unique organism, scientists have identified and now understand the role of many genes in frog development, providing insight into vertebrate development.

Key terms

embryology: the study of developing embryos

fate map: a map created by following the adult fate of embryonic cells

model organism: an organism well suited for genetic research because it has a well-known genetic history, a short life cycle, and genetic variation between individuals in the population

transgenic organism: an organism that contains a gene not normally expressed in its genome

THE ORGANISM

The African clawed frog, *Xenopus laevis*, is in the class *Amphibia*, order *Anura*, suborder *Opisthocoela*, family *Pipidae*, and genus *Xenopus*. This genus includes five other species that inhabit silt-filled ponds throughout much of southern Africa. Members of this species share a distinctive habitat and morphology. The organism's name alone provides insight into its structure and habitats: The root *xeno* stems from Greek for "strange," while *pus* is from the Greek for "foot" and *laevis* is Latin for "slippery." *Xenopus laevis* is entirely aquatic, a feature that makes it unique among the members of the genus, feeding and breeding under water. It is believed that they evolved from terrestrial anurans, organisms that are aquatic as tadpoles but are terrestrial as adults. Migration across land from pond to pond has been observed but is limited by distance and time of year (occurring during the rainy season) because out of water, the frogs will dry out and die within a day. In instances of extreme drought, adult frogs will bury themselves in the mud and wait until the next rainfall.

Xenopus laevis is mottled greenish-brown on its dorsal surface and yellowish-white on its ventral surface. In appearance, these frogs are flattened dorsoventrally, with dorsally oriented eyes as adults. The members of the genus are collectively known as platannas, from the word "plathander," meaning flat-handed. Three toes of the hind limbs are clawed, and a line of specialized sensory organs (the lateral line organs) is found on both the dorsal and ventral surfaces and encircles the eyes. The breeding season for *X. laevis* depends on temperature and rainfall. The tadpoles are herbivorous, feeding on algae, whereas the adults are carnivorous, feeding on worms, crustaceans, and other creatures living in the mud.

A MODEL ORGANISM

A model organism is defined as one that breeds quickly, is easily managed in the laboratory, and has large numbers of offspring or broods. *Xenopus laevis* meets these requirements nicely. An interesting feature of this organism is its responsiveness to human chorionic gonadotropin, a hormone secreted by the placenta and present in the urine of pregnant women. When exposed to the hormone, female frogs will spawn (lay eggs). As a result of this phenomenon, *X. laevis* was once used as an indicator in human pregnancy tests, whereby the female frogs were injected with human female urine. At present, researchers take advantage of this phenomenon to produce large numbers of offspring by injecting frogs with the hormone. Another characteristic that makes *X. laevis* a good model organism is that it is hardy and can survive in captivity for long periods of time with relatively low mortality rates.

A final requirement for an animal model to be useful is that research on the animal should add to the understanding of biological principles in other organisms. *Xenopus laevis* is widely used in the field of developmental biology. For many decades, amphibian embryologists used salamander embryos, such as *Triturus*, and embryos of the frog *Rana* species. As mentioned above, amphibian embryos have several advantages over other organisms: amphibian embryos are large, can be obtained in large numbers, and can be maintained easily and inexpensively in the laboratory. However, one disadvantage of traditional amphibian species is that they are seasonal breeders. As a result, investigators cannot conduct experiments throughout the year on most amphibians. *Xenopus laevis* is a notable exception, because it can be induced to breed year-round.

As the fertilized *X. laevis* zygote develops, the yolk-laden cytoplasm, known as the vegetal pole, is oriented downward by gravity. The rest of the cytoplasm, termed the animal pole, orients itself upward. The animal pole is the main portion of the cell, giving rise to the embryo proper. Cell division, or cleavage of cells, in the animal pole increases the number of cells greatly. Movement and migration of these cells, under the influences of interactions with neighboring cells, give rise to a multilaminar embryo that includes the ectoderm (which gives rise to skin and nervous system), the mesoderm (which gives rise to muscle), and the endoderm (which gives rise to many of the "tubes" of the organism, such as the intestines and the respiratory tract).

By following embryos from the very earliest stages, researchers have been able to create "fate maps" of fertilized eggs, which can be used to predict adult derivatives of specific regions in a developing embryo. Early researchers introduced many different techniques to create these kinds of maps. One technique involves destroying single cells during early development and following the development of the embryo to see what tissue is altered. Other methods include transplantation of individual cells or small groups of cells into a host organism and following the fate of the transplanted tissue. Much of what is now known about the interactions between cells in developing vertebrate embryos has come from *X. laevis*. The early work of embryologists Hans Spemann and

Pieter Nieuwkoop has been supported with molecular techniques, and many genes have been identified that control nearly every aspect of *Xenopus* development. A few examples include the *Xenopus Brachury* gene (*Xbra*), which is involved in the establishment of the dorsal-ventral axis; *Xenopus ventral* (*vent1*), which aids in the differentiation of ventral mesoderm and epidermal structures; and *Xenopus nodal-related 1* (*Xnr1*), a gene that is responsible for the specification of the left-right axis.

Xenopus embryos possess a number of advantages that have allowed investigators to study many aspects of developmental biology. One of the struggles that early researchers faced was the lack of dependable techniques for creating transgenic embryos to study the functions and role of individual genes. One can isolate and clone the genes of *Xenopus* and inject RNA into zygotes. RNA, however, is an unstable molecule and relatively short-lived. Therefore, the study of molecular events in the embryo after the period when the embryonic genes are turned on remained problematic. Attempts to inject cloned DNA to be expressed in the embryo were complicated by the fact that it does not integrate into the frog genomic chromosomes during cleavage. Exogenous DNA is then unequally distributed in embryonic cells and, therefore, is always expressed in random patterns. In 1996, Kristen L. Kroll and Enrique Amaya developed a technique to make stable transgenic *Xenopus* embryos. This technique has the potential to boost the utility of *Xenopus* tremendously. One significant advantage of using transgenic frogs over transgenic mice is that one can produce first-generation transgenics, making it unnecessary to wait until the second generation to examine the effects of the exogenous gene on development.

The transgenic technique has several steps, and each step is full of problems. Because exogenous DNA is not incorporated into the zygotic genome, Kroll and Amaya decided to attempt to introduce it into sperm nuclei. Sperm nuclei are treated with the enzyme lysolecithin to remove the plasma membrane prior to incubation with the linearized DNA plasmid containing the exogenous gene. The sperm nuclei are then incubated with restriction enzyme to introduce nicks in the nuclear DNA. The nicks facilitate incorporation of the plasmid DNA. The nuclei are then placed in an interphase egg extract, which causes the nuclei to swell as if they were male pronuclei. This technique has been used in many laboratories to introduce into the frog genes that are not normally expressed, allowing the researcher to study the function of these genes.

The National Institutes of Health is supporting the Trans-NIH *Xenopus* Initiative, specifically developed to support research in the areas of genomics and genetics in *Xenopus* research. While there is still much to be learned from these unique organisms, it is clear that the advantages of this animal model far outweigh the disadvantages. With continued work in laboratories around the world, scientists may soon fully understand the genetics involved in vertebrate development. *Xenopus laevis* is ideally suited to provide critical breakthroughs in embryonic body patterning and cell fate determination, later development and the formation of organs, and cell biological and biochemical processes.

FURTHER READING

"African Clawed Frog." *Encyclopedia of Invasive Species: From Africanized Honey Bees to Zebra Mussels.* Eds. Susan L. Woodward, Joyce Ann Quinn. Santa Barbara: ABC-CLIO, 2011. Digital file.

Brown, A. L. *The African Clawed Toad Xenopus laevis: A Guide for Laboratory Practical Work.* London: Butterworths, 1970. Print.

Gurdon, J. B., et al. "Use of Frog Eggs and Oocytes for the Study of Messenger RNA and Its Translation in Living Cells." *Nature* 233 (1971): 177–182. Print.

Jaworski, Jacob M. *Animal Science and Issues.* New York: Nova, 2011. Digital file.

Kroll, K. L., and E. Amaya. "Transgenic *Xenopus* Embryos from Sperm Nuclear Transplantations Reveal FGF Signaling Requirements During Gastrulation." *Development* 122.10 (1996): 3173–3183. Print.

Kubiak, Jacek Z., Malgorzata Kloc. *Xenopus Development.* Ames: Wiley, 2014. Digital file.

Nieuwkoop, P. D., J. Faber, and M. W. Kirschner. *Normal Table of Xenopus laevis (Daudin): A Systematical and Chronological Survey of the Development from the Fertilized Egg Till the End of Metamorphosis.* New York: Garland, 1994. Print.

Seidman, S., and H. Soreq. *Transgenic Xenopus: Microinjection Methods and Developmental Neurobiology.* Totowa: Humana, 1997. Print.

Wiechmann, Allan F., and Celeste E. Wirsig-Wiechmann. *Color Atlas of Xenopus laevis Histology.* Boston: Kluwer, 2003. Print.

Xenotransplants

CATEGORY: Genetic engineering and biotechnology

Significance: Xenotransplants are transplants of organs or cellular tissue between different species of animals, such as between pigs and humans.

KEY TERMS

hyperacute rejection: when a transplanted organ or tissue is immediately (within minutes) rejected by the body of the transplant recipient

neural crest cells: embryonic cells that eventually form part of the nervous system and other tissues

stem cells: multipotent cells that can differentiate into a diverse range of specialized cells

transgenic: involving the deliberate incorporation of foreign genes into an animal, such as human genes incorporated into the pig genome

xenosis: the transmission of infectious agents between species

HISTORY

The idea of xenotransplants is actually quite old. During the eighteenth century, for example, transfusions of sheep's blood were believed to be therapeutic for certain human illnesses. As the science of organ transplants between humans progressed, researchers became increasingly interested in experimenting with using animals as donors. Organ transplantation is an accepted medical treatment in humans, but there are not enough donor organs from humans available to treat every patient who could benefit from the procedure. In 2013, more than 120,000 people in the United States were waiting for an organ, according to the US Department of Health and Human Services. As the demand for transplant surgery grows, the pool of available donor organs shrinks in relation. One of the ethical dilemmas inherent in human organ transplant is that, in most cases, for one person to receive a transplant, another person must die. Bone marrow, partial liver, and kidney transplants are among the few exceptions; donors can usually donate bone marrow, a lobe of their liver, or one kidney and still survive. Nevertheless, for most organs the dilemma remains.

Researchers are interested in using organs harvested from compatible animals, eliminating both the need to wait for a compatible human donor and the shortage of usable organs. This is one form of xenotransplant, and it could eliminate the shortage of donor organs. However, researchers have encountered two major barriers to xenotransplantation; organ rejection by the human body's immune system and the risk of xenosis, or the transmission of infectious agents, like viruses, between species.

Early research focused on potential donor animals that were similar to humans—that is, primates such as baboons and chimpanzees. Perhaps the most publicized example of such a xenotransplant was the 1984 Baby Fae case, in which doctors in California transplanted a baboon heart into a newborn human infant who otherwise had no chance for survival. The infant survived for several days before succumbing to complications. In 1993, a baboon liver was transplanted to a patient with liver failure. The patient lived for seventy days before dying of an infection. Researchers quickly learned that primates were not ideal candidates for organ donation; not only might the human body reject these organs, but primate organs are small in comparison to those of humans. Chimpanzee kidneys, for example, are too small to perform adequately in an adult human.

Researchers then turned their attention to pigs as possible donors. Swine make ideal donor candidates because they are physically large enough to have organs that can sustain humans, have a short gestation cycle, produce large litters of offspring, and, because they are routinely raised for meat production, are viewed as expendable by the general public. Pig heart valves are already routinely used in humans, with thousands implanted annually, and pig skin is often grafted onto burns. In a clinical trial, pig pancreas cells were injected into patients with Type I (juvenile) diabetes mellitus and several patients required less insulin afterward. People with liver failure have also been hooked up to pigs' livers to keep them alive until a human liver was available for transplant.

In preliminary trials in humans conducted in the 1990s, neural crest cells (embryonic cells that eventually form part of the nervous system) from fetal pigs were injected into the brains of patients who had experienced a stroke or who had Parkinson's disease. While a few patients had side effects that could have been the result of this treatment, some patients also seemed to get better. Later, another clinical trial was conducted in patients with Parkinson's disease. In this trial, all patients underwent a surgical procedure, but only half of the eighteen patients in the study had pig cells injected into their brains, while the other half did not. Neither the patients nor the neurologists who evaluated the patients for improvement knew who had gotten the cell treatment. When the trial was complete, the results showed that there was no difference between patients who got the cells and those who did not, indicating that the pig cells did not improve Parkinson's disease.

Despite the possible benefit of using pig cells to treat some human diseases, the use of larger organs from pigs has been less successful. Transplant recipients experienced hyperacute rejection; that is, their bodies immediately reacted to the foreign tissue by shutting off the flow of blood to it.

TRANSGENIC PIGS

In 1992, researchers in the United Kingdom announced the creation of Astrid, the first transgenic pig. A transgenic animal is one who has been genetically modified with genes from another species. Since then, several groups have worked to create pigs with organs that have been genetically modified to be human compatible so that they are not rejected by the human immune system. Another goal of this kind of research is to create pigs with organs that are not susceptible to pig viruses.

ETHICAL AND MEDICAL CONCERNS

Xenotransplantation presents a number of ethical and medical dilemmas. The possibility that a virus, harmless to the donor animal, might be transmitted to the human host and then prove fatal is a major concern. Scientists worry that a potentially deadly disease epidemic could result from using organs or other tissue from either swine or primates. While many researchers are confident that careful screening of donor animals would eliminate or minimize such risks, critics remain convinced that it is possible a virus could lie dormant and undetected in animals, causing problems only after the transplants occurred. Baboons, for example, carry a virus that has the potential to cause cancer in humans.

In addition to the medical issues raised, many bioethicists question the morality of using animals as a source of "spare parts" for humans. They are particularly troubled by the idea of genetically altering a species such as swine in order to make their organs more compatible with human hosts. Proponents of xenotransplants counter these arguments by noting that humans have selectively bred animals for various purposes for thousands of years to eliminate certain characteristics while enhancing others. In addition,

animals such as swine are already routinely slaughtered for human consumption.

Finally, there is the problem of human perceptions. While many people support the idea of xenotransplants on the genetic or cellular level, they are less enthusiastic about possible organ transplants. That is, while a majority of people surveyed said they would have no problem accepting a xenotransplant if it were part of gene therapy, far fewer were interested in possibly receiving a pig's heart if the need arose. If researchers do achieve successful xenotransplants using such organs, however, public perceptions could change. It is easy to question a medical procedure when it is still theoretical; it becomes much more difficult to do so after it becomes a reality.

IMPACT

An immediate and plentiful source of organs from swine could improve and save many human lives. Overcoming the immunological problems and infectious disease risks are serious barriers to xenotransplantation, and remain active areas of research. Creating transgenic pigs with human-compatible organs is a main thrust of research in xenotransplantation. However, human stem cells from unused embryos or adult stem cells is a competing line of research that may offer an alternative source of organs for transplantation, or a means to repair diseased ones.

Nancy Farm Männikkö, Ph.D.;
updated by Nancy E. Price, Ph.D.

FURTHER READING

"United States Decides Close Tabs Must Be Kept on Xenotransplants." *Nature* 8 June 2000: 606–07. Print.

Bassett, Pamela. *Emerging Markets in Tissue Engineering: Angiogenesis, Soft and Hard Tissue Regeneration, Xenotransplant, Wound Healing, Biomaterials, and Cell Therapy.* Southborough: D & MD Reports, 1999. Print.

Bloom, E. T., et al. "Xenotransplantation: The Potential and the Challenges." *Critical Care Nurse* 19 (1999): 76–83. Print.

Boneva, R. S., and T. M. Folks. "Xenotransplantation and Risks of Zoonotic Infections." *Annals of Medicine* 36 (2004): 504–17. Print.

Cowan, Peter J., et al. "Kidney Xenotransplantation." *Kidney Intl.* 85.2 (2014): 265–75. Print.

Cruz, J., et al. "Ethical Challenges of Xenotransplantation." *Transplant Proceedings* 32 (2000): 2687. Print.

Daar, A. S. "Xenotransplants: Proceed with Caution." *Nature* 5 March 1998: 11. Print.

Fishman, Jay A., et al. "Xenotransplantation-Associated Infectious Risk: A WHO Consultation." *Xenotransplantation* 19.2 (2012): 72–81. Print.

Ghebremariam, Y. T., et al. "Intervention Strategies and Agents Mediating the Prevention of Xenorejection." *Annals of the New York Academy of Science* 1056 (2005): 123–43. Print.

Griesemer, Adam, et al. "Xenotransplantation: Immunological Hurdles and Progress Toward Tolerance." *Immunological Reviews* 258.1 (2014): 241–58. Print.

Hagelin, J. "Public Opinion Surveys About Xenotransplantation." *Xenotransplantation* 11 (2004): 551–58. Print.

Inui, Akio. *Epigenetic Risks of Cloning.* Boca Raton: CRC Press, 2006. Print.

Persson, M. D., et al. "Xenotransplantation Public Perceptions: Rather Cells than Organs." *Xenotransplantation* 10 (2003): 72–79. Print.

See also: Animal cloning; Cancer; Cloning; Cloning: Ethical issues; Gene therapy: Ethical and economic issues; Genetic engineering: Historical development; Heart disease; Immunogenetics; In vitro fertilization and embryo transfer; Model organism: Mus musculus; Model organism: Xenopus laevis; Organ transplants and HLA genes; Stem cells; Synthetic antibodies; Totipotency; Transgenic organisms.

Xeroderma pigmentosum and genetics

CATEGORY: Diseases and syndromes

ALSO KNOWN AS: Melanosis lenticularis progressiva; Kaposi disease; atrophoderma pigmentosum; XP

DEFINITION

Xeroderma pigmentosum is a group of rare skin disorders characterized by extreme sensitivity to sunlight (photosensitivity), with possible ocular and neurologic involvement. An inherited disease, it results from a defect in the genes involved in the repair of DNA damage caused by ultraviolet light.

RISK FACTORS

A child born to parents who each carry a copy of the defective DNA repair gene responsible for this disorder has a 25 percent chance of being affected. The disorder usually manifests at age one to two years and affects both sexes across ethnic groups, although a higher incidence is reported in Japan and the Middle East. Typically, it results from mutations in genes *XPA, ERCC3, XPC, ERCC2, DDB2, ERCC4, ERCC5,* and *ERCC1*—involved in DNA repair—or in the gene *POLH* that encodes an enzyme (a specialized polymerase) that replicates ultraviolet-damaged DNA.

a child with XP, found during medical camp in mid western hills of Nepal. By Himynameislax, via Wikimedia Commons

An eight year old girl from Guatemala with Xeroderma pigmentosum. This left lateral view of the face shows the diffuse nature of the hyperpigmented lentigos on the face and neck, as well as demonstrating again the corneal damage and para-nasal hyperkeratosis. By James Halpern, Bryan Hopping and Joshua M Brostoff, via Wikimedia Commons

Etiology and Genetics

Xeroderma pigmentosum is an autosomal recessive disease that manifests as hypersensitivity to the sun's ultraviolet rays. Exposure to ultraviolet light induces the formation of pyrimidine dimers by favoring the cross-linking of adjacent pyrimidine bases present in DNA. These structures distort the DNA double helix, thus preventing replication and gene expression. Normally, several distinct enzymes, involved in a process termed "nucleotide excision repair," work in concert to remove the lesion. The resulting gap is then filled in by a DNA polymerase that restores the original base sequence.

Persons with xeroderma pigmentosum carry a mutation in any of the known genes that specify the enzymes that participate in nucleotide excision repair. Several genetic subtypes of the disorder exist. They differ in disease severity and frequency of occurrence and are classified according to the defective repair gene involved. Thus, the classic form of xeroderma pigmentosum, known as XPA, results from a mutation in gene *XPA*. The other subtypes, designated XPB through XPH, are defective in other DNA repair genes and a variant form, known as XPV, is defective in gene *POLH*. Subgroups XPA and XPC encompass about half of xeroderma pigmentosum cases, with very rare cases reported of XPB, XPE, and XPH.

Accumulation of damaged DNA causes progressive degenerative alterations of the skin, thus greatly increasing the likelihood of mutagenesis and skin cancers, such as basal cell carcinoma, squamous cell carcinoma, or melanoma. Classic XPA, which shows the lowest level of DNA repair, is more likely to be associated with progressive neurologic complications. Individuals with subtypes XPB, XPD, XPF, XPG, and XPH show varying degrees of neurologic abnormalities, whereas individuals with subtypes XPC, XPE, and XPV generally do not. Although form XPV is clinically indistinguishable from classic XPA, it is genetically distinct from the other subtypes. In fact, XPV cells have the ability to repair DNA damage induced by ultraviolet light but lack the specialized polymerase that replicates ultraviolet-damaged DNA.

Symptoms

Persons with xeroderma pigmentosum typically experience unusually severe sunburn with skin redness and blistering after only brief exposure to sunlight. The condition is characterized by excessive skin dryness, pigmentary changes, skin atrophy, lesions termed solar keratoses, and a 2,000-fold risk of developing sunlight-induced skin cancer before age twenty. Eye damage from ultraviolet radiation causes photophobia and irritation in about 80 percent of cases and may lead to ocular tumors. Neurologic complications are present in 20 to 30 percent of cases and include poor coordination, deafness, developmental delay, and mental retardation.

Screening and Diagnosis

Clinical diagnosis usually is based on a visual examination of the skin and eyes and on a history of photosensitivity, freckling, and skin tumors in young children. A blood test or skin biopsy can reveal a DNA repair defect. For persons with a family history of xeroderma pigmentosum, prenatal tests, including amniocentesis, are available, as are genetic counseling and genetic testing to determine carrier status for individuals with subtypes XPA and XPC.

Treatment and Therapy

Currently, no treatment for xeroderma pigmentosum exists. Disease management consists of preventing sun-induced damage and ensuring the prompt removal of precancerous and cancerous lesions. Premalignant solar keratoses may be removed by cryotherapy or dermabrasion. More aggressive tumors, such as melanoma, may require radiation and chemotherapy in addition to surgical excision. Retinoid therapy, moisturizers, and vitamin D supplements are recommended. Topical lotion containing a DNA repair enzyme has been reported to have reduced the development of solar keratoses and basal cell carcinoma in clinical trials.

Prevention and Outcomes

Avoidance of all sources of ultraviolet radiation, including fluorescent lights, can improve outcome. Protective clothing, a wide-brimmed hat, ultraviolet-absorbing sunglasses, and a sunscreen with high sun-protection factor are mandatory when outdoors. Medications that increase sensitivity to sunlight should be used with caution and tobacco smoking avoided. Regular checkups by a dermatologist (every three months) and an ophthalmologist (annually) are important for disease surveillance. By taking measures that reduce deadly skin cancer, affected persons with no neurologic complications can achieve a normal life span.

Anna Binda, Ph.D.

FURTHER READING

DiGiovanna, John J., and Kenneth H. Kraemer. "Shining a Light on Xeroderma Pigmentosum." *Journ. of Investigative Dermatology* 132.3 (2012): 785–96. Print.

Karp, Gerald. "DNA Replication and Repair." *Cell and Molecular Biology: Concepts and Experiments*. 5th ed. Hoboken: Wiley, 2008. Print.

Ono, Ryusuke, et al. "Three School-Aged Cases of Xeroderma Pigmentosum Variant Type." *Photodermatology, Photoimmunology & Photomedicine* 29.3 (2013): 132–39. Print.

Snustad, D. Peter, and Michael J. Simmons. "Mutation, DNA Repair, and Recombination." *Principles of Genetics*. 5th ed. Hoboken: Wiley, 2009. Print.

Tamura, Deborah, et al. "Living With Xeroderma Pigmentosum: Comprehensive Photoprotection for Highly Photosensitive Patients." *Photodermatology, Photoimmunology & Photomedicine* 30.2/3 (2014): 146–52. Print.

Webb, Sandra. "A Patient's Journey: Xeroderma Pigmentosum." *British Medical Journal* 336 (2008): 444–46. Print.

See also: Albinism; Chediak-Higashi syndrome; Epidermolytic hyperkeratosis; Hermansky-Pudlak syndrome; Ichthyosis; Melanoma; Palmoplantar keratoderma.

X-linked periventricular heterotopia

CATEGORY: Diseases and syndromes

ALSO KNOWN AS: Heterotopia periventricular X-linked dominant; Periventricular nodular heterotopia 1; Heterotopia familial nodular; Nodular heterotopia bilateral periventricular; NHBP; Bilateral periventricular nodular heterotopia; BPNH; PVNH; *FLNA*-related periventricular nodular heterotopia

DEFINITION

X-linked periventricular heterotopia (PVNH) is a genetic disorder in which nerve cells in the brain do not migrate properly during early fetal development (between about the 6th and 24th week of pregnancy. Disorders of this type are known as neuronal migration disorders ("heterotopia" meaning "out of place", and periventricular refers to the areas of the brain surrounding the fluid-filled cavities known as the "ventricles").

It is characterized by the presence of clumps or clusters of neurons near the brain's ventricles. Most individuals with this genetic disorder are female. It is often, but not always, lethal in males. Symptoms typically begin with seizures in the middle teen years although some develop seizures during childhood. Intelligence is usually normal, although mild intellectual disability, including difficulty with reading and spelling may occur. Individuals appear to be at increased risk for stroke and other vascular/coagulation problem. Some people also have hyperflexible joints and vascular anomalies (aortic dilation and other), symptoms also seen in the Ehlers-Danlos syndrome. PVNH is caused by mutations in the *FNLA* gene and is usually inherited in an X-linked dominant fashion. Treatment is dependent on the signs and symptoms present in each individual and may include anti-seizure medications.

The Ehlers-Danlos variant (PVNH4) or Ehlers-Danlos syndrome (EDS) with periventricular heterotopia is now considered to be the same as X-linked periventricular heterotopia type 1 (PVNH1) and it is not part of the EDS subtypes under the new 2017 classification of EDS.

RISK FACTORS

The main known risk factor is having a family member who has PVNH found to be secondary to mutations in either the *FNLA* or *ARFGEF2* gene.

ETIOLOGY AND GENETICS

In most cases, PVNH is caused by mutations in the *FLNA* gene. This gene provides instructions for producing the protein filamin A, which helps build the network of protein filaments that gives structure to cells and allows them to change shape and move. Certain mutations in the *FLNA* gene result in an impaired FLNA protein that cannot perform this function, disrupting the normal migration patterns of neurons during brain development.

PVNH can also be caused by mutations in the *ARFGEF2* gene. This gene provides instructions for making a protein that is involved in the movement (trafficking) of small sac-like structures (called vesicles) within the cell. Vesicle trafficking is important in controlling the migration of neurons during the development of the brain. Mutations in the *ARFGEF2* gene may disrupt this function, which could result in the abnormal neuronal migration seen in periventricular heterotopia.

Researchers believe that mutations in the FLNA or ARFGEF2 genes may also result in weakening of the attachments (adhesion) between cells that form the lining of the ventricles. A weakened ventricular lining could allow some neurons to form clumps around the ventricles of the brain while others migrate normally to the exterior of the brain, as seen in periventricular heterotopia.

In a very few cases, periventricular heterotopia has been associated with abnormalities in chromosome 5 inherited in an autosomal dominant manner. In each case, the affected individual had extra genetic material caused by an abnormal duplication of part of this chromosome. It is not known how this duplicated genetic material results in the signs and symptoms of periventricular heterotopia.

Most cases of PVNH are inherited in an X-linked manner. The condition is prenatally or neonatally lethal in most males; therefore, the majority of affected individuals are female. About 50 percent of affected females inherit the pathogenic variant from their mother and at least 50 percent have a *de novo* pathogenic variant. For women with *FLNA*-related PVNH, the risk of passing the pathogenic variant to each child is 50 percent. Because of the high rate of prenatal lethality in males, most sons born to women with *FLNA*-related PVNH are unaffected. Several families with PVNH have also been shown to inherit the disorder in an autosomal recessive fashion; however, this is much less common.

SIGNS AND SYMPTOMS

The signs and symptoms of PVNH usually begin in the teenage years with seizures. Although intelligence is usually normal in individuals with this condition, some may have mild intellectual disability, including difficulties with reading and spelling. There may also be a greater risk for cardiovascular abnormalities, stroke, and other blood vessel and/or blood clotting problems. More common abnormalities may include:

- Cardiovascular defects such as patent ductus arteriosus, dilatation (and possibly eventual rupture and sudden death) of the thoracic aorta, atrial and ventricular septal defects, and abnormalities of heart valves.
- Congenital strabismus (muscle weakness in one eye)

- Shortened digits (fingers and toes)
- Hyperflexible joints
- Pulmonary (lung) disease
- Skin that is too elastic

Less commonly, individuals with X-linked periventricular heterotopia may have other brain findings, gastrointestinal symptoms, and musculoskeletal symptoms similar to those with Ehlers-Danlos syndrome.

Males with this condition experience much more severe symptoms than females, and in most cases die before birth.

SCREENING AND DIAGNOSIS

The development of new onset seizures during the teenage years and a history suggesting others with PVNH or other genetic disorders that are X-linked may lead a clinician to suspect the possibility of PVNH as the underlying problem. The diagnosis of *FLNA*-related PVNH is established by the identification of:

- Characteristic head MRI findings of clumps of misplaced groups of neurons along the linings of the ventricles of the brain beneath an otherwise normal appearing brain cortex; and
- Heterozygous pathogenic variants in the *FLNA* gene in females or hemizygous pathogenic variants in the *FLNA* gene in males. In many, this may be identified using single-gene testing; however, if no pathogenic variant is found, a multi-gene panel may be recommended.

If the pathogenic variant in the family is known, molecular genetic testing can be used to clarify the genetic status of at-risk relatives. If the pathogenic variant in the family is not known, head MRI can be used to clarify the disease status of at-risk relatives.

After the diagnosis is confirmed, it is often recommended to echocardiography and MRI imaging studies to screen for various potential heart and blood vessel abnormalities.

Prenatal diagnosis by molecular genetic testing is possible if the pathogenic variant has been identified in an affected relative.

Given the risk for vascular disease in neurologically asymptomatic individuals, it is appropriate to screen and evaluate the older and younger at-risk relatives of an affected individual in order to identify as early as possible those who would benefit from initiation of treatment and preventive measures.

TREATMENT AND THERAPY

Treatment of epilepsy generally follows principles for a seizure disorder caused by a known structural brain abnormality. If imaging tests of the heart and major blood vessels reveal abnormalities in heart valves, the ascending aorta or other cardiac-related structures, the patient is usually referred to medical and surgical specialists to help manage those defects and to possibly recommend surgical repair.

If a female with PVNH wishes to have children, management generally includes a careful evaluation of prescribed anti-seizure medications and the potential risk for a future fetus. There are currently no guidelines regarding the most appropriate surveillance for and management of cardiac, vascular, and connective tissue problems during pregnancy.

There are several case reports of individuals with *FLNA*-related PVNH who have pulmonary disease resembling bronchopulmonary dysplasia. Although rare, this has led to lung transplantation in several of these young children.

PREVENTION AND OUTCOMES

There is no available method to prevent PVNH, per se. At the same time, effective medical and surgical management of the associated seizure, heart, and blood vessel problems can prevent complications and early death. Many affected individuals demonstrate normal intellect but typically have seizures that will need to be managed throughout their lives. Untreated heart and blood vessel defects may lead to very early death. Although early mortality is much more common in affected males, there are case reports of a few male patients living well past the teen years.

Gary M Flashner MS MD

FURTHER READING

Cardoso C, Boys A, Parrini E, Mignon-Ravix C, McMahon JM, Khantane S, Bertini E, Pallesi E, Missirian C, Zuffardi O, Novara F, Villard L, Giglio S, Chabrol B, Slater HR, Moncla A, Scheffer IE, Guerrini R. "Periventricular heterotopia, mental retardation, and epilepsy associated with 5q14.3-q15 deletion". *Neurology.* 2009;72:784–92

Clapham KR, Yu TW, Ganesh VS, Barry B, Chan Y, Mei D, Parrini E, Funalot B, Dupuis L, Nezarati MM, du Souich C, van Karnebeek C, Guerrini R, Walsh CA. "FLNA genomic rearrangements cause periventricular nodular heterotopia". Neurology. 2012;78:269–78. de Wit MC, de Coo IF, Halley DJ, Lequin MH, Mancini GM. "Movement disorder and neuronal migration disorder due to ARFGEF2 mutation". *Neurogenetics.* 2009;10:333–6.

Lange M, Kasper B, Bohring A, Rutsch F, Kluger G, Hoffjan S, Spranger S, Behnecke A, Ferbert A, Hahn A, Oehl-Jaschkowitz B, Graul-Neumann L, Diepold K, Schreyer I, Bernhard MK, Mueller F, Siebers-Renelt U, Beleza-Meireles A, Uyanik G, Janssens S, Boltshauser E, Winkler J, Schuierer G, Hehr U. "47 patients with *FLNA* associated periventricular nodular heterotopia", *Orphanet Journal of Rare Diseases* 2015 **10**:134

Reinstein E, Frentz S, Morgan T, García-Miñaúr S, Leventer RJ, McGillivray G, Pariani M, van der Steen A, Pope M, Holder-Espinasse M, Scott R, Thompson EM, Robertson T, Coppin B, Siegel R, Bret Zurita M, Rodríguez JI, Morales C, Rodrigues Y, Arcas J, Saggar A, Horton M, Zackai E, Graham JM, Rimoin DL, Robertson SP. "Vascular and connective tissue anomalies associated with X-linked periventricular heterotopia due to mutations in Filamin A". *Eur J Hum Genet.* 2013;21:494–502

Sheen VL, Dixon PH, Fox JW, Hong SE, Kinton L, Sisodiya SM, Duncan JS, Dubeau F, Scheffer IE, Schachter SC, Wilner A, Henchy R, Crino P, Kamuro K, DiMario F, Berg M, Kuzniecky R, Cole AJ, Bromfield E, Biber M, Schomer D, Wheless J, Silver K, Mochida GH, Berkovic SF, Andermann F, Andermann E, Dobyns WB, Wood NW, Walsh CA. "Mutations in the X-linked filamin 1 gene cause periventricular nodular heterotopia in males as well as in females". *Hum Mol Genet.* 2001;10:1775–83

WEB SITES OF INTEREST

https://rarediseases.info.nih.gov/diseases/7371/x-linked-periventricular-heterotopia
https://www.ncbi.nlm.nih.gov/books/NBK1213/
https://ghr.nlm.nih.gov/condition/periventricular-heterotopia#genes
https://www.omim.org/entry/300049

See also: Ehlers-Danlos Syndrome, Fragile X Syndrome, Tuberous Sclerosis

XYY syndrome

CATEGORY: Diseases and syndromes
ALSO KNOWN AS: 47, XYY syndrome; YY syndrome; XYY Karyotype; Jacobs syndrome

DEFINITION

Males with XYY syndrome bear an extra Y chromosome in each cell. The syndrome occurs at fertilization and represents one of several human sex chromosome abnormalities. It causes intellectual and developmental symptoms in some cases, but other than unusually tall stature, does not present other physical features.

RISK FACTORS

Only males are at risk for XYY syndrome. Most cases of the disorder are not inherited but result from a random event during the formation of sperm cells.

ETIOLOGY AND GENETICS

All normal human cells contain forty-six chromosomes consisting of twenty-three pairs; one member of each pair is contributed by the female parent and one by the male. Of these forty-six chromosomes, two chromosomes, designated X and Y, are known as the sex chromosome pair. Individuals with an XX pair are female, while those with an XY pair are male. Unlike the other twenty-two chromosome pairs, the X and Y chromosomes are strikingly different from each other in both size and function. While they chromosome is primarily concerned with maleness, the X chromosome contains information important to both genders.

During formation of sperm and eggs in the testes and ovaries, respectively, a unique form of nuclear division, known as meiosis (or reductional division), occurs during cell division that halves the chromosome number from forty-six to twenty-three. Sperm and eggs thus carry only one member of each pair of chromosomes, and the original number will be restored during fertilization. Because females have an XX pair, their eggs can have only an X chromosome, while males, having an XY pair, produce sperm bearing an X or a Y chromosome.

A common genetic error during sperm or egg production is known as nondisjunction, which is the improper division of chromosomes between the daughter cells. Nondisjunction in the production of either gamete can result, at fertilization, in embryos without the normal forty-six chromosomes. XYY syndrome is one of several of these aneuploid conditions (possession of one or a few more or less than the normal number of chromosomes) that involve the sex chromosome pair. While Klinefelter syndrome (an XXY male) and Turner syndrome (an X female) are more widely studied and recognized genetic diseases, the XYY male occurs with a frequency of 1 in 1,000 male births in the United States. Caused by a Y-bearing sperm fertilizing a normal X-bearing egg, the XYY embryo develops along a seemingly normal route and, unlike most other sex chromosome diseases, is not apparent at birth. The only physical clue is unusually tall stature; otherwise, an affected male will be normal in appearance. The XYY male is also fertile, unlike those with aneuploidies involving other combinations of sex chromosomes, which usually result in sterility.

SYMPTOMS

Boys with XYY syndrome are usually tall, have difficulties with language, and may have slightly lower intelligence quotients (IQs) than other members of their families. They may also develop learning disabilities, hyperactivity, attention deficit disorder, and minor behavioral disorders. A small percentage will have autism spectrum disorder. How having an extra Y chromosome gives rise to these features is not fully understood.

Interest in the association between aggression and the Y chromosome began in the years following World War II. Both psychologists and geneticists began intensive scrutiny of the genes that were located on the male sex chromosome. Men with multiple copies of they chromosome thus became the subjects of much of this research. Genetic links to violent, aggressive, and even criminal behavior were found, although many argued that below-average intelligence played a greater role. Many males with XYY syndrome do perform lower than average on standard intelligence tests and have a greater incidence of behavioral problems. The majority, how ever, lead normal lives and are indistinguishable from XY males.

The controversy surrounding this research began with a study at Harvard University that began in the early 1960's and ended in 1973 because of pressure from both public and scientific communities. The researchers screened all boys born at a Boston hospital, identifying those with sex chromosomal

Karyotype from a male with 47,XYY

© Clinical Tools, Inc.

XYY. public domain via wikimedia commons

This diagram shows the chromosomal nondisjunction in the father that can result in XYY syndrome in his son. The two X chromosomes separate correctly (one per sperm cell), but the shorter Y chromosomes do not separate, which results in one cell with two chv. public domain via wikimedia commons

abnormalities. Because the parents of XYY boys were told of their children's genetic makeup and the possibility of lower intelligence and bad behavior, critics claimed that the researchers had biased the parents against their sons, causing the parents to treat the children differently. The environment would thus play a greater role than genetics in their behavior. Subsequent research has shown that the original hypothesis is at least partially accurate. There is a disproportionately large number of XYY males in prison populations, and they are usually of subaverage intelligence compared to other prisoners. It must be emphasized, however, that the majority of XYY males show neither low intelligence nor criminal behavior.

Scientists, doctors, geneticists, and psychologists now agree that the extra Y chromosome does cause above-normal height, reading and math difficulties, and, in some cases, severe acne, but the explanation of the high prevalence of XYY men in prison populations has changed its focus from genes to environment. Large body size during childhood, adolescence, and early adulthood will no doubt cause people to treat these individuals differently, and they may in turn have learned to use their size defensively. Aggressive behavior, coupled with academic difficulties, may lead to further problems. Clearly, however, the majority of XYY males do well. The issue would be

much easier to resolve if a YY or Y male existed, but because lack of an X chromosome results in spontaneous miscarriage, no YY or Y male embryo could ever survive.

SCREENING AND DIAGNOSIS

Identification of this disorder after a child is born requires that the child receive genetic testing or screening and is often discovered accidentally as a consequence of results from another genetic test. A pregnant woman's cells can be examined by either amniocentesis or chorionicvillus sampling to determine if her child will have XYY syndrome. In amniocentesis, a sample of cells is taken from the amniotic fluid; chorionicvillus sampling examines cells in the placenta.

TREATMENT AND THERAPY

Men with XYY syndrome may require help in school to deal with learning disabilities and behavioral difficulties. Speech, physical, and occupational therapies can also prove beneficial. The support of family members is another important element in helping men cope with this disorder.

PREVENTION AND OUTCOMES

There is no cure for XYY syndrome. However, help in school and a supportive family can reduce the educational and behavioral problems associated with the disorder. Most males with XYY syndrome lead normal lives.

Connie Rizzo, M.D., Ph.D.; updated by Deanna M. Neff, M.P.H.

FURTHER READING

Campos-Acevedo LD, Ibarra-Ramirez M, de Jesús Lugo-Trampe J, de Jesús Zamudio-Osuna M, Torres-Muñoz I, Del Roble Velasco-Campos M. "Dosage of Sex Chromosomal Genes in Blood Deposited on Filter Paper for Neonatal Screening of Sex Chromosome Aneuploidy. Genet Test Mol Biomarkers". 2016;20(12):786–790.

Chen H. XYY Syndrome. "Atlas of Genetic Diagnosis and Counseling, Second Edition". US: Springer; 2012; 2221–2224. Provides an over view of the syndrome, including its genetics, clinical features, diagnostic tests, and genetic counseling issues.

Gruchy N, Blondeel E, Le Meur N, Joly-Hélas G, Chambon P, Till M. "Pregnancy outcomes in prenatally diagnosed 47, XXX and 47, XYY syndromes: a 30–year French, retrospective, multicentre study. Prenat Diagn". 2016;36(6):523–9.

Mader, Sylvia S. "Human Reproductive Biology". 3d ed. Dubuque, Iowa: McGraw-Hill Higher Education, 2005. Provides an excellent introduction to cell division, genetics, and sex from fertilization through birth. Illustrations, bibliography, index.

Simpson, Joe Leigh, and Sherman Elias. "Sex Chromosomal Polysomies (47,XXY; 47,XY Y; 47,XXX), Sex Reversed (46,XX) Males, and Disorders of the Male Reproductive Ducts." In "Genetics in Obstetrics and Gynecology". 3d ed. Philadelphia: Saunders, 2003. Describes how XYY syndrome and other genetic anomalies arise, how they are identified, and the implications of these genetic disorders for patients.

Tamarin, Robert H. "Principles of Genetics". Boston: McGraw-Hill, 2002. A well-written reference text on genetics with complete discussions on aneuploidy, the sex chromosomes, genes, and abnormalities. Includes a thorough reading list, illustrations, maps (some color), index.

Vernice, Mirta, and Anna Cremante. "Life Span Development in XY Y." In "Life Span Development in Genetic Disorders: Behavioral and Neurobiological Aspects". New York: Nova Biomedical Books, 2008. Charts how persons with genetic disorders progress through their life span, from infancy through old age. Discusses the diagnosis and treatment of XYY and other genetic disorders.

WEB SITES OF INTEREST

Association for X and Y Chromosome Variations (AXYS)
http://www.genetic.org

Resources on X and Y anomalies and ways to donate toward research.

Chromosome Disorder Outreach
http://www.chromodisorder.org
Education, advocacy, information, and support.

Genetics Home Reference: 47, XYY Syndrome
http://ghr.nlm.nih.gov/condition

=47XYYsyndrome
A fact sheet on the disorder, describing what it is and the genes related to it. Offers links to additional information.

Johns Hopkins University, Division of Pediatric Endocrinology: Syndromes of Abnormal Sex Differentiation
http://www.hopkinschildrens.org/intersex

Site provides a guide to the science and genetics of sex differentiation, with information about syn dromes of sex differentiation.

Klinefelter Syndrome and Associates (KS&A), Inc.: XYY Syndrome
http://www.genetic.org/knowledge/support/action/201
KS&A provides information and support to per sons who have one or more extra X or Y chromosomes. Its Web site offers access to a range of information about XYY syndrome.

See also: Aggression; Androgen insensitivity syndrome; Behavior; Criminality; Intelligence; Klinefelter syndrome; Metafemales; Nondisjunction and aneuploidy; Steroid hormones; X chromosome in activation.

Z

Zellweger syndrome

CATEGORY: Diseases and syndromes

ALSO KNOWN AS: Zellweger syndrome spectrum (ZSS) (including infantile Refsum disease and neonatal adrenoleukodystrophy); cerebrohepatorenal syndrome; peroxisomal biogenesis disorder; ZWS; ZS; Zellweger leukodystrophy

DEFINITION

The Zellweger syndrome spectrum (ZSS) includes a group of disorders caused by a deficiency in peroxisomal biogenesis. Insufficient peroxisomal function results in multisystem organ dysfunction and subsequent death, typically in childhood.

RISK FACTORS

The ZSS disorders are inherited in an autosomal recessive manner. Individuals with mutations in both copies of any one of the twelve different *PEX genes* known to be associated with ZSS disorders are affected. Full siblings of these individuals have a 25 percent risk of being affected. Males and females are affected with equal frequency. Cases of ZSS disorders have been observed worldwide; no particular ethnic preponderance has been noted. It is estimated to occur in 1 in 50,000 people.

ETIOLOGY AND GENETICS

Peroxisomes are small, membrane-bound organelles found in cells throughout the body. They are involved in a variety of metabolic processes, including the breakdown of toxic substances, such as hydrogen peroxide, and the production of bile acids, necessary for digestion of dietary fats. Peroxisomes are also involved in degradation of very long chain fatty acids (VLCFAs) in a process known as beta-oxidation, essential for energy production. Peroxisomes play a role in the synthesis of certain types of lipids, such as plasmalogens, which are important components of cell membranes in certain tissues (such as the brain).

Proteins necessary for peroxisome function and membrane formation are made within the cell, then transported into existing peroxisomes. Importing these essential proteins prompts growth and division, resulting in the formation of new peroxisomes. In the ZSS disorders, these proteins are unable to be transported into peroxisomes, resulting in decreased biogenesis and function. Diseases affecting peroxisomes are called peroxisome biogenesis disorders.

ZSS disorders are caused by mutations in the PEX genes, which encode these essential proteins, known as peroxins. Though approximately 29 PEX genes have been identified, ZSS disorders have been associated with mutations in only 12 (located at the following chromosomal positions): PEX1 (7q21q22) PEX2 or PXMP3 (8q21.1), PEX3(6q23q24), PEX5(12p13.3), PEX6 (6p21.1), PEX10(1p36.32), PEX12 (17q12), PEX13(2p15), PEX14(1p36.2), PEX16 (11p12p11.2), PEX19 (1q22), and PEX26 (22q11.2). In some cases, the particular gene involved and the type of mutations present are predictive of the ultimate effect on biogenesis and can be associated with clinical severity. Mutations in PEX1 is the most common cause of ZSS, affecting nearly 70 percent of individuals with the disease.

SYMPTOMS

Though once considered separate entities, it is now known that Zellweger syndrome (ZS), neonatal adrenoleukodystrophy (NALD), and infantile Refsum disease (IRD) share a common etiology and represent differing degrees of severity along the Zellweger syndrome spectrum. There is little distinction between these conditions, although historically, severely affected infants were characterized as having ZS and those surviving more than one year and making some type of developmental progress were thought to have NALD or IRD. Zellweger syndrome affects many areas of the body including the skeleton, liver, heart, and kidneys.

The ZSS disorder typically appears during childhood; though extremely rare, presentation in adulthood has been reported. Affected neonates often present with severe hypotonia, failure to thrive, seizures, and liver dysfunction. Some are noted to have distinctive facial features (flattened face, high forehead, and broad nasal bridge) and neuronal migration defects. Bony stippling may also be seen on radiographs. Older children may have additional issues such as hearing loss and/or retinal dystrophy. Affected individuals are noted to have decreased levels of docosahexaenoic acid (DHA), thought to be important in brain development, as well as decreased bile acids, important in normal digestion. Liver dysfunction can result in coagulation problems, and renal failure, thought to be due to renal cysts, can also occur. Severely affected individuals usually make no developmental progress; individuals with milder disease have a wide range of intellectual abilities, with most exhibiting developmental delays. Loss of previously acquired skills occurs in some due to progressive leukodystrophy.

SCREENING AND DIAGNOSIS

Distinctive facial features are often the first sign. Analysis of levels of VLCFAs in the plasma is a useful initial screening test. Affected individuals typically have elevated concentrations of C26:0 and C26:1 and elevated C24/C22 and C26/C22 ratios. Measurements of plasmalogens, phytanic and pristanic acids, pipecolic acid, and plasma bile acids are also helpful in diagnosing ZSS and distinguishing this from other peroxisomal disorders. Confirmation of abnormalities noted on blood samples should be performed on cultured fibroblasts. Ultrasound to look for cysts on the kidneys or enlarged liver may be performed. Documentation of causative mutations in one of the 12 PEX genes associated with ZSS can also further confirm the diagnosis. Carrier and pre-natal testing are possible if the family mutation is known.

TREATMENT and Therapy

Treatment for ZSS disorders remains largely symptomatic by a team of pediatric specialists Treatment focuses on feeding and nutrition, hearing, vision, and management of seizures, liver dysfunction and orthopedic issues. Cow's milk is often avoided to reduce exposure to phytanic acid. Supplementation with bile acids, deficient in ZSS, is currently under investigation and has been shown, anecdotally, to benefit patients. Supplemental DHA has been proposed as a treatment for ZSS, but its clinical effects for growth and liver function have not been proven. Liver transplantation has been attempted in few cases, though long-term clinical outcomes are currently unavailable.

PREVENTION AND OUTCOMES

Most severely affected individuals die before one year of age. Evidence suggests that, of those that survive beyond this point with an apparently stable course, most will survive through early childhood, and survival into young adulthood has been documented. Death in older individuals is typically the result of respiratory complications and/or liver/renal failure.

There is no effective means of prevention for the ZSS disorders. Prenatal testing is typically available for those in which the causative mutations in the index case have been identified or the biochemical abnormalities have been demonstrated on cultured fibroblasts. Individuals with a family history of these disorders should be offered genetic counseling.

Erin Rooney Riggs, M.S.; updated by Deanna M. Neff, M.P.H.

X-Ray image, Neonate with congenital hyperextended knee plus Zellweger-Syndrome By Kinderradiologie Olgahospital Klinikum Stuttgart (Own work), via Wikimedia Commons

Simple diagram of peroxisome. Agateller at the English language Wikipedia, via Wikimedia Commons

FURTHER READING

Ebberink M S, Mooijer PAW, Gootjes J, Koster J, Wanders RJA, Waterham HR. "Genetic classification and mutational spectrum of more than 600 patients with a Zellweger syndrome spectrum disorder. Hum. Mutat". 2011;32: 59–69.

Poll-The, B., et al. "Peroxisome Biogenesis Disorders with Prolonged Survival: Phenotypic Expression in a Cohort of 31 Patients." "American Journal of Medical Genetics" 126A, no. 4 (2004): 333–338.

Steinberg, S., et al. "Peroxisome Biogenesis Disorders." "Biochimica et Biophysica Acta" 1763 (2006):1733–1748.

Wanders, R., et al. "Peroxisomal Disorders I: Biochemistry and Genetics of Peroxisome Biogenesis Dis orders." "Clinical Genetics" 67, no. 2 (2005): 107–133.

WEB SITES OF INTEREST

GeneReviews: Peroxisome Biogenesis Disorders, Zellweger Syndrome Spectrum

http://www.ncbi.nlm.nih.gov/bookshelf/br.fcgi?book=gene&part=pbd

Genetic and Rare Diseases Information Center
https://rarediseases.info.nih.gov/diseases

Genetics Home Reference
https://ghr.nlm.nih.gov/condition

Global Foundation for Peroxisomal Disorders
http://www.thegfpd.org

National Institute of Neurological Disorders and Stroke: Zellweger Syndrome
http://www.ninds.nih.gov/disorders/zellweger/zellweger.htm

United Leukodystrophy Foundation
http://www.ulf.org/types/Zellweger.html

See also: Adrenoleukodystrophy; Alexander disease; Alzheimer's disease; Amyotrophic lateral sclerosis; Arnold-Chiari syndrome; Ataxia telangiectasia; Canavan disease; Cerebrotendinous xanthomatosis; Charcot-Marie-Tooth syndrome; Chediak-Higashi syndrome; Dandy-Walker syndrome; Deafness; Epi lepsy; Essential tremor; Friedreich ataxia; Huntington's disease; Jansky-Bielschowsky disease; Joubert syndrome; Kennedy disease; Krabbé disease; Leigh syndrome; Leukodystrophy; Limb girdle muscular dystrophy; Maple syrup urine disease; Metachromatic leukodystrophy; Myoclonic epilepsy associated with ragged red fibers (MERRF); Narcolepsy; Nemaline myopathy; Neural tube defects; Neurofi bromatosis; Parkinson disease; Pelizaeus-Merzbacher disease; Pendred syndrome; Periodic paralysis syndrome; Prion diseases: Kuru and Creutzfeldt-Jakob syndrome; Refsum disease; Sandhoff disease; San filippo syndrome; Spinal muscular atrophy; Spino cerebellar ataxia; Vanishing white matter disease.

Appendixes

Appendixes

BIOGRAPHICAL DICTIONARY
OF IMPORTANT GENETICISTS

Adams, Jerry McKee (1940-): His research focus is on the genetics of haemopoietic cell differentiation and malignancy. He was a pioneer developer, with Professor Suzanne Cory, his wife, of the gene cloning techniques used to clone mammalian genes successfully. He also codiscovered the mechanism by which antibody genes combine to help the body fight infections.

Allis, Charles David (1951-): His research on covalent modifications of histone tails including acetylation, phosphorylation, ubiquitination, and methylation is the basis for the histone code that may be responsible for the epigenetic regulation of genetic information or gene expression (transcription) from the DNA code.

Alport, Cecil A. (1880-1959): English-born geneticist and physician who first identified a genetic disorder named after him, Alport syndrome, in a British family in the 1920's. This condition, the second most common inherited cause of kidney failure, usually affects young men but can also affect women and older people.

Alström, Carl-Henry (1907-1993): Swedish psychiatrist who first described Alström syndrome, an inherited condition characterized by a progressive loss of vision and hearing, dilated cardiomyopathy, obesity, Type II diabetes mellitus, and short stature.

Altman, Sidney (1939-): Won the 1989 Nobel Prize in Chemistry, with Thomas R. Cech. Working independently, Altman and Cech discovered that RNA, like proteins, can act as a catalyst; moreover, they found that when ribosomal RNA participates in translation of messenger RNA (mRNA) and the synthesis of polypeptides, it acts as a catalyst in some steps.

Ames, Bruce (1928-): He is a recipient of the 1998 National Medal of Science award and inventor of the test for determining if a chemical or compound is a mutagen. The test is named after him, the Ames Test. Ames is also known for his research on cancer and aging.

Anfinsen, Christian B. (1916-1995): Won the 1972 Nobel Prize in Chemistry. Anfinsen, studying the three-dimensional structure of the enzyme ribonuclease, proved that its conformation was determined by the sequence of its amino acids and that to construct a complete enzyme molecule no separate structural information was passed on from the DNA in the cell's nucleus.

Arber, Werner (1929-): First to isolate enzymes that modify DNA and enzymes that cut DNA at specific sites. Such restriction enzymes were critical in the developing field of molecular biology. Arber was awarded the 1978 Nobel Prize in Physiology or Medicine.

Aristotle (384-322 b.c.e.): Greek philosopher and scientist. Aristotle's De Generatione was devoted in part to his theories on heredity. Aristotle believed that the semen of the male contributes a formgiving principle (eidos), while the menstrual blood of the female is shaped by the eidos. The philosophy implied it was the father only who supplied form to the offspring.

Attardi, Giuseppe (1923-2008): Italian American molecular biologist who was awarded the 1998 Gairdner Foundation International Award for his pioneering contribution to the understanding of the structure of the human mitochondrial genome and its role in human disease.

Auerbach, Charlotte (1899-1994): German-born geneticist who fled to England following the rise of the Nazi Party. Demonstrated that the mutations produced by mustard gases and other chemicals in Drosophila (fruit flies) were similar to those induced by X rays, suggesting a common mechanism.

Avery, Oswald Theodore (1877-1955): Immunologist and biologist who determined DNA to be the genetic material of cells. Avery's early work involved classification of the pneumococci, the common cause of pneumonia in the elderly. In 1944, he reported that the genetic information in these bacteria is DNA.

Bailey, Catherine Hayes (1921-2014): By applying methods of selective breeding, she developed new varieties of fruits.

Baltimore, David (1938-): Along with Howard Temin, Baltimore isolated the enzyme RNAdirected DNA polymerase (reverse transcriptase), demonstrating the mechanism by which RNA tumor viruses can integrate their genetic material into the cell chromosome. Baltimore was awarded the 1975 Nobel Prize in Physiology or Medicine.

Barr, Murray Llewellyn (1908-1995): Canadian geneticist who discovered the existence of the Barr (Barr's) body, an inactive X chromosome found in cells from a female. The existence or absence of the body has been used in determining the sex of the individual from whom the cell originated.

Bateson, William (1861-1926): Plant and animal geneticist who popularized the earlier work of Gregor Mendel. In his classic Mendel's Principles of Heredity (1909), Bateson introduced much of the modern terminology used in the field of genetics. Bateson suggested the term "genetics" (from the Greek word meaning "descent") to apply to the field of the study of heredity.

Beadle, George Wells (1903-1989): Beadle's studies of the bread mold Neurospora demonstrated that the function of a gene is to encode an enzyme. Beadle and Edward Tatum were awarded the 1958 Nobel Prize in Physiology or Medicine for their one gene-one enzyme hypothesis.

Beckwith, Jonathan R. (1935-): Determined role of specific genes in regulating bacterial cell division. During the 1960's, he was among the first to isolate a specific gene. Beckwith is also known as a social activist in his arguments for the use of science for improvement of society.

Bell, Julia (1879-1979): British geneticist who applied statistical analysis in understanding hereditary medical disorders of the nervous system and limbs.

Benacerraf, Baruj (1920-2011): Won the 1980 Nobel Prize in Physiology or Medicine, with Jean Dausset and George D. Snell. Benacerraf, Dausset, and Snell each explained the genetic components of the major histocompatibility complex (MHC), the key to a person's immune system, and how the system produces antibodies to such a wide variety of foreign molecules and pathogens, such as viruses, fungi, and bacteria.

Berg, Paul (1926-): Developed DNA recombination techniques for insertion of genes in chromosomes. The techniques became an important procedure in understanding gene function and for the field of genetic engineering. Berg was awarded the 1980 Nobel Prize in Chemistry.

Bishop, John Michael (1936-): Determined that oncogenes, genetic information initially isolated from RNA tumor viruses, actually originate in normal host cells. Bishop was awarded the 1989 Nobel Prize in Physiology or Medicine for his discovery.

Bluhm, Agnes (1862-1943): German physician whose controversial theories on improvement of the "Aryan race" through eugenics and fertility selection provided a basis for Nazi race theories. Among other aspects of her theory was the use of enforced sterilization.

Boring, Alice Middleton (1883-1955): Confirmed existing theories of the chromosomal basis of heredity. Her professional career consisted primarily of serving as a biology teacher to students in China between the world wars.

Borlaug, Norman (1914-2009): Winner of the 1970 Nobel Peace Prize. Borlaug was a key figure in the Green Revolution in agriculture. Working as a geneticist and plant physiologist in a joint Mexican-American program, he developed strains of high-yield, short-strawed, disease-resistant wheat. His goal was to increase crop production and alleviate world hunger.

Botstein, David (1942-): Developed methods of localized mutagenesis for understanding the relationship between the structure and function of proteins. His development of a linkage map involving human genes contributed to the progress of the Human Genome Project.

Boyer, Herbert W. (1936-): His isolation of restriction enzymes that produced a staggered cut on the DNA allowed for creation of so-called "sticky ends," which allowed DNA from different sources or species to be spliced together.

Brenner, Sydney (1927-): Molecular geneticist whose observations of mutations in nematodes (long, unsegmented worms) helped in understanding the design of the nervous system. Brenner was among the first to clone specific genes. He was awarded the Nobel Prize in Physiology or Medicine in 2002.

Bridges, Calvin Blackman (1889-1938): American geneticist whose research on the sex-linked traits in the fruit fly led to the hypothesis, which was eventually proved, that the chromosomes contain genes.

Brink, Royal Alexander (1897-1984): Plant geneticist and breeder at the University of Wisconsin-Madison. His effort led to the development of the Wisconsin maize breeding program, and he created new varieties of clover and alfalfa. Brink was elected to the National Academy of Sciences.

Brown, Michael S. (1941-): By studying the role of cell receptors in uptake of lipids from the blood,

Brown discovered the genetic defect in humans associated with abnormally high levels of cholesterol. He was awarded the 1985 Nobel Prize in Physiology or Medicine.

Buchwald, Manuel (1940-   ): Canadian human molecular geneticist who is a part of the team that owns the U.S. patent for "methods of detecting cystic fibrosis gene by nucleic acid hybridization."

Burnet, Frank Macfarlane (1899-1985): Proposed a theory of clonal selection to explain regulation of the immune response. Burnet was awarded the 1960 Nobel Prize in Physiology or Medicine.

Cairns, John (1922-   ): British virologist whose investigations of rates and mechanisms of DNA replication helped to lay the groundwork in studying the replication process.

Capecchi, Mario Renato (1937-   ): Molecular geneticist who studied the homeobox genes in the mouse. He was a cowinner of the 2007 Nobel Prize in Physiology or Medicine for the discoveries of principles for introducing specific gene modifications in mice by the use of embryonic stem cells.

Carroll, Christiane Mendrez (1937-1978): French geneticist and paleontologist most noted for her taxonomic interpretations of early reptiles.

Cech, Thomas R. (1947-   ): Won the 1989 Nobel Prize in Chemistry, with Sidney Altman. Working independently, Cech and Altman discovered that RNA, like proteins, can act as a catalyst; moreover, Cech found that when ribosomal RNA participates in translation of mRNA and the synthesis of polypeptides, it acts as a catalyst in some steps.

Chargaff, Erwin (1905-2002): Determined that the DNA composition in a cell is characteristic of that particular organism. His discovery of base ratios, in which the concentration of adenine is equal to that of thymine, and guanine to that of cytosine, provided an important clue to the structure of DNA.

Church, George (1954-   ): American molecular geneticist who developed the first commercial genome sequence. He is also the architect of the Human Genome Project and the Personal Genome Project.

Clarke, Sir Cyril Astley (1907-2000): British physician and geneticist and a Fellow of the Royal College of Physicians of London. His pioneering research on Rh disease of the newborn led to the development of prevention techniques.

Cohen, Stanley Norman (1935-   ): Developed the techniques for transfer of DNA between species, a major factor in the process of genetic engineering.

Collins, Francis Sellers (1950-   ): In 1989, Collins identified the gene that, when mutated, results in the genetic disease cystic fibrosis. Collins was instrumental in the identification of a number of genes associated with genetic diseases.

Correns, Carl Erich (1864-1935): German botanist who confirmed Gregor Mendel's laws through his own work on the garden pea. Correns was one of several geneticists who rediscovered Mendel's work in the early 1900's. Crick, Francis Harry Compton (1916-2004): Along with James Watson, Crick determined the double-helix structure of DNA. Crick was awarded the Nobel Prize in Physiology or Medicine in 1962.

Darlington, Cyril (1903-1981): British geneticist who demonstrated changes in chromosomal patterns which occur during meiosis, leading to an understanding of chromosomal distribution during the process. He also described a role played by crossing over, or genetic exchange, in changes of patterns.

Darwin, Charles Robert (1809-1882): Naturalist whose theory of evolution established natural selection as the basis for descent with modification, more commonly referred to as evolution. His classic work on the subject, On the Origin of Species by Means of Natural Selection (1859), based on his five-year voyage during the 1830's on the British ship HMS Beagle, summarized the studies and observations that initially led to the theory. Darwin's pangenesis theory, first noted in The Variation of Animals and Plants Under Domestication (1868), later became the basis for the concept of the gene.

Darwin, Erasmus (1731-1802): British physician, inventor, and writer. In his classic Zoonomia, he advanced a theory of the role of the environment on genetic changes in organisms. A similar theory was later developed by Jean-Baptiste Lamarck. Darwin was the grandfather of both Charles Darwin and Francis Galton.

Dausset, Jean (1916-2009): Won the 1980 Nobel Prize in Physiology or Medicine, with Baruj Benacerraf and George D. Snell. Dausset, Benacerraf, and Snell each explained the genetic components of the major histocompatibility complex (MHC), the key to a person's immune system, and how the system produces antibodies to such a wide variety of foreign molecules and pathogens, such as viruses, fungi, and bacteria.

Delbrück, Max (1906-1981): Leading figure in the application of genetics to bacteriophage research, and later, with Phycomyces, a fungal organism. His bacteriophage course, taught for decades at Cold Spring Harbor, New York, provided training for a generation of biologists. He was awarded the 1969 Nobel Prize in Physiology or Medicine.

Demerec, Milislav (1895-1966): Croatian-born geneticist who was among the scientists who brought the United States to the forefront of genetics research. Demerec's experiments, based on the genetics of corn, addressed the question of what a gene represents. His work with bacteria included the determination of mechanisms of antibiotic resistance, as well as the existence of operons, closely linked genes which are coordinately regulated. Demerec was director of the biological laboratories in Cold Spring Harbor, New York, for many years among the most important sites of genetic research.

De Vries, Hugo (1848-1935): Dutch botanist whose hypothesis of intracellular pangenesis postulated the existence of pangenes, factors which determined characteristics of a species. De Vries established the concept of mutation as a basis for variation in plants. In 1900, de Vries was one of several scientists who rediscovered Mendel's work.

Dobzhansky, Theodosius (1900-1975): Russianborn American geneticist who established evolutionary genetics as a viable discipline. His book Genetics and the Origin of Species (1937) represented the first application of Mendelian theory to Darwinian evolution.

Doherty, Peter C. (1940-): Australian geneticist who, with Rolf Zinkernagel, described the mechanism of the cell-mediated immune defense system of the body. They were awarded the 1996 Nobel Prize in Physiology or Medicine for their discoveries.

Dulbecco, Renato (1914-2012): Among the first to study the genetics of tumor viruses. Dulbecco was awarded the 1975 Nobel Prize in Physiology or Medicine.

Ferguson, Margaret Clay (1863-1951): Plant geneticist whose use of Petunia as a model helped explain life cycles of various plants. Also noted for her description of the life cycle of pine trees.

Fink, Gerald R. (1940-): Isolation of specific mutants in yeast allowed the use of genetics in understanding biochemical mechanisms in that organism.

Fisher, Ronald Aylmer (1890-1962): British biologist whose application of statistics provided a means by which use of small sampling size could be applied to larger interpretations. Fisher's breeding of small animals led to an understanding of genetic dominance. He later applied his work to the study of inheritance of blood types in humans.

Franklin, Rosalind Elsie (1920-1958): British crystallographer whose X-ray diffraction studies helped confirm the double-helix nature of DNA. Franklin's work, along with that of Maurice Wilkins, was instrumental in confirming the structure of DNA as proposed by James Watson and Francis Crick. Franklin's early death precluded her receiving a Nobel Prize for her research.

Galton, Francis (1822-1911): British scientist who was an advocate of eugenics, the belief that human populations could be improved through "breeding" of desired traits. Galton was also the first to observe that fingerprints were unique to the individual.

Garnjobst, Laura Flora (1895-1977): Following her training under Nobel laureate Edward Tatum at both Stanford and Yale, Garnjobst spent her career in the study of genetics of the mold Neurospora.

Garrod, Archibald Edward (1857-1936): Applying his work on alkaptonuria, Garrod proposed that some human diseases result from a lack of specific enzymes. His theory of inborn errors of metabolism, published in 1908, established the genetic basis for certain hereditary diseases.

Gartler, Stanley Michael (1923-): He described the polymorphic nature of some types of protein and, with Walter Nelson-Rees, discovered the contamination of cell lines by HeLa cells.

Gartner, Carl Friedrich von (1772-1850): German plant biologist and geneticist. Though Gartner did not generalize as to the significance of his work, his results provided the experimental basis for questions later developed by Gregor Mendel and Charles Darwin.

Giblett, Eloise R. (1921-2009): Discoverer of numerous genetic markers useful in defining blood groups and serum proteins. In the 1970's, Giblett discovered that certain immunodeficiency diseases result from the absence of certain enzymes necessary for immune cell development.

Gilbert, Walter (1932-): Developed method of sequencing DNA. With Paul Berg and Frederick Sanger, awarded the 1980 Nobel Prize in Chemistry.

Gilman, Alfred G. (1941-2015): Discovered the role of "G" proteins in regulating signal transduction in eukaryotic cells. With Martin Rodbell, won the Nobel Prize in Physiology or Medicine for 1994.

Goldschmidt, Richard B. (1878-1958): Germanborn geneticist who proposed that the chemical makeup of the chromosome determines heredity rather than the quantity of genes. He theorized that large mutations, or "genetic monsters," were important in generation of new species.

Goldstein, Joseph L. (1940-): Won the 1985 Nobel Prize in Physiology or Medicine, with Michael S. Brown. Brown and Goldstein conducted extensive research in the regulation of cholesterol in humans. They showed that in families with a history of high cholesterol, individuals who carry two copies of a mutant gene (homozygotes) have cholesterol levels several times higher than normal and those who have one mutant gene (heterozygotes) have levels about double normal. Their discoveries proved invaluable in managing heart disease and other cholesterol-related ailments.

Griffith, Frederick (1877-1941): British microbiologist who in 1928 reported the existence of a "transforming principle," an unknown substance that could change the genetic properties of bacteria. In 1944, Oswald Avery determined the substance to be DNA, three years after Griffith was killed during the German bombing of London.

Gruhn, Ruth (1907-1988): German geneticist who applied mathematical principles in the breeding of poultry and pigs. Haeckel, Ernst Heinrich (1834-1919): German zoologist whose writings were instrumental in the dissemination of Charles Darwin's theories. Haeckel's "biogenetic law," since discarded, stated that "ontogeny repeats phylogeny," suggesting that embryonic development mirrors the evolutionary relationship of organisms.

Haldane, John Burdon Sanderson (1892-1964): British physiologist and geneticist who proposed that natural selection, and not mutation per se, was the driving force of evolution. Haldane was the first to determine an accurate rate of mutation for human genes, and he later demonstrated the genetic linkage of hemophilia and color blindness.

Hanafusa, Hidesaburo (1929-2009): Japaneseborn scientist who played a key role in elucidating the role of oncogenes found among the RNA tumor viruses in transforming mammalian cells.

Hanawalt, Philip C. (1931-): In 1963, discovered the existence of a repair mechanism associated with DNA replication in bacteria. He later found a similar mechanism in eukaryotic cells. Hanawalt's later work included development of the technique of site mutagenesis in gene mapping.

Hardy, Godfrey Harold (1877-1947): British mathematician who, along with Wilhelm Weinberg, developed the Hardy-Weinberg law of population genetics. In a 1908 letter to the journal Science, Hardy used algebraic principles to confirm Mendel's theories as applied to populations, an issue then currently in dispute.

Hartwell, Leland H. (1939-): Discovered genes that regulate the movement of eukaryotic cells through the cell cycle. With Tim Hunt and Sir Paul Nurse, won the Nobel Prize in Physiology or Medicine in 2001.

Haynes, Robert Hall (1931-1998): Canadian molecular biologist who carried out much of the early work in the understanding of DNA repair mechanisms.

Hershey, Alfred Day (1908-1997): Molecular biologist who played a key role in understanding the replication and genetic structure of viruses. His experiments with Martha Chase confirmed that DNA carried the genetic information in some viruses. Hershey was awarded the 1969 Nobel Prize in Physiology or Medicine.

Herskowitz, Ira (1946-2003): His studies of gene conversion pathways in yeast led to an understanding of gene switching in control of mating types.

Hertwig, Paula (1889-1983): German embryologist who studied the effects of radiation on embryonic development of fish and animals.

Hippocrates (c. 460-377 b.c.e.): Greek physician who proposed the earliest theory of inheritance. Hippocrates believed that "seed material" was carried by body humors to the reproductive organs.

Hogness, David S. (1925-): One of the first to clone a gene from Drosophila (fruit flies). His technique of chromosomal "walking" allowed for the isolation of any known gene based on its ability to mutate. Also involved in identification of homeotic genes, genes which regulate development of body parts.

Holley, Robert William (1922-1993): Determined the sequence of nucleotide bases in transfer RNA (tRNA), the molecule that carries amino acids to ribosomes for protein synthesis. Holley's work provided a means for demonstrating the reading of the genetic code. He was awarded the Nobel Prize in Physiology or Medicine in 1968.

Horvitz, H. Robert (1947-): Harvard neurobiologist whose study of cell regulation in the nematode Caenorhabditis led to the discovery of genes that regulate cell death during embryonic development. With Sydney Brenner and John Sulston, he was awarded the Nobel Prize in Physiology or Medicine in 2002.

Hunt, R. Timothy (1943-): Discovered the existence and role of proteins called cyclins, which regulate the cell cycle in eukaryotic cells. With Leland Hartwell and Sir Paul Nurse, won the Nobel Prize in Physiology or Medicine in 2001.

Jacob, Francois (1920-2013): French geneticist and molecular biologist who, along with Jacques Monod, elucidated a mechanism of gene and enzyme regulation in bacteria. The Jacob-Monod theory of gene regulation became the basis for understanding a wide range of genetic processes; they were awarded the 1965 Nobel Prize in Physiology or Medicine.

Jaenisch, Rudolf (1942-): German geneticist and pioneer of transgenic research including the creation of transgenic mice in the study of cancer and neurological disorders. Rudolf is a leader in the field of therapeutic cloning, and he created the first transgenic mice.

Jeffreys, Sir Alec (1950-): British biochemist who discovered the existence of introns in mammalian genes. His study of the pattern of repeat sequences in DNA was shown to be characteristic of individuals, and became the theoretical basis for DNA fingerprinting and DNA profiles.

Johannsen, Wilhelm L. (1857-1927): Danish botanist who introduced the term "genes," derived from "pangenes," factors suggested by Hugo de Vries to determine hereditary characteristics in plants. Johannsen also introduced the concepts of phenotype and genotype to distinguish between physical and hereditary traits.

Kabat, Elvin Abraham (1914-2000): Pioneer of modern quantitative immunochemistry who described the structure of antibodies as gamma globulins and the structural variation of their combining sites. He was also involved in the characterization of the structures of blood group antigens.

Kenyon, Cynthia (1955-): Discovered the role of specific genes in regulation of cell migration and the aging process in the nematode Caenorhabditis, helping to clarify similar processes in more highly evolved eukaryotic organisms.

Kerr, Warwick Estevam (1922-): Brazilian entomologist and geneticist who applied genetics to the sex determination of bees. Through his research, he created Africanized bees by the hybridization of the African bee and the Italian bee and was responsible for the 1957 release of his experimental, Africanized bee queens, often called "killer bees."

Khorana, Har Gobind (1922-2011): Developed methods for investigating the structure of DNA and deciphering the genetic code. Khorana synthesized the first artificial gene in the 1960's. He was awarded the Nobel Prize in Physiology or Medicine in 1968.

King, Helen Dean (1869-1955): By selective breeding of rodents, developed a method for production of inbred strains of animals for laboratory studies. The methodology was later applied to development of more desirable breeds of horses.

King, Mary-Claire (1946-): American human geneticist who identified breast cancer genes and demonstrated the genetic similarity of the chimpanzees to humans.

Klug, Aaron (1759-1853): Won the 1982 Nobel Prize in Chemistry. Klug used X-ray crystallography to investigate biochemical structures, especially that of viruses. He was able to link the assembly of viral protein subunits with specific sites on viral RNA, which helped in fighting viruses that cause disease in plants and, more basically, in understanding the mechanism of RNA transfer of genetic information. He also determined the structure of transfer RNA (tRNA), which has a shape similar to that of a bent hairpin.

Knight, Thomas Andrew (1759-1853): Plant biologist who first recognized the usefulness of the garden pea for genetic studies because of its distinctive traits. Knight was the first to characterize dominant and recessive traits in the pea, though, unlike Gregor Mendel, he never determined the mathematical relationships among his crosses.

Kölreuter, Josef Gottlieb (1733-1806): Forerunner of Gregor Mendel, Kölreuter demonstrated the sexual nature of plant fertilization, in which characteristics were derived from each member of the parental generation in equivalent amounts.

Kornberg, Arthur (1918-2007): Carried out the first purification of DNA polymerase, the enzyme that replicates DNA. His work on the synthesis of biologically active DNA in a test tube culminated with his being awarded the 1959 Nobel Prize in Physiology or Medicine.

Kossel, Albrecht (1853-1927): Won the 1910 Nobel Prize in Physiology or Medicine. Isolated and described molecular constituents of the cell's nucleus, notably cytosine, thymine, and uracil. These molecules later proved to be constituents of the codons in DNA and RNA. Thus, Kossel's research prepared the way for understanding the biochemistry of genetics.

Lamarck, Jean-Baptiste (1744-1829): French botanist and evolutionist who introduced many of the earliest concepts of inheritance. Lamarck proposed that hereditary changes occur as a result of an organism's needs; his theory of inherited characteristics, since discredited, postulated that organisms transmit acquired characteristics to their offspring.

Leder, Philip (1934-): Along with Marshall Nirenberg, identified the genetic code words for amino acids. His later work has involved the transplantation of human oncogenes into mice, for the purpose of studying the effects of such genes in development of cancer.

Lederberg, Joshua (1925-2008): Established the occurrence of sexual reproduction in bacteria. Lederberg demonstrated that genetic manipulation of the DNA during bacterial conjugation could be used to map bacterial genes. He was awarded the 1958 Nobel Prize in Physiology or Medicine.

Lejeune, Jérôme Jean Louis Marie (1926-1994): French pediatrician and geneticist who discovered the link of diseases to chromosome abnormalities and the link between inadequate intake of folic acid in pregnancy and neural tube defects. He also described trisomy, an extra copy of a chromosome (as with chromosome 21, or Down syndrome).

Levene, Phoebus Aaron (1869-1940): American biochemist who determined the components found in DNA and RNA. Levene described the presence of ribose sugar in RNA and of 2'-deoxyribose in DNA, thereby differentiating the two molecules. He also identified the nitrogen bases found in nucleic acid, though he was never able to determine the acid's molecular structure.

Lewis, Edward B. (1918-2004): Through the use of X-ray-induced mutations in Drosophila (fruit flies), Lewis was able to discover and map genes that regulate embryonic development. Among Lewis's discoveries was the existence of homeotic genes, genes that regulate development of body parts. Along with Christiane Nüsslein-Volhard and Eric Wieschaus, awarded the Nobel Prize in Physiology or Medicine in 1995.

Linnaeus, Carolus (1707-1778): Swedish naturalist and botanist most noted for establishing the modern method for classification of plants and animals. In his Philosophia Botanica (1751; The Elements of Botany, 1775), Linnaeus proposed that variations in plants or animals are induced by environments such as soil.

Luria, Salvador E. (1912-1991): Pioneer in understanding replication and genetic structure in viruses. The Luria-Delbrück fluctuation test, developed by Luria and Max Delbrück, demonstrated that genetic mutations precede environmental selection. Luria was awarded the 1969 Nobel Prize in Physiology or Medicine.

Lwoff, André (1902-1994): French biochemist and protozoologist. Lwoff's early work demonstrated that vitamins function as components of living organisms. He is best known for demonstrating that the genetic material of bacteriophage can become part of the host bacterium's DNA, a process known as lysogeny. Lwoff was awarded the 1965 Nobel Prize in Physiology or Medicine.

Lykken, David Thoreson (1928-2006): He was a behavioral geneticist and a principal investigator on the Minnesota Twin Family Study, which seeks to identify the genetic and environmental influences on the development of psychological traits in identical and fraternal twins through a birth record-based registry.

Lyon, Mary Francis (1925-2014): British cytogeneticist who proposed what became known as the Lyon hypothesis, that only a single X chromosome is active in a cell. Any other X chromosomes are observed as Barr bodies.

McClintock, Barbara (1902-1992): Demonstrated the existence in plants of transposable elements, or transposons, genes that "jump" from one place on a chromosome to another. The process was discovered to be widespread in nature. McClintock was awarded the 1983 Nobel Prize in Physiology or Medicine.

Macklin, Madge Thurlow (1893-1962): Developed a method to apply statistical analysis to understanding congenital diseases in human families. Her arguments were used to introduce genetics as a component of the curriculum in medical schools. Her support of eugenics for improvement of humans later made her views controversial.

McKusick, Victor A. (1921-2008): Cataloged and indexed many of the genes responsible for disorders that are passed in Mendelian fashion.

Margulis, Lynn (1938-2011): Developed the endosymbiont theory, which suggests that internal eukaryotic organelles, such as mitochondria and chloroplasts, originated as free-living prokaryotic ancestors. She proposed that free-living bacteria became incorporated in a larger, membrane-bound structure and developed a symbiotic relationship within the larger cell.

Mendel, Johann Gregor (1822-1884): The "father of genetics," Mendel was an Austrian monk whose studies on the transmission of traits in the garden pea established the mathematical basis of inheritance. Mendel's pioneering theories, including such fundamental genetic principles as the law of segregation and the law of independent assortment, were published in 1866 but received scant attention until the beginning of the twentieth century.

Meselson, Matthew Stanley (1930-): Demonstrated the nature of DNA replication, in which the two parental DNA strands are separated, each passing into one of the two daughter molecules. Also noted as a social activist.

Meyerowitz, Elliot M. (1951-): Discovered roles played by specific genes in differentiation of the plant Arabidopsis, as well as genes which regulate flowering in plants.

Miescher, Johann Friedrich (1844-1895): In 1869, Miescher discovered and purified DNA from cellfree nuclei obtained from white blood cells and gave the name "nuclein" to the extract. The substance was later known as nucleic acid.

Mintz, Beatrice (1921-): Noted for studies of the role of gene control in differentiation of cells and disease in humans. Developed a mouse model for the understanding of melanoma development in humans.

Monod, Jacques Lucien (1910-1976): French geneticist and molecular biologist who, with François Jacob, demonstrated a method of gene regulation in bacteria that came to be known as the Jacob-Monod model. Jacob and Monod were jointly awarded the 1965 Nobel Prize in Physiology or Medicine.

Moore, Stanford (1913-1982): Won the 1972 Nobel Prize in Chemistry, with William H. Stein. Moore and Stein supplemented Christian Anfinsen's research by identifying the sequence of amino acids in ribonuclease, a clue to the structure of the gene responsible for it.

Morgan, Lilian Vaughan (1870-1952): Discovered the attached X and ring X chromosomes in Drosophila (fruit flies). Later contributed to studying the effects of polio vaccines in primates. Married to Thomas Hunt Morgan.

Morgan, Thomas Hunt (1866-1945): Considered the father of modern genetics, an embryologist whose studies of fruit flies (Drosophila melanogaster) established the existence of genes on chromosomes. Through his selective breeding of flies, Morgan also established concepts such as gene linkage, sexlinked characteristics, and genetic recombination. Won the 1933 Nobel Prize in Physiology or Medicine.

Müller, Hermann Joseph (1890-1967): Geneticist and colleague of Thomas Hunt Morgan. Muller's experimental work with fruit flies established the gene as the site of mutation. His work with X rays demonstrated a means of artificially introducing mutations into an organism. Won the 1946 Nobel Prize in Physiology or Medicine.

Mullis, Kary Banks (1944-): Devised the polymerase chain reaction (PCR), a method for duplicating small quantities of DNA. The PCR procedure became a major tool in research in the fields of genetics and molecular biology. Mullis was awarded the 1993 Nobel Prize in Chemistry.

Nathans, Daniel (1928-1999): Applied the use of restriction enzymes to the study of genetics. Nathans developed the first genetic map of SV40, among the first DNA viruses shown to transform normal cells into cancer. Nathans was awarded the 1978 Nobel Prize in Physiology or Medicine.

Neel, James Van Gundia (1915-2000): Considered to be the father of human genetics. Among his discoveries was the recognition of the genetic basis of sickle-cell disease. He was also noted for his study of the aftereffects of radiation on survivors of the atomic attack on Hiroshima and Nagasaki in World War II. He was the first to propose what was referred to as the thrifty-gene hypothesis, the idea that potentially lethal genes may have been beneficial to the human population earlier in evolution.

Neitz, Jay (1953-): Ophthalmologist and color vision researcher in the field of functional genomics. With his wife Maureen, codiscovered the genes responsible for color blindness and defined examples of nervous system defect for which the DNA can be used to predict the occurrence and the severity of color blindness.

Neitz, Maureen (1957-): Ophthalmologist and color vision researcher who codiscovered the genes responsible for color blindness and defined examples of nervous system defect for which the DNA can be used to predict the occurrence and the severity of color blindness.

Nelson, Oliver Evans, Jr. (1920-2001): During the 1950's, carried out the first structural analysis of a gene in higher plants (corn), at the same time confirming the existence of transposable elements. His later work demonstrated the genetic significance of enzymatic defects in maize.

Neufeld, Elizabeth F. (1928-): French-born biochemist who found that many mucopolysaccharide storage diseases resulted from the absence of certain metabolic enzymes. Her work opened the way for prenatal diagnosis of such diseases.

Nirenberg, Marshall Warren (1927-2010): Molecular biologist who was among the first to decipher the genetic code. He later demonstrated the process of ribosome binding in protein synthesis and carried out the first cell-free synthesis of protein. Nirenberg was awarded the 1968 Nobel Prize in Physiology or Medicine.

Nurse, Sir Paul M. (1949-): British scientist who discovered the role of chemical modification (phosphorylation) in regulation of the cell cycle. With Tim Hunt and Leland Hartwell, he was awarded the Nobel Prize in Physiology or Medicine in 2001.

Nüsslein-Volhard, Christiane (1942-): German biologist whose genetic studies in Drosophila (fruit flies) led to the discovery of genes that regulate body segmentation in the embryo. Along with Edward Lewis and Eric Wieschaus, won the Nobel Prize in Physiology or Medicine in 1995.

Ochoa, Severo (1905-1993): Won the 1959 Nobel Prize in Physiology or Medicine, with Arthur Kornberg. Ochoa and Kornberg isolated enzymes involved in the synthesis of DNA and RNA, representing the first steps in decoding the biochemical instructions preserved in the structure of genes.

Ohno, Susumu (1928-2000): Asian American geneticist and evolutionary biologist. In 1970, he postulated that gene duplication plays an important role in molecular evolution and that the vertebrate genome is a result of duplications of the entire genome. He also proposed that the gene content of the mammalian species has been conserved over species not only in DNA content but also in the genes themselves—that is, nearly all mammalian species have conserved the X chromosome from their primordial X chromosome of a common ancestor (Ohno's law).

Olson, Maynard V. (1943-): Studied basepair polymorphisms in the human genome and their significance to evolution. In 1987, with David Burke, Olson developed a new type of cloning vector, artificial chromosomes, that filled the need created by the Human Genome Project to clone very large insert DNAs (hundreds of thousands to millions of base pairs in length).

Patau, Klaus (1908-1975): German-born American geneticist who first reported a congenital disorder associated with the presence of an extra copy of chromosome 13 in 1960. The extra chromosome 13 causes numerous physical and mental abnormalities in a condition known as Patau syndrome or Bartholin-Patau syndrome, after Thomas Bartholin, a French physician who described the clinical picture associated with trisomy 13 in 1656.

Pauling, Linus (1901-1994): American chemist who received the Nobel Prize in Chemistry in 1954 for his work on the nature of the chemical bond and the 1962 Nobel Peace Prize for his antinuclear activism. His 1950's investigations of protein structure contributed to the determination of the structure of DNA.

Punnett, Reginald C. (1875-1967): English biologist who collaborated with William Bateson in a series of important breeding experiments that confirmed the principles of Mendelian inheritance. Punnett also introduced the Punnett square, the standard graphical method of depicting hybrid crosses.

Rahbar, Samuel (1929-2012): Iranian director at the University of Tehran, who became known as the most important immunologist in the Muslim world.

Roberts, Richard J. (1943-): Discovered that genes in eukaryotic cells and animal viruses are often discontinuous, with intervening sequences between segments of genetic material. With Phillip Sharp, Roberts received the Nobel Prize in Physiology or Medicine in 1993.

Rodbell, Martin (1925-1998): Discovered the role of membrane-bound "G" proteins in regulation of signal transduction in eukaryotic cells. With Alfred Gilman, awarded the Nobel Prize in Physiology or Medicine in 1994.

Rowley, Janet (1925-2013): Cytogeneticist who developed the staining techniques for observation of cell structures. She demonstrated the role of chromosomal translocation as the basis for chronic myeloid leukemia, the first example of translocation as a cause of cancer.

Rubin, Gerald M. (1950-): Major figure in developing a structure/functional relationship of genes in Drosophila (fruit flies) through the use of insertion mutagenesis to inactivate specific genes.

Russell, Elizabeth Shull (1913-2001): Contributed to the understanding of the role played by specific genes in creating coat variations in animals. Her later work involved the identification of genetic defects in the aging process and in the development of diseases such as muscular dystrophy.

Russell, William (1910-2003): Pioneer in the genetic effects of radiation at Oak Ridge National Laboratory whose testing of mice led to standards for acceptable levels of human exposure to radiation. Winner of the 1976 Fermi Award.

Sager, Ruth (1918-1997): During the 1950's, demonstrated the existence of nonchromosomal heredity, also known as cytoplasmic inheritence, and hence the role of cytoplasmic genes in organelle development. Later involved in study of tumor suppressor and breast cancer genes.

Sageret, Augustin (1763-1851): French botanist who discovered the ability of different traits to segregate independently in plants.

Sanger, Frederick (1918-2013): Determined the method for sequencing DNA. His method separated the strands of DNA and then rebuilt them in stages that allowed the terminal nucleotides to be identified. This made it possible to sequence the entire genomes of organisms. With Paul Berg and Walter Gilbert, Sanger received the 1980 Nobel Prize in Chemistry.

Sharp, Phillip A. (1944-): Discovered that genes in eukaryotic cells or animal viruses are discontinuous, with segments divided by sections separated by intervening sequences of genetic material. With Richard Roberts, received the Nobel Prize in Physiology or Medicine in 1993.

Simpson, George Gaylord (1902-1984): American paleontologist who applied population genetics to the study of the evolution of animals. Simpson was instrumental in establishing a neo-Darwinian theory of evolution (the rejection of Jean-Baptiste Lamarck's inheritance of acquired characteristics) during the early twentieth century.

Singer, Maxine (1931-): Applied the use of the newly discovered restriction enzymes in formation of recombinant DNA. Singer is most noted as a "voice of calm" in the debate over genetic research, emphasizing the application of such research and the self-policing of scientists carrying out such work.

Smith, Hamilton Othanel (1931-): Pioneered the purification of restriction enzymes, winning the 1978 Nobel Prize in Physiology or Medicine, with Werner Arber and Daniel Nathans. Arber and the team of Nathans and Smith separately described the restriction-modification system by studying bacteria and bacteriophages; the system involves the action of site-specific endonuclease and other enzymes that cleave DNA into segments.

Smith, Michael (1932-2000): Won the 1993 Nobel Prize in Chemistry. Smith developed site-directed mutagenesis, a means for reconfiguring genes in order to create altered proteins with distinct properties. Smith's genetic engineering tool made it possible to treat genetic disease and cancer and to create novel plant strains.

Snell, George D. (1903-1996): Snell's discovery of the H-2 histocompatibility complex, which regulates the immune response in mice, led to the later discovery of the equivalent HLA complex in humans. Awarded the Nobel Prize in Physiology or Medicine in 1980.

Sonneborn, Tracy Morton (1905-1981): Discovered crossbreeding and mating types in paramecia, integrating the genetic principles as applied to multicellular organisms with single-celled organisms such as protozoa.

Spector, David L. (1952-): Through research on live cell imaging of gene expression and noncoding RNAs, developed a live-cell gene expression system to visualize a stably integrated regulatable genetic locus and follow in real-time transcription of that locus, including visualization of its mRNA and protein products in living cells.

Spemann, Hans (1869-1941): Won the 1935 Nobel Prize in Physiology or Medicine. By transplanting bits of one embryo into a second, viable embryo, Spemann compiled evidence that an "organizer center" directs the development of an embryo and that different parts of the organizer governed distinct portions of the embryo. His experiments provided clues to the genetic control of growth from the earliest stages of an organism.

Spencer, Herbert (1820-1903): English philosopher influenced by the work of Charles Darwin. Spencer proposed the first general theory of inheritance, postulating the existence of self-replicating units within the individual which determine the traits. Spencer is more popularly known as the source of the notion of "survival of the fittest" as applied to natural selection.

Stanley, Wendell Meredith (1904-1971): American biochemist who was the first to crystallize a virus (tobacco mosaic virus), demonstrating its protein nature. Stanley was later a member of the team that determined the amino acid sequence of the TMV protein. Stanley spent the last years of his long career studying the relationship of viruses and cancer.

Stein, William H. (1911-1980): Won the 1972 Nobel Prize in Chemistry, with Stanford Moore. Stein and Moore supplemented Christian Anfinsen's research by identifying the sequence of amino acids in ribonuclease, a clue to the structure of the gene responsible for it.

Stevens, Nettie Maria (1861-1912): Discovered the existence of the specific chromosomes that determine sex, now known as the X and Y chromosomes. Described the existence of chromosomes as paired structures within the cell.

Strobell, Ella Church (1862-1920): Developed the technique of photomicroscopy for analysis of chromosomal theory.

Sturtevant, Alfred Henry (1891-1970): Colleague of Thomas Hunt Morgan and among the pioneers in application of the fruit fly (Drosophila) in the study of genetics. In 1913, Sturtevant constructed the first genetic map of a fruit fly chromosome. His work became a major factor in chromosome theory. In the 1930's, his work with George Beadle led to important observations of meiosis.

Sulston, John E. (1942-): Developed the first map of cell lineages in the model nematode Caenorhabditis, leading to the discovery of the first gene associated with programmed cell death. Sulston was also part of the team that sequenced the worm's genome. With Sydney Brenner and H. Robert Horvitz, he was awarded the Nobel Prize in Physiology or Medicine in 2002.

Sutton, Walter Stanborough (1877-1916): Biologist and geneticist who demonstrated the role of chromosomes during meiosis in gametes, and demonstrated their relationship to Gregor Mendel's laws. Sutton observed that chromosomes form homologous pairs during meiosis, with one member of each pair appearing in gametes. The particular member of each pair was subject to Mendel's law of independent assortment.

Tammes, Jantine (1871-1947): Dutch geneticist who demonstrated that the inheritance of continuous characters, traits that have a range of expression, could be explained in a Mendelian fashion. She developed a multiple allele hypothesis that helped explain some of the data.

Tan Jiazhen (C. C. Tan; 1909-2008): Considered the father of Chinese genetics. In a career spanning more than seven decades, Tan studied genetic structure and variation in a wide range of organisms. His most important work involved the study of evolution of genetic structures in Drosophila (fruit flies), as well as the concept of mosaic dominance in the beetle.

Tatum, Edward Lawrie (1909-1975): Along with George Beadle, Tatum demonstrated that the function of a gene is to encode an enzyme. Beadle and Tatum were awarded the 1958 Nobel Prize in Physiology or Medicine for their one gene-one enzyme hypothesis.

Temin, Howard Martin (1934-1994): Proposed that RNA tumor viruses replicate by means of a DNA intermediate. Temin's theory, initially discounted, became instrumental in revealing the process of infection and replication by such viruses. He later isolated the replicating enzyme, the RNA-directed DNA polymerase (reverse transcriptase). He was awarded the 1975 Nobel Prize in Physiology or Medicine, along with David Baltimore, for this work.

Todd, Alexander Robertus (1907-1997): Won the 1957 Nobel Prize in Chemistry. As part of wideranging research in organic chemistry, Todd revealed how ribose and deoxyribose bond to the nitrogenous bases on one side of a nucleotide unit and to the phosphate group on the other side. These discoveries provided necessary background for work by others that explained the structure of the DNA molecule.

Tonegawa, Susumu (1939-): Discovered the role of genetic rearrangement of DNA in lymphocytes, which plays a key role in generation of antibody diversity.

In 1987, awarded the Nobel Prize in Physiology or Medicine.

Varmus, Harold Elliot (1939-): Elucidated the molecular mechanisms by which retroviruses (RNA tumor viruses) transform cells. Varmus was awarded the 1989 Nobel Prize in Physiology or Medicine.

Waelsch, Salome Gluecksohn (1907-2007): Studied the role genes play in abnormal cell differentiation and congenital abnormalities. Born in Germany, she fled to the United States from the Nazis in 1933. Her 1938 publication of the role of genes in the T (tailless) phenotype in mice is considered a genetic classic.

Waterston, Robert (1943-): Identified many of the genes that regulate muscle development in the nematode Caenorhabditis, as well as contributing to the sequence of the genome. His sequencing work was also applied in the Human Genome Project led by Francis Collins.

Watson, James Dewey (1928-): Along with Francis Crick, determined the double-helix structure of DNA. Together with Crick and Maurice Wilkins, Watson was awarded the 1962 Nobel Prize in Physiology or Medicine for their work in determining the structure of DNA.

Weinberg, Robert Allan (1942-): Molecular biologist who isolated the first human oncogene, the ras gene, associated with a variety of cancers, including those of the colon and brain. Weinberg later isolated the first tumor-suppressor gene, the retinoblastoma gene. Weinberg is considered one of the leading researchers in understanding the role played by oncogenes in development of cancer.

Weinberg, Wilhelm (1862-1937): German obstetrician who demonstrated that hereditary characteristics of humans such as multiple births and genetic diseases were subject to Mendel's laws of heredity. The mathematical application of such characteristics, published simultaneously (and independently) by Godfrey Hardy, became known as the Hardy-Weinberg equilibrium. The equation demonstrates that dominant genes do not replace recessive genes in a population; gene frequencies would not change from one generation to the next if certain criteria such as random mating and lack of natural selection were met.

Weismann, August (1834-1914): German zoologist noted for his chromosome theory of heredity.

Weismann proposed that the source of heredity is in the nucleus only and that inheritance is based on transmission of a chemical or molecular substance from one generation to the next. Weismann's theory, which rejected the inheritance of acquired characteristics, came to be called neo-Darwinism. Though portions of Weismann's theory were later disproved, the nature of the chromosome was subsequently demonstrated by Thomas Hunt Morgan and his colleagues.

Wieschaus, Eric F. (1947-): Wieschaus's studies of genetic control in Drosophila (fruit flies) led to the discovery of genes that regulate cell patterns and shape in the embryo. Along with Edward Lewis and Christiane Nüsslein-Volhard, he was awarded the Nobel Prize in Physiology or Medicine in 1995.

Wilkins, Maurice Hugh Frederick (1916-2004): Studies on the X-ray diffraction patterns exhibited by DNA confirmed the double-helix structure of the molecule. Wilkins was a colleague of Rosalind Franklin, and it was their work that confirmed the nature of DNA as proposed by James Watson and Francis Crick. Wilkins was awarded the Nobel Prize for Physiology and Medicine in 1962, along with Watson and Crick.

Wilmut, Ian (1944-): Scottish embryologist and leader of a research team at the Roslin Institute near Edinburgh. In 1996, Wilmut and his colleagues succeeded in cloning an adult sheep, Dolly, the first adult mammal to be successfully produced by cloning.

Wilson, Edmund Beecher (1856-1939): His study of chromosomes in collaboration with Nettie Stevens led to the discovery of the X and Y chromosomes, playing a key role in the foundation of modern genetics. His later work involved the study of development and differentiation of the fertilized egg.

Witkin, Evelyn Maisel (1921-): Through her studies of induced or spontaneous mutations in bacterial DNA, discovered processes of enzymatic repair of DNA.

Woese, Carl R. (1928-2012): Based on his studies of ribosomal RNA differences in prokaryotes and eukaryotes, proposed that all life-forms exist in one of three domains: Bacteria, Archaea ("ancient" bacteria), and Eukarya (eukaryotic organisms, from microscopic plants to large animals). Woese expanded his theory in arguing that the Archaea represent the earliest form of life on Earth and that they later formed a branch which became the eukaryotes.

Wright, Sewall (1889-1988): Discovered genetic drift of genetic traits. The "Sewall Wright" effect, the random drift of characters in small populations, was explained by the random loss of genes, even in the absence of natural selection.

Yanofsky, Charles (1925-): Confirmed that the genetic code involved groups of three bases by demonstrating colinearity of the bases and amino acid sequences. He applied this work in demonstrating similar colinearity of mutations in the tryptophan operon and changes in amino acid sequences.

Zinder, Norton (1928-2012): With Joshua Lederberg, discovered the role of bacteriophage in transduction, the movement of genes from one host to another by means of viruses. Zinder was also noted for his discovery of RNA bacteriophage and his work on the molecular genetics of such agents.

Zinkernagel, Rolf Martin (1944-): Swiss geneticist who, with Peter C. Doherty, described the mechanism of the cell-mediated immune defense system of the body. They were awarded the 1996 Nobel Prize in Physiology or Medicine for their discoveries concerning the specificity of the cell-mediated immune defense.

Richard Adler, Ph.D.;
updated by Oladayo Oyelola, Ph.D., S.C. (ASCP)

NOBEL PRIZES FOR DISCOVERIES IN GENETICS

1910

Albrecht Kossel (German). Isolated and described molecular constituents of the cell's nucleus, notably cytosine, thymine, and uracil. These molecules later proved to be constituents of the codons in deoxyribonucleic acid (DNA) and ribonucleic acid (RNA). Thus, Kossel's research prepared the way for understanding the biochemistry of genetics.

1933

Thomas Hunt Morgan (American). Experimenting with the fruit fly Drosophila melanogaster, Morgan discovered that the mechanism for the Mendelian laws of heredity lies in the chromosomes inside the nucleus of cells and that specific genes on the chromosomes govern specific somatic traits in the flies. He confirmed the accuracy of Gregor Mendel's laws and ended a controversy over their physiological source.

1935

Hans Spemann (German). By transplanting bits of one embryo into a second, viable embryo, Spemann compiled evidence that an "organizer center" directs the development of an embryo and that different parts of the organizer governed distinct portions of the embryo. His experiments provided clues to the genetic control of growth from the earliest stages of an organism.

1946

Hermann J. Muller (American). Muller proved that X rays damage genes by altering their structure: radiation-induced mutation. Consequently, X rays also modify the structure of chromosomes. The mutations most often produce recessive and harmful traits in the irradiated organism.

1958

George Beadle and Edward Tatum (both American). In research on the fungus Neurospora crassa, Beadle and Tatum found that biotin was essential to cultivating certain mutant strains of the fungus; this fact demonstrated that genes regulate the synthesis of specific cellular chemicals, one or more of these genes being mutated in the biotin-dependent strain.

1958

Joshua Lederberg (American). Lederberg showed that the bacterium Escherichia coli, although not able to reproduce sexually, is capable of genetic recombination between chromosomes from different cells through a process called conjugation.

1959

Severo Ochoa (Spanish) and Arthur Kornberg (American). Ochoa and Kornberg isolated enzymes involved in the synthesis of DNA and RNA, representing the first steps in decoding the biochemical instructions preserved in the structure of genes.

1960

Frank Macfarlane Burnet (Australian) and Peter Brian Medawar (British). Burnet proposed a theory of clonal selection, confirmed by Medawar, to explain regulation of the immune response.

1962

Francis Crick (British), James Watson (American), and Maurice Wilkins (British). Using X-ray diffraction analysis and molecular modeling, Wilkins, Crick, and Watson found that DNA is structured in a double helix. They were able to identify the specific three-dimensional structure that is the basis for the ability of DNA to be replicated and transcribed.

1965

François Jacob and Jacques Monod (both French). Studying enzyme action, Jacob and Monod proved that messenger ribonucleic acid (mRNA) carries instructions from the nucleus to ribosomes, where molecules are assembled for use in the body, and they distinguished structural genes from regulatory genes.

1965

André Lwoff (French). Lwoff proposed that viral DNA can become active after invading cells and cause the cells to divide out of control, producing cancerous tumors.

1968

Robert W. Holley (American), Har Gobind Khorana (Indian), and Marshall W. Nirenberg (American). Working separately, Holley, Khorana, and Nirenberg deciphered the genetic code in RNA and DNA. Their work anticipated DNA sequencing and genetic engineering.

1969

Max Delbrück (German), Alfred D. Hershey (American), and Salvador E. Luria (Italian). In joint studies of bacteriophages and their bacterial hosts, Delbrück, Hershey, and Luria described the conformation of bacteriophage DNA, showed that different strains exchange genetic information, and proved that bacterial DNA mutated to confer protection from attack, demonstrating that bacterial heredity is based on genetic exchange. The discovery explained why bacteria gradually become resistant to pharmaceuticals.

1975

David Baltimore and Howard M. Temin (both American). Working separately, Baltimore and Temin discovered reverse transcriptase, the enzyme that inserts viral DNA into cellular DNA, which can cause cancer, They also identified retroviruses, a class of virus that includes the human immunodeficiency virus (HIV) that causes acquired immunodeficiency syndrome (AIDS).

1975

Renato Dulbecco (Italian). Dulbecco described how tumor viruses cause cellular transformation in somatic cells by suppressing the regulatory system that controls division; the cells then divide out of control.

1978

Werner Arber (Swiss), Daniel Nathans (American), and Hamilton O. Smith (American). Arber and the team of Nathans and Smith separately described the restriction-modification system by studying bacteria and bacteriophages; the system involves the action of site-specific endonuclease and other enzymes that cleave DNA into segments.

1980

Baruj Benacerraf (Venezuelan), Jean Dausset (French), and George D. Snell (American). Benacerraf, Dausset, and Snell each explained the genetic components of the major histocompatibility complex (MHC), the key to a person's immune system, and how the system produces antibodies to such a wide variety of foreign molecules and pathogens, such as viruses, fungi, and bacteria.

1983

Barbara McClintock (American). McClintock investigated the genetics of maize (corn) and discovered a new mechanism of gene modification: Some "jumping genes" (now called transposable elements or transposons) move to new sites on chromosomes and either suppress nearby structural genes or inactivate suppressor genes. The discovery was a major breakthrough in understanding novel, non-Mendelian types of genetic variation.

1985

Michael S. Brown and Joseph L. Goldstein (both American). Brown and Goldstein conducted extensive research in the regulation of cholesterol in humans. They showed that in families with a history of high cholesterol, individuals who carry two copies of a mutant gene (homozygotes) have cholesterol levels several times higher than normal and those who have one mutant gene (heterozygotes) have levels about double normal. Their discoveries proved invaluable in managing heart disease and other cholesterol-related ailments.

1987

Susumu Tonegawa (Japanese). Tonegawa explained the diversity of antibodies by showing that the antigen-sensitive part of each antibody is created by segments of three genes; since the segments from each gene can vary in length, the possible combinations from three genes can produce billions of distinct antibodies.

1989

J. Michael Bishop and Harold E. Varmus (both American). Bishop and Varmus discovered that oncogenes (genes that play a role in initiating cancer) originate in normal cells and control cellular growth and are not solely derived from retroviruses, as previously thought. Their work greatly influenced subsequent studies of tumor development.

1993

Richard J. Roberts (British) and Phillip A. Sharp (American). Roberts and Sharp separately studied the relationship between DNA and RNA. They discovered that portions of a human gene can be divided among several DNA segments, called introns, separated by noncoding segments called exons. This discovery became important to genetic engineering and to understanding the mechanism for hereditary diseases.

1994

Alfred G. Gilman and Martin Rodbell (both American). Gilman and Rodbell discovered the role of "G" proteins in regulating signal transduction in eukaryotic cells.

1995

Edward B. Lewis (American). Lewis found that an array of master genes governs embryo development.

1995

Christiane Nüsslein-Volhard (German) and Eric F. Wieschaus (American). Nüsslein-Volhard and Wieschaus worked together to extend Lewis's investigations into the genetic control of embryo development through studies of fruit flies. They isolated more than five thousand participating genes and distinguished four types of "master" control genes: gap, pair-rule, segment polarity, and even-skipped.

1996

Peter C. Doherty (Australian) and Rolf Zinkernagel (Swiss). Doherty and Zinkernagel described the mechanism of the cell-mediated immune defense.

2001

Leland H. Hartwell (American), R. Timothy Hunt (British), and Paul M. Nurse (British). Hartwell, Hunt, and Nurse conducted research on the regulation of cell cycles. Hartwell identified a class of genes that controls the cycle, including a gene that initiates it. Nurse cloned and described the genetic model of a key regulator, cyclin-dependent kinase, while Hunt discovered cyclins, a class of regulatory proteins.

2002

Sydney Brenner (American). Brenner used the transparent nematode *Caenorhabditis elegans* to establish a simple model organism for studying how genes control the development of organs.

2002

John E. Sulston (British). Sulston studied cell division and cell lineages in *Caenorhabditis elegans* following Brenner's methods. He demonstrated that genetic control of specific lineages includes programmed cell death, called apoptosis, as part of the regulatory process, and he isolated the protein that degrades the DNA of dead cells.

2002

H. Robert Horvitz (American). Using Brenner's *Caenorhabditis elegans* model, Horvitz discovered the first two "death genes" which instigate cell death. He further found that another gene helps protect cells from cell death.

2004

Richard Axel and Linda B. Buck (both American). Working as collaborators in Axel's laboratory, the two researchers discovered the extensive gene family which encodes odorant receptors in rats. They initially determined that more than one hundred related gene products are involved in detection of odors. Ultimately, Axel and Buck were able to identify approximately 1,000 different genes, constituting nearly 3 percent of the total genetic material in the cell, which encode odor receptors on the surface of cells in the nasal epithelium.

2005

Barry J. Marshall and J. Robin Warren (both Australian). Historically, peptic ulcers were successfully treated using standard procedures that inhibited acid production but routinely returned in more than 50 percent of patients. Warren, a pathologist, had observed the presence of an unusual curveshaped bacterium in the stomach of these patients. Marshall began a clinical collaboration with Warren in which they demonstrated the relationship between a newly discovered bacterium, *Helicobacter pylori*, and inflammation leading to ulcers. Infection may lead to stomach cancer as well. Warren and Marshall developed ulcer treatment that included the use of antibiotics to eliminate the infectious agents. For most patients, antibiotics prevented recurrence. Because *Helicobacter* is found in some 50 percent of humans and not all persons develop ulcers, it is believed that genetic factors regulate the response to colonization by these bacteria.

2006

Andrew Z. Fire and Craig C. Mello (both American). Earlier work by researchers had demonstrated that gene expression could be silenced in cells following the insertion of RNA sequences corresponding to messenger RNA (mRNA) transcribed from genes. Mello termed this process RNA interference (RNAi). The mechanism was unknown. Fire and Mello discovered that the process utilized doublestranded RNA (dsRNA), which caused the degradation of mRNA and resulted in what they called posttranslational gene silencing. Using the nematode *Caenorhabditis elegans* as a test organism, they observed that injection of specific dsRNA into cells was followed by cleavage of the double-stranded RNA into short small interfering RNA (siRNA) fragments, which led to the degradation of the mRNA. The process was subsequently shown to be a common method of gene regulation in both plants and animals.

2007

Mario Capecchi (American), Sir Martin Evans (British), and Oliver Smithies (American). Working independently, the laureates developed the methodology used for isolating and growing embryonic stem cells and for introducing genetic changes within those cells. Evans isolated cells from the blastocyst obtained from pregnant mice, subsequently growing those cells in laboratory cultures. Capecchi and Smithies developed a mechanism to insert specific genes into such embryonic cells, creating genetically modified mice. Their work led to the use of "knockout" mice, genetically modified animals in which specific sites on DNA could be inactivated in order to better understand the function of those genes.

2008

Harald zur Hausen (German). Zur Hausen demonstrated that certain variants of human papillomaviruses (HPV) were the etiological agents of cervical cancer and confirmed his suspicions by isolating HPV DNA from cervical cancer tissue. His work ultimately led to a better understanding of how cell division is regulated, as well as development of HPV vaccines.

2008

Françoise Barre-Sinoussi and Luc Montagnier (both French). Barre-Sinoussi and Montagnier isolated HIV, the etiological agent of AIDS. Their work led to methods for the detection of the virus in blood and lymph nodes, as well as a better understanding of how viral replication results in depression of the immune system.

2009

Elizabeth H. Balckburn, Carol W. Greider and Jack W. Szostak Blackburn, Greider and Szostak solved how chromosomes can be completely copied during cell divisions and how they are protected by their telomeres and the enzyme that forms them – telomerase - against degradation. The activity level and structure of telomerase result in cell changes causing or leading to disease. This discovery has stimulated the development of new therapeutic strategies for certain inherited diseases and cancer.

2010

Robert G. Edwards Edwards developed in-vitro fertilization (IVF), a procedure where conception occurs outside the human body. The egg is removed from a woman, fertilized in a test tube and then returned to her body for development. This procedure has helped millions of infertile couples conceive.

2011

Bruce A. Beutler, Jules A. Hoffmann and Ralph M. Steinman Beutler and Hoffmann discovered receptor proteins that recognize attacks by bacteria and other microorganisms and then activate the body's innate immunity. This is the body's first immune response. Steinman discovered the dendritic cells of the immune system as well as how they activate and regulate adaptive immunity. This occurs later in the body's immune response as microorganisms are eliminated. These discoveries provide new insights into disease mechanisms, thus allowing scientists greater opportunities to develop prevention and therapy strategies in dealing with infections, cancer and inflammatory diseases.

2012

Sir John B. Gurdon and Shinya Yamanaka Gurdon and Yamanaka discovered that mature, specialized cells could be reprogrammed to become pluripotent stem cells (immature cells) that are capable of being developed into all types of cells in the body. This discovery has changed how cell development and specialization are studied. Scientists can now reprogram human cells, thereby creating new avenues to study disease and develop better methods for diagnosis and therapy.

2013

James E. Rothman, Randy W. Schekman, and Thomas C. Sudhof Rothman, Schekman and Sudhof discovered the control system for the transport and delivery of cellular cargo. Schekman discovered a set of genes that were required for vesicle traffic, Rothman found the protein machinery that allows vesicles to fuse with their targets to permit the transfer of cargo, while Sudhof revealed how signals instruct vesicles to release their cargo with precision. Disturbances in this system contribute to conditions such as neurological diseases, diabetes and immunological disorders.

2014

John O'Keefe, May-Britt Moser and Edvard I. Moser O'Keefe, Moser and Moser discovered place and grid cells in the brain. These cells make it possible to determine a body's position in space and to allow us to navigate our way through a complex environment. It has encouraged research into other cognitive processes such as memory, thinking and planning.

2015

William C. Campbell, Satoshi Omura and Touyou Tu Campbell and Omura discovered a novel therapy drug, Avermectin, to fight diseases such as River Blindness and Lymphatic Filariasis, as well as the expanding number of new diseases caused by roundworm parasites. Tu discovered a new therapy drug, Artemisinin, that has significantly decreased the mortality rate associated with Malaria.

2016

Yoshinori Ohsumi Ohsumi was able to explain autophagy – the process whereby a cell degrades itself and recycles the cellular components in it. This process is important to the body because it provides an essential response to stress upon the body in instances such as starvation and infection. It is also an important process during embryo development and cell differentiation as well as countering the effects of aging. Disruptions in this process can lead to disease so being able to target this process could lead to new therapies.

2017

Hall, Rosbash & Young Hall, Rosbash and Young discovered the molecular mechanisms that control the body's internal biological clock - its circadian rhythm. We now know how plants, animals and humans have adapted their biological rhythms so they synchronize such important functions as behavior, hormone levels, sleep, body temperature and metabolism with the Earth's revolutions. There are indications that chronic misalignment between our lifestyle and our biological clocks increases the risk for various diseases.

CHEMISTRY
1957

Alexander Robertus Todd (British). As part of wide-ranging research in organic chemistry, Todd revealed how ribose and deoxyribose bond to the nitrogenous bases on one side of a nucleotide unit and to the phosphate group on the other side. These discoveries provided necessary background for work by others that explained the structure of the DNA molecule.

1972

Christian B. Anfinsen (American). Anfinsen, studying the three-dimensional structure of the enzyme ribonuclease, proved that its conformation was determined by the sequence of its amino acids and that to construct a complete enzyme molecule, no separate structural information was passed on from the DNA in the cell's nucleus.

1972

Stanford Moore and William H. Stein (both American). Moore and Stein supplemented Anfinsen's research by identifying the sequence of amino acids in ribonuclease, a clue to the structure of the gene responsible for it.

1980

Paul Berg (American). Berg invented procedures for removing a gene from a chromosome of one species and inserting it into the chromosome of an entirely different species, enabling him to study how the genetic information of the contributing organism interacts with the host's DNA. The recombinant DNA technology, sometimes called gene splicing, became fundamental to the genetic engineering of transgenic species.

1980

Walter Gilbert (American) and Frederick Sanger (British). Gilbert and Sanger independently developed methods for determining the sequence of nucleic acids in DNA, thus decoding the genetic information. Gilbert's method cuts DNA into small units that reveal their structure when exposed to specific chemicals; Sanger's method separates the strands of DNA and then rebuilds them in stages that allow the terminal nucleotides to be identified. Their methods later made it possible to sequence the entire genomes of organisms.

1982

Aaron Klug (British). Klug used X-ray crystallography to investigate biochemical structures, especially those of viruses. He was able to link the assembly of viral protein subunits with specific sites on viral RNA, which helped in fighting viruses that cause disease in plants and, more basically, in understanding the mechanism of RNA transfer of genetic information. He also determined the structure of transfer RNA (tRNA), which has a shape similar to that of a bent hairpin.

1989

Sidney Altman (Canadian) and Thomas R. Cech (American). Working independently, Altman and Cech discovered that RNA, like proteins, can act as a catalyst; moreover, Cech found that when ribosomal RNA participates in translation of mRNA and the synthesis of polypeptides, it acts as a catalyst in some steps.

1993

Kary B. Mullis (American). Mullis invented polymerase chain reaction (PCR), a method for swiftly making millions of copies of DNA. PCR soon became an important tool in genetic engineering, DNA fingerprinting, and medicine.

1993

Michael Smith (British). Smith developed sitedirected mutagenesis, a means for reconfiguring genes in order to create altered proteins with distinct properties. Smith's genetic engineering tool made it possible to treat genetic disease and cancer and to create novel plant strains.

2004

Aaron Ciechanover (Israeli), Avram Hershko (Israeli), and Irwin Rose (American). The laureates were awarded for their work toward a better understanding of how cells regulate the hydrolysis (breakdown) of proteins. The researchers observed that proteins are "tagged" with a molecule called ubiquitin, which signals protein degradation complexes (proteosomes). The proteosomes in turn carry out the degradation process. In this manner, analogous to quality control, defective proteins are removed. A variety of cell processes, including DNA repair and cell division, are regulated in this manner. Genetic defects in the degradation process may lead to certain forms of cancer.

2006

Roger D. Kornberg (American). Kornberg was honored for his contribution toward the understanding of transcription regulation in eukaryotic cells such as yeast, plant, or animal cells. His work began with developing a system using extracts from the yeast Saccharomyces to study cell components involved in DNA expression. He subsequently discovered a complex of mediator proteins involved in regulating transcription in these cells. Combining the technique of X-ray crystallography with electron microscopy, Kornberg was able to produce a molecular model of the interactions. He was following in the footsteps of his father, Arthur Kornberg, a Nobel laureate in 1959 for his work in molecular biology.

2008

Osamu Shimomura, Martin Chalfie, and Roger Y. Tsien (all American). The laureates were honored for their discovery and development of green fluorescent proteins (GFP). During the early 1960's, Shimomura isolated and purified GFPs from jellyfish, molecules he named aequorin, which had the property of fluorescing in the presence of ultraviolet light. He subsequently isolated the chromophore, the fluorescent component from the molecule. During the 1980's, Chalfie received a cloned copy of the GFP gene, which he inserted into the cells of the nematode Caenorhabditis, resulting in the organism acquiring the ability to fluoresce. Tsien further applied the procedures originating with Chalfie to use GFPs and similar fluorescent molecules attached to proteins in the brains of mice, creating, in effect, molecular tags. With this procedure, it became possible to identify and follow gene products within cells by observing the color patterns in regions of the brain, termed "brainbow" by Tsien and colleagues.

2009

Venkatraman Ramakrishan, Thomas A. Steitz and Ada E. Yonath Ramakrishan, Steitz and Yonath have used x-ray crystallography to ascertain the position for each of the hundreds of thousands of atoms that form the body's ribosome, the producer of proteins based on the information in its DNA that controls the chemistry in all living organisms. Since many of today's antibiotics cure diseases by blocking bacteria's ribosomes, the understanding of how ribosomes function becomes important in the development of new antibiotics.

2010

Richard F. Heck, Ei-ichi Negishi and Akira Suzuki Heck, Negishi and Suzuki are responsible for the development of the chemical tool palladium-catalyzed cross coupling that provides chemists with the ability to create complex chemicals. This discovery will pave the way for the creation of new medicines and revolutionary commercial materials.

2011

Dan Shechtman Shechtman using an electron microscope discovered that atoms in the crystal he was studying were packed in a pattern that could not be repeated, defying the accepted laws of nature. Scientists have used his discovery to find other quasicrystals in nature and produced even more in the lab that they are experimenting with for commercial use in items such as frying pans and diesel engines.

2012

Robert J. Lefkowitz and Brian K. Kobilka Lefkowitz and Kobilka are responsible for uncovering the inner workings of the important family of G-protein-coupled receptors. These receptors allow cells to sense their environments, interact and adapt to new situations via hormone communications. This discovery impacts the study of medications because almost half of all medications are effective because they target G-protein-coupled receptors.

2013

Martin Karplus, Michael Levitt and Arieh Warshel Karplus, Levitt and Warshel pioneered the use of powerful computer programs to understand and predict various chemical processes by incorporating both classical and quantum physics. These technological advances have made it possible for chemists to observe and understand lightning-quick chemical reactions.

2014

Eric Betzig, Stefan W. Hell and William E. Moerner Betzig, Hell and Moerner are responsible for the development of super-resolved fluorescence microscopy – nanoscopy - that allows for the observance of the pathways of individual molecules found inside living cells. Nanoscopy is presently used worldwide producing new knowledge on a daily basis.

2015

Tomas Lindahl, Paul Modrich and Aziz Sancar Lindahl, Modrich and Sancar uncovered the process whereby cells repair damaged DNA at the molecular level to safeguard their genetic information. This discovery has important ramifications regarding the development of new treatments for cancer.

2016

Jean-Pierre Sauvage, Sir J. Fraser Stoddart and Bernard L. Feringa Sauvage, Stoddart and Feringa designed and produced molecular machines whereby they can now control the movement of molecules, inducing them to perform a task once energy is added. It is anticipated that molecular machines will be used to develop new materials, sensors and energy storage systems.

2017

Jaques Dubochet, Joachim Frank and Richard Henderson Dubochet, Frank and Henderson are responsible for the development of cryo-electron microscopy – which simplifies and allows for the three-dimensional imaging of biomolecules – images researchers have never seen before. This discovery has an enormous impact on the understanding of life's chemistry and in the development of pharmaceuticals.

TIME LINE OF MAJOR DEVELOPMENTS IN GENETICS

12,000 b.c.e.

With the transition from hunter-gatherer societies to agrarian civilizations, humans begin domesticating plants and animals through artificial selection, in some cases coupled with intentional hybridization for certain traits. Domesticated plants and animals become the basis that allows advanced civilizations to develop.

c. 350-322 b.c.e.

Aristotle writes and teaches on nature of living organisms, including their reproduction, hybridization, and classification.

c. 1283

Zakariya al-Qazwini (or Kazwini) writes 4Aja'ib almakhluqat wa ghara'ib al-mawjudat (on the marvels of nature and of the singularities of created things), in which he refers to sexual reproduction in the date palm, comparing it to sexual reproduction in humans.

1651

William Harvey publishes Exercitationes de Generatione Animalium (Anatomical Exercitations, Concerning the Generation of Living Creatures, 1653), in which he suggests that animals must originate in an egg.

1677

Antoni van Leeuwenhoek describes sperm and eggs and collects evidence that helps refute the theory of spontaneous generation.

1694

German botanist Rudolph Jakob Camerer (Camerarius) publishes De Sexu Plantarum Epistola (a letter on sex in plants), in which he presents experimental evidence on sexual reproduction in flowering plants.

1751

Carl von Linné (Carolus Linnaeus) publishes Plantae Hybridae (plant hybrids), in which he records his observation on plant hybrids, among them interspecific hybrids.

1759

In his doctoral dissertation, Kaspar Friedrich Wolff revives the hypothesis of epigenesis, which states that the complex structures of chickens develop from initially homogeneous, structureless areas of the embryo, and not from a pre-formed homunculus.

1761-1766

Joseph Gottlieb Kölreuter publishes a series of three papers titled "Vorläufige Nachricht von einigen das Geschlecht der Pflanzen betreffenden Versuchen und Bebachtungen" (preliminary report of some experiments and observations concerning sex in plants), which documents studies on fertilization and hybridization in a wide range of plant species.

1798

Thomas Robert Malthus publishes An Essay on the Principle of Population, in which he analyzes population growth and relates it to the struggle for existence, setting the stage for Charles Darwin's theory of natural selection.

1798

Edward Jenner publishes his findings on vaccination against smallpox in "Inquiry into the Cause and Effects of the Variolae Vaccinae." Jenner used the cowpox virus as a vaccine to induce immunity against the genetically and structurally similar, but lethal, virus that causes smallpox in humans.

1809

Jean-Baptiste Lamarck publishes Philosophie Zoologique (Zoological Philosophy, 1914), in which he sets forth his ideas on evolution, particularly his hypothesis of the inheritance of acquired characteristics. Although his notion that acquired traits alter the inherited constitution and are transmitted to the next generation was later dismissed in favor of Darwinian natural selection, Lamarck's book makes the link between evolution and inherited traits that lays a foundation for later evolutionary theory. Lamarck would have a significant influence on Darwin's development of the theory of natural selection.

1823

Thomas Andrew Knight presents "Some Remarks on the Supposed Influences of the Pollen, in Cross-Breeding, on the Colour of the Seed-Coats of Plants and the Qualities of their Fruits" to the Royal Horticultural Society. His experiments with the garden pea include hybrids, testcrosses, and reciprocal crosses. He documents dominance, parental equivalence, and the true-breeding nature of plants with a recessive phenotype but does notice mathematical patterns of the type Gregor Mendel would later observe.

1838-1839

Theodor Schwann (1838) and Matthias Jakob Schleiden (1839) propose the cell theory that all organisms are composed of cells.

1839

Gerardus Johannes Mulder publishes "On the Composition of Some Animal Substances," which provides chemical analysis of a fibrous material precipitated from cells. He calls this material "protein" (which means "of first importance") and believes it is the most important of the known components of living matter.

1839

Carl Friedrich von Gärtner publishes Experiments and Observations on Hybrid Production in the Plant Kingdom, documenting nearly ten thousand plant hybridization experiments. He noted repeated observations of dominance and uniformity in firstgeneration hybrids followed by variability in subsequent generations. Gärtner's work strongly influenced Darwin, who referred to it in On the Origin of Species by Means of Natural Selection, and Mendel, who cited it seventeen times in his 1866 paper and familiarized himself with Knight's work with the garden pea through Gärtner's citations of it.

1852

Franz Unger publishes Botanical Letters, in which he proposes that new species can arise through new combinations of inherited characteristics. As a professor at the University of Vienna, he is nearly dismissed for teaching evolution. Mendel is one of his students.

1854

Louis Pasteur begins research into fermentation. His "pasteurization" process is originally proposed as a means of preserving beer and wines. Through his work, Pasteur makes the important discovery that "life must be derived from life."

1855

Rudolph Virchow extends the cell theory of Schwann and Schleiden, proposing that all cells arise from previous cells (Omnis cellula e cellula).

1855-1857

Alfred Russel Wallace publishes On the Law Which Has Regulated the Introduction of New Species; later, in 1857, he sends Darwin a manuscript, "On the Tendency of Varieties to Depart Indefinitely from the Original Type." Today Wallace is recognized as having developed the theory of natural selection along with Darwin.

1859

Charles Darwin publishes On the Origin of Species by Means of Natural Selection: Or, The Preservation of Favoured Races in the Struggle for Life (usually referred to as On the Origin of Species) in 1859, in which he sets forth his theory of natural selection. Inheritance is a key element of Darwin's theory but is not fully understood at the time. Once genetics was studied as a discipline, it became clear that genetics is the foundation for explaining evolution through natural selection.

1862

The Organic Act establishes the U.S. Department of Agriculture (USDA). As one of its functions, the USDA is responsible for the collection of new and valuable seeds and plants and the distribution of them to agriculturists. The preservation and dissemination of agriculturally important plants is a necessity for maintaining and increasing the world's food supply.

1863

Gregor Mendel reads a German translation of Darwin's On the Origin of Species and makes marginal notes in it.

1865-1866

Gregor Mendel presents a paper titled "Versuche über Pflanzen-Hybriden" (experiments in plant hybrids) in 1865 to the Natural History Society of Brünn and publishes it in the society's Proceedings in 1866. His paper summarizes his experimental data on hybridization and his interpretations of those data to establish the theory of inheritance. Major components of this theory are now known as the principles of segregation, independent assortment, dominance, and parental equivalence. The first two are unique to Mendel's work, the latter two having been recognized by previous hybridists but explained by Mendel's theory. Although his work was cited several times following its publication, its importance was largely unrecognized until it was rediscovered in 1900 and became the foundation for the science of genetics. 1866 Ernst Haeckel develops the hypothesis that hereditary information is transmitted by the cell nucleus.

1866-1873

Gregor Mendel corresponds with Karl von Nägeli in a series of ten letters regarding plant hybridization experiments. These letters were preserved and later became an invaluable resource documenting how Mendel approached experimental design.

1868-1871

Charles Darwin publishes "the provisional hypothesis of pangenesis" as the mechanism of inheritance in his two-volume work Plants and Animals Under Domestication. Darwin's cousin, Francis Galton, publishes a paper in 1871, "Experiments in Pangenesis," which, on the basis of blood transfusion experiments in rabbits, offers strong experimental evidence refuting pangenesis.

1869

Francis Galton publishes Hereditary Genius, on the heredity of intelligence, which lays the foundation for the eugenics movement.

1869

Friedrich Miescher isolates "nuclein" from the nuclei of white blood cells. This substance is later found to consist of the nucleic acids DNA and RNA.

1870

Gregor Mendel publishes a paper on hybridization in hawkweed (Hieracium), an apomict, and concludes that principles of inheritance he discovered in the pea and the bean are not universal in the plant kingdom.

1876

Oskar Hertwig, a student of Ernst Haeckel, demonstrates the fertilization of an ovum in a sea urchin, thus establishing one of the basic principles of sexual reproduction: the union of egg and sperm cells.

1878-1882

In research published in 1878 and 1880, Walther Flemming describes cell division and the partitioning of chromosomes and names the process "mitosis." In 1882, he determines that chromosomes are split longitudinally during mitosis.

1883

Francis Galton founds the field of eugenics with the publication of Inquiries into Human Faculty and Its Development. The notion that the human species can be genetically improved by artificial selection perpetuates racism and provides a supposed scientific rationale for subsequent eugenic programs.

1883

Wilhelm Roux proposes, on the basis of experimental evidence, that mitosis must result in equal sharing of chromosomal particles by the daughter cells and describes the process.

1883

Edouard van Beneden studies the processes of meiosis and fertilization in the parasitic worm Ascaris. Van Beneden observes that meiosis halves the chromosome number in the resulting gametes and that fertilization restores the original chromosome number in the zygote.

1883

Emil Hansen develops a method for isolating and propagating pure yeast culture from a single cell, and it is adopted at Denmark's Carlsberg Brewery. The ability to propagate and maintain pure strains of organisms— genetically identical strains, or clones— will prove pivotal to future genetic research.

1885

August Weismann publishes Die Continuitat des Keimplasmas als Grundlage einer Theorie der Vererbung (the continuity of germ-plasm as the foundation of a theory of heredity), in which he maintains that only the germ cells, not somatic cells, can transmit hereditary information from one generation to the next; his experiments refuted the Larmarckian notion of inheritance of acquired characteristics.

1887-1889

In a series of articles, Émile Maupas describes the relationship of sexual conjugation and cellular senescence in protozoans.

1887-1890

Theodor Boveri investigates and describes chromosomes and their behavior, noting that they are preserved through the process of cell division and that sperm and egg contribute equal numbers of chromosomes to the zygote.

1889

Richard Altmann renames "nuclein" (isolated by Miescher in 1869) "nucleic acid."

1889

Francis Galton publishes a book titled Natural Inheritance in which he rejects blending inheritance and coins the term "particulate inheritance." He proposes that traits displaying continuous variation are governed by "a fine mosaic too minute for its elements to be distinguished in a general view."

1894

Albrecht Kossel identifies thymine, completing his identification of all four bases in DNA. He named it after the thymus gland from which it was isolated. 1896 Edmund B. Wilson publishes The Cell in Development and Heredity, in which he discusses the role of cells and chromosomes in inherited traits.

1897

Eduard Buchner shows that biochemical reactions that normally take place within living cells can proceed in cell extracts. He discovers that yeast extracts can convert glucose to ethyl alcohol. Buchner's was one of the first in vitro experiments on biochemical reactions. Performing such experiments outside the body allowed researchers to control conditions and to observe the effects of individual variables.

1899

The Royal Horticultural Society holds a meeting in Chiswick, London, in which William Bateson calls for research on discontinuous variations. The meeting is renamed the First International Conference of Genetics, later renamed the International Congress of Genetics, currently held every five years.

1900

Carl Correns, Hugo de Vries, and Erich Tschermak von Seysenegg independently rediscover Mendelian principles with experiments similar to Mendel's but not as extensive. Although de Vries soon abandons Mendelism, Correns and Tschermak continue experimentation on heredity, confirming Mendelian principles. Mendelian theory soon provides a framework for observations at the time in cytology, cellular biology, plant hybridization, and biochemistry.

1901

Karl Landsteiner discovers human blood groups.

1901

Clarence McClung describes the role of the X chromosome in determining sex in insects.

1902

W. F. R. Weldon publishes a paper titled "Mendel's Law of Alternative Inheritance in Peas," in which he subjects some of Mendel's data to Karl Pearson's recently developed (1900) chi-square statistical test. Weldon concludes that Mendel's data are exceptionally close to expectation. William Bateson responds with a booklet titled Mendel's Principles of Heredity: A Defence. A bitter debate ensues between Bateson and Weldon over the relevance of Mendelian inheritance.

1902

William Bateson, Reginald Punnett, Edith Saunders, Carl Correns, Erich Tschermak, Lucien Cuénot, and others begin to confirm Mendelian inheritance in numerous plant and animal species.

1902

Austrian botanist Gottlieb Haberlandt advances the cell theory with his idea of totipotentiality (later called totipotency): Cells contain all the genetic information necessary to develop into an entire, multicellular organism. Therefore, an individual plant cell is capable of developing into an entire plant.

1902

In an article titled "The Incidence of Alkaptonuria: A Study in Chemical Individuality," Sir Archibald Garrod proposes that alkaptonuria is an "inborn error of metabolism," due to the absence of a "ferment" (enzyme), and that it is inherited as a recessive trait in accordance with Mendel's principles. In this article, Garrod provides the first evidence of a specific relationship between genes and enzymes as well as Mendelian inheritance in humans.

1902

Theodor Boveri recognizes the correlation between Mendel's principles of inheritance and current studies of cellular biology; he deduces the haploid nature of sperm and egg cells (that each has equal numbers of chromosomes) and determines, by experimenting with sea urchin sperm and egg cells, that each must contribute half the total number of chromosomes to offspring for their normal development.

1903

Working independently of Boveri, Walter Sutton comes to similar conclusions using grasshoppers. Both Boveri and Sutton have formed the chromosomal theory of heredity. Mendel's principles of segregation and independent assortment coincided with Sutton's observations of how chromosomes segregated during cell division. This provided a cellular explanation for Mendel's observations.

1903

William Ernest Castle is appointed an assistant professor at Harvard University, where he directs one of the most ambitious genetics programs in the United States. He was the first to conduct genetic experiments on the fruit fly but is best known for his research on rodent genetics. In 1909, he is appointed director of the Bussey Institute at Harvard. His laboratory produces some of the most influential mammalian geneticists of the twentieth century, including L. C. Dunn, Clarence Little, Sewall Wright, and George Snell.

1903

Phoebus A. T. Levene discovers a distinction between some nucleic acid preparations in the amounts of thymine and uracil that they contain. Research will eventually show that thymine is a component of DNA and uracil a component of RNA.

1905

William Bateson coins the term "genetics" to describe the science of heredity in a letter to Adam Sedgwick.

1905

Nettie Stevens and Edmund Wilson independently describe the inheritance of sex chromosomes in relation to sex determination in insects. Their observations enhance Boveri and Sutton's evidence supporting the chromosomal theory of heredity.

1907

The first mandatory sterilization law intended to enforce eugenics is passed in Indiana. Mandatory sterilization and antimiscegenation laws will be passed throughout the United States and other countries over the next several decades as scientists, dignitaries, government leaders, the wealthy, and well-educated members of society embrace the eugenics movement. Outspoken proponents of eugenics will include Alexander Graham Bell, Theodore Roosevelt, Charles Davenport, Leonard Darwin, Ronald Fisher, and Winston Churchill, among many others.

1908

William Bateson and Reginald C. Punnett discover a case of gene linkage but fail to interpret it correctly when they observe a violation of the Mendelian principle of independent assortment, noting two traits in sweet pea that do not assort independently.

1908

George Shull self-pollinates corn plants for several generations to produce true-breeding inbred lines, notes the effect of heterosis in hybrid plants, and offers a genetic explanation for inbreeding depression.

1908

Godfrey Hardy and Wilhelm Weinberg independently discover mathematical relationships between genotypic and phenotypic frequencies in populations. Known as the Hardy-Weinberg law, the rules governing these mathematical relationships help researchers understand the dynamics of population genetics and the evolution of species.

1909

Wilhelm Johannsen, working on the statistical analysis of continuous variation, expands the modern genetic vocabulary, coining the terms "gene," "genotype," and "phenotype."

1909

Hermann Nilsson-Ehle's studies of kernel color in wheat indicate this is a polygenic trait. This was one of the first demonstrations that several genes could influence a single trait. His experiments showed that each gene contributes to the trait in an additive fashion.

1909

Carl Correns discovers a class of exceptions to Mendelian inheritance, one of the first examples of extranuclear inheritance. The idea that other cellular organelles besides the nucleus carry DNA was not recognized for decades. However, Correns's experiments in the plant Mirabilis jalapa showed inheritance of leaf color via the DNA in the chloroplasts.

1909

Phoebus A. T. Levene determines that the sugar in RNA is ribose.

1910

Thomas Hunt Morgan further establishes the chromosomal theory of heredity after investigating a white-eyed fruit fly and finding that the trait does not segregate exactly according to Mendelian principles but rather is influenced by the sex of the fly. This fly experiment becomes the cornerstone upon which theories of Mendelian, chromosomal, and sexual inheritance are built into a cohesive whole. Morgan also establishes the "Fly Room" at Columbia University, where he and his students will conduct groundbreaking experiments using Drosophila for the next quarter century. He will win the Nobel Prize in Physiology or Medicine in 1933.

1910

Albrecht Kossel wins the Nobel Prize in Physiology or Medicine for earlier work isolating and describing molecular constituents of the cell's nucleus, notably guanine (which had earlier been described by Piccard, but not as a constituent of nucleic acids), adenine, cytosine, thymine, and uracil.

1910

The Eugenics Records Office is established at Cold Spring Harbor Laboratory under the direction of geneticist Charles B. Davenport.

1911

Peyton Rous produces cellfree extracts from chicken tumors that, when injected, can induce tumors in other chickens. The tumor-producing agent in the extract is later found to be a virus. Thus, Rous has discovered a link between cancer and viruses. He wins the Nobel Prize in Physiology or Medicine in 1966.

1912-1913

The first International Eugenics Conference is held in London in 1912. Some of the earliest books on genetics, including Heredity and Eugenics by William Ernest Castle and others (1912), Mendelism by Reginald C. Punnett (1912), and Mendel's Principles of Heredity by William Bateson (1913), each conclude praising eugenics as a bright future for human society.

1913

Alfred H. Sturtevant, an undergraduate student studying under Thomas Hunt Morgan, publishes the first gene linkage map: five linked genes on the X chromosome of Drosophila melanogaster. He develops a method of gene mapping that would standardize genetic mapping of genes and genetic markers relative to one another on chromosomes.

1913

Eleanor Carothers reports her discovery of the chromosomal basis of independent assortment. By examining grasshopper chromosomes, Carothers observed the segregation of the X chromosome relative to a heteromorphic pair of autosomes during meiosis. This observation was consistent with Mendel's principle of independent assortment.

1913

Rollins A. Emerson and Edward M. East demonstrate the multiple genes in corn can influence a single trait and that their pattern of inheritance can be explained by Mendelian principles.

1914

Calvin Blackman Bridges uses the phenomenon of primary nondisjunction (a fault in cell division resulting in the failure of chromosomes to separate during metaphase I) to confirm that genes are carried on chromosomes.

1914-1919

In 1914, William Castle publishes a study on artificial selection in hooded rats, demonstrating the ability of selection to genetically alter phenotypic expression of a recessive trait. By 1919, he interprets his results as the effect of modifier genes, each of which has a minor effect on the phenotype conferred by a single gene with a major effect.

1915

The Mechanism of Mendelian Heredity, by Thomas Hunt Morgan, Alfred Sturtevant, Hermann J. Muller, and Calvin Bridges, is published, establishing Drosophila as a model organism for genetics research and describing fundamentals of gene mapping.

1915

In a letter to Charles Davenport, editor of the Journal of Heredity, Thomas Hunt Morgan privately expresses his doubts about the eugenics movement and refuses to take part in it. He delays his public opposition, however, until his Nobel speech in 1934.

1916

Edward M. East publishes an extensive analysis of controlled experiments on the inheritance of corolla length in tobacco and concludes that his observations are best explained by Mendelian inheritance of multiple genes with alleles that do not display dominance.

1916

Research on the major histocompatibility complex begins with Clarence Little and E. E. Tyzzer's experiments transplanting tumors between mice.

1917

Félix d'Herelle discovers bacteriophages, viruses that infect bacteria. Bacteriophages later played important roles in early genetics research, including confirmation that DNA is the hereditary material and their use as vectors in recombinant DNA applications.

1917

Ojvind Winge publishes "The Chromosomes: Their Number and General Importance," which describes the relationship between chromosome doubling and allopolyploidy in plants.

1917

Eleanor Carothers extends her 1913 observations of independent assortment of chromosomes to more than two pairs of chromosomes.

1917

In an article titled "Elimination of Feeblemindedness," Reginald Punnett mathematically demonstrates the futility of mandatory sterilization for reducing the frequency of recessive genetic disorders. Nonetheless, mandatory sterilization of individuals possessing genetic disorders thought to be recessive, such as "feeblemindedness," continues for decades to come.

1917

Calvin Bridges determines that the ratio of X chromosomes to autosomes determines sex in Drosophila, with no influence of the Y chromosome on sex determination in this species.

1921

The second International Eugenics Conference is held in New York under the theme "Eugenics is the self-direction of human evolution."

1922

Lillian Vaughan Sampson Morgan publishes her research on attached-X females in Drosophila, which carry a Y chromosome, confirming Bridges's proposed mechanism of sex determination. The attached-X chromosome becomes an important tool for Drosophila research.

1924

Donald Jones publishes the results of experiments on inbred-line development and F1 hybrid production in corn, establishing a genetic basis for inbreeding depression and heterosis.

1924

J. B. S. Haldane publishes the first of a series of articles on the genetic basis of natural selection, initiating the merger of Mendelian genetics with Darwinian evolution, which would later be called the "modern synthesis."

1925

Alfred Sturtevant documents unequal crossing over between duplicated chromosomal segments at the Bar locus in Drosophila.

1925-1926

Sturtevant discovers position effect: An inversion may place a gene in another location in the chromosome, removing the gene from its regulatory elements and altering its expression. He also provides genetic data best explained by chromosomal inversion.

1926

Nicolai Vavilov, a Soviet geneticist who studied under Bateson, publishes his theory of centers of origin, which proposes that the centers of origin for domesticated plant species are the regions where the genetic diversity for those species is the greatest. From 1917 to 1940, he carries out a series of more than one hundred expeditions throughout the world to collect and preserve the genetic diversity of the world's food plants. These extraordinary efforts are the beginning of the worldwide establishment of gene banks to conserve and utilize genetic diversity for plant and animal breeding.

1927

The Buck v. Bell eugenics case reaches the U.S. Supreme Court. A woman from Virginia, Carrie Bell, challenges her legally mandated sterilization. In an 8-1 decision, the Supreme Court upholds the lower court rulings that Bell must be sterilized. In the majority opinion, Chief Justice Oliver Wendell Holmes, Jr., writes, "The principle that sustains compulsory vaccination is broad enough to cover cutting the Fallopian tubes." This case establishes precedent in support of eugenic mandatory sterilization laws.

1927-1928

Hermann J. Muller and Lewis Stadler independently discover that X rays induce inherited mutations, demonstrating the mutagenic effect of ionizing radiation. Muller works with Drosophila and publishes his work in 1927, whereas Stadler works with barley and publishes his work in 1928. Muller receives the Nobel Prize in Physiology or Medicine for this work in 1946.

1928

Frederick Griffith discovers the "transforming principle" in experiments targeted at developing a vaccine for pneumonia. The hereditary material has not yet been identified, but later experiments by Oswald Avery et al. in 1944 indicate that the transforming principle discovered by Griffith is DNA.

1929

Phoebus Levene determines the chemical structure of the sugar deoxyribose in the nucleic acid that would be named DNA on the basis of this discovery.

1929

Clarence Little helps found the Jackson Memorial Laboratory in Bar Harbor, Maine, which will become one of the most influential genetics research institutions in North America, particularly in mouse (mammalian) genetics, and cancer research.

1930

Ronald Aylmer Fisher publishes The Genetical Theory of Natural Selection, which will become one of the most influential works of the modern synthesis.

1931

Harriet Creighton and Barbara McClintock discover that a physical exchange between chromosomes in corn is associated with recombination of genes mapped to that chromosome, confirming that crossing over is responsible for recombination of linked genes. Curt Stern uses a similar approach to document a physical exchange in the X chromosome of Drosophila.

1931

Sewall Wright publishes a lengthy article titled "Evolution in Mendelian Populations," which establishes genetic drift as an important factor in evolution, and is another key publication in the modern synthesis.

1932-1934

The third and final International Eugenics Conference is held in New York in 1932. Nazi implementation of extreme eugenic measures in 1933 and the subsequent atrocities of the Holocaust are the start of the eugenics movement's downfall. Thomas Hunt Morgan, who has quietly opposed eugenics since 1915, publicly renounces it in his 1934 Nobel Prize acceptance speech.

1933

Theophilus Painter discovers polytene chromosomes in Drosophila salivary glands. These special chromosomes, resulting from numerous rounds of DNA replications without separation, are large, with distinct banding patterns. They are used extensively in mapping genes to specific regions of the chromosome.

1933

Theodosius Dobzhansky publishes an article on chromosomal evolution in Drosophila pseudoobscura. Dobzhansky and Alfred Sturtevant will, over a fortyyear period, publish 43 articles under the collective title "Genetics of Natural Populations," firmly establishing the modern synthesis.

1934

John Desmond Bernal examines protein structure by using X-ray crystallography.

1935

Phoebus Levene correctly determines the chemical structure of single-stranded DNA, building on his previous discoveries of deoxyribose and the structure of the nucleotide. However, he incorrectly presumes that the molecule consists of repeating tetranucleotides, with equal proportions of T, C, A, and G.

1935

Hans Spemann wins the Nobel Prize in Physiology or Medicine. By transplanting bits of one embryo into a second, viable embryo, Spemann compiled evidence that an "organizer center" directs the development of an embryo and that different parts of the organizer governed distinct portions of the embryo. His experiments provided clues to the genetic control of growth from the earliest stages of an organism.

1935-1964

Trofim Denisovich Lysenko and Isaak Izrailevich Prezent initiate in 1935 a campaign against traditional geneticists in the Soviet Union, branding them as "kulak-wreckers and saboteurs." Lysenko resurrects Larmarckism as the "true" theory of genetics. The movement becomes known as Lysenkoism and receives Joseph Stalin's approval. Vavilov leads the opposition, for which he is arrested and imprisoned in 1941. He dies of maltreatment in prison in 1943. Several Soviet geneticists are also imprisoned for their refusal to support Lysenkoism, and they also die in prison or are executed. Lysenkoism is forced on Soviet geneticists until Nikita Khrushchev's forced resignation in 1964.

1936

Ronald Aylmer Fisher publishes an exhaustive analyses of Mendel's work, including reconstruction of Mendel's experiments and subjection of Mendel's data to chi-square analysis. Fisher concludes that Mendel's experiments are especially well described, literal, and conducted exactly as Mendel presented them, and that Mendel is a supporter of Darwin. Fisher points out, however, that Mendel's data are exceptionally close to expectation, and speculates that they may have been cooked by an assistant. This latter conclusion sparked the Mendel- Fisher controversy in the 1960's, which has continued to the present.

1937

Theodosius Dobzhansky publishes Genetics and the Origin of Species. He shows that, in natural and experimental populations of Drosophila species, frequency changes and geographic patterns of variation in chromosome variants are consistent with the effects of natural selection. This book is another cornerstone of the modern synthesis.

1937

George Beadle and Boris Ephrussi, on the basis of mutational analysis in two genes and tissue transplantation experiments, determine the order of two enzymes in a biochemical pathway in Drosophila.

1939

R. J. Gautheret demonstrates the first successful culture of isolated plant tissues as a continuously dividing callus tissue.

1940

Clarence P. Oliver discovers in Drosophila that a gene is not a point on a chromosome but rather a segment divisible by crossing over.

1940

Karl Landsteiner and A. S. Wiener describe the Rh blood groups.

1941

George Wells Beadle and Edward Tatum, working with a bread mold, Neurospora, publish results indicating that genes mediate cellular chemistry through the production of specific enzymes: the "one gene-one enzyme" experiment. This establishes the use of fungi as model systems to study genetics. Beadle and Tatum will receive the Nobel Prize in Physiology or Medicine in 1958.

1941-1942

The siege of Leningrad places Nicolai Vavilov's seed collections in peril. The curators of the collection, although they are starving along with tens of thousands of people, make a pact that they will not eat the seeds in the collections. Nine of them voluntarily starve to death, sacrificing their lives to preserve the genetic diversity collected by Vavilov.

1943-1944

The Rockefeller Foundation, in collaboration with the Mexican government, initiates the Mexican Agricultural Program. This program relies extensively on plant breeding, coupled with other improved agricultural practices, to increase Mexico's wheat, corn, and bean production. It is one of a series of projects that over a period of decades result in the Green Revolution, a dramatic increase in staple food production in less developed countries in Latin America and Asia. Norman Borlaug, who founded the wheat breeding programs in Mexico, India, and Pakistan, will receive the Nobel Peace Prize in 1970 for his contributions to the Green Revolution.

1944

Oswald T. Avery, Colin MacLeod, and Maclyn McCarty purify DNA and identify it as the "transforming principle" in the pneumococcal bacteria of Frederick Griffith's work. Although this experiment provides solid evidence that DNA is the hereditary material, most scientists still do not suspect that the conclusion may apply to other organisms.

1945

R. D. Owen conducts studies with two sets of cattle twins which demonstrate that their blood antigens could have come only from the opposite sires. These findings suggest the reciprocal passage of ancestral red blood cells. Owen's work has significant implications for immunology.

1945

Max Delbrück, Salvador Luria, and Alfred Hershey work on bacteriophage as a model system to study the mechanism of heredity. Delbrück organizes a course at Cold Spring Harbor, New York, to introduce researchers to the methods of working with bacteriophage. His course will be taught for twenty-six years, helping countless researchers to understand the use of bacteria and bacteriophages as model organisms in genetic investigations. Delbrück, Luria, and Hershey will later share the 1969 Nobel Prize in Physiology or Medicine.

1946

Joshua Lederberg and Edward Tatum discover genetic recombination through conjugation in bacteria. This discovery demonstrates that the genetic material may be transferred from one bacterial cell to another, and may recombine in the recipient cell, albeit by different mechanisms than those employed by the eukaryotes. Lederberg will win the Nobel Prize in Physiology or Medicine in 1958; Tatum and Beadle will also share in the 1958 prize for their work with cellular chemistry, enzymes, and genetics.

1946

Theodosius Dobzhansky publishes Heredity, Race, and Society, a book refuting the eugenics movement on the basis of genetic principles.

1949

Linus Pauling determines that sickle-cell anemia is the result of a change in the structure and chemical properties of hemoglobin. His investigations into protein structure contribute to determination of the structure of DNA. He will receive the Nobel Prize in Chemistry in 1954.

1949

Murray Barr and E. G. Bertram identify a condensed body of chromatin present in the nucleus of female mammalian cells. It will later be identified as an inactivated X chromosome and named the Barr body.

1950

Barbara McClintock publishes her conclusions that certain chromosomal elements in corn can be excised and inserted elsewhere in the chromosome. The name of this phenomenon is transposition, and the mobile elements were later termed "transposable elements," or transposons. McClintock's ideas were far ahead of her time. Her work will not be widely recognized until more evidence of transposition surfaces decades later. She will win the Nobel Prize in Physiology or Medicine in 1983.

1950

Bernard Davis shows that cell-to-cell contact is required for bacterial conjugation, ruling out transformation, of the type studied by Frederick Griffith and Oswald Avery et al., as an explanation of the Lederberg and Tatum experiments. Conjugation and transformation are two separate processes that allow bacterial genetic recombination.

1950-1951

Erwin Chargaff discovers consistent one-to-one ratios of adenine to thymine and of guanine to cytosine in DNA, suggesting a possible chemical relationship between these base pairs. Chargaff's observations become an important clue in determining the double-helical structure of DNA.

1950-1951

Maurice Wilkins obtains an X-ray diffraction image of the A form of DNA in 1950, which indicates that the crystalline molecule is symmetrical and helical. Rosalind Franklin obtains in 1951 a clear X-ray diffraction image of the B form (the form assumed by the vast majority of DNA in cells), which reveals important aspects of cellular DNA structure, among them its dimensions, helical shape, regular repeating subunits, and positioning of the sugar-phosphate backbones on the outside and bases on the inside of the molecule. Franklin's image, dubbed Photo 51, would be a key piece of evidence for deciphering the structure of DNA.

1952

Joshua Lederberg, Esther Lederberg, and Norton Zinder discover transduction, the transfer of genetic information between bacterial cells via a viral vector. Using Escherichia coli and a bacteriophage called P1, they show that transduction can be used to map genes on the bacterial chromosome.

1952

Alfred Hershey and Martha Chase use radioactive isotopes and bacteriophage infection of bacterial cells to demonstrate that bacteriophage's genetic material is DNA and not protein. This experiment is another key piece of evidence confirming that DNA is the hereditary material.

1952

Investigations into bacteriophage by Salvador Luria and Mary L. Human, and independently by Jean J. Weigle, lay the groundwork for the discovery of restriction endonucleases.

1953

James Watson and Francis Crick propose a model for the double-helical structure of DNA in a brief manuscript published in Nature, "Molecular Structure of Nucleic Acids: A Structure for Deoxyribose Nucleic Acid." This elegant and concise paper describes the structure of the B form of DNA and suggests a mode of replication. Watson and Crick, along with Maurice Wilkins, will receive the Nobel Prize in Physiology or Medicine in 1962. Rosalind Franklin, whose X-ray diffraction work was a major component in the discovery, will not share in the prize, having died several years earlier of cancer, possibly a result of her work with X rays.

1955

Seymour Benzer maps more than 2,400 mutations in a gene by observing bacteriophage recombination. He discovers a lower limit for the units of recombination, which he shows correspond to the individual nucleotides in DNA, a powerful correlation between DNA structure and a genetic phenomenon.

1956

Joe Hin Tjio and Albert Levan determine the chromosome number in humans to be forty-six. Until that time, the chromosome number was thought to be forty-eight. The advances that Tjio and Levan pioneered were instrumental in obtaining good chromosome preparations, allowing for significant advances in the field of cytogenetics.

1956

Elie Wollman and François Jacob map seven genes in the E. coli genome based on the relative times at which genes enter a recipient bacterial cell during conjugation. Time-of-entry mapping becomes the standard method for mapping genes in E. coli, the most researched bacterial model organism. 1956-1958 Arthur Kornberg purifies the enzyme DNA polymerase from Escherichia coli. This is the enzyme responsible for DNA replication, making it possible to synthesize DNA in vitro. Kornberg, along with Severo Ochoa, will win the Nobel Prize in Physiology or Medicine in 1959.

1957

Vernon M. Ingram determines that a single amino acid substitution in the beta subunit of hemoglobin is the cause of sickle-cell anemia, clarifying the alteration in protein structure discovered by Pauling in 1949.

1957

Heinz Fraenkel-Conrat and B. Singer show that tobacco mosaic virus contains RNA—the first concrete evidence that RNA, in addition to DNA, serves as the genetic material.

1957

In a landmark address to the British Society of Experimental Biology titled "On Protein Synthesis," Francis Crick articulates both the sequence hypothesis (the order of bases on a section of DNA encodes the amino acid sequence in a protein) and the "central dogma" of molecular genetics (genetic information moves from DNA to RNA to proteins, but not from proteins back to DNA).

1957

Alexander Robertus Todd wins the Nobel Prize in Chemistry. As part of wide-ranging research in organic chemistry, Todd revealed how ribose and deoxyribose bond to the nitrogenous bases on one side of a nucleotide unit and to the phosphate group on the other side. These discoveries provide a foundation for work by others that explains the structure of the DNA molecule.

1958

Matthew Meselson and Franklin Stahl, in what has been dubbed "the most elegant experiment in biology," use light and heavy isotopes of nitrogen to demonstrate that bacterial DNA replicates in a semiconservative manner: Each strand of the molecule serves as a template for the synthesis of a new, complementary strand, a hypothesis proposed by Watson and Crick in their seminal 1953 paper.

1959

Jérôme Lejeune discovers that Down syndrome is the result of an extra chromosome, evidence that genetic disorders in humans could be the result of changes in chromosome number.

1961

Sol Spiegelman and Benjamin Hall discover that single-stranded DNA will hydrogen bond to its complementary RNA. The discovery of the ability of DNA and RNA to form an association contributed to determining how genes are expressed.

1961

In a series of experiments, Jacques Monod, François Jacob, Sydney Brenner, Matthew Meselson, François Gros, and Francis Crick discover messenger RNA (mRNA), discovering that it is the molecule that carries information from DNA to the ribosome for protein synthesis. This discovery was critical to the understanding of protein synthesis and hence gene expression. Monod and Jacob will win the 1965 Nobel Prize in Physiology or Medicine for this work.

1961-1966

Marshall Nirenberg and Heinrich Matthaei discover the first sequence of three bases of RNA that encode an amino acid using RNA homopolymers: UUU encodes phenylalanine. Severo Ochoa used random RNA heteropolymers to narrow the possibilities of the genetic code. By 1963, Nirenberg have identified the nucleotide composition, albeit not the nucleotide order, of thirty-five codons, using data from his and other laboratories. In 1965, Nirenberg and Philip Leder develop a three-nucleotide "mini-RNA" method that allowed them to identify fifty of the sixty-four codons. In 1966, H. Gobind Khorana identifies the final fourteen codons using repeating RNA heteropolymers. Robert W. Holley, in 1965, sequences a yeast transfer RNA (tRNA), which led to the discovery of the tRNA function in transferring the genetic-code information in mRNA into a sequence of amino acids. Nirenberg, Khorana, and Holley will receive the Nobel Prize in Physiology or Medicine in 1968 for their contributions to understanding protein synthesis.

1962

Mary Lyon hypothesizes that during development, one of the two X chromosomes in normal mammalian females is inactivated at random, clarifying the function of the Barr body, discovered by Murray Barr in 1949. Her hypothesis is known as the Lyon hypothesis.

1962

Werner Arber finds bacteria that are resistant to infection by bacteriophage. It appears that some cellular enzymes destroy phage DNA, while others modify the bacterial DNA to prevent self-destruction. Several years later, Arber, Stuart Linn, Matthew

Meselson, and Robert Yuan isolate the first restriction endonuclease and identify the modification of bacterial DNA as methylation. By this time, scientists are looking at how DNA regulates, and is regulated by, cellular activities in a new discipline, molecular genetics. Arber will win the Nobel Prize in Physiology or Medicine in 1978.

1963-1964

Evidence published in 1963 by Margit Nass and Sylvan Nass, who used chemical methods coupled with electron microscopy, points to the presence of DNA in chick embryo mitochondria. In 1964, Gottfried Schatz, E. Halsbrunner, and H. Tuppy purify yeast mitochondria and show that they contain significant amounts of DNA. These discoveries offer a plausible explanation for extranuclear inheritance observed in fungi, plants, and animals.

1964

Robin Holliday proposes a model for the recombination of DNA. Although recombination, or crossing over, is not a new idea, the molecular mechanism underlying the exchange between two homologous molecules of DNA was not known. Holliday's model explains the phenomenon and will become the basis for more detailed models in later years.

1964

John B. Gurdon transfers nuclei from toad tadpole intestinal cells into toad eggs whose native nuclei had been ablated. A small percentage of these eggs develop into adults, genetic clones of the original tadpole. This same year, F. C. Steward and coworkers regenerate whole plants from undifferentiated carrot callus cell culture. These experiments introduce animal and plant cloning.

1965

André Lwoff shares the Nobel Prize in Physiology or Medicine with Monod and Jacob. Lwoff earlier demonstrated that the genetic material of bacteriophage can become part of the host bacterium's DNA, a process known as lysogeny. 1965-1967 Sydney Brenner and colleagues identify the three stop codons.

1966

Victor McKusick publishes the first catalog of single genes that govern variation for traits in humans, Mendelian Inheritance in Man, which continues to

be published in subsequent editions, including an online version.

1966

The International Rice Research Institute (IRRI) releases IR8, a short-stature rice variety derived from IRRI's rice breeding program. This new rice outperforms all previous varieties of rice and is widely adopted in rice-growing regions throughout the world. This event is one in a series known collectively as the Green Revolution.

1967

Mary Weiss and Howard Green introduce a method for physical chromosome mapping of human genes using somatic cell hybridization of human and mouse cells.

1967

Scientists in several laboratories isolate DNA ligase, the enzyme that joins DNA molecules.

1968

Reiji Okazaki reports the discovery of short fragments of DNA, later known as Okazaki fragments, evidence of discontinuous synthesis of the lagging DNA strand.

1970

Morton Mandel and Akiko Higa discover a method to increase the efficiency of bacterial transformation. They make the cells "competent" to take up DNA by treating bacteria with calcium chloride and then heat-shocking the cells. Introducing foreign DNA into cells was a key to the success of recombinant DNA methods.

1970

H. Gobind Khorana and twelve associates synthesize the first artificial gene: a gene encoding alanine transfer RNA in yeast.

1970

David Baltimore and Howard Temin independently discover reverse transcriptase, an enzyme used by viruses to generate a complementary DNA copy of their RNA. The reverse transcriptase enzyme becomes a key tool in genetic engineering, for which Baltimore and Temin will win the 1975 Nobel Prize in Physiology or Medicine.

1970

Hamilton O. Smith isolates the first restriction endonuclease, HindII, that cuts at a specific DNA sequence—the first "site-specific restriction enzyme." Daniel Nathans uses this enzyme to create a restriction map of the virus SV40. The use of restriction enzymes, those that cut DNA, allowed for the detailed mapping and analysis of genes. It also was pivotal for recombinant DNA techniques, including the production of transgenic organisms. Nathans and Smith will win the Nobel Prize in Physiology or Medicine in 1978 for their work on restriction enzymes.

1972

Paul Berg is the first to create a recombinant DNA molecule. He shows that restriction enzymes can be used to cut DNA in a predictable manner and that these DNA fragments can be joined together with fragments from different organisms. He will be awarded the Nobel Prize in Physiology or Medicine in 1980.

1972

Stanford Moore and William H. Stein win the Nobel Prize in Chemistry for earlier work identifying the sequence of amino acids in ribonuclease, a clue to the structure of the gene that encodes it.

1973

Joseph Sambrook and other researchers at Cold Spring Harbor improve the method of separating DNA fragments based on size, a technique called agarose gel electrophoresis. This method makes it possible to achieve an accurate interpretation of the information in DNA.

1973

Stanley Cohen and Herbert Boyer develop recombinant DNA technology by producing the first recombinant plasmid in bacteria. Plasmids—small, circular pieces of DNA—occur naturally in bacteria. Using tools of molecular biology, Cohen and Boyer inserted a new, or "foreign," piece of DNA into a genetically engineered plasmid, which then propagated itself, along with the foreign DNA, in bacterial cells. The process of replicating foreign DNA in bacteria is eventually named molecular cloning.

1975

The Asilomar Conference is held in response to increasing concerns over safety and ethics of recombinant DNA technology. Convening in Pacific Grove, California, under the auspices of the National Institutes of Health, 140 prominent international researchers and academicians air their opinions about recombinant DNA experimentation and advocate adoption of ethical guidelines. NIH later issues guidelines for recombinant DNA research to minimize potential hazards if genetically altered bacteria were released into the environment. The guidelines will be relaxed by 1981.

1975

Mary-Claire King and Allan Wilson report, based on results of a survey of protein and nucleic acid studies, that the average human protein is more than 99 percent identical to that of chimpanzees, which is confirmed by later research.

1975

Edward Southern develops a method for transferring DNA from an agarose gel to a solid membrane. This technique, known as Southern blotting, becomes one of the most important methods in recombinant DNA research.

1975

Renato Dulbecco, David Baltimore, and Howard Temin receive the Nobel Prize in Physiology or Medicine for their work on the interaction between tumor viruses and the genetic material of the cell.

1975

David Pribnow compares the sequences in the promoter regions of several bacterial genes and finds a conserved DNA sequence in them, which is later named the Pribnow box.

1976

Herbert Boyer and Robert Swanson form Genentech, a company devoted to the development and promotion of biotechnology and applications of genetic engineering.

1976

Susumu Tonegawa discovers the genetic mechanism for generation of antibody diversity. The DNA of antibody-encoding genes of immune cells is rearranged in a countless array of different combinations. This explains how millions of different antibodies can be produced from a very small number of genes.

Tonegawa will win the Nobel Prize in Physiology or Medicine in 1987.

1977

Allan Maxam and Walter Gilbert develop a method to determine the nucleotide sequence of a segment of DNA. This same year, Frederick Sanger develops a different method, chain termination (dideoxy) sequencing. Although both the Gilbert-Maxam and the Sanger methods are effective, the Sanger method predominates because it is less complex and does not require toxic chemicals. Gilbert and Sanger will both receive the Nobel Prize in Physiology or Medicine in 1980.

1977

James Alwine develops Northern blotting, a variant of Southern blotting but with RNA instead of DNA.

1977

The U.S. Court of Customs and Patent Appeals rules that an inventor can patent genetically engineered microorganisms. The first patent granted for a recombinant organism, an oil-degrading bacterium, will be awarded in 1980. The legality and ethics of patenting recombinant organisms and other biological systems are highly controversial.

1977

Herbert Boyer synthesizes the human hormone somatostatin in Escherichia coli—the first successful use of recombinant DNA to produce a protein encoded by a eukaryotic gene in bacteria. Before recombinant DNA methods became available, isolation of mammalian somatostatin required a half million sheep brains to produce 5 milligrams of the hormone. Now, with the use of recombinant DNA, only two gallons of bacterial culture are required to produce the same amount.

1977

Phillip A. Sharp and Richard Roberts independently discover that genes in adenovirus contain intervening sequences that are not present in the mRNAs encoded by those genes. Later, the DNA segments that persist in the mRNA are named exons, and the intervening sequences removed during processing of the mRNA are named introns. Sharp and Roberts will win the 1993 Nobel Prize in Physiology or Medicine for this discovery.

1978

M. L. Goldberg and D. S. Hogness and collaborators discover a conserved promoter sequence about twenty-five nucleotide pairs upstream of the transcription startpoint in genes encoding histones in Drosophila melanogaster. This sequence is later named the TATA box and is a transcription factor binding site present in the promoters of most eukaryotic genes.

1978

Herbert Boyer generates a synthetic version of the human insulin gene and inserts it into Escherichia coli cells, which produce human insulin. Development of this technology leads to commercial production of recombinant human insulin for treatment of diabetes.

1978

P. C. Steptoe and R. G. Edwards successfully use in vitro fertilization and artificial implantation in humans. Louise Brown, the first "test-tube baby," is born July 25. The process gives hope to many childless couples who, prior to this development, have been unable to conceive. It also raises concerns from ethicists and others over both the potential effects on the individual child's long-term health and social implications.

1980

A team headed by David Botstein discovers variation among individuals for the lengths of DNA fragments generated by digestion of DNA with restriction enzymes. These fragments that vary in size are named "restriction fragment length polymorphisms" (RFLPs), and they become an important tool for genetic analysis, paternity identification, DNA fingerprinting, and genetic testing for mutant alleles that cause genetic disorders.

1980

Jon W. Gordon produces the first transgenic mouse.

1980

The U.S. Supreme Court votes 5-4 that living organisms can be patented under federal law, and Ananda M. Chakrabarty receives the first patent for a genetically engineered organism, a form of bacteria, Pseudomona originosa, that can decompose crude oil for use in cleaning up oil spills.

1980

George Snell, Baruj Benacerraf, and Jean Dausset receive the Nobel Prize in Physiology or Medicine for their research on the genes encoding proteins of the major histocompatibility complex (MHC), a key component of the mammalian immune system.

1981

J. Michael Bishop and Harold Varmus discover that oncogenes (genes that play a role in initiating cancer) originate in normal cells as genes that control cellular growth and are not solely derived from retroviruses, as previously speculated. Their work influences subsequent studies of tumor development. Varmus and Bishop will win the Nobel Prize in Physiology or Medicine in 1989.

1982

Jorge Yunis and Om Prakash publish a comparison of G-banded human, chimpanzee, gorilla, and orangutan chromosomes. Although the chromosomes of all four species align well with one another, analysis reveals major structural differences among the aligned chromosomes which distinguish the species. These include evidence of a fusion that formed human chromosome 2, inversions, and translocations. The human and chimpanzee karyotypes are the most similar, differing by a fusion and nine inversions.

1982

The U.S. government approves commercialization of the first genetically engineered product, human insulin, dubbed Humulin. The production of pharmaceuticals through recombinant DNA technology is becoming a driving force behind both the drug industry and agriculture.

1982

Aaron Klug wins the Nobel Prize in Chemistry. Klug used X-ray crystallography to investigate biochemical structures, especially those of viruses. He linked the assembly of viral protein subunits with specific sites on viral RNA, which helped in fighting viruses that cause disease in plants and, more basically, in understanding the mechanism of RNA transfer of genetic information. He also determined the structure of transfer RNA (tRNA), which has a shape similar to that of a bent hairpin.

1983

Nancy Wexler, Michael Conneally, and James Gusella determine the chromosomal region of the gene that is mutated in people who have Huntington's disease. They are unable to locate the gene itself; it will be discovered ten years later.

1983

Thomas Cech and Sidney Altman independently discover catalytic RNA. The idea that RNA can have an enzymatic function changes researchers' views on the role of this molecule, leading to important new theories about the evolution of life. Cech and Altman will win the 1989 Nobel Prize in Chemistry.

1983

Bruce Cattanach provides evidence of genomic imprinting in mice. The phenomenon of imprinting is the differential targeting of genes for regulation in male and female gametes. This leads to differential expression of these genes during embryonic development.

1983

John Sulston, Sydney Brenner, and H. Robert Horvitz describe the cell lineage of the nematode Caenorhabditis elegans. The fixed developmental pattern of this small worm provides researchers with insights into how cell fate is determined during development and how cells influence the fates of neighboring cells. Sulston, Brenner, and Horvitz will win the 2002 Nobel Prize in Physiology or Medicine.

1983

Nina Fedoroff leads a team that clones the Ac and Ds elements in corn, transposable elements studied in depth more than thirty years earlier by Barbara McClintock. Characterization of these elements at the molecular level explains McClintock's observations.

1983-1984

William Bender's laboratory isolates and characterizes the molecular details of Drosophila homeotic genes. William McGinnis and J. Weiner discover that the base sequences of the homeotic genes they examined contain a highly similar sequence in a 180-base region. They term the conserved 180-base sequence a "homeobox." These regulatory genes direct the differentiation of body parts in animals.

1983-1985

Kary B. Mullis invents the polymerase chain reaction (PCR). This revolutionary method of copying DNA from extremely small amounts of material changes the way molecular research is done in only a few short years. It also becomes important in medical diagnostics and forensic analysis. Mullis will win the Nobel Prize in Chemistry in 1995.

1984

The Plant Gene Expression Center, a collaborative effort between academia and the U.S. Department of Agriculture, is established to research plant molecular biology, sequence plant genomes, and develop genetically modified plants.

1985

Michael S. Brown and Joseph L. Goldstein win the Nobel Prize in Physiology or Medicine for their work on the regulation of cholesterol in humans. They showed that in families with a history of high cholesterol, individuals who are homozygous for a mutant allele have cholesterol levels several times higher than normal, and those who are heterozygous for the mutant allele have levels about double normal.

1985-1987

Alec Jeffreys publishes methods for DNA fingerprinting as a way to positively link a sample of DNA with that of an individual. In a high-profile rapemurder case in England, DNA fingerprinting excludes a suspect who had been coerced into confessing and later identifies the actual perpetrator.

1985-1987

Robert Sinsheimer, Renato Dulbecco, and Charles DeLisi begin investigating the possibility of sequencing the entire human genome. DeLisi, head of the Department of Energy's Office of Health and Environmental Research, seeks federal funding. After the invention of automated sequencing, the National Research Council and later the Office of Technology Assessment support the idea.

1986

Leroy Hood, a biologist at the California Institute of Technology, constructs a prototype of the automated DNA sequencer, the most important advance in DNA sequencing technology since Gilbert and Maxam, and Sanger, developed their sequencing

methods in the 1970's. Automated sequencing replaces radioactive labels for identifying the four DNA bases with colored fluorescent dyes. Each of the four DNA bases is coded with a different dye to eliminate the need to run separate reactions. Laser and computer technology are integrated at the end stage to gather data. The result is safer, more accurate, and more rapid DNA sequencing.

1986

R. M. Myers, K. Tilly, and T. Maniatis use a saturation mutagenesis procedure to test the effect of mutations in the promoter region of the mouse beta-major globin gene. Mutations in the conserved TATA and CAAT boxes significantly alter transcription, whereas most mutations elsewhere do not, evidence that that these conserved regions have an important functional role in the initiation of transcription.

1987

Rebecca L. Cann, Mark Stoneking, and Allan C. Wilson propose on the basis of RFLP analysis of mitochondrial DNA from humans of diverse geographic origins that a single female, who lived in Africa about 200,000 years ago, is the common ancestor of the mitochondrial DNA of all living humans, the so-called "mitochondrial Eve" hypothesis.

1987

Frostban, a genetically engineered bacterium designed to prevent freezing, is tested on strawberries in California. These bacteria are released under controlled conditions outdoors, where it is hoped they will grow on the strawberries and prevent the fruit from being damaged by frost early in the growing season. The environmental release of recombinant organisms is an important and controversial step in the application of genetic engineering.

1987

Calgene receives a patent for a DNA sequence that extends the shelf life of genetically modified tomatoes.

1987

Carol Greider and Elizabeth Blackburn, using the model organism Tetrahymena (a protozoan), report evidence that telomeres are regenerated by an enzyme called telomerase with an RNA component. Based on the action of DNA polymerase, telomeres (located at the tips of chromosomes) should become shorter during each round of cell division. Telomerase, however, is found to extend telomere DNA, restoring the telomeres. Research in this field sparks interest in the possibility that declining levels of telomerase may contribute to aging and that the expression of this enzyme in tumor cells may be a factor in cancer.

1988

The Human Genome Organization (HUGO) is founded to coordinate and collect data from international efforts to sequence the human genome.

1988

The U.S. Congress establishes the National Center for Biotechnology Information (NCBI) as a division of the National Library of Medicine at the National Institutes of Health as a clearinghouse for molecular genetic information.

1988

The Food and Drug Administration (FDA) approves the sale of recombinant TPA (tissue plasminogen activator) as a treatment for blood clots. TPA shows promise in helping victims recovering from heart attack and stroke.

1989

Francis Collins, Lap-Chee Tsui, and researchers at Toronto's Hospital for Sick Children use chromosome walking and jumping to locate and isolate the CF gene, which codes the cystic fibrosis transmembrane conductance regulator (CFTR) protein. Mutations in this gene are responsible for cystic fibrosis.

1990

Maynard Olsen, Leroy Hood, Charles Cantor, and David Botstein publish "A Common Language for Physical Mapping of the Human Genome," in which they propose the use of "sequence tagged sites" to coordinate human genome sequencing efforts across laboratories. Their proposal is widely adopted and contributes to collaboration in the genome sequencing and assembly effort.

1990

Madan K. Bhattacharyya, Alison M. Smith, T. H. Noel Ellis, Cliff Hedley, and Cathie Martin publish

the first molecular characterization of a gene Mendel studied, the gene that governs seed shape in garden pea. They find that the mutation that causes wrinkled seeds is a transposable element insertion.

1990

Gene therapy for severe combined immunodeficiency (SCID) is tested in clinical trials and becomes one of the first successful applications of somatic cell gene therapy. The first patient is a four-year-old girl who was born without a functioning immune system as a result of a faulty gene that makes an enzyme called ADA (adenosine deaminase).

1990

The Human Genome Project officially begins, headed by James Watson, under the auspices of the National Institutes of Health, National Center for Human Genome Research. The project is to be completed by the year 2005. The ambitious project is designed to sequence and assemble the entire euchromatic portion of the human genome and annotate it with identification of its genes and other features. Also included as part of the Human Genome Project is genome sequencing of several model organisms.

1990

At the Plant Gene Expression Center, biologist Michael Fromm announces the use of a high-speed "gene gun" to transform corn. Gene guns are used to inject genetic material directly into cells via DNAcoated microparticles.

1991

J. Craig Venter of the National Institutes of Health demonstrates the use of automated sequencing and expressed sequence tags (ESTs)—cloned sequences of complementary DNA (cDNA) molecules stored in "libraries"—to identify genes and their functions rapidly and accurately.

1991

Steven T. Warren and coworkers discover that most mutations responsible for fragile X syndrome are trinucleotide repeat expansions. Several other genetic disorders, including Huntington's disease, are found to also be a consequence of trinucleotide expansions.

1991

Scientists at the Howard Hughes Medical Institute, Yale University School of Medicine determine the DNA sequence of the ancient chromosome fusion site in human chromosome 2 and find that it was a head-to-head fusion within the telomeres of the two chromosomes.

1992

One of the first major accomplishments of the Human Genome Project is publication of an RFLP linkage map of human chromosomes with 1,416 mapped markers spanning 92 percent of the genome. Also, by 1992, physical maps of chromosome 21 and the Y chromosome had been completed with overlapping contigs in the euchromatic regions.

1992

The National Research Council in the United States publishes standards for the use of DNA technology in forensic science.

1992

The GenBank database, which will become the principal centralized database for deposition of DNA sequences, is transferred from the Department of Energy to the National Center for Biotechnology Information (NCBI).

1993

The gene that is mutated in people who have Huntington's disease is isolated and sequenced, ten years after its chromosomal region was first identified. Fifty-eight scientists collaborated on the project. The mutations responsible for Huntington's disease are trinucleotide expansion mutations within the protein-encoding portion of the gene.

1993

Michael Smith wins the Nobel Prize in Chemistry for developing "site-directed mutagenesis," a means of reconfiguring genes to produce altered proteins with distinct properties.

1994

The FDA approves the bovine hormone known as BST or BGH. The hormone is made from recombinant bacteria containing a genetically engineered version of the gene encoding BST. When injected into cows, the hormone increases milk production by up to 20 percent. Many supermarkets and manufacturers of dairy products refuse to carry or use milk from BST-injected cows.

1994

The FDA gives approval for the marketing of the Flavr Savr tomato. This genetically altered tomato can be ripened on the vine before being picked and transported. Because the spoilage process is prolonged, the tomatoes have longer shelf lives. The product is not successful, due in part to public concerns over genetically modified foods and in part to the mediocre quality of the tomato variety used as the recipient for the modified gene.

1994

Alfred G. Gilman and Martin Rodbell receive the Nobel Prize in Physiology or Medicine for discovering the role of "G" proteins in regulating signal transduction in eukaryotic cells.

1995

A mutation in the gene BRCA1, found by Mark Skolnick and others, is implicated in breast cancer. More than any other gene previously identified, this discovery has potential for assessing inherited breast cancer risk.

1995

J. Craig Venter of The Institute for Genome Research (TIGR) announces completion of the first DNA sequence of a nonviral, self-replicating, freeliving organism, the bacterium Haemophilus influenzae, using "whole-genome random sequencing," nicknamed "shotgun" sequencing. This method, which precludes the need for a preliminary physical map of the genome, speeds the sequencing of other organisms significantly.

1995

Sequencing of the bacterium with the smallest known genome, Mycoplasma genitalium, is completed.

1995

Edward B. Lewis, Christiane Nüsslein-Volhard, and Eric Wieschaus win the Nobel Prize in Physiology or Medicine for their work on the genetic control of early development in Drosophila.

1995

Nüsslein-Volhard completes a genetic mutation project in zebrafish. Following her earlier work with Drosophila, Nüsslein-Volhard used similar techniques to begin an intensive study of development in a vertebrate system. This involved screening thousands of mutant individuals to determine if any had developmental defects.

1996

Kristen L. Kroll and Enrique Amaya develop a technique to produce stable transgenic Xenopus (frog) embryos.

1996

A group of more than six hundred researchers sequences the DNA of the yeast Saccharomyces cereviseae, the first eukaryotic organism to have its genome sequenced.

1996

Monsanto introduces genetically engineered soybeans that are resistant to the herbicide glyphosate (Roundup). So-called Roundup-Ready soybeans become one of the most successful genetically engineered agricultural products. Roundup-Ready corn, cotton, and canola soon follow.

1997

Ian Wilmut at the Roslin Institute in Scotland announces the successful cloning of a sheep. The clone is named Dolly, the first mammal cloned from a nucleus extracted from a cell of an adult animal.

1997

The United Nations Educational, Scientific, and Cultural Organization (UNESCO) adopts the Universal Declaration on the Human Genome and Human Rights.

1997

The genomic sequence of the bacterium Escherichia coli is reported by Frederick Blattner and colleagues. Although E. coli is not the first complete bacterial sequence reported, because of the importance of E. coli, this event is a key step in genomic science.

1997

An eight-year court battle between the University of California and Eli Lilly & Co. over the ownership of rights to genetically engineered human insulin is settled on appeal in Lilly's favor. The litigants have spent more than $30 million in the dispute.

1998

The genome of the bacterium Mycobacterium tuberculosis is sequenced.

1998

Celera Genomics is founded by former National Institutes of Health researcher J. Craig Venter. Its mission is to sequence the human genome in the private sector, relying on high-throughput automated sequencers and shotgun sequencing.

1998

The genome of the nematode Caenorhabditis elegans is the first genome of a multicellular organism to be sequenced.

1998

The Human Genome Project completes physical mapping of human chromosomes.

1999

Laboratory tests suggest that the pollen of corn genetically engineered to contain a protein derived from the bacterium Bacillus thuringiensis (Bt) endangers monarch butterfly caterpillars. Although later evidence calls the finding into question, it prompts controversy over the environmental impact of transgenic plants.

1999

The first human death attributable to gene therapy during clinical trial is reported when an eighteen-year-old participant in a trial on gene therapy for hereditary ornithine transcarbamylase (OTC) deficiency dies of multiorgan failure caused by a severe immunological reaction to the disarmed adenovirus vector used in the trial.

1999

The publicly funded Berkeley Drosophila Genome Project and privately funded Celera Genomics have separately sequenced the Drosophila melanogaster genome using different methods. The two projects join forces to annotate the genome, saving the federal government approximately $10 million. They jointly report the results the following year in the May

24 issue of Science. Of the fly's 13,601 genes, a significant number are similar in sequence to human genes.

1999

The first human chromosome, chromosome 22, is completely sequenced.

2000

At a meeting in Montreal, Canada, the United Nations Convention on Biological Diversity approves the Cartegena Protocol on Biosafety, which sets the criterion internationally for patenting genetically modified organisms, including agricultural products.

2000

Chromosome 21, the smallest human chromosome, is completely sequenced; it is the second human chromosome to be completed.

2000

It is estimated that more than two-thirds of the processed foods in U.S. markets contain genetically modified ingredients, mostly products derived from soybeans or corn.

2000

The environmental organization Friends of the Earth reveals that materials derived from StarLink, a genetically engineered corn variety meant only for animal fodder, are present in food products sold in the United States. The news ignites public debate over the use of genetically modified food crops.

2000

At a press conference, a team of more than three hundred scientists from throughout the world announces that they have sequenced the genome of a plant, the model organism Arabidopsis thaliana.

2000

U.S. president Bill Clinton and British prime minister Tony Blair, via videolink, announce completion of the first draft of the human genome. Accompanying Clinton are Francis Collins, representing the publicly funded Human Genome Project, and J. Craig Venter representing privately funded Celera Genomics. A tenuous and limited agreement for collaboration has been reached between the public and private projects.

2001

Complete sequencing of human chromosomes 20 and 14 is published.

2001

The first working drafts of the human genome sequence are published in Science (which reports the results from the private company Celera Genomics, headed by J. Craig Venter) and in Nature (reporting the results from the publicly funded Human Genome Project). The number of protein-encoding genes is estimated to be about 30,000, which is less than previously thought but is later shown to be a significant overestimate in more refined drafts of the genome. Other key features include the observation that 43 percent of the human genome consists of transposable elements, many genes reside in clusters of similar genes, derived from duplication of preexisting genes, mutations occur more often in males than in females, and a few hundred of the estimated 30,000 human genes originated as horizontally transferred bacterial genes.

2001

Researchers complete the genomic sequence for rice, Oryza sativa, the first food crop to have its genome sequenced.

2001

Scientists report that genetic material from transgenic corn has mysteriously turned up in the genome of native corn species near Oaxaca, Mexico. Mexico banned transgenic crops three years earlier, and the closest known crop was located beyond the range of windborne pollen, an indication that transgenic corn is illegally produced in Mexico.

2001

Leland H. Hartwell, R. Timothy Hunt, and Paul M. Nurse win the Nobel Prize in Physiology or Medicine for their research on the regulation of cell cycles. Hartwell identified a class of genes that controls the cycle, including a gene that initiates it. Nurse cloned and described the genetic model of a key regulator, cyclin dependent kinase (cdk), and Hunt discovered cyclins, a class of regulatory proteins.

2002

The mouse genome sequence is completed, using the shotgun method; it is compared with the draft of the human genome and found to have a high degree of synteny (segments with groups of similar genes in the same spatial arrangement).

2003

Dolly, the first mammal cloned from an adult cell, is euthanized after suffering advanced arthritis and lung disease. Researchers speculate about whether cloned animals age prematurely.

2003

D. Torrents, M. Suyama, E. Zdobnov, and P. Bork identify the total number of pseudogenes (nonfunctional copies of genes) in the human genome as 19,724, almost as many as the number of genes. Approximately 70 percent are processed pseudogenes derived from reverse transcription of mRNAs. They consider their methods to be conservative and suspect that the actual number of pseudogenes is much higher.

2003-2004

The Human Genome Project announces a completed draft of the euchromatic portion of the human genome in April, 2003, two years ahead of schedule. An article describing this draft is published in 2004. Among its most notable findings is a more definitive estimate of the number of proteinencoding genes at "19,238 known genes and 2,188 predicted genes," considerably lower than the estimate of 30,000 genes in the 2001 draft.

2005

The first draft of the chimpanzee genome is published. Among the many discoveries associated with this accomplishment, is the observation that the human and chimpanzee genomes are more than 98 percent similar in aligned regions (more than 99 percent within protein-coding sequences). There is evidence of positive and negative selection, and the evolution of genes in both species is highly correlated. This genome serves as an outgroup for examination of human population genetics.

2005

454 Life Sciences introduces next-generation high-throughput DNA sequencing based on a new technology that allows researchers to sequence 400- 600 million nucleotides with 400-500 nucleotide read lengths at high accuracy in a single run. The technology is especially beneficial for genomic projects because it allows rapid large-scale sequencing at a fraction of the time and cost of previous automated sequencing methods.

2006

Andrew Fire and Craig Mello receive the Nobel Prize in Physiology or Medicine for their research on RNA interference (RNAi). RNAi is hailed as one of the most significant discoveries in molecular biology, and this Nobel Prize is considered to be an unusually early award because of its significance. In an attempt beginning in 1986 to produce transgenic petunia plants with overly pigmented purple flowers, Richard Jorgensen had found that the transgenic plants have white flowers with no pigment. In 1998, he explained the phenomenon as a consequence of RNA molecules that interfere with gene expression. This same year, Fire and Mello unravel the causes of this same phenomenon in C. elegans and name the mechanism RNAi. Over the ensuing years, RNAi becomes a promising tool for studying gene expression and for treatment of a wide array of genetically based diseases, disorders, and cancers.

2007

The first draft of the rhesus macaque genome is published, offering genome-wide comparison of three primate genomes (human, chimpanzee, and rhesus macaque).

2007

Mario R. Capecchi, Martin J. Evans, and Oliver Smithies receive the Nobel Prize in Physiology or Medicine "for their discoveries of principles for introducing specific gene modifications in mice by the use of embryonic stem cells." This technology, dubbed gene knockout technology, allows researchers to target specific genes and deactivate them as a way of studying their functions, and has revealed much about mammalian gene expression and function.

2008

A team led by Svante Pääbo publishes the sequence of the Neanderthal mitochondrial genome, noting that the sequence has no evidence of human-Neanderthal hybridization.

2009

Completion of Neanderthal nuclear genome sequencing and annotation is announced. Nancy Morvillo, Ph.D., and Christina J. Moose; updated by Daniel J. Fairbanks, Ph.D.

2009

The long awaited Genetic Information Non-discrimination Act (GINA) is enacted into law and becomes the first federal legislation of its kind. GINA prohibits health insurance and employment discrimination on the basis of genetic information. Unfortunately, GINA contains many loop holes. It does not protect individuals from genetic discrimination for life insurance, disability, or long-term care coverage and only applies to individuals who are asymptomatic among other limitations. Some states have individually adapted GINA to include more stringent regulations.

2009-2010

In the years 2009 and 2010, there was sudden progress in the discovery of DNA sequence variants associated with risk of common complex diseases thanks in part to the launch of the Human Genome Project and the advent of genome-wide association studies (GWAS).

2010

The first published data from the 1000 Genomes Project became available and included the most comprehensive map of genomic variants which is thought to cover 95% of all genetic variants in any person on Earth. The 1000 Genomes Project was launched in 2008 and was a 5-year endeavor that finished in 2012. The objective was to sequence the entire genome of 1000 healthy individuals and catalogue different genetic variants.

2010

Society began to see a rise in the creation and availability of direct to consumer (DTC) genetic testing targeting potential risk for common complex diseases; rather than primarily ancestry screening which had been available for many years based on uniparentally inherited genetic material from mitochondria and/or the Y chromosome.

2011

The completed orangutan genome sequence is published. Orangutans share 97 percent of their genome in common with humans.

2012

National Institutes of Health (NIH) Human Microbiome Project defines the bacterial make up of healthy adults. Some researchers believe that knowing this information will help us understand how changes in the microbiome are associated with and/or cause disease.

2012

The first ever pharmaceutical treatment designed to correct an underlying genetic defect was introduced for cystic fibrosis, a severe multisystem disease that has a wide spectrum of symptoms and is associated with significant morbidity and mortality. Variants in the gene, CFTR, are associated with this disease and hundreds have been identified since the discovery of the gene in 1989. Although it is only effective for a single mutation found in approximately 4-5% of affected individuals, at the time this drug was proof that understanding the genetic mechanism of disease can improve quality of life.

2013

Actress Angelina Jolie authored an opinion piece in the New York Times disclosing her BRCA 1 mutation positive status. The increased media attention caused an increased demand for genetic testing for cancer risk, and a major national 3rd party payer began requiring the involvement of genetics professionals in the ordering of specific genetic tests. This event was dubbed the "The Angelina effect."

2013

Since the discovery and isolation of the BRCA1 and BRCA2 genes in 1994 and 1995, the genetic testing laboratory, Myriad Genetics, was the only laboratory through which patients could obtain testing for hereditary breast and ovarian cancer due to patents held on the genes. However, on June 13, 2013, after the landmark trial regarding gene patenting, Association for Molecular Pathology v. Myriad Genetics, the US Supreme Court announced that genes cannot be patented because they are naturally occurring.

2013

Direct to consumer genetic testing has been available to the general population for many years and, as previously noted, the number of available tests began to increase in 2010. However, in 2013, the FDA instructed several major direct to consumer genetic testing companies to cease all testing due to the lack of demonstrated reliability as predictive tests for medical risk factors.

2014

This was the year of the stem cell. Prior to 2014, stem cell research had only been conducted through animal trials. However, this was a banner year for stem cell research due to the start of human trials by scientists around the world. A team in France began trials which introduced cardiac progenitor cells in heart failure patients. In England, researchers where having some success with stem cell therapy for stroke victims. In California, an FDA-approved trial involving the implantation of pancreatic progenitor cells restored some insulin production for individuals affected by type 1 diabetes. These are just a few examples of the many breakthroughs in stem cell research during 2014 that set the stage for the potential to further develop life-changing treatments in the future.

2015

The FDA began granting limited approval for direct to consumer genetic testing that was deemed to have demonstrated adequate clinical utility with the caveat that DTC companies make genetic counseling available to customers.

2015

During the State of the Union Address, President Barack Obama announced the launch of the Precision Medicine Initiative. Its aim is to make advances in medicine tailored to the individual by collecting genetic and health information from 1 million people. The Precision Medicine Initiative put forth the Mission Statement: "*To enable a new era of medicine through research, technology, and policies that empower patients, researchers, and providers to work together toward development of individualized care.*"

2015

Two promising drugs for the treatment of Duchenne Muscular dystrophy are in development. This treatment will likely only provide a reduction in symptoms for a small percentage of affected boys with a particular gene mutation. However, due to the severity of the disease, advocacy groups pushed for the drugs to be made available to all affected individuals, regardless of genotype, on the small chance that it may slow progression of the disease.

2015

Researchers in Guangzhou China announced they had conducted gene-modification using the CRISPER gene editing technique to correct a defect in the beta-globin gene in a human embryo. This was a terrible failure and resulted in scientists from around the world calling for a halt on altering human embryos that were intended for birth.

2016

The world's first so called "three-parent baby" was born in Mexico. This child received its nuclear DNA from the biologic/intended parents and mitochondrial DNA from another woman. Mitochondrial DNA is exclusively maternally inherited and due to the nature of genetic disease caused by mutations in mitochondrial DNA, some at risk women may not be able to have unaffected offspring. The technique used in the conception of this child in Mexico is thought to have important clinical applications that could allow women who are carriers of (or affected by) mitochondrial conditions to have healthy biological children.

2016

Britain becomes the only country where embryos can be legally modified and transferred to a woman's uterus with the intention of resulting in pregnancy. As of the time of this publication, genetic modification of embryos that are intended for use to achieve a pregnancy is not legal in the United States.

2016

FDA approves a drug for the treatment of spinal muscular atrophy, the most common genetic disease that causes mortality in infants. Researchers are hopeful that this particular type of drug can be modified for the treatment of other genetic conditions in the future.

2017

Donald J. Trump was inaugurated as the 45th president of the United States of America. President

Trump has begun to implement substantial changes to the modern American healthcare system which will likely have implications for the long-term goals of the genetics community.

2017

Canadian Parliament adopts Bill S-201, an Act to Prohibit and Prevent Genetic Discrimination. This act requires the government to create a Genetic Non-Discrimination Act, amend the Canada Labour Code, and amend the Canadian Human Rights Act.

2017

It is difficult to predict the future of genetics and genomics. However, the hope is that by the year 2020, targeted cancer treatments, medications for complex diseases, and other therapies will be personalized based on each individual's genetic information.

Nancy Morvillo, Ph.D., and Christina J. Moose;
2010 edition updated by Daniel J. Fairbanks, Ph.D.
2017 edition updated by Meredith K. Jones, MS, LCGC

GLOSSARY

A: the abbreviation for adenine, a purine nitrogenous base found in the structure of both DNA and RNA.

acentric chromosome: a chromosome that does not have a centromere and that is unable to participate properly in cell division; often the result of a chromosomal mutation during recombination.

acquired characteristic: a change in an individual organism brought about by its interaction with its environment.

acrocentric chromosome: a chromosome with its centromere near one end. *See also* metacentric chromosome; telocentric chromosome.

activator: a protein that binds to DNA, thus increasing the expression of a nearby gene.

active site: the region of an enzyme that interacts with a substrate molecule; any alteration in the three-dimensional shape of the active site usually has an adverse effect on the enzyme's activity.

adaptation: the evolution of a trait by natural selection, or a trait that has evolved as a result of natural selection.

adaptive advantage: increased reproductive potential in offspring as a result of passing on favorable genetic information.

adenine (A): a purine nitrogenous base found in the structure of both DNA and RNA.

adenosine deaminase deficiency: a fatal immunodeficiency disorder caused by an insufficiency of the enzyme adenosine deaminase; death commonly occurs when the infant is a few months old.

adenosine triphosphate (ATP): the major energy molecule of cells, produced either through the process of cellular respiration or fermentation; it is also a component of DNA and RNA.

adenovirus: a group of viruses that cause respiratory illnesses, such as the common cold; they have been genetically altered and used for treatment of cancer and cystic fibrosis.

adult stem cell: an undifferentiated cell found among differentiated cells in a tissue or organ of an adult organism.

agarose: a chemical substance derived from algae and used to create gels for the electrophoresis of nucleic acids.

aggression: behavior directed toward causing harm to others.

Agrobacterium tumefaciens: a species of bacteria that causes disease in some plants and is able to transfer genetic information, in the form of Ti plasmids, into plant cells; modified Ti plasmids can be used to produce transgenic plants.

Alagille syndrome: a genetic disorder of the liver of infants and young children whereby bile builds up in the liver because the bile ducts are abnormally narrow or absent; the child may present with jaundice, fatty deposits under the skin, facial deformities, growth retardation, and heart, kidney, eye, and vertebrae abnormalities.

albinism: the absence of pigment such as melanin in eyes, skin, hair, scales, or feathers or of chlorophyll in plant leaves and stems.

albino: a genetic condition in which an individual does not produce the pigment melanin in the skin; other manifestations of the trait may be seen in the pigmentation of the hair or eyes; albino individuals occur in many animals and plants and are due to the absence of a variety of different pigments.

alcoholism: a medical diagnosis given when there is repeated use of alcohol over the course of at least a year, despite the presence of negative consequences; tolerance, withdrawal, uncontrolled use, unsuccessful efforts to quit, considerable time spent getting or using the drug, and a decrease in other important activities because of the use are part of this condition.

algorithm: a mathematical rule or procedure for solving a specific problem.

alkaptonuria: a genetic disorder, first characterized by geneticist Archibald Garrod, in which a compound called homogentisic acid accumulates in the cartilage and is excreted in the urine of affected individuals, turning both the cartilage and the urine black (the name of the disorder literally means "black urine"); the specific genetic defect involves an inability to process by-products of phenylalanine and tyrosine metabolism.

allele frequency: the proportion of all the genetic variants at a locus within a population of organisms.

allele: a form of a gene at a locus; each locus in an individual's chromosomes has two alleles, which may be the same or different.

allergy: an abnormal immune response to a substance that does not normally provoke an immune response or that is not inherently dangerous to the body (such as plant pollens, dust, or animal dander).

allopatric speciation: a model of speciation in which parts of a population may become geographically isolated, effectively preventing interbreeding, and over time may develop differences that lead to reproductive isolation and the development of a new species.

allopolyploid: a type of polyploid species that contains genomes from more than one ancestral species.

altruism: behavior that benefits others at the evolutionary (reproductive) cost of the altruist.

Alu sequence: a repetitive DNA sequence of unknown function, approximately three hundred nucleotides long, scattered throughout the genome of primates; the name comes from the presence of recognition sites for the restriction endonuclease Alu I in these sequences.

Alzheimer's disease: a degenerative brain disorder, usually found among the elderly, characterized by brain lesions leading to loss of memory, personality changes, and deterioration of higher mental functions.

amber codon: a stop codon (UAG) found in messenger RNA (mRNA) molecules that signals termination of translation.

ambiguous genitalia: external sexual organs that are not clearly male or female.

Ames test: a test devised by molecular biologist Bruce Ames for determining the mutagenic or carcinogenic properties of various compounds based on their ability to affect the nutritional characteristics of the bacterium *Salmonella typhimurium*.

amino acid: a nitrogen-containing compound used as the building block of proteins (polypeptides); in nature, there are twenty amino acids that can be used to build proteins.

aminoacyl tRNA: a transfer RNA (tRNA) molecule with an appropriate amino acid molecule attached; in this form, the tRNA molecule is ready to participate in translation.

amniocentesis: a procedure in which a small amount of amniotic fluid containing fetal cells is withdrawn from the amniotic sac surrounding a fetus; fetal cells, found in the fluid, are then tested for the presence of genetic abnormalities.

amniotic fluid: the fluid in which the fetus is immersed during pregnancy.

amyloid plaques: protein deposits in the brain formed by fragments from amyloid precursor proteins; amyloid plaques are characteristic of Alzheimer's disease.

anabolic steroids: drugs derived from androgens and inappropriately used to enhance performance in sports.

anabolism: the part of the cell's metabolism concerned with synthesis of complex molecules and cell structures.

anaphase: the third phase in the process of mitosis; in anaphase, sister chromatids separate at the centromere and migrate toward the poles of the cell.

anaphylaxis: a severe, sometimes fatal allergic reaction often characterized by swelling of the air passages, leading to inability to breathe.

ancient DNA: DNA isolated from archaeological artifacts or fossils; it is typically extensively degraded.

androgen receptors: molecules in the cytoplasm of cells that join with circulating male hormones.

androgens: steroid hormones that cause masculinization.

anencephalus: a neural tube defect characterized by the failure of the cerebral hemispheres of the brain and the cranium to develop normally.

aneuploid: a cell or individual with one or a few missing or extra chromosomes.

angstrom: a unit of measurement equal to one ten-millionth of a millimeter; a DNA molecule is 20 angstroms wide.

animal cloning: the process of generating a genetic duplicate of an animal starting with one of its differentiated cells.

animal model: an animal that has a disorder that is similar to a human disorder; scientists can then study the disorder and transfer genes into the animals to test therapies.

annealing: the process by which two single-stranded nucleic acid molecules are converted into a doublestranded molecule through hydrogen bonding between complementary base pairs.

anthrax: an acute bacterial disease caused by *Bacillus anthracis* that affects animals and humans and that is especially deadly in its pulmonary form.

antibiotic: any substance produced naturally by a microorganism that inhibits the growth of other microorganisms; antibiotics are important in the treatment of bacterial infections.

antibody: an immune protein (immunoglobulin) that specifically recognizes an antigen; produced by B cells of the immune system.

anticipation: a phenomenon whereby as a genetic disorder is passed on to the next generation, the symptoms of the genetic disorder become apparent at an earlier age with each generation. In most cases, an increase of severity of symptoms is also noted.

anticodon: the portion of a transfer RNA (tRNA) molecule that is complementary in sequence to a codon in a messenger RNA (mRNA) molecule; because of this complementarity, the tRNA molecule can bind briefly to mRNA during translation and direct the placement of amino acids in a polypeptide chain.

antigen: any molecule that is capable of being recognized by an antibody molecule or of provoking an immune response.

antigenic drift or shift: minor changes in the H and N proteins of the influenza virus that enable the virus to evade the immune system of a potential host.

antioxidant: a molecule that preferentially reacts with free radicals, thus keeping them from reacting with other molecules and causing cellular damage.

antiparallel: a characteristic of the Watson-Crick double-helix model of DNA, in which the two strands of the molecule can be visualized as oriented in opposite directions; this characteristic is based on the orientation of the deoxyribose molecules in the sugar-phosphate backbone of the double helix.

antirejection medication: drugs developed to counteract the human body's natural immune system's reaction to transplanted organs.

antisense RNA: a small RNA molecule that is complementary to the coding region of a messenger RNA (mRNA) and when bound to the mRNA prevents it from being translated.

antisense: a term referring to any strand of DNA or RNA that is complementary to a coding or regulatory sequence, for example, the strand opposite the coding strand (the sense strand) in DNA is called the antisense strand.

antitoxin: a vaccine containing antibodies against a specific toxin.

Apo-B: a protein essential for cholesterol transport.

apoptosis: cell "suicide" occurring after a cell is too old to function properly, as a response to irreparable genetic damage, or as a function of genetic programming; apoptosis prevents cells from developing into a cancerous state and is a natural event during many parts of organismal development.

archaea: the domain of life that includes diverse prokaryotic organisms distinct from the historically familiar bacteria and which often require severe conditions for growth, such as high temperatures, high salinity, or lack of oxygen.

artificial selection: selective breeding of desirable traits, typically in domesticated organisms.

ascomycetes: organisms of the phylum Ascomycota, a group of fungi known as the sac fungi, which are characterized by a saclike structure, the ascus.

ascospore: a haploid spore produced by meiosis in ascomycete fungi.

ascus: a reproductive structure, found in ascomycete fungi, that contains ascospores.

asexual reproduction: reproduction of cells or organisms without the transfer or reassortment of genetic material; results in offspring that are genetically identical to the parent.

assortative mating: mating that occurs when individuals make specific mate choices based on the phenotype or appearance of others.

ataxia telangiectasia: a genetic disorder caused by the ataxia-telangiectasia mutated gene; the portion of the brain that controls motor movement and speech deteriorates. The affected child commonly has normal or above normal intelligence, develops slurred speech and poor balance, and has delayed motor development . Telangiectasias develop in the corners of the eyes and on the surfaces of the cheeks and ears. These children are also at risk for cancer, such as acute lymphocytic leukemia and lymphoma. Many children also have a weakened immune system making them prone to infection. Ataxia telangiectasia is commonly fatal before age twenty.

ATP synthase: the enzyme that synthesizes ATP.

ATP: *See* adenosine triphosphate.

autoimmune disorders: chronic diseases that arise from a breakdown of the immune system's ability to distinguish between the body's own cells (self) and foreign substances, leading to an individual's immune system attacking the body's own organs or tissues.

autoimmune response: an immune response of an organism against its own cells.

automated fluorescent sequencing: a modification of dideoxy termination sequencing that uses fluorescent markers to identify the terminal nucleotides, allowing the automation of sequencing.

autopolyploid: a type of polyploid species that contains more than two sets of chromosomes from the same species.

autosomal dominant allele: an allele of a gene (locus) on one of the nonsex chromosomes that is always expressed, regardless of the form of the other allele at the same locus.

autosomal recessive allele: an allele of a gene (locus) that will be expressed only if there are two identical copies at the same locus.

autosomal trait: a trait that typically appears just as frequently in either sex because an autosomal chromosome, rather than a sex chromosome, carries the gene.

autosomes: non-sex chromosomes; humans have forty-four autosomes.

auxotrophic strain: a mutant strain of an organism that cannot synthesize a substance required for growth and therefore must have the substance supplied in the growth medium.

azoospermia: the absence of spermatozoa in the semen.

B cells: a class of white blood cells (lymphocytes) derived from bone marrow and responsible for antibody-directed immunity.

B lymphocytes: *See* B cells.

B memory cells: descendants of activated B cells that are long-lived and that synthesize large amounts of antibodies in response to a subsequent exposure to the antigen, thus playing an important role in secondary immunity.

B-DNA: the predominant form of DNA in solution and in the cell; a right-handed double helix most similar to the Watson-Crick model. *See also* Z-DNA.

Bacillus thuringiensis *(Bt):* a species of bacteria that produces a toxin deadly to caterpillars, moths, beetles, and certain flies.

backcross: a cross involving offspring crossed with one of the parents. *See also* cross.

bacterial artificial chromosomes (BACs): cloning vectors used to clone large DNA fragments (up to 500 kb) that can be readily inserted in a bacterium, such as *Escherichia coli.*

bacteriophage: a virus that infects bacterial cells; often simply called a phage.

baculovirus: a type of virus that is capable of causing disease in a variety of insects.

Barr body: a darkly staining structure primarily present in female cells, believed to be an inactive X chromosome; used as a demonstration of the Lyon hypothesis.

base pair (bp): often used as a measure of the size of a DNA fragment or the distance along a DNA molecule between markers; both the singular and plural are abbreviated bp.

base pairing: the process by which bases link up by hydrogen bonding to form double-stranded molecules of DNA or loops in RNA; in DNA, adenine (A) always pairs with thymine (T), and cytosine (C) pairs with guanine (G); in RNA, uracil (U) replaces thymine.

base: a chemical subunit of DNA or RNA that encodes genetic information; in DNA, the bases are adenine (A), cytosine (C), guanine (G), and thymine (T); in RNA, thymine is replaced by uracil (U).

beta-amyloid peptide: the main constituent of the neuritic plaques in the brains of Alzheimer's patients.

bidirectional replication: a characteristic of DNA replication involving synthesis of DNA in both directions away from an origin of replication.

binary fission: cell division in prokaryotes in which the plasma membrane and cell wall grow inward and divide the cell in two.

biochemical pathway: the steps in the production or breakdown of biological chemicals in cells; each step usually requires a specific enzyme.

bioethics: the study of human actions and goals in a framework of moral standards relating to use and abuse of biological systems.

bioinformatics: the application of information technology to the management of biological information to organize data and extract meaning; a hybrid discipline that combines elements of computer science, information technology, mathematics, statistics, and molecular genetics.

biological clocks: genetically and biochemically based systems that regulate the timing and/or duration of biological events in an organism; examples of processes controlled by biological clocks include circadian rhythms, cell cycles, and migratory restlessness.

biological determinism: the concept that all characteristics of organisms, including behavior, are determined by the genes the organism possesses;

it is now generally accepted that the characteristics of organisms are determined both by genes and environment.

biological weapon: a delivery system or "weaponization" of such pathological organisms as bacteria and viruses to cause disease and death in people, animals, or plants.

biometry: the measurement of biological and psychological variables.

biopesticides: chemicals or other agents derived from or involving living organisms that can be used to control the population of a pest species.

bioremediation: biologic treatment methods to clean up contaminated water and soils.

biotechnology: the use of biological molecules or organisms in industrial or commercial products and techniques.

bioterrorism: use of organisms as instruments or weapons of terror; for example, deliberate introduction of smallpox, anthrax, or other diseases in civilian populations.

blastocyst: a preimplantation embryo consisting of a hollow ball of two layers of cells.

blind proficiency test: a competency assessment in which laboratory personnel are unaware that it is taking place.

blood type: one of the several groups into which blood can be classified based on the presence or absence of certain molecules called antigens on the red blood cells.

blotting: the transfer of nucleic acids or proteins separated by gel electrophoresis onto a filter paper, which allows access by molecules that will interact with only one specific sequence or molecule.

brachycephaly: the shape of a skull shorter than typical for its species. It is perceived as a desirable trait in some domesticated dog and cat breeds, such as Pugs, and can be normal or abnormal in other animal species. In humans, the cephalic disorder is known as flat head syndrome, and results from premature fusion of the coronal sutures (see craniosynostosis) or from external deformation (see plagiocephaly). The coronal suture is the fibrous joint that unites the frontal bone with the two parietal bones of the skull. The parietal bones form the top and sides of the skull. This feature can be seen in Down syndrome.

BRCA1 and BRCA2 genes: the best known examples of genes associated with inherited breast cancers.

Bt toxin: a toxic compound naturally synthesized by bacterium *Bacillus thuringiensis,* which kills insects.

C terminus: the end of a polypeptide with an amino acid that has a free carboxyl group.

C-value: the characteristic genome size for a species.

C: the abbreviation for cytosine, a pyrimidine nitrogenous base found in the structure of both DNA and RNA.

CAG expansion: a mutation-induced increase in the number of consecutive CAG nucleotide triplets in the coding region of a gene.

callus: a group of undifferentiated plant cells growing in a clump.

cAMP: *See* cyclic adenosine monophosphate.

cancer: a disease in which there is unrestrained growth and reproduction of cells, loss of contact inhibition, and, eventually, metastasis (the wandering of cancer cells from a primary tumor to other parts of the body); invasion of various tissues and organs by cancer cells typically leads to death.

candidate gene: a gene suspected of causing a specific disease.

capsid: the protective protein coating of a virus particle.

carcinogen: any physical or chemical cancer-causing agent.

carrier screening: specialized testing to see whether an individual carries a mutated gene for a specific condition.

carrier: a healthy individual who has one normal allele and one defective allele for a recessive genetic disease.

catabolism: the part of the cell's metabolism concerned with the breakdown of complex molecules, usually as an energy-generating mechanism.

catabolite repression: a mechanism of operon regulation involving an enzyme reaction's product used as a regulatory molecule for the operon that encodes the enzyme; a kind of feedback inhibition.

cDNA library: a collection of clones produced from all the RNA molecules in the cells of a particular organism, often from a single tissue. *See also* complementary DNA.

cDNA: *See* complementary DNA.

ceiling principle: a method for estimating the frequency in which a DNA's profile occurs in a population containing a variety of ethnic groups.

cell culture: growth and maintenance of cells or tissues in laboratory vessels containing a precise mixture of nutrients and hormones.

cell cycle: the various growth phases of a cell, which include (in order) G1 (gap phase 1), S (DNA synthesis), G2 (gap phase 2), and M (mitosis).

cell differentiation: a process during which a cell becomes specialized as a specific type of cell, such as a neuron, or undergoes programmed cell death (apoptosis).

cell line: a cell culture maintained for an indeterminate time.

cell signaling: communication between cells that occurs most commonly when one cell releases a specific "signaling" molecule that is received and recognized by another cell.

centiMorgan (cM): a unit of genetic distance between genes on the same chromosome, equal to a recombination frequency of 1 percent; also called a map unit, since these distances can be used to construct genetic maps of chromosomes.

central dogma: a foundational concept in modern genetics stating that genetic information present in the form of DNA can be converted to the form of messenger RNA (or other types of RNA) through transcription and that the information in the form of mRNA can be converted into the form of a protein through translation.

centriole: a eukaryotic cell structure involved in cell division, possibly with the assembly or disassembly of the spindle apparatus during mitosis and meiosis; another name for this organelle is the microtubule organizing center (MTOC).

centromere: a central region where a pair of chromatids are joined before being separated during anaphase of mitosis or meiosis; also, the region of the chromatids where the microtubules of the spindle apparatus attach.

checkpoint: the time in the cell cycle when molecular signals control entry to the next phase.

chemical mutagens: chemicals that can directly or indirectly create mutations in DNA.

chi-square analysis: a nonparametric statistical analysis of data from an experiment to determine how well the observed data correlate with the expected data.

chiasma: the point at which two homologous chromosomes exchange genetic material during the process of recombination; the word literally means "crosses," which refers to the appearance of these structures when viewed with a microscope.

chloroplast DNA (cpDNA): circular DNA molecules found in multiple copies in chloroplasts; they contain some of the genes required for chloroplast functions.

chloroplast: the cellular organelle in plants responsible for photosynthesis.

cholera: an intestinal disease caused by the bacteria *Vibrio cholerae,* which is often spread by water contaminated with human waste.

chorion: an embryonic structure that develops into the placenta; cells from this structure have the same genetic composition as the fetus and are sampled during chorionic villus testing.

chorionic villus sampling: a procedure in which fetal cells are obtained from an embryonic structure called the chorion and analyzed for the presence of genetic abnormalities in the fetus.

chromatid: one half of a chromosome that has been duplicated in preparation for mitosis or meiosis; each chromatid is connected to its sister chromatid by a centromere.

chromatin: the form chromosomes take when not undergoing cell division; a complex of fibers composed of DNA, histone proteins, and nonhistone proteins.

chromatography: a separation technique involving a mobile solvent and a stationary, adsorbent phase.

chromosome jumping: similar to chromosome walking, but involving larger fragments of DNA and thus resulting in faster analysis of longer regions of DNA. *See also* chromosome walking.

chromosome map: a diagram showing the locations of genes on a particular chromosome; generated through analysis of linkage experiments involving those genes.

chromosome mutation: a change in chromosome structure caused by chromosome breakage followed by improper rejoining; examples include deletions, insertions, inversions, and translocations.

chromosome puff: an extremely unwound or uncoiled region of a chromosome indicative of a transcriptionally active region of the chromosome.

chromosome rearrangement (or genomic rearrangement): a type of chromosome abnormality involving a change in the structure of the native chromosome. Such changes may involve several different classes of events, like deletions, duplications, inversions, and translocations.

chromosome theory of inheritance: a concept, first proposed by geneticists Walter Sutton and Theodor Boveri, that genes are located on chromosomes and that the inheritance and movement of chromosomes during meiosis explain Mendelian principles on the cellular level.

chromosome walking: a molecular genetics technique used for analysis of long DNA fragments; the name comes from the technique of using previously cloned and characterized fragments of DNA to "walk" into uncharacterized regions of the chromosome that overlap with these fragments. *See also* chromosome jumping.

chromosome: the form in which genetic material is found in the nucleus of a cell; composed of a single DNA molecule that is extremely tightly coiled, usually visible only during the processes of mitosis and meiosis.

circadian rhythm: a cycle of behavior, approximately twenty-four hours long, that is expressed independent of environmental changes.

cirrhosis: a disease of the liver, marked by the development of scar tissue that interferes with organ function, that can result from chronic alcohol consumption.

cistron: a unit of DNA that is equivalent to a gene; it encodes a single polypeptide.

clinical trial: an experimental research study used to determine the safety and effectiveness of a medical treatment or drug.

clinodactyly: the curvature of a digit (a finger or toe) in the plane of the palm, most commonly the fifth finger (the "little finger") towards the adjacent fourth finger (the "ring finger"). It is a fairly common isolated anomaly which often goes unnoticed, but also occurs in combination with other abnormalities in certain genetic syndromes.

clone: a molecule, cell, or organism that is a perfect genetic copy of another.

cloning vector: a DNA molecule that can be used to transport genes of interest into cells, where these genes can then be copied.

cloning: the technique of making a perfect genetic copy of an item such as a DNA molecule, a cell, or an entire organism.

codominance: a genetic condition involving two alleles at a locus in a heterozygous organism; each of these alleles is fully expressed in the phenotype of the organism.

codon: a group of three nucleotides in messenger RNA (mRNA) that represent a single amino acid in the genetic code; this is mediated through binding of a transfer RNA (tRNA) anticodon to the codon during translation.

color blindness: an inherited condition in people whose eyes lack one or more of the three color receptors.

comparative genomic hybridization (CGH) array: (also microarray-based comparative genomic hybridization, matrix CGH, array CGH, aCGH) is a molecular cytogenetic technique for the detection of chromosomal copy number changes on a genome wide and high-resolution scale.

complementary base pairing: hydrogen bond formation in DNA and RNA that occurs only between cytosine and guanine (in both DNA and RNA) or between adenine and thymine (in DNA) or adenine and uracil (in RNA).

complementary DNA (cDNA): a DNA molecule that is synthesized using messenger RNA (mRNA) as a template and that is catalyzed by the enzyme reverse transcriptase.

complementation testing: performing a cross between two individuals with the same phenotype to determine whether or not the mutations occur within the same gene.

composite transposon: a transposable element that contains genes other than those required for transposition.

comprehensive genomic testing: allows for the estimation of disease risk years to decades before any disease even exists, or even whether a healthy fetus is at higher risk for developing a disease in adolescence or adulthood. Individuals who are more susceptible to disease in the future can be offered lifestyle advice or medication with the aim of preventing the predicted illness. Current genetic testing guidelines supported by the health care professionals discourage purely predictive genetic testing of minors until they are competent to understand the relevancy of genetic screening so as to allow them to participate in the decision about whether or not it is appropriate for them. Genetic screening of newborns and children in the field of predictive medicine is deemed appropriate if there is a compelling clinical reason to do so, such as the availability of prevention or treatment as a child that would prevent future disease.

concerted evolution: a process in which the members of a gene family evolve together.

concordance: the presence of a trait in both members of a pair of twins.

cones: the light-sensitive structures in the retina that are the basis for color vision.

congenital defect: a defect or disorder that occurs during prenatal development.

conjugation: a form of genetic transfer among bacterial cells involving the F pilus.

consanguine: of the same blood or origin; in genetics, the term implies the sharing of genetic traits or characteristics from the same ancestors (as cousins, for example).

consensus sequence: a sequence with no or only slight differences commonly found in DNA molecules from various sources, implying that the sequence has been actively conserved and plays an important role in some genetic process.

contig: shows regions on a chromosome where neighboring portions of DNA overlap; the map provides information about a large segment of a genome by looking at a series of overlapping clones .

cordocentesis: removing a sample of blood for prenatal testing from the umbilical cord using ultrasound guidance.

cosmid: a cloning vector partially derived from genetic sequences of lambda, a bacteriophage; cosmids are useful in cloning relatively large fragments of DNA.

craniofacial syndromes: birth defects of the face or head. Some, like cleft lip and palate, are among the most common of all birth defects. Others are very rare. Most of them affect how a person's face or head looks. These conditions may also affect other parts of the body. Treatment depends on the type of problem. Plastic and reconstructive surgery may help the person's appearance.

craniosynostosis: a congenital defect involving the skull bones of an infant; the bones are fused together at birth requiring surgical intervention to allow for normal brain development.

cross: the mating of individuals to produce offspring by sexual reproduction.

crossing over: the exchange of genetic material between two homologous chromosomes during prophase I of meiosis, providing an important source of genetic variation; also called "recombination" or crossover.

CT scan: uses a computer linked to an x-ray machine to make a series of detailed pictures of areas inside the body. The pictures are taken from different angles and are used to create 3-dimensional (3-D) views of tissues and organs. A dye may be injected into a vein or swallowed to help the tissues and organs show up more clearly. A CAT scan may be used to help diagnose disease, plan treatment, or find out how well treatment is working. Also called computed tomography scan, computerized axial tomography scan, computerized tomography, and CT scan.

cultivar: a variety of plant developed through controlled breeding techniques.

cyclic adenosine monophosphate (cAMP): an important cellular molecule involved in cell signaling and regulation pathways.

cyclins: a group of eukaryotic proteins with characteristic patterns of synthesis and degradation during the cell cycle; part of an elaborate mechanism of cell cycle regulation, and a key to the understanding of cancer.

cystic fibrosis: the most common recessive lethal inherited disease among Caucasians in the United States and the United Kingdom.

cytogenetics: the study of chromosome number and structure, including identification of abnormalities.

cytokines: soluble intercellular molecules produced by cells such as lymphocytes that can influence the immune response.

cytokinesis: the division of the cytoplasm, typically occurring in concert with nuclear division (mitosis or meiosis).

cytoplasmic inheritance: *See* extranuclear inheritance.

cytosine (C): a pyrimidine nitrogenous base found in the structure of both DNA and RNA.

cytoskeleton: the structure, composed of microtubules and microfilaments, that gives shape to a eukaryotic cell, enables some cells to move, and assists in such processes as cell division.

dalton: a unit of molecular weight equal to the mass of a hydrogen atom; cellular molecules such as proteins are often measured in terms of a kilodalton, equal to 1,000 daltons.

daughter cells: cells that result from cell division.

de novo: an alteration in a gene that is present for the first time in one family member as a result of a mutation in a germ cell (egg or sperm) of one of the parents or in the fertilized egg itself.

deamination: the removal of an amino group from an organic molecule.

degenerate: refers to a property of the genetic code via which two or more codons can code for the same amino acid.

degradation: the act of chemically or physically breaking down DNA.

deletion: a type of chromosomal mutation in which a genetic sequence is lost from a chromosome, usually through an error in recombination.

denaturation: changes in the physical shape of a molecule caused by changes in the immediate environment, such as temperature or pH level; denaturation usually involves the alteration or breaking of various bonds within the molecule and is important in DNA and protein molecules.

deoxyribonucleic acid (DNA): the genetic material found in all cells; DNA consists of nitrogenous bases (adenine, guanine, cytosine, and thymine), sugar (deoxyribose), and phosphate.

deoxyribose: a five-carbon sugar used in the structure of DNA.

diabetes: a syndrome in which the body cannot metabolize glucose appropriately.

diakinesis: a subphase of prophase I in meiosis in which chromosomes are completely condensed and position themselves in preparation for metaphase.

dicentric chromosome: a chromosome with two centromeres, usually resulting from an error of recombination.

dideoxy termination sequencing: *See* Sanger sequencing.

differentiation: the series of changes necessary to convert an embryonic cell into its final adult form, usually with highly specialized structures and functions.

dihybrid: an organism that is hybrid for each of two genes—for example, *AaBb;* when two dihybrid organisms are mated, the offspring will appear in a 9:3:3:1 ratio with respect to the traits controlled by the two genes.

diphtheria: an acute bacterial disease caused by *Corynebacterium diphtheriae,* symptoms are primarily the result of a toxin released by the bacteria.

diploid: a cell or organism with two complete sets of chromosomes, usually represented as $2N$, where N stands for one set of chromosomes, for example, humans have two sets of twenty-three chromosomes in their somatic cells, making them diploid.

diplotene: a subphase of prophase I in meiosis in which synapsed chromosomes begin to move apart and the chiasmata are clearly visible.

discontinuous replication: replication on the lagging strand of a DNA molecule, resulting in the formation of Okazaki fragments. *See also* Okazaki fragments.

discontinuous variation: refers to a set of related phenotypes that are distinct from one another, with no overlapping.

discordant: a condition where a set of twins does not display the same characteristics.

disjunction: the normal division of chromosomes that occurs during meiosis or mitosis, the related term "nondisjunction" refers to problems with this process.

disomy: a case in which both copies of a chromosome come from a single parent, rather than (as is usual) one being maternal and one being paternal.

dizygotic: developed from two separate zygotes, fraternal twins are dizygotic because they develop from two separate fertilized ova (eggs).

DNA fingerprinting: a DNA test used by forensic scientists to aid in the identification of criminals or to resolve paternity disputes, which involves looking at known, highly variable DNA sequences; more correctly called DNA genotyping.

DNA footprinting: a molecular biology technique involving DNA-binding proteins that are allowed to bind to DNA; the DNA is then degraded by DNases, and the binding sites of the proteins are revealed by the nucleotide sequences protected from degradation.

DNA gyrase: a bacterial enzyme that reduces tension in DNA molecules that are being unwound during replication; a type of cellular enzyme called a topoisomerase.

DNA library: a collection of cloned DNA fragments from a single source, such as a genome, chromosome, or set of messenger RNA (mRNA) molecules; most common examples are genomic and cDNA libraries.

DNA ligase: a cellular enzyme used to connect pieces of DNA together; important in genetic engineering procedures.

DNA polymerase: the cellular enzyme responsible for making new copies of DNA molecules through replication of single-stranded DNA template molecules or, more rarely, using an RNA template molecule as in the case of RNA-dependent DNA polymerase or reverse transcriptase.

DNA replication: synthesis of new DNA strands complementary to template strands resulting in new double-stranded DNA molecules comprising the old template and the newly synthesized strand joined by hydrogen bonds; described as a semiconservative process in that half (one strand) of the original template is retained and passed on.

DNA: *See* deoxyribonucleic acid.

DNase: refers to a class of enzymes, deoxyribonucleases, which specifically degrade DNA molecules.

domain: the highest-level division of life, sometimes called a superkingdom.

dominant: an allele or a trait that will mask the presence of a recessive allele or trait.

dosage compensation: an equalization of gene products that can occur whenever there are more or fewer genes for specific traits than normal.

double helix: a model of DNA structure proposed by molecular biologists James Watson and Francis Crick; the major features of this model are two strands of DNA wound around each other and connected by hydrogen bonds between complementary base pairs.

Down syndrome: a genetic defect caused by possession of an extra copy of chromosome 21; symptoms include mental retardation, mongoloid facial features, and premature aging.

down-regulation: generally used in reference to gene expression and refers to reducing the amount that a gene is transcribed and/or translated; up-regulation is the opposite.

downstream: in relation to the left-to-right direction of DNA whose nucleotides are arranged in sequence with the 5' carbon on the left and the 3' on the right, downstream is to the right.

drug resistance: a phenomenon in which pathogens no longer respond to drug therapies that once controlled them; resistance can arise by recombination, by mutation, or by several methods of gene transfer, and is made worse by misuse of existing drugs.

duplication: a type of chromosomal mutation in which a chromosome region is duplicated because of an error in recombination during prophase I of meiosis; thought to play an important role in gene evolution.

dwarfism: the condition of adults of short stature who are less than 50 inches in height, which can be caused by genetic factors, endocrine malfunction, acquired conditions, or growth hormone deficiency; many dwarfs prefer to be called "little people."

dye blobs: an artifact that may occur during short tandem repeats testing.

dysplasia: abnormal cell or tissue growth or development.

E. coli: See *Escherichia coli.*

Edwards syndrome: a genetic disorder in which there is an extra copy of chromosome 18; infants with this disorder commonly have small eyes, deformed ears, heart defects, and severe intellectual impairment. These children rarely live longer than 1 year; also known as trisomy 18.

electron transport chain: a series of protein complexes that use high-energy electrons to do work such as pumping H+ ions out of the mitochondrial matrix into the intermembrane space as a way of storing energy that is then used by ATP synthase to make ATP.

electrophoresis: *See* gel electrophoresis.

embryo: the term for a complex organism (particularly humans) during its earliest period of development, the stage of development that begins at fertilization and ends with the eighth week of development, after which the embryo is called a fetus.

embryology: the study of developing embryos.

embryonic stem cell: a cell derived from an early embryo that can replicate indefinitely in vitro and can differentiate into other cells of the developing embryo.

emerging disease: a disease whose incidence in humans or other target organisms has increased.

empiric risk: estimated risk for an individual developing a certain condition based on observations of other families affected by the condition.

endemic: prevalent and recurring in a particular geographic region; for example, an organism that is specific to a particular region is characterized as endemic to that region.

endocrine gland: a gland that secretes hormones into the circulatory system.

endonuclease: an enzyme that degrades a nucleic acid molecule by breaking phosphodiester bonds within the molecule.

endosymbiotic hypothesis: a hypothesis stating that mitochondria and chloroplasts were once freeliving bacteria that entered into a symbiotic relationship with early pre-eukaryotic cells; structural and genetic similarities between these organelles and bacteria provide support for this hypothesis.

enhancer: a region of a DNA molecule that facilitates the transcription of a gene, usually by stimulating the interaction of RNA polymerase with the gene's promoter.

enzyme replacement therapy: replaces an enzyme that is deficient or absent in the body. Usually, this is done by giving the patient an intravenous (IV) infusion of a solution containing the enzyme.

enzyme: a protein that acts as a catalyst to speed up or facilitate a specific biochemical reaction in a cell.

epigenesis: the formation of differentiated cell types and specialized organs from a single, homogeneous fertilized egg cell without any preexisting structural elements.

Epilepsy: a group of neurological disorders characterized by epileptic seizures. Epileptic seizures are episodes that can vary from brief and nearly undetectable to long periods of vigorous shaking. These episodes can result in physical injuries including occasionally broken bones. In epilepsy, seizures tend to recur and as a rule, have no immediate underlying cause.

epistasis: a genetic phenomenon in which a gene at one locus influences the expression of a second gene at another locus, usually by masking the effect of the second gene; however, only one trait is being controlled by these two genes, so epistasis is characterized by modified dihybrid ratios.

equational division: refers to meiosis II, in which the basic number of chromosome types remains the same although sister chromatids are separated from one another; after equational division occurs, functional haploid gametes are present.

Escherichia coli: a bacterium widely studied in genetics research and extensively used in biotechnological applications.

estrogens: steroid hormones or chemicals that stimulate the development of female sexual characteristics and control the female reproductive cycle.

ethidium bromide: a chemical substance that inserts itself (intercalates) into the DNA double helix; when exposed to ultraviolet light, ethidium bromide fluoresces, making it useful for the visualization of DNA molecules in molecular biology techniques.

etiology: the cause or causes of a disease or disorder.

euchromatin: chromatin that is loosely coiled during interphase; thought to contain transcriptionally active genes.

eugenics: a largely discredited field of genetics that seeks to improve humankind by selective breeding; can be positive eugenics, in which individuals with desirable traits are encouraged or forced to breed, or negative eugenics, in which individuals with undesirable traits are discouraged or prevented from breeding.

eukaryote: a cell with a nuclear membrane surrounding its genetic material (a characteristic of a true nucleus) and a variety of subcellular, membrane-bound organelles; eukaryotic organisms include all known organisms except bacteria, which are prokaryotic. See also prokaryote.

euploid: the normal number of chromosomes for a cell or organism.

eusociality: an extreme form of altruism and kin selection in which most members of the society do not reproduce but rather feed and protect their relatives; bees, for example, are eusocial.

euthanasia: the killing of suffering individuals; sometimes referred to as "mercy" killing.

exogenous gene: a gene produced or originating from outside an organism.

exome studies: Exome sequencing, also known as whole exome sequencing (WES), is a transcriptomics technique for sequencing all of the protein-coding genes in a genome (known as the exome).

exon: a protein-coding sequence in eukaryotic genes, usually flanked by introns.

exonuclease: an enzyme that degrades a nucleic acid molecule by breaking phosphodiester bonds at either end of the molecule.

expressed sequence tags (ESTs): an STS (sequence tagged site) that has been derived from a cDNA library.

expression vector: a DNA cloning vector designed to allow genetic expression of inserted genes via promoters engineered into the vector sequence.

expressivity: the degree to which a genotype is expressed as a phenotype.

extranuclear inheritance: inheritance involving genetic material located in the mitochondria or chloroplasts of a eukaryotic cell; also known as maternal inheritance (because these organelles are generally inherited from the mother) and cytoplasmic inheritance (because the organelles are found in the cell's cytoplasm rather than its nucleus).

extreme halophiles: microorganisms that require extremely high salt concentrations for optimal growth.

F pilus: also called the fertility pilus; a reproductive structure found on the surface of some bacterial cells that allows the cells to exchange plasmids or other DNA during the process of conjugation.

F2 generation: second filial generation; offspring produced from a mating of Fi generation individuals.

familial Mediterranean fever: a genetic inflammatory disorder of the abdominal cavity, affecting people of Mediterranean descent, that causes abdominal pain and recurrent fevers; also known as recurrent polyseroserositis.

fate map: a description of the adult fate of embryonic cells.

faulty gene: a gene that does not function properly.

fertilization: the fusion of two cells (egg and sperm) in sexual reproduction.

fetus: a prenatal human between the embryonic state and birth. The fetal stage of development tends to be taken as beginning at the gestational age of eleven weeks, i.e. nine weeks after fertilization. In biological terms, however, prenatal development is a continuum, with no clear defining feature distinguishing an embryo from a fetus. The use of the term "fetus" generally implies that an embryo has developed to the point of being recognizable as a human; this is the point usually taken to be the ninth week after fertilization. A fetus is also characterized by the presence of all the major body organs, though they will not yet be fully developed and functional and some not yet situated in their final anatomical location.

Fi generation: first filial generation; offspring produced from a mating of P (parental) generation individuals.

fitness: a measure of the ability of a genotype or individual to survive and reproduce; when fitness is compared to other genotypes or individuals it is called relative fitness.

fluorescence in situ hybridization (FISH): an extremely sensitive assay for determining the presence of deletions on chromosomes, which uses a fluorescence-tagged segment of DNA that binds to the DNA region being studied.

foreign DNA: DNA taken from a source other than the host cell that is joined to the DNA of the cloning vector; also known as "insert DNA."

forensic genetics: the use of genetic tests and principles to resolve legal questions.

formylmethionine (fMet): the amino acid used to start all bacterial proteins; it is attached to the initiator transfer RNA (tRNA) molecule.

frame-shift mutation: a DNA mutation involving the insertion or deletion of one of several nucleotides that are not in multiples of three, resulting in a shift of the codon reading frame; usually produces nonfunctional proteins. *See also* open reading frame; reading frame.

fraternal twins: twins that develop and are born simultaneously but are genetically unique, being produced from the fertilization of two separate eggs; a synonymous term is "dizygotic twins."

free radical: *See* oxygen free radical.

G0: a point in the cell cycle at which a cell is no longer progressing toward cell division; can be considered a "resting" stage.

G: the abbreviation for guanine, a purine nitrogenous base found in the structure of both DNA and RNA.

gamete: a sex cell, either sperm or egg, containing half the genetic material of a normal cell.

gel electrophoresis: a technique of molecular biology in which biological molecules are placed into a gel-like matrix (such as agarose or polyacrylamide) and then subjected to an electric current; using this technique, researchers can separate molecules of varying sizes and properties.

GenBank: a comprehensive, annotated collection of publicly available DNA sequences maintained by the National Center for Biotechnology Information and available through its Web site.

gene amplification: a rise in the number of copies of a DNA sequence for a particular protein without a proportional rise in others; this process takes place in tumor cells.

gene expression: the combined biochemical processes, called "transcription" and "translation," that convert the linearly encoded information in the bases of DNA into the three-dimensional structures of proteins.

gene families: multiple copies of the same or similar genes in the same genome; the copies can be identical and tandemly repeated, or they may differ slightly and be scattered on the same or different chromosomes.

gene flow: movement of alleles from one population to another by the movement of individuals or gametes.

gene frequency: the occurrence of a particular allele present in a population, expressed as a percentage of the total number of alleles present for the locus.

gene pool: the complete assortment of genes present in the gametes of the members of a population that are eligible to reproduce.

gene silencing: any form of genetic regulation in which the expression of a gene is completely repressed, either by preventing transcription (pretranscriptional gene silencing) or after a messenger RNA (mRNA) has been transcribed (posttranscriptional gene silencing).

gene therapy: any procedure to alleviate or treat the symptoms of a disease or condition by genetically altering the cells of the patient.

gene transfer: the movement of fragments of genetic information, whole genes, or groups of genes between organisms.

gene: a portion of a DNA molecule containing the genetic information necessary to produce a molecule of messenger RNA (via the process of transcription) that can then be used to produce a protein (via the process of translation); also includes regions of DNA that are transcribed to RNA that does not get translated, but carries out other roles in the cell.

genetic code: the correspondence between the sequence of nucleotides in DNA or messenger RNA (mRNA) molecules and the amino acids in the polypeptide a gene codes for.

genetic counseling: a discipline concerned with analyzing the inheritance patterns of a particular genetic defect within a given family, including the determination of the risk associated with the presence of the genetic defect in future generations and options for treatment of existing genetic defects.

genetic drift: chance fluctuations in allele frequencies within a population, resulting from random variation in the number and genotypes of offspring produced by different individuals.

genetic engineering: a term encompassing a wide variety of molecular biology techniques, all concerned with the modification of genetic characteristics of cells or organisms to accomplish a desired effect.

genetic load: the average number of the recessive deleterious (lethal or sublethal) alleles in individuals in a population.

genetic map: a "map" showing distances between genes in terms of recombination frequency; using DNA sequence data, a physical map with distance in base pairs can also be produced.

genetic marker: a distinctive DNA sequence that shows variation in the population and can therefore potentially be used for identification of individuals and for discovery of disease genes.

genetic screening: the testing of individuals for disease-causing genes or genetic disease.

genetic testing: the use of the techniques of genetics research to determine a person's risk of developing, or status as a carrier of, a disease or other disorder.

genetically modified (GM) foods: foods produced through the application of recombinant DNA technology, whereby genes from the same or different species are transferred and expressed in crops that do not naturally harbor those genes.

genetically modified organism (GMO): an organism produced by using biotechnology to introduce a new gene or genes, or new regulatory sequences for genes, into it for the purpose of giving the organism a new trait, usually to adapt the organism to a new environment, provide resistance to pest species, or enable the production of new products from the organism. *See also* transgenic organism.

genetics: an area of biology involving the scientific study of heredity.

genome: all of the DNA in the nucleus or in one of the organelles, such as a chloroplast or mitochondrion.

genomic imprinting: a genetic phenomenon in which the phenotype associated with a particular allele depends on which parent donated the allele.

genomic library: a collection of clones that includes the entire genome of a single species as fragments ligated to vector DNA.

genomics: that branch of genetics dealing with the study of genetic sequences, including their structure and arrangement.

genotype: the genetic characteristics of a cell or organism, expressed as a set of symbols representing the alleles present at one or more loci.

germ cells: reproductive cells such as eggs and sperm.

germ-line gene therapy: a genetic modification in gametes or fertilized ova so all cells in the organism will have the change, which potentially can be passed on to offspring.

germ-line mutation: a heritable change in the genes of an individual's reproductive cells, often linked to hereditary diseases.

Gi checkpoint: a point in the cell cycle at which a cell commits either to progressing toward cell division (by replicating its DNA and eventually engaging in mitosis) or to entering the Go phase, thereby withdrawing from the cell cycle either temporarily or permanently.

glossoptosis: involves the downward displacement or retraction of the tongue. It may cause non-fusion of the hard palate causing cleft palate. It is one of the features of Pierre Robin sequence and Down syndrome.

gonad: an organ that produces reproductive cells and sex hormones; termed ovaries in females and testes in males.

Green Revolution: the introduction of scientifically bred or selected varieties of grain (such as rice, wheat, and maize) that, with high enough inputs of fertilizer and water, can greatly increase crop yields.

guanine (G): a purine nitrogenous base found in the structure of both DNA and RNA.

H substance: a carbohydrate molecule on the surface of red blood cells; when modified by certain monosaccharides, this molecule provides the basis of the ABO blood groups.

haplodiploidy: a system of sex determination in which males are haploid (developing from unfertilized eggs) and females are diploid.

haploid: refers to a cell or an organism with one set of chromosomes; usually represented as the *N* number of chromosomes, with 2N standing for the diploid number of chromosomes.

haploinsufficiency: protein produced by a single gene copy is insufficient for normal function.

haplotype: a sequential set of genes on a single chromosome inherited together from one parent; the other parent provides a matching chromosome with a different set of genes.

Hardy-Weinberg law: a concept in population genetics stating that, given an infinitely large population that experiences random mating without mutation or any other such affecting factor, the frequency of particular alleles will reach a state of equilibrium, after which their frequency will not change from one generation to the next.

HeLa cells: the first human tumor cells shown to form a continuous cell line; they were derived from a cervical cancer tumor removed from a woman known as Henrietta Lacks.

helicase: a cellular enzyme that breaks hydrogen bonds between the strands of the DNA double helix, thus unwinding the helix and facilitating DNA replication.

helper T cells: a class of white blood cells (lymphocytes) derived from bone marrow that prompts the production of antibodies by B cells in the presence of an antigen.

hematopoietic cell transplantation (HCT): a procedure that involves infusion of hematopoietic stem cells (hematopoietic progenitor cells) to reconstitute the hematopoietic system of a patient. It suppresses the patient's immune system to prevent rejection.

hemizygous: characterized by having a gene present in a single copy, such as any gene on the X chromosome in a human male.

hemoglobin: a molecule made up of two alpha and two beta amino acid chains whose precise chemical and structural properties normally allow it to bind with oxygen in the lungs and transport it to other parts of the body.

hemophilia: an X-linked recessive disorder in which an individual's blood does not clot properly because of a lack of blood-clotting factors; as in all X-linked recessive traits, the disease is most common in males, the allele for the disease being passed from mother to son.

heredity: the overall mechanism by which characteristics or traits are passed from one generation of organisms to the next; genetics is the scientific study of heredity.

heritability: a proportional measure of the extent to which differences among organisms within a population for a particular characteristic result from genetic rather than environmental causes (a measure of nature versus nurture).

hermaphrodite: an individual who has both male and female sex organs.

heterochromatin: a highly condensed form of chromatin, usually transcriptionally inactive.

heterochrony: a change in the timing or rate of development of characters in an organism relative to those same events in its evolutionary ancestors.

heteroduplex: a double-stranded molecule of nucleic acid with each strand from a different source, formed either through natural means such as recombination or through artificial means in the laboratory.

heterogametic sex: the particular sex of an organism that produces gametes containing two types of sex chromosome; in humans, males are the heterogametic sex, producing sperm that can carry either an X chromosome or a Y chromosome.

heterogeneous nuclear RNA (hnRNA): an assortment of RNA molecules of various types found in the nucleus of the cell and in various stages of processing prior to their export to the cytoplasm.

heterozygote: an individual with two different alleles at a gene locus.

heterozygous: composed of two alleles that are different, for example Aa; synonymous with "hybrid."

highly conserved sequence: A DNA sequence that is similar among different organisms.

Hirschsprung's disease: genetic disorder in which the nerve cells in the colon do not develop properly leading to constipation and abdominal distention; neonates suffering from this disorder may not have a bowel movement and may vomit bile. Surgical intervention is the treatment of choice.

histones: specialized proteins in eukaryotic cells that bind to DNA molecules and cause them to become more compact; thought to be involved in regulation of gene expression as well.

HLA: *See* human leukocyte antigens.

hnRNA: *See* heterogeneous nuclear RNA.

holandric: refers to a trait passed from father to son via a sex chromosome such as the Y chromosome in human males.

homeobox: a DNA sequence encoding a highly basic protein known as a homeodomain; a homeodomain functions as a transcription factor and is thought to help regulate major events in the embryonic development of higher organisms.

homeotic gene: a gene that helps determine body plan early in development; the products of homeotic genes are transcription factors that control the expression of other genes.

homogametic sex: the particular sex of an organism that produces gametes containing only one type of sex chromosome; in humans, females are the homogametic sex, producing eggs with X chromosomes.

homologous: refers to chromosomes that are identical in terms of types of genes present and the location of the centromere; because of their high degree of similarity, homologous chromosomes can synapse and recombine during prophase I of meiosis.

homology: similarity resulting from descent from a common evolutionary ancestor.

homozygote: an individual with two identical alleles at a gene locus.

homozygous: characterized by a genotype composed of two alleles at the same locus that are the same, for example *AA* or *aa;* synonymous with "purebred."

human artificial chromosome: an agent constructed similarly to a human chromosome, that is used to transfer large segments of human DNA.

Human Genome Project: a multiyear genetic research endeavor to sequence the entire human genome, as well as the genomes of related organisms; the human genome sequence was officially completed in 2003.

human leukocyte antigens (HLAs): molecules found on the surface of cells that allow the immune system to differentiate between foreign, invading cells and the body's own cells.

hybrid: any cell or organism with genetic material from two different sources, through either natural processes such as sexual reproduction or more artificial processes such as genetic engineering.

hybridization: a process of base pairing involving two single-stranded nucleic acid molecules with complementary sequences; the extent to which two unrelated nucleic acid molecules will hybridize is often used as a way to determine the amount of similarity between the sequences of the two molecules.

hybridoma: a type of hybrid cancer cell created by artificially joining a cancer cell with an antibodyproducing cell; hybridomas have useful applications in immunological research.

hydrogen bond: a bond formed between molecules containing hydrogen atoms with positive charges and molecules containing atoms such as nitrogen or oxygen that can possess a negative charge; a relatively weak but important bond in nature that, among other things, connects water molecules, allows DNA strands to base-pair, and contributes to the three-dimensional shape of proteins.

identical twins: a pair of genetically identical offspring that develop from a single fertilized egg; also known as monozygotic twins.

immune system: the system in the body that normally responds to foreign agents by producing antibodies and stimulating antigen-specific lymphocytes, leading to destruction of these agents.

immunotherapy: uses substances to stimulate or suppress the immune system to help the body fight cancer, infection, and other diseases. Some types of immunotherapy only target certain cells of the immune system. Others affect the immune system in a general way. Types of immunotherapy include cytokines, vaccines, bacillus Calmette-Guerin (BCG), and some monoclonal antibodies.

in situ hybridization: the process of base pairing a sequence of DNA to metaphase chromosomes on a microscope slide.

in vitro fertilization: a fertilization that occurs unnaturally in a laboratory or other controlled environment.

in vitro: literally, "in glass"; an event occurring in an artificial setting such as in a test tube, as opposed to inside a living organism.

in vivo: literally, "in the living"; an event occurring in a living organism, as opposed to an artificial setting.

inborn error of metabolism: a genetic defect in one of a cell's metabolic pathways, usually at the level of an enzyme, that causes the pathway to malfunction; results in phenotypic alterations at the cellular or organismal level.

inbreeding depression: a reduction in the health and vigor of offspring from closely related individuals, a common and widespread phenomenon among nonhuman organisms.

inbreeding: mating between genetically related individuals.

incidence: the frequency in which a disorder appears in a given population.

inclusive fitness: an individual's total genetic contribution to future generations, comprising both direct fitness, which results from individual reproduction, and indirect fitness, which results from the reproduction of close relatives.

incomplete dominance: a phenomenon involving two alleles, neither of which masks the expression of the other; instead, the combination of the alleles in the heterozygous state produces a new phenotype that is usually intermediate to the phenotypes produced by either allele alone in the homozygous state.

independent assortment: a characteristic of standard Mendelian genetics referring to the random assortment or shuffling of alleles and chromosomes that occurs during meiosis I; independent assortment is responsible for the offspring ratios observed in Mendelian genetics.

inducer: a molecule that activates some bacterial operons, usually by interacting with regulatory proteins bound to the operator region.

induction: a process in which a cell or group of cells signals an adjacent cell or group of cells to pursue a different developmental pathway and so become differentiated from neighboring cells.

informed consent: the right of patients to know the risks of medical treatment and to determine what is done to their bodies, including the right to accept or refuse treatment based on this information.

inherited: genetic transfer from parents to children.

initiation codon: also called the "start codon," a codon, composed of the nucleotides AUG, that signals the beginning of a protein-coding sequence in a messenger RNA (mRNA) molecule; in the genetic code, AUG always represents the amino acid methionine.

insert DNA: *See* foreign DNA.

insertion sequence: a small, independently transposable genetic element.

insertion: a process whereby a DNA sequence is abnormally inserted into a gene, disrupting the normal function and structure of the gene and leading to a chromosomal abnormality.

intelligence quotient (IQ): the most common measure of intelligence; it is based on the view that there is a single capacity for complex mental work and that this capacity can be measured by testing.

intercalary deletion: a type of chromosome deletion in which DNA has been lost from within the chromosome (as opposed to a terminal deletion involving a region of DNA lost from the end of the chromosome).

interference: in genetic linkage, a mathematical expression that represents the difference between the expected and the observed number of double recombinant offspring; this can be a clue to the physical location of linked genes on the chromosome.

interphase: the period of the cell cycle in which the cell is preparing to divide, consisting of two distinct growth phases (Gi and G2) separated by a period of DNA replication (S phase).

introgression: the transfer of genes from one species to another or the movement of genes between species (or other well-marked genetic populations) mediated by backcrossing.

intron: an intervening sequence within eukaryotic DNA, transcribed as part of a messenger RNA (mRNA) precursor but then removed by splicing before the mRNA molecule is translated; introns are thought to play an important role in the evolution of genes.

inversion: a chromosomal abnormality resulting in a region of the chromosome where the normal order of genes is reversed.

isotope: an alternative form of an element with a variant number of neutrons in its atomic nucleus; isotopes are frequently radioactive and are important tools for numerous molecular biology techniques.

jumping: *See* chromosome jumping.

junk DNA: a disparaging (and now known to be inaccurate) characterization of the noncoding DNA content of a genome.

karyokinesis: division of a cell's nuclear contents, as opposed to cytokinesis (division of the cytoplasm). *See also* cytokinesis.

karyotype: the complete set of chromosomes possessed by an individual, usually isolated during metaphase and arranged by size and type as a method of detecting chromosomal abnormalities.

kilobase (kb): a unit of measurement for nucleic acid molecules, equal to 1,000 bases or nucleotides.

kinase: an enzyme that catalyzes phosphate addition to molecules.

kinetochore: a chromosome structure found in the region of the centromere and used as an attachment point for the microtubules of the spindle apparatus during cell division.

Klinefelter syndrome: a human genetic disorder in males who possess an extra X chromosome; Klinefelter males have forty-seven chromosomes instead of the normal forty-six and suffer from abnormalities such as sterility, body feminization, and mental retardation.

knockout: the inactivation of a specific gene within a cell (or whole organism, as in the case of knockout mice) to determine the effects of loss of function of that gene.

lactose: a disaccharide that is an important part of the metabolism of many bacterial species; lactose metabolism in these species is genetically regulated via the *lac* operon.

lagging strand: in DNA replication, the strand of DNA being synthesized in a direction opposite to that of replication fork movement; this strand is synthesized in a discontinuous fashion as a series of Okazaki fragments later joined together. *See also* Okazaki fragments.

Lamarckianism: the theory, originally proposed by Jean-Baptiste Lamarck, that traits acquired by an organism during its lifetime can be passed on to offspring.

lambda (Λ) phage: a bacteriophage that infects bacteria and then makes multiple copies of itself by taking over the infected bacteria's cellular machinery.

lateral gene transfer: the movement of genes between organisms; also called horizontal gene transfer.

leading strand: in DNA replication, the strand of DNA being synthesized in the same direction as the movement of the replication fork; this strand is synthesized in a continuous fashion.

leptotene: a subphase of prophase I of meiosis in which chromosomes begin to condense and become visible.

lethal allele: an allele capable of causing the death of an organism; a lethal allele can be recessive (two copies of the allele are required before death results) or dominant (one copy of the allele produces death).

leucine zipper: an amino acid sequence, found in some DNA-binding proteins, characterized by leucine residues separated by sets of seven amino acids; two molecules of this amino acid sequence can combine via the leucine residues and "zip" together, creating a structure that can then bind to a specific DNA sequence.

library: a cloned collection of DNA created from a specific organism.

linkage mapping: a form of genetic mapping that uses recombination frequencies to estimate the relative distances between linked genes.

linkage: a genetic phenomenon involving two or more genes inherited together because they are physically located on the same chromosome; Gregor Mendel's principle of independent assortment does not apply to linked genes, but genotypic and phenotypic variation is possible through crossing over.

locus *(pl.* **loci):** the specific location of a particular gene on a chromosome.

LOD score: statistical calculation of whether two gene sites (loci) are likely to be located near one another on a chromosome and be genetically linked; also known as logarithm of the odds score.

lymphocytes: sensitized cells of the immune system that recognize and destroy harmful agents via antibody and cell-mediated responses that include B lymphocytes from the bone marrow and T lymphocytes from the thymus.

Lyon hypothesis: a hypothesis stating that one X chromosome of the pair found in all female cells must be inactivated in order for those cells to be normal; the inactivated X chromosome is visible by light microscopy and stains as a Barr body.

lysis: the breaking open of a cell.

lysogeny: a viral process involving repression and integration of the viral genome into the genome of the host bacterial cell.

macrocephaly: a condition in which the head is abnormally large. This includes the scalp, the cranial bone, and the contents of the cranium. Macrocephaly may be pathological, but many people with abnormally large heads or large skulls are healthy. Pathologic macrocephaly may be due to megalencephaly (enlarged brain), hydrocephalus (water on the brain), cranial hyperostosis (bone overgrowth), and other conditions.

major histocompatibility complex (MHC): a group of molecules found on the surface of cells, allowing the immune system to differentiate between foreign, invading cells and the body's own cells; in humans, this group of molecules is called HLAs (human leukocyte antigens). *See also* human leukocyte antigens.

malformation: an inherited organ defect that occurs during fetal development.

map unit: *See* centiMorgan.

maternal inheritance: *See* extranuclear inheritance.

Maxam-Gilbert sequencing: a method of base-specific chemical degradation to determine DNA sequence; this method has largely been supplanted by the Sanger method. *See also* Sanger sequencing.

megakaryocyte: a large bone marrow cell that has a nucleus containing many lobes; the cell functions to produce platelets.

meiosis: a process of cell division in which the cell's genetic material is reduced by half and sex cells called gametes are produced; important as the basis of sexual reproduction.

melanism: the opposite of albinism, a condition that leads to the overproduction of melanin.

melting: a term sometimes used to describe the denaturation of a DNA molecule as it is heated in solution; as the temperature rises, hydrogen bonds between the DNA strands are broken until the double-strand molecule has been completely converted into two single-strand molecules.

Mendelian genetics: the genetics of traits that show simple inheritance patterns; based on the work of Gregor Mendel, a nineteenth century monk who studied the genetics of pea plants.

Mental retardation: a developmental disability that first appears in children under the age of 18. It is defined as an intellectual functioning level (as measured by standard tests for intelligence quotient) that is well below average and significant limitations in daily living skills (adaptive functioning).

messenger RNA (mRNA): a type of RNA molecule containing the genetic information necessary to produce a protein through the process of translation; produced from the DNA sequence of a gene in the process of transcription.

metabolic pathway: a series of enzyme-catalyzed reactions leading to the breakdown or synthesis of a particular biological molecule.

metabolism: the collection of biochemical reactions occurring in an organism.

metacentric chromosome: a chromosome with the centromere located at or near the middle of the chromosome. *See also* acrocentric chromosome; telocentric chromosome.

metafemale: a term used to describe *Drosophila* (fruit fly) females that have more X chromosomes than sets of autosomes (for example, a female that has two sets of autosomes and three X chromosomes); also used in reference to human females with more than two X chromosomes.

metaphase: the second phase in the process of mitosis, involving chromosomes lined up in the middle of the cell on a line known as the equator.

methylation: the process of adding a methyl chemical group (one carbon atom and three hydrogen atoms) to a particular molecule, such as to the base portion of a nucleotide in a DNA nucleotide.

metric trait: *See* quantitative trait.

microarray: a flat surface on which 10,000 to 100,000 tiny spots of short DNA molecules (oligonucleotides) are fixed and are used to detect the presence of DNA or RNA molecules that are homologous to the oligonucleotides.

microcephaly: a medical condition in which the brain does not develop properly resulting in a smaller than normal head. Microcephaly may be present at birth or it may develop in the first few years of life. Often people with the disorder have an intellectual disability, poor motor function, poor speech, abnormal facial features, seizures, and dwarfism.

micrognathia: a condition where the jaw is undersized. It is also sometimes called "mandibular hypoplasia". It is common in infants, but is usually self-corrected during growth, due to the jaws' increasing in size. It may be a cause of abnormal tooth alignment and in severe cases can hamper feeding. It can also, both in adults and children, make intubation difficult, either during anesthesia or in emergency situations.

microsatellite DNA: a type of variable number tandem repeat (VNTR) in which the repeated motif is 1 to 6 base pairs; also called a simple sequence repeat (SSR) or a short tandem repeat (STR).

microtubule organizing center (MTOC): *See* centriole.

microtubule: a cell structure involved in the movement and division of chromosomes during mitosis and meiosis; part of the cell's cytoskeleton, microtubules can be rapidly assembled and disassembled.

minimal media: an environment that contains the simplest set of ingredients that a microorganism can use to produce all the substances required for reproduction and growth.

minisatellite DNA: a type of variable number tandem repeat (VNTR) in which the repeated motif is 12 to 500 base pairs in length.

miscegenation: sexual activity or marriage between members of two different human races.

mismatch repair: a cellular DNA repair process in which improperly base-paired nucleotides are enzymatically removed and replaced with the proper nucleotides.

missense mutation: a DNA mutation that changes an existing amino acid codon in a gene to some other amino acid codon; depending on the nature of the change, this can be a harmless or a serious mutation (for example, sickle-cell disease in humans is the result of a missense mutation).

mitochondrial genome (mtDNA): DNA found in mitochondria, which contains some of the genes that code for proteins involved in energy metabolism; it is a circular molecule similar in structure to the genome of bacteria.

mitochondrion: the organelle responsible for production of ATP through the process of cellular respiration in a eukaryotic cell; sometimes referred to as the "powerhouse of the cell."

mitosis: a process of cell division in which a cell's duplicated genetic material is evenly divided between two daughter cells, so that each daughter cell is genetically identical to the original parent cell.

model organism: an organism well suited for genetic research because it has a well-known genetic history, a short life cycle, and genetic variation between individuals in the population.

modern synthesis: the merging of the Darwinian mechanisms for evolution with Mendelian genetics to form the modern fields of population genetics and evolutionary biology; also called the neo-Darwinian synthesis.

molecular clock hypothesis: a hypothesis that predicts that amino acid changes in proteins and nucleotide changes in DNA are approximately constant over time.

molecular cloning: the process of splicing a piece of DNA into a plasmid, virus, or phage vector to obtain many identical copies of that DNA.

molecular genetics: the branch of genetics concerned with the central role that molecules, particularly the nucleic acids DNA and RNA, play in heredity.

monoclonal antibodies: identical antibodies (having specificity for the same antigen) produced by a single type of antibody-producing cell, either a B cell or a hybridoma cell line; important in various types of immunology research techniques.

monoculture: the agricultural practice of growing the same cultivar on large tracts of land.

monohybrid: an organism that is hybrid with respect to a single gene (for example, Aa); when two monohybrid organisms are mated, the offspring will generally appear in a 3:1 ratio involving the trait controlled by the gene in question.

monosomy: a genetic condition in which one chromosome from a homologous chromosome pair is missing, producing a 2n-1 genotype; usually causes significant problems in the phenotype of the organism.

monozygotic: developed from a single zygote; identical twins are monozygotic because they develop from a single fertilized ovum that splits in two.

morphogen: a protein or other molecule made by cells in an egg that creates a concentration gradient affecting the developmental fate of surrounding cells by altering their gene expression or their ability to respond to other morphogens.

morphogenesis: the induction and formation of organized body parts or organs.

mosaicism: a condition in which an individual has two or more cell populations derived from the same fertilized ovum, or zygote, as in sex chromosome mosaics, in which some cells contain the usual XY chromosome pattern and others contain extra X chromosomes.

MRI scan: a procedure in which radio waves and a powerful magnet linked to a computer are used to create detailed pictures of areas inside the body. These pictures can show the difference between normal and diseased tissue. Magnetic resonance imaging makes better images of organs and soft tissue than other scanning techniques, such as computed tomography (CT) or x-ray. Magnetic resonance imaging is especially useful for imaging the brain, the spine, the soft tissue of joints, and the inside of bones. Also called MRI, NMRI, and nuclear magnetic resonance imaging.

mRNA: *See* messenger RNA.

mtDNA: *See* mitochondrial genome.

MTOC: *See* centriole.

multi-gene testing: tests that use next-generation sequencing to test multiple genes simultaneously. Also called multi-gene test and multiple-gene test.

multifactorial: characterized by a complex interaction of genetic and environmental factors.

multiple alleles: a genetic phenomenon in which a particular gene locus is represented by more than two alleles in a population; the greater the number of alleles, the greater the genetic diversity.

mutagen: any chemical or physical substance capable of increasing mutations in a DNA sequence.

mutant: a trait or organism different from the normal, or wild-type, trait or organism seen commonly in nature; mutants can arise either through expression of particular alleles in the organism or through spontaneous or intentional mutations in the genome.

mutation: a change in the genetic sequence of an organism, usually leading to an altered phenotype.

N terminus: the end of a polypeptide with an amino acid that has a free amino group.

natural selection: a process involving genetic variation on the genotypic and phenotypic levels that contributes to the success or failure of various species in reproduction; thought to be the primary force behind evolution.

negative eugenics: improving human stocks through the restriction of reproduction by individuals with inferior traits or who are known to carry alleles for inferior traits.

neural tube: the embryonic precursor to the spinal cord and brain, which normally closes at small openings, or neuropores, by the twenty-eighth day of gestation in humans.

neurofibromatosis: a genetic disorder whereby tumors develop along peripheral nerves. The tumors may cause disfiguration, hearing and vision loss, and learning disabilities.

Neuronal migration disorder: a heterogenous group of disorders that, it is supposed, share the same etiopathological mechanism: a variable degree of disruption in the migration of neuroblasts during neurogenesis. The neuronal migration disorders are cerebral dysgenesis, brain malformations caused by primary alterations during neurogenesis; on the other hand, brain malformations are highly diverse and refer to any insult to the brain during its formation and maturation due to intrinsic or extrinsic causes that ultimately will alter the normal brain anatomy. However, there is some controversy in the terminology because virtually any malformation will involve neuroblast migration, either primarily or secondarily.

neurotransmitter: a chemical that carries messages between nerve cells.

neutral mutation: a mutation in a gene, or some other portion of the genome, that is considered to have no effect on the fitness of the organism.

neutral theory of evolution: Motoo Kimura's theory that nucleotide substitutions in the DNA often have no effect on fitness, and thus changes in allele frequencies in populations are caused primarily by genetic drift.

Niemann-Pick disease, Type C: a fatal genetic disorder involving the inability to metabolize cholesterol and other lipids within the cell, causing cholesterol to accumulate in the spleen and liver and excessive amounts of other lipids to accumulate in the brain.

noncoding DNA: a strand of DNA that is unable to make protein because it lacks the necessary information.

nondisjunction: the improper division of chromosomes during anaphase of mitosis or meiosis, resulting in cells with abnormal numbers of chromosomes and sometimes seriously altered phenotypes.

nonhistone proteins: a heterogeneous group of acidic or neutral proteins found in chromatin that may be involved with chromosome structure, chromatin packaging, or the control of gene expression.

nonsense codon: another term for a termination or stop codon (UAA, UAG, or UGA).

nonsense mutation: a DNA mutation that changes an existing amino acid codon in a message to one of the three termination, or stop, codons; this results in an abnormally short protein that is usually nonfunctional.

Northern blot: a molecular biology procedure in which a labeled single-stranded DNA probe is exposed to cellular RNA immobilized on a filter; under the proper conditions, the DNA probe will seek out and bind to its complementary sequence in the RNA molecules if such a sequence is present.

nuclease: an enzyme that degrades nucleic acids by breaking the phosphodiester bond that connects nucleosides.

nucleic acid: the genetic material of cells, found in two forms: deoxyribonucleic acid (DNA) and ribonucleic acid (RNA); composed of repeating subunits called nucleotides.

nucleocapsid: a viral structure including the capsid, or outer protein coat, and the nucleic acid of the virus.

nucleoid: a region of a prokaryotic cell containing the cell's genetic material.

nucleolus: a eukaryotic organelle located in the nucleus of the cell; the site of ribosomal RNA (rRNA) synthesis.

nucleoside: a building block of nucleic acids, composed of a sugar (deoxyribose or ribose) and one of the nitrogenous bases: adenine (A), cytosine (C), guanine (G), thymine (T), or uracil (U).

nucleosome: the basic unit molecule of chromatin, composed of a segment of a DNA molecule that is bound to and wound around histone molecules; DNA with nucleosomes appears as beads on a string when viewed by electron microscopy.

nucleotide: a building block of nucleic acids, composed of a sugar (deoxyribose or ribose), one of the nitrogenous bases (adenine, cytosine, guanine, thymine, or uracil) and one or more phosphate groups.

nucleus: the "control center" of eukaryotic cells, where the genetic material is separated from the rest of the cell by a membrane; site of DNA replication and transcription.

nullisomy: a genetic condition in which both members of a homologous chromosome pair are absent; usually, embryos with this type of genetic defect are not viable.

ochre codon: a stop codon (UAA) found in messenger RNA (mRNA) molecules that signals termination of translation.

Okazaki fragments: short DNA fragments, approximately two thousand or fewer bases in length, produced during discontinuous replication of the "lagging" strand of a DNA molecule.

oligonucleotide: a short molecule of DNA, generally fewer than twenty bases long and usually synthesized artificially; an important tool for numerous molecular biology procedures, including sitedirected mutagenesis.

oncogene: any gene capable of stimulating cell division, thereby being a potential cause of cancer if unregulated; found in all cells and in many cancer-causing viruses.

oncovirus: a group of retroviruses that form tumors; these viruses have been associated with leukemia and sarcoma in animals and may also cause them in humans.

oogenesis: the process of producing eggs in a sexually mature female organism; another term for meiosis in females.

opal codon: a stop codon (UGA) found in messenger RNA (mRNA) molecules; signals termination of translation.

open reading frame (ORF): a putative proteincoding DNA sequence, marked by a start codon at one end and a stop codon at the other end.

operator: a region of a bacterial operon serving as a control point for transcription of the operon; a regulatory protein of some type usually binds to the operator.

operon: a genetic structure found only in bacteria, whereby a set of genes are controlled together by the same control elements; usually these genes have a common function, such as the genes of the lactose operon in *Escherichia coli* for the metabolism of lactose.

oxygen free radical: a highly reactive form of oxygen in which a single oxygen atom has a free, unpaired electron; free radicals are common byproducts of chemical reactions.

P generation: parental generation; the original individuals mated in a genetic cross.

p53 **gene:** a gene that typically controls the cell cycle, protecting the cell from damage; cancer cells may develop if this gene mutates and no longer protects the cell.

pachytene: a subphase of prophase I in meiosis in which tetrads become visible.

palindrome: in general, a word that reads the same forward and backward (such as the words "noon" and "racecar"); in genetics, a DNA sequence that reads the same on each strand of the DNA molecule, although in opposite directions because of the antiparallel nature of the double helix; most DNA palindromes serve as recognition sites for restriction endonucleases.

pandemic: a worldwide outbreak of a disease.

paracentric inversion: an inversion of a chromosome's sequence that does not involve the centromere, taking place on a single arm of the chromosome.

parthenogenesis: production of an organism from an unfertilized egg.

Patau syndrome: genetic disorder in which there is an extra copy of chromosome 13; individuals born with this condition commonly have malformed, low set ears, severe intellectual impairment, kidney and heart defects, and microcephaly. Also known as trisomy 13.

paternal: coming from the father.

pedigree: a diagram of a particular family, showing the relationships between all members of the family and the inheritance pattern of a particular trait or genetic defect; especially useful for research into human traits that may otherwise be difficult to study.

penetrance: a quantitative term referring to the percentage of individuals with a certain genotype that also exhibit the associated phenotype.

peptide bond: a bond found in proteins; occurs between the carboxyl group of one amino acid and the amino group of the next, linking them together.

pericentric inversion: an inversion of a chromosome's sequence involving the centromere.

PET scan: a procedure in which a small amount of radioactive glucose (sugar) is injected into a vein, and a scanner is used to make detailed, computerized pictures of areas inside the body where the glucose is taken up. Because cancer cells often take up more glucose than normal cells, the pictures can be used to find cancer cells in the body. Also called PET scan.

pharmacogenomics: the branch of human medical genetics that evaluates how an individual's genetic makeup influences his or her response to drugs.

phenotype: the physical appearance or biochemical and physiological characteristics of an individual, which is determined by both heredity and environment.

phenotypic plasticity: the ability of a genotype to produce different phenotypes when exposed to different environments.

phosphodiester bond: in DNA, the phosphate group connecting one nucleoside to the next in the polynucleotide chain.

photoreactivation repair: a cellular enzyme system responsible for repairing DNA damage caused by ultraviolet light; the system is activated by light.

phylogeny: often called an evolutionary tree, the branching patterns that show evolutionary relationships, with the taxa on the ends of the branches.

pilus: a hairlike reproductive structure possessed by some species of bacterial cells that allows them to engage in a transfer of genetic material known as conjugation.

Plagiocephaly: a condition characterized by an asymmetrical distortion (flattening of one side) of the skull. It is characterized by a flat spot on the back or one side of the head caused by remaining in a supine position for too long.

plasmid: a small, circular DNA molecule commonly found in bacteria and responsible for carrying various genes, such as antibiotic resistance genes; important as a cloning vector for genetic engineering.

pleiotropy: a genetic phenomenon in which a single gene has an effect on two or more traits.

-ploid, -ploidy: a suffix that refers to a chromosome set; humans have two sets of chromosomes and are referred to as being diploid, whereas some plants may have four sets, called tetraploid. Other terms include "autoploidy" and "polyploidy." *See also* allopolyploid; aneuploid; autopolyploid; diploid; euploid; haplodiploidy; haploid; polyploid; triploid.

pluripotency: the ability of a cell to give rise to all the differentiated cell types in an embryo.

point mutation: a DNA mutation involving a single nucleotide.

polar body: a by-product of oogenesis used to dispose of extra, unnecessary chromosomes while preserving the cytoplasm of the developing ovum.

polycistronic: characterizing messenger RNA (mRNA) molecules that contain coding sequences for more than one protein, common in prokaryotic cells.

polydactyly: a genetic disorder where the embryo develops extra fingers or toes.

polygenic inheritance: expression of a trait depending on the cumulative effect of multiple genes; human traits such as skin color, obesity, and intelligence are thought to be examples of polygenic inheritance.

polymerase chain reaction (PCR): a technique of molecular biology in which millions of copies of a single DNA sequence can be artificially produced in a relatively short period of time; important for a wide variety of applications when the source of DNA to be copied is either scarce or impure.

polymerase: a cellular enzyme capable of creating a phosphodiester bond between two nucleotides, producing a polynucleotide chain complementary to a single-stranded nucleic acid template; the enzyme DNA polymerase is important for DNA replication, and the enzyme RNA polymerase is involved in transcription.

polymorphism: the presence of many different alleles for a particular locus in individuals of the same species.

polypeptide: a single chain of amino acids connected to one another by peptide bonds; all proteins are polypeptides, but a protein may comprise one or more polypeptide molecules.

polyploid: a cell or organism that possesses multiple sets of chromosomes, usually more than two.

polysome: a group of ribosomes attached to the same messenger RNA (mRNA) molecule and producing the same protein product in varying stages of completion.

population genetics: the study of how genes behave in populations; often a highly mathematical branch of genetics in which evolutionary processes are modeled.

population: a group of organisms of the same species in the same place at the same time and thus potentially able to mate; populations are the basic unit of speciation.

positional cloning: a gene mapping technique used to locate a specific gene that causes a disorder when evidence is lacking about the biochemical nature of the disorder; also known as reverse genetics.

positive eugenics: selecting individuals to reproduce who have desirable genetic traits, as seen by those in control.

post-translational modification: chemical alterations to proteins after they have been produced at a ribosome that alters their properties.

prenatal testing: testing that is done during pregnancy to examine the chromosomes or genes of a fetus to detect the presence or absence of a genetic disorder.

prevalence: the percentage of people in a given population that are affected by a disorder at that particular time.

primary immunodeficiency: a genetic disorder involving a defect in the immune system, leaving the affected individual prone to infection; the defect may involve a single cell or one or more components of the immune system; more than 150 primary immunodeficiency disorders have been identified.

primer: a short nucleic acid molecule used as a beginning point for the enzyme DNA polymerase as it replicates a single-stranded template.

prion: an infectious agent composed solely of protein; thought to be the cause of various human and animal diseases characterized by neurological degeneration, including scrapie in sheep, mad cow disease in cattle, and Creutzfeldt-Jakob disease in humans.

probe: in genetics research, typically a single-stranded nucleic acid molecule or antibody that has been labeled in some way, either with radioactive isotopes or fluorescent dyes; this molecule is then used to seek out its complementary nucleic acid molecule or protein target in a variety of molecular biology techniques such as Southern, Northern, or Western blotting.

product rule: a rule of probability stating that the probability associated with two simultaneous yet independent events is the product of the events' individual probabilities.

prokaryote: a cell that lacks a nuclear membrane (and therefore has no true nucleus) and membrane-bound organelles; bacteria are the only known prokaryotic organisms.

promoter: a region of a gene that controls transcription of that gene; a physical binding site for RNA polymerase.

pronucleus: nucleus of a sperm or an egg before fertilization; when fertilization occurs the pronucleus of the egg and sperm join together to form the nucleus of the embryo that contains chromosomes from both the egg and the sperm.

prophase: the first phase in the process of mitosis or meiosis, in which the nuclear membrane disappears, the spindle apparatus begins to form, and chromatin takes on the form of chromosomes by becoming shorter and thicker.

propositus: the individual in a human pedigree who is the focus of the pedigree, usually by being the first person who came to the attention of the geneticist.

protease: enzyme required to digest protein.

protein: a biological molecule composed of amino acids linked together by peptide bonds; used as structural components of the cell or as enzymes; the term "protein" can refer to a single chain of amino acids or to multiple chains of amino acids functioning in a concerted way, as in the molecule hemoglobin.

proteomics: the study of which proteins are expressed in different types of cells, tissues, and organs during normal and abnormal conditions.

proto-oncogene: a gene, found in eukaryotic cells, that stimulates cell division; ordinarily, expression of this type of gene is tightly controlled by the cell, but in cancer cells, proto-oncogenes have been converted into oncogenes through alteration or elimination of controlled gene expression.

pseudodominance: a genetic phenomenon involving a recessive allele on one chromosome that is automatically expressed because of the deletion of its corresponding dominant allele on the other chromosome of the homologous pair.

pseudogenes: DNA sequences derived from partial copies, mutated complete copies, or normal copies of functional genes that have lost their control sequences and therefore cannot be transcribed; may originate by gene duplication or retrotransposition and are apparently nonfunctional regions of the genome that may evolve at a maximum rate, free from the evolutionary constraints of natural selection.

pseudohermaphrodite: individual born with either ambiguous genitalia or external genitalia that are the opposite of the chromosomal sex.

punctuated equilibrium: a model of evolutionary change in which new species originate abruptly and then exist through a long period of stasis; important as an explanation of the stepwise pattern of species change seen in the fossil record.

purine: either of the nitrogenous bases adenine or guanine; used in the structure of nucleic acids.

pyrimidine: any of the nitrogenous bases cytosine, thymine, or uracil; used in the structure of nucleic acids.

quantitative trait loci (QTLs): genomic regions that affect a quantitative trait, generally identified via DNA-based markers.

quantitative trait: a trait, such as human height or weight, that shows continuous variation in a population and can be measured; also called a metric trait.

reaction norm: the relationship between environment and phenotype for a given genotype.

reading frame: refers to the manner in which a messenger RNA (mRNA) sequence is interpreted as a series of amino acid codons by the ribosome; because of the triplet nature of the genetic code, a typical messenger RNA (mRNA) molecule has three possible reading frames, although usually only one of these will actually code for a functional protein.

receptors: molecules to which signaling molecules bind in target cells.

recessive: a term referring to an allele or trait that will only be expressed if another, dominant, trait or allele is not also present.

reciprocal cross: a mating that is the reverse of another with respect to the sex of the organisms that possess certain traits; for example, if a particular cross were tall male H short female, then the reciprocal cross would be short male H tall female.

reciprocal translocation: a two-way exchange of genetic material between two nonhomologous chromosomes, resulting in a wide variety of genetic problems depending on which chromosomes are involved in the translocation.

recombinant DNA: DNA molecules that are the products of artificial recombination between DNA molecules from two different sources; important as a foundation of genetic engineering.

recombination: an exchange of genetic material, usually between two homologous chromosomes; provides one of the foundations for the genetic reassortment observed during sexual reproduction.

reductional division: refers to meiosis I, in which the amount of genetic material in the cell is reduced by half through nuclear division; it is at this stage that the diploid cell is converted to an essentially haploid state.

reductionism: the explanation of a complex system or phenomenon as merely the sum of its parts.

replication: the process by which a DNA or RNA molecule is enzymatically copied.

replicon: a region of a chromosome under control of a single origin of replication.

replisome: a multiprotein complex that functions at the replication fork during DNA replication; it contains all the enzymes and other proteins necessary for replication, including DNA polymerase.

repressor: a protein molecule capable of preventing transcription of a gene, usually by binding to a regulatory region close to the gene.

resistance plasmid (R plasmid): a small, circular DNA molecule that replicates independently of the bacterial host chromosome and encodes a gene for antibiotic resistance.

restriction endonuclease: a bacterial enzyme that cuts DNA molecules at specific sites; part of a bacterial cell's built-in protection against infection by viruses; an important tool of genetic engineering.

restriction enzyme: *See* restriction endonuclease.

restriction fragment length polymorphism (RFLP): a genetic marker, consisting of variations in the length of restriction fragments in DNA from individuals being tested, allowing researchers to compare genetic sequences from various sources; used in a variety of fields, including forensics and the Human Genome Project.

retrotransposon (retroposon): a DNA sequence that is transcribed to RNA and reverse transcribed to a DNA copy able to insert itself at another location in the genome.

retrovirus: a virus that carries reverse transcriptase that converts its RNA genome into a DNA copy that integrates into the host chromosome.

reverse transcriptase: a form of DNA polymerase, discovered in retroviruses, that uses an RNA template to produce a DNA molecule; the name indicates that this process is the reverse of the transcription process occurring naturally in the cell.

reverse transcription polymerase chain reaction (RT-PCR): a technique, requiring isolated RNA, for quickly determining if a gene or a small set of genes are transcribed in a population of cells.

RFLP analysis: *See* restriction fragment length polymorphism.

Rh factor: a human red blood cell antigen, first characterized in rhesus monkeys, that contributes to blood typing; individuals can be either Rh positive (possessing the antigen on their red blood cells) or Rh negative (lacking the antigen).

ribonucleic acid (RNA): a form of nucleic acid in the cell used primarily for genetic expression through transcription and translation; in structure, it is virtually identical to DNA, except that ribose is used as the sugar in each nucleotide and the nitrogenous base thymine is replaced by uracil; present in three major forms in the cell: messenger RNA (mRNA), transfer RNA (tRNA), and ribosomal RNA (rRNA).

ribose: a five-carbon sugar used in the structure of ribonucleic acid (RNA).

ribosomal RNA (rRNA): a type of ribonucleic acid in the cell that constitutes some of the structure of the ribosome and participates in the process of translation.

ribosome: a cellular structure, composed of ribosomal RNA (rRNA) and proteins, that is the site of translation.

ribozyme: an RNA molecule that can function catalytically as an enzyme.

RNA interference (RNAi): an artificial technique using small, interfering RNAs that cause gene silencing by binding to the part of a messenger RNA (mRNA) to which they are complementary, thus blocking translation.

RNA polymerase: the cellular enzyme required for making an RNA copy of genetic information contained in a gene; an integral part of transcription.

RNA: *See* ribonucleic acid.

RNase: refers to a group of enzymes, ribonucleases, capable of specifically degrading RNA molecules.

rRNA: *See* ribosomal RNA.

Sanger sequencing: also known as dideoxy termination sequencing, a method using nucleotides that are missing the 3' hydroxyl group in order to terminate the polymerization of new DNA at a specific nucleotide; the most common sequencing method, used almost exclusively.

segregation: a characteristic of Mendelian genetics, resulting in the division of homologous chromosomes into separate gametes during the process of meiosis.

semiconservative replication: a characteristic of DNA replication, in which every new DNA molecule is actually a hybrid molecule, being composed of a parental, preexisting strand and a newly synthesized strand.

sequence-tagged sites: a short sequence of DNA that occurs once in the genome; the location and sequence of this DNA segment are known and can be easily found using polymerase chain reaction when particular primers are used.

severe immunodeficiency: a primary disorder of the immune system characterized by a severe defect in the T- and B-lymphocyte systems; infants born with this disorder commonly develop a severe sometimes life-threatening infection, such as meningitis, pneumonia, or bloodstream infection within the first few months of life.

sex chromosome: a chromosome carrying genes responsible for determination of an organism's sex; in humans, the sex chromosomes are designated X and Y

sex-influenced inheritance: inheritance in which the expression of autosomal traits is influenced or altered relative to the sex of the individual possessing the trait; pattern baldness is an example of this type of inheritance in humans.

sex-limited inheritance: inheritance of traits expressed in only one sex, although these traits are usually produced by non-sex-linked genes (that is, they are genes located on autosomes instead of sex chromosomes).

sex-linked: disorder that is inherited through one of the sex chromosomes, the X or Y chromosomes.

sexual reproduction: reproduction of cells or organisms involving the transfer and reassortment of genetic information, resulting in offspring that can be phenotypically and genotypically distinct from either of the parents; mediated by the fusion of gametes produced during meiosis.

Shine-Dalgarno sequence: a short sequence in prokaryotic messenger RNA (mRNA) molecules complementary to a sequence in the prokaryotic ribosome; important for proper positioning of the start codon of the mRNA relative to the P site of the ribosome.

short interspersed sequences (SINES): short repeats of DNA sequences scattered throughout a genome.

shotgun cloning: a technique by which random DNA fragments from an organism's genome are inserted into a collection of vectors to produce a library of clones, which can then be used in a variety of molecular biology procedures.

sigma factor: a molecule that is part of RNA polymerase molecules in bacterial cells; allows RNA polymerase to select the genes that will be transcribed.

signal transduction: all of the molecular events that occur between the arrival of a signaling molecule at a target cell and its response; typically involves a cascading series of reactions that can eventually determine expression of many dozens of genes.

single nucleotide polymorphism (SNP): differences at the individual nucleotide level among individuals.

single-gene testing: a type of medical test that identifies changes in chromosomes, genes, or proteins. The results of a genetic test can confirm or rule out a suspected genetic condition or help determine a person's chance of developing or passing on a genetic disorder. Single gene disorders are genetic conditions caused by a mutation of a specific gene. Single gene disorders are often heritable (they run in families), and therefore, individuals with a family history of a single gene disorder may be at risk for passing the condition onto their children.

site-directed mutagenesis: a molecular genetics procedure in which synthetic oligonucleotide molecules are used to induce carefully planned mutations in a cloned DNA molecule.

small nuclear RNA (snRNA): small, numerous RNA molecules found in the nuclei of eukaryotic cells and involved in splicing of messenger RNA (mRNA) precursors to prepare them for translation.

snRNA: *See* small nuclear RNA.

sociobiology: the study of social structures, organizations, and actions in terms of underlying biological principles.

solenoid: a complex, highly compacted DNA structure consisting of many nucleosomes packed together in a bundle.

somatic cell: any cell in the body, excluding the reproductive cells.

somatic mutation: a mutation occurring in a somatic, or nonsex, cell; because of this, somatic mutations cannot be passed to the next generation.

Southern blot: a molecular biology technique in which a labeled single-stranded DNA probe is exposed to denatured cellular DNA immobilized on a filter; under the proper conditions, the DNA probe will seek out and bind to its complementary sequence among the cellular DNA molecules, if such a sequence is present.

speciation: the process of evolutionary change that leads to the formation of new species.

species: a group of organisms that can interbreed with one another but not with organisms outside the group; generally, members of a particular species share the same gene pool; defining a species is still controversial and remains a debated concept.

spermatogenesis: the process of producing sperm in a sexually mature male organism; another term for meiosis in males.

spindle apparatus: a structure, composed of microtubules and microfilaments, important for the proper orientation and movement of chromosomes during mitosis and meiosis; appears during prophase and begins to disappear during anaphase.

splice site: a genetic mutation that inserts, deletes or changes a number of nucleotides in the specific site at which splicing takes place during the processing of precursor messenger RNA into mature messenger RNA.

spliceosome: a complex of nuclear RNA and protein molecules responsible for the excision of introns from messenger RNA (mRNA) precursors before they are translated.

spontaneous mutation: a mutation that arises naturally and not as a result of exposure to mutagens.

SRY gene: the sex-determining region of the Y chromosome; a gene encoding a protein product called testis determining factor (TDF), responsible for conversion of a female embryo to a male embryo through the development of the testes.

stem cell: an undifferentiated cell that retains the ability to give rise to other, more specialized cells.

stutter: polymerase chain reaction (PCR) amplification product that arises as a result of strand slippage during PCR ; it is one or more repeat units less than the sample's allele.

suicide gene: a gene that when expressed in a cell becomes lethal to the cell; suicide genes make cancer cells vulnerable to chemotherapy.

sum rule: a rule of probability theory stating that the probability of either of two mutually exclusive events occurring is the sum of the events' individual probabilities.

supercoil: a complex DNA structure in which the DNA double helix is itself coiled into a helix; usually observed in circular DNA molecules such as bacterial plasmids.

sympatric speciation: the genetic divergence of populations, not separated geographically, that eventually results in formation of new species.

synapsis: the close association of homologous chromosomes occurring during early prophase I of meiosis; during synapsis, recombination between these chromosomes can occur.

Syndactyly: This is a condition wherein two or more digits are fused together. It occurs normally in some mammals, such as the siamang and diprotodontia, but is an unusual condition in humans.

T: the abbreviation for thymine, a pyrimidine nitrogenous base found in the structure of DNA; in RNA, thymine is replaced by uracil.

tandem mass spectrometry: also known as MS/MS or MS2, involves multiple steps of mass spectrometry selection, with some form of fragmentation occurring in between the stages. The resulting ions are then separated and detected in a second stage of mass spectrometry (MS2).

Taq polymerase: DNA polymerase from the bacterium *Thermus aquaticus;* an integral component of polymerase chain reaction.

tautomerization: a spontaneous internal rearrangement of atoms in a complex biological molecule that often causes the molecule to change its shape or its chemical properties.

taxon *(pl.* **taxa):** a general term used by evolutionists to refer to a type of organism at any level in a classification of organisms.

telocentric chromosome: a chromosome with a centromere at the end. *See also* acrocentric chromosome; metacentric chromosome.

telomere: the end of a eukaryotic chromosome, protected and replaced by the cellular enzyme telomerase.

telophase: the final phase in the process of mitosis or meiosis, in which division of the cell's nuclear contents has been completed and division of the cell itself occurs.

template: a single-stranded DNA molecule (or RNA molecule) used to create a complementary strand of nucleic acid through the activity of a polymerase.

teratogen: any chemical or physical substance, such as thalidomide, that creates birth defects in offspring.

testcross: a mating involving an organism with a recessive genotype for desired traits crossed with an organism that has an incompletely determined genotype; the types and ratio of offspring produced allow geneticists to determine the genotype of the second organism.

tetrad: a group of four chromosomes formed as a result of the synapsis of homologous chromosomes that takes place early in meiosis.

tetranucleotide hypothesis: a disproven hypothesis, formulated by geneticist P. A. Levene, stating that DNA is a structurally simple molecule composed of a repeating unit known as a tetranucleotide (composed, in turn, of equal amounts of the bases adenine, cytosine, guanine, and thymine).

thermal cycler: a machine that can rapidly heat and cool reaction tubes; used for performing PCR reactions.

theta structure: an intermediate structure in the bidirectional replication of a circular DNA molecule; the name comes from the resemblance of this structure to the Greek letter theta.

thymine (T): a pyrimidine nitrogenous base found in the structure of DNA; in RNA, thymine is replaced by uracil.

thymine dimer: a pair of thymine bases in a DNA molecule connected by an abnormal chemical bond induced by ultraviolet light; prevents DNA replication in the cell unless it is removed by specialized enzymes.

topoisomerases: cellular enzymes that relieve tension in replicating DNA molecules by introducing single- or double-stranded breaks into the DNA molecule; without these enzymes, replicating DNA becomes progressively more supercoiled until it can no longer unwind, and DNA replication is halted.

totipotent: the ability of a cell to produce an entire adult organism through successive cell divisions and development; as cells become progressively differentiated, they lose this characteristic.

trait: a phenotypic characteristic that is heritable.

transcription factor: a protein that is involved in initiation of transcription but is not part of the RNA polymerase.

transcription: the cellular process by which genetic information in the form of a gene in a DNA molecule is converted into the form of a messenger RNA (mRNA) molecule; dependent on the enzyme RNA polymerase.

transduction: DNA transfer between cells, with a virus serving as the genetic vector.

transfer RNA (tRNA): a type of RNA molecule necessary for translation to occur properly; provides the basis of the genetic code, in which codons in a messenger RNA (mRNA) molecule are used to direct the sequence of amino acids in a polypeptide; contains a binding site for a particular amino acid and a region complementary to a messenger RNA (mRNA) codon (an anticodon).

transformation: the process by which a normal cell is converted into a cancer cell; also refers to the change in phenotype accompanying entry of foreign DNA into a cell, such as in bacterial cells being used in recombinant DNA procedures.

transgenic organism: an organism possessing one or more genes from another organism, such as mice that possess human genes; important for the study of genes in a living organism, especially in the study of mutations within these genes. *See also* genetically modified organism (GMO).

transition mutation: a DNA mutation in which one pyrimidine (cytosine or thymine) takes the place of another, or a purine (adenine or guanine) takes the place of another.

translation: the cellular process by which genetic information in the form of a messenger RNA (mRNA) molecule is converted into the amino acid sequence of a protein, using ribosomes and RNA molecules as accessory molecules.

translocation: the movement of a chromosome segment to a nonhomologous chromosome as a result of an error in recombination; also refers to the movement of a messenger RNA (mRNA) codon from the A site of the ribosome to the P site during translation.

transposable element: *See* transposon.

transposon: a DNA sequence capable of moving to various places in a chromosome, discovered by geneticist Barbara McClintock; transposons are thought to be important as mediators of genetic variability in both prokaryotes and eukaryotes.

transversion: a DNA mutation in which a pyrimidine (cytosine or thymine) takes the place of a purine (adenine or guanine), or vice versa.

triploid: possessing three complete sets of chromosomes, or 3N; important in the development of desirable characteristics in the flowers or fruit of some plants; triploids are often sterile.

trisomy: a genetic condition involving one chromosome of a homologous chromosome pair that has been duplicated in some way, giving rise to a 2N + 1 genotype and causing serious phenotypic abnormalities; a well-known example is trisomy 21, or Down syndrome, in which the individual possesses three copies of chromosome 21 instead of the normal two copies.

tRNA: *See* transfer RNA.

tumor-suppressor genes: any of a number of genes that limit or halt cell division under certain circumstances, thereby preventing the formation of tumors in an organism; two well-studied examples are the retinoblastoma gene and the *p53* gene; mutations in tumor-suppressor genes can lead to cancer.

Turner syndrome: a human genetic defect in which an individual has only forty-five chromosomes, lacking one sex chromosome; the sex chromosome present is an X chromosome, making these individuals phenotypically female, although with serious abnormalities such as sterility and anatomical defects.

Turribrachycephaly: having a high prominent forehead.

Ultrasound: a procedure that uses high-energy sound waves to look at tissues and organs inside the body. The sound waves make echoes that form pictures of the tissues and organs on a computer screen (sonogram). Ultrasound may be used to help diagnose diseases, such as cancer. It may also be used during pregnancy to check the fetus (unborn baby) and during medical procedures, such as biopsies. Also called ultrasonography.

uracil (U): a pyrimidine nitrogenous base found in the structure of RNA; in DNA, uracil is replaced by thymine.

variable number tandem repeat (VNTR): a repetitive DNA sequence of approximately fifty to one hundred nucleotides; important in the process of forensic identification known as DNA fingerprinting.

vector: a DNA molecule, such as a bacterial plasmid, into which foreign DNA can be inserted and then transported into a cell for further manipulation; important in a wide variety of recombinant DNA techniques.

Villefranche **nomenclature:** *Ehlers-Danlos* syndrome is a group of disorders that affect the connective tissues that support the skin, bones, blood vessels, and many other organs and tissues. Defects in connective tissues cause the signs and symptoms of Ehlers-Danlos syndrome, which vary from mildly loose joints to life-threatening complications. Previously, there were more than 10 recognized types of Ehlers-Danlos syndrome, differentiated by Roman numerals. In 1997, researchers proposed a simpler classification that reduced the number of major types to six and gave them descriptive names: the classical type (formerly types I and II), the hypermobility type (formerly type III), the vascular type (formerly type IV), the kyphoscoliosis type (formerly type VIA), the arthrochalasia type (formerly types VIIA and VIIB), and the dermatosparaxis type (formerly type VIIC). This six-type classification, known as the Villefranche nomenclature, is still commonly used. The types are distinguished by their signs and symptoms, their underlying genetic causes, and their patterns of inheritance. Since 1997, several additional forms of the condition have been described. These additional forms appear to be rare, affecting a small number of families, and most have not been well characterized.

virions: mature infectious virus particles.

viroids: naked strands of RNA, 270 to 380 nucleotides long, that are circular and do not code for any proteins that are able to cause disease in susceptible plants, many of them economically important. *See also* virusoids.

virus: a microscopic infectious particle composed primarily of protein and nucleic acid; bacterial viruses, or bacteriophages, have been important tools of study in the history of molecular genetics.

virusoids: similar to viroids, microscopic infectious particles composed primarily of protein and nucleic acid; unlike viroids, virusoids are packaged in the protein coat of other plant viruses, referred to as helpers, and are therefore dependent on the other virus. *See also* viroids.

VNTR: *See* variable number tandem repeat.

walking: *See* chromosome walking.

Western blot: a molecular biology technique involving labeled antibodies exposed to cellular proteins immobilized on a filter; under the proper conditions, the antibodies will seek out and bind to the proteins for which they are specific, if such proteins are present.

wild-type: interacting with more than one messenger RNA (mRNA) codon by virtue of the inherent flexibility present in the third base of the anticodon; first proposed by molecular biologist Francis Crick.

Wolfram syndrome: an autosomal recessive disorder, caused by a mutation in a gene responsible for the production of the wolfram protein, resulting in the functional loss of the protein. Patients who suffer from this neurodegenerative disorder typically develop diabetes insipidus, diabetes mellitus, blindness, and deafness. Also known as DIDMOAD, an acronym for diabetes insipidus, diabetes mellitus, optic atrophy, and deafness.

X linkage: a genetic phenomenon involving a gene located on the X chromosome; the typical pattern of X linkage involves recessive alleles, such as that for hemophilia, which exert their effects when passed from mother to son and are more likely to be exhibited by males than females.

X-ray diffraction: a method for determining the structure of molecules that infers structure by the way crystals of molecules scatter X rays as they pass through.

xenotransplants: transplants of organs or cellular tissue between different species of animals, such as between pigs and humans.

Y linkage: a genetic phenomenon involving a gene located on the Y chromosome; as a result, such a condition can be passed only from father to son.

yeast artificial chromosome (YAC): a cloning vector that has been engineered with all of the major genetic characteristics of a eukaryotic chromosome so that it will behave as such during cell division; YACs are used to clone extremely large DNA fragments from eukaryotic cells and are an integral part of the Human Genome Project.

Z-DNA: a zigzag form of DNA in which the strands form a left-handed helix instead of the normal right-handed helix of B-DNA; Z-DNA is known to be present in cells and is thought to be involved in genetic regulation. *See also* B-DNA.

zinc finger: an amino acid sequence, found in some DNA-binding proteins, that complexes with zinc ions to create polypeptide "fingers" that can then wrap around a specific portion of a DNA molecule.

zygote: a diploid cell produced by the union of a male gamete (sperm) with a female gamete (egg); through successive cell divisions, the zygote will eventually give rise to the adult form of the organism.

zygotene: a subphase of prophase I of meiosis involving synapsis between homologous chromosomes.

Randall K. Harris, Ph.D, and Bryan Ness, Ph.D.;
updated by Collette Bishop Hendler, R.N., M.S.

BIBLIOGRAPHY

GENERAL

Andreasen, Nancy C., ed. *Research Advances in Genetics and Genomics: Implications for Psychiatry.* Washington, D.C.: American Psychiatric Publishing, 2005.

Audesirk, Teresa, Gerald Audesirk, and Bruce E. Myers. *Biology: Life on Earth.* 6th ed. Upper Saddle River, N.J.: Prentice Hall, 2001.

Bailey, Philip S., Jr., Christina A. Bailey, and Robert J. Ouellette. *Organic Chemistry.* New York: Prentice Hall, 1997.

Banaszak, Leonard J. *Foundations of Structural Biology.* San Diego: Academic Press, 2000.

Barash, David P. *Revolutionary Biology: The New, GeneCentered View of Life.* New Brunswick, N.J.: Transaction Publishers, 2003.

Berg, Paul, and Maxine Singer. *Dealing with Genes: The Language of Heredity.* Mill Valley, Calif.: University Science Books, 1992.

Brenner, Sydney, and Jeffrey K. Miller, eds. *Encyclopedia of Genetics.* New York: Elsevier, 2001.

Campbell, Neil A., and Jane B. Reece. *Biology.* 6th ed. San Francisco: Benjamin Cummings, 2002.

Carey, Gregory. *Human Genetics for the Social Sciences.* Thousand Oaks, Calif.: Sage Publications, 2003.

Clark, David P., and Lonnie D. Russell. *Molecular Biology Made Simple and Fun.* 2d ed. Vienna, Ill.: Cache River Press, 2000.

Compston, Alastair, et al. *McAlpine's Multiple Sclerosis.* Sydney: Elsevier/Churchill Livingstone, 2005.

Cummings, Michael. *Human Heredity: Principles and Issues.* Australia: Brooks/Cole Cengage Learning, 2009.

DeBusk, Ruth M. *Genetics: The Nutrition Connection.* Chicago: American Dietetic Association, 2003.

Diagram Group. *Genetics and Cell Biology on File.* Rev. ed. New York: Facts On File, 2003.

Entine, Jon. *Abraham's Children: Race, Identity, and the DNA of the Chosen People.* New York: Grand Central, 2007.

Fairbanks, Daniel J., and W. Ralph Anderson. *Genetics: The Continuity of Life.* New York: Brooks/Cole, 1999.

Finch, Caleb Ellicott. *Longevity, Senescence, and the Genome.* Reprint. Chicago: University of Chicago Press, 1994.

Goldstein, David B. *Jacob's Legacy: A Genetic View of Jewish History.* New Haven, Conn.: Yale University Press, 2008.

Hartl, Daniel L. *Genetics: Analysis of Genes and Genomes.* 5th ed. Boston: Jones and Bartlett, 2001.

Hartwell, L. H., et al. *Genetics: From Genes to Genomes.* 2d ed. New York: McGraw-Hill, 2003.

Hill, John, et al. *Chemistry and Life: An Introduction to General, Organic, and Biological Chemistry.* 6th ed. New York: Prentice Hall, 2000.

Jones, Steve Y. *The Descent of Men.* Boston: Houghton Mifflin, 2003.

King, Robert C., and William D. Stansfield. *A Dictionary of Genetics.* 6th ed. New York: Oxford University Press, 2001.

Klug, William S. *Essentials of Genetics.* 3d ed. Upper Saddle River, N.J.: Prentice Hall, 1999.

Lerner, K. Lee. *World of Genetics.* Detroit: Gale Research, 2001.

Lewin, Benjamin. *Genes VII.* New York: Oxford University Press, 2001.

Madigan, Michael T., John M. Martinko, and Jack Parker. *Brock Biology of Micro-organisms.* 10th ed. Upper Saddle River, N.J.: Prentice Hall, 2003.

Marks, Jonathan. *What It Means to Be 98 Percent Chimpanzee: Apes, People, and Their Genes.* Berkeley: University of California Press, 2002.

Micklos, David A., Greg A. Freyer, and David A. Crotty. *DNA Science: A First Course.* Cold Spring Harbor, N.Y.: Cold Spring Harbor Laboratory Press, 2003.

Moore, David S. *Dependent Gene: The Fallacy of Nature vs. Nurture.* New York: W. H. Freeman, 2001.

Moore, John A. *Science as a Way of Knowing.* 1993. Reprint. Cambridge, Mass.: Harvard University Press, 1999.

Raven, Peter H., and George B. Johnson. *Biology.* 6th ed. New York: W. H. Freeman/Worth, 1999.

Reeve, Eric C. R. *Encyclopedia of Genetics.* Chicago: Fitzroy Dearborn, 2001.

Relethford, John H., and John Relethford. *Reflections of Our Past: How Human History Is Revealed in Our Genes.* Boulder, Colo.: Westview Press, 2003.

Ridley, Matt. *Nature Via Nurture: Genes, Experience, and What Makes Us Human.* London: Fourth Estate, 2003.

Robinson, Richard, ed. *Genetics.* New York: Macmillan, 2002.

Russell, Peter J. *Genetics.* San Francisco: Benjamin Cummings, 2002.

Salter, Frank. *On Genetic Interests: Family, Ethnicity, and Humanity in an Age of Mass Migration.* Frankfurt am Main, Germany: Peter Lang, 2003.

Simon, Anne. *The Real Science Behind "The X-Files": Microbes, Meteorites, and Mutants.* New York: Simon & Schuster, 1999.

Singer, Maxine, and Paul Berg, eds. *Exploring Genetic Mechanisms.* Sausalito, Calif.: University Science Books, 1997.

Starr, Cecie. *Biology: Concepts and Applications.* 5th ed. New York: Brooks/Cole, 2003.

Sykes, Brian. *Adam's Curse: A Future Without Men.* London: Bantam, 2003.

Tamarin, Robert H. *Principles of Genetics.* Boston: McGraw-Hill, 2002.

Tortora, Gerard. *Microbiology: An Introduction.* 7th ed. San Francisco: Benjamin Cummings, 2001.

Weaver, Robert F., and Philip W. Hedrick. *Genetics.* 3d ed. New York: McGraw-Hill, 1997.

Wells, Spencer. *The Journey of Man: A Genetic Odyssey.* London: Penguin, 2003.

AGRICULTURE AND GENETICALLY MODIFIED FOODS

Altieri, Miguel A. *Genetic Engineering in Agriculture.* Chicago: LPC Group, 2001.

Anderson, Luke. *Genetic Engineering, Food, and Our Environment.* White River Junction, Vt.: Chelsea Green, 1999.

Avery, Dennis T. *Saving the Planet with Pesticides and Plastic: The Environmental Triumph of High-Yield Farming.* 2d ed. Indianapolis: Hudson Institute, 2000.

Carozzi, Nadine, and Michael Koziel, eds. *Advances in Insect Control: The Role of Transgenic Plants.* Bristol, Pa.: Taylor & Francis, 1997.

Chrispeels, Maarten J., and David E. Sadava. *Plants, Genes, and Crop Biotechnology.* Boston: Jones and Bartlett, 2003.

Engel, Karl-Heinz, et al. *Genetically Modified Foods: Safety Aspects.* Washington, D.C.: American Chemical Society, 1995.

Entwhistle, Philip F., Jenny S. Cory, Mark J. Bailey, and Steven R. Higgs. *"Bacillus thuringiensis," an*

Environmental Biopesticide: Theory and Practice. New York: Wiley, 1994.

Fedoroff, Nina, and Nancy Marie Brown. *Mendel in the Kitchen: A Scientist's View of Genetically Modified Foods.* Washington, D.C.: Joseph Henry Press, 2004.

Galun, Esra, and Adina Breiman. *Transgenic Plants.* London: Imperial College Press, 1997.

Goodman, David, et al. *From Farming to Biotechnology: A Theory of Agro-Industrial Development.* New York: Basil Blackwell, 1987.

Hall, Franklin R., and Julius J. Menn, eds. *Biopesticides: Use and Delivery.* Totowa, N.J.: Humana Press, 1999.

Henry, Robert J. *Practical Applications of Plant Molecular Biology.* New York: Chapman & Hall, 1997.

Hindmarsh, Richard, and Geoffrey Lawrence, eds. *Recoding Nature: Critical Perspectives on Genetic Engineering.* Sydney: UNSW Press, 2004.

Koul, Opender, and G. S. Dhaliwal, eds. *Microbial Biopesticides.* New York: Taylor & Francis, 2002.

Krimsky, Sheldon, et al., eds. *Agricultural Biotechnology and the Environment: Science, Policy, and Social Issues.* Urbana: University of Illinois Press, 1996.

Lambrecht, Bill. *Dinner at the New Gene Cafe: How Genetic Engineering Is Changing What We Eat, How We Live, and the Global Politics of Food.* New York: Thomas Dunne Books, 2001.

Lurquin, Paul F. *The Green Phoenix: A History of Genetically Modified Plants.* New York: Columbia University Press, 2001.

Rissler, Jane, and Margaret Mellon. *The Ecological Risks of Engineered Crops.* Cambridge, Mass.: MIT Press, 1996.

Winston, Mark L. *Travels in the Genetically Modified Zone.* Cambridge, Mass.: Harvard University Press, 2002.

Zohary, Daniel, and Maria Hopf. *Domestication of Plants in the Old World: The Origin and Spread of Cultivated Plants in West Asia, Europe, and the Nile Valley.* 3d ed. New York: Oxford University Press, 2001.

BACTERIAL GENETICS

Adelberg, Edward A., ed. *Papers on Bacterial Genetics.* Boston: Little, Brown, 1966.

Birge, Edward A. *Bacterial and Bacteriophage Genetics.* 5th ed. New York: Springer, 2006.

Brock, Thomas D. *The Emergence of Bacterial Genetics.* Cold Spring Harbor, N.Y: Cold Spring Harbor Laboratory Press, 1990.

Carlberg, David M. *Essentials of Bacterial and Viral Genetics.* Springfield, Ill.: Charles C Thomas, 1976.

Dale, Jeremy. *Molecular Genetics of Bacteria.* New York: John Wiley & Sons, 1994.

Day, Martin J. *Plasmids.* London: Edward Arnold, 1982.

Dean, Alastair Campbell Ross, and Sir Cyril Hinshelwood. *Growth, Function, and Regulation in Bacterial Cells.* Oxford, England: Clarendon Press, 1966.

De Bruijn, Frans J., et al., eds. *Bacterial Genomes: Physical Structure and Analysis.* New York: Chapman & Hall, 1998.

Dorman, Charles J. *Genetics of Bacterial Virulence.* Oxford, England: Blackwell Scientific, 1994.

Drlica, Karl, and Monica Riley, eds. *The Bacterial Chromosome.* Washington, D.C.: American Society for Microbiology, 1990.

Fry, John C., and Martin J. Day, eds. *Bacterial Genetics in Natural Environments.* London: Chapman & Hall, 1990.

Goldberg, Joanna B., ed. *Genetics of Bacterial Polysaccharides.* Boca Raton, Fla.: CRC Press, 1999.

Jacob, Franyois, and Elie L. Wollman. *Sexuality and the Genetics of Bacteria.* New York: Academic Press, 1961.

Joset, Franyoise, et al. *Prokaryotic Genetics: Genome Organization, Transfer, and Plasticity.* Boston: Blackwell Scientific Publications, 1993.

Miller, Jeffrey H. *A Short Course in Bacterial Genetics: A Laboratory Manual and Handbook for Escherichia coli and Related Bacteria.* Cold Spring Harbor, N.Y: Cold Spring Harbor Laboratory Press, 1999.

Murray, Patrick, ed. *Manual of Clinical Microbiology.* Washington, D.C.: ASM Press, 2003.

Park, Simon. *Molecular Genetics of Bacteria.* Chichester, England: John Wiley & Sons, 2005.

Schumann, Wolfgang, S. Dusko Ehrlich, and Naotake Ogasawara, eds. *Functional Analysis of Bacterial Genes: A Practical Manual.* New York: Wiley, 2001.

Siezen, Roland J., et al., eds. *Lactic Acid Bacteria: Genetics, Metabolism, and Applications.* 7th ed. Boston: Kluwer Academic, 2002.

Snyder, Larry, and Wendy Champness. *Molecular Genetics of Bacteria.* Washington, D.C.: ASM Press, 1997.

Summers, David K. *The Biology of Plasmids.* Malden, Mass.: Blackwell, 1996.

Thomas, Christopher M., ed. *The Horizontal Gene Pool: Bacterial Plasmids and Gene Spread.* Amsterdam: Harwood Academic, 2000.

U.S. Congress. Office of Technology Assessment. *New Developments in Biotechnology—Field-Testing Engineered Organisms: Genetic and Ecological Issues.* Washington, D.C.: National Technical Information Service, 1988.

Vaughan, Pat, ed. *DNA Repair Protocols: Prokaryotic Systems.* Totowa, N.J.: Humana Press, 2000.

BIOETHICS AND SOCIAL POLICY

Becker, Gerhold K., and James P. Buchanan, eds. *Changing Nature's Course: The Ethical Challenge of Biotechnology.* Hong Kong: Hong Kong University Press, 1996.

Bonnicksen, Andrea L. *Crafting a Cloning Policy: From Dolly to Stem Cells.* Washington, D.C.: Georgetown University Press, 2002.

Boylan, Michael, and Kevin E. Brown. *Genetic Engineering: Science and Ethics on the New Frontier.* Upper Saddle River, N.J.: Prentice Hall, 2001.

Brannigan, Michael C., ed. *Ethical Issues in Human Cloning: Cross-Disciplinary Perspectives.* New York: Seven Bridges Press, 2001.

Bulger, Ruth Ellen, Elizabeth Heitman, and Stanley Joel Reiser, eds. *The Ethical Dimensions of the Biological and Health Sciences.* 2d ed. New York: Cambridge University Press, 2002.

Caplan, Arthur. *Due Consideration: Controversy in the Age of Medical Miracles.* New York: Wiley, 1997.

Chadwick, Ruth, et al., eds. *The Ethics of Genetic Screening.* Boston: Kluwer Academic, 1999.

Chapman, Audrey R., ed. *Perspectives on Genetic Patenting: Religion, Science, and Industry in Dialogue.* Washington, D.C.: American Association for the Advancement of Science, 1999.

Charon, Rita, and Martha Montello, eds. *Stories Matter: The Role of Narrative in Medical Ethics.* New York: Routledge, 2002.

Comstock, Gary L., ed. *Life Science Ethics.* Ames: Iowa State Press, 2002.

Danis, Marion, Carolyn Clancy, and Larry R. Churchill, eds. *Ethical Dimensions of Health Policy.* New York: Oxford University Press, 2002.

Davis, Bernard D., ed. *The Genetic Revolution: Scientific Prospects and Public Perceptions.* Baltimore: Johns Hopkins University Press, 1991.

De Waal, Franz. *Good Natured: The Origins of Right and Wrong in Humans and Other Animals.* Cambridge, Mass.: Harvard University Press, 1996.

Doherty, Peter, and Agneta Sutton, eds. *Man-Made Man: Ethical and Legal Issues in Genetics.* Dublin: Four Courts Press, 1997.

Espejo, Roman, ed. *Biomedical Ethics: Opposing Viewpoints.* San Diego: Greenhaven Press, 2003.

Evans, John Hyde. *Playing God? Human Genetic Engineering and the Rationalization of Public Bioethical Debate.* Chicago: University of Chicago Press, 2002.

Gonder, Janet C., Ernest D. Prentice, and LillyMarlene Russow, eds. *Genetic Engineering and Animal Welfare: Preparing for the Twenty-first Century.* Greenbelt, Md.: Scientists Center for Animal Welfare, 1999.

Grace, Eric S. *Biotechnology Unzipped: Promises and Reality.* Washington, D.C.: National Academy Press, 1997.

Harpignies, J. P. *Double Helix Hubris: Against Designer Genes.* Brooklyn, N.Y.: Cool Grove Press, 1996.

Holland, Suzanne, Karen Lebacqz, and Laurie Zoloth, eds. *The Human Embryonic Stem Cell Debate: Science, Ethics, and Public Policy (Basic Bioethics).* Cambridge, Mass.: MIT Press, 2001.

Hubbard, Ruth, and Elijah Wald. *Exploding the Gene Myth: How Genetic Information Is Produced and Manipulated by Scientists, Physicians, Employers, Insurance Companies, Educators, and Law Enforcers.* Boston: Beacon Press, 1999.

Kass, Leon R. *Life, Liberty, and the Defense of Dignity: The Challenge for Bioethics.* San Francisco: Encounter Books, 2002.

Kevles, Daniel J. *In the Name of Eugenics: Genetics and the Uses of Human Heredity.* Cambridge, Mass.: Harvard University Press, 1995.

Kristol, William, and Eric Cohen, eds. *The Future Is Now: America Confronts the New Genetics.* Lanham, Md.: Rowman & Littlefield, 2002.

Leroy, Bonnie, Dianne M. Bartels, and Arthur L. Caplan, eds. *Prescribing Our Future: Ethical Challenges in Genetic Counseling.* New York: Aldine de Gruyter, 1993.

Long, Clarisa, ed. *Genetic Testing and the Use of Information.* Washington, D.C.: AEI Press, 1999.

MacKinnon, Barbara, ed. *Human Cloning: Science, Ethics, and Public Policy.* Urbana: University of Illinois Press, 2000.

May, Thomas. *Bioethics in a Liberal Society: The Political Framework of Bioethics Decision Making.* Baltimore: Johns Hopkins University Press, 2002.

O'Neill, Onora. *Autonomy and Trust in Bioethics.* New York: Cambridge University Press, 2002.

Post, Stephen G., ed. *Encyclopedia of Bioethics.* New York: Macmillan Reference USA, 2003.

Rantala, M. L., and Arthur J. Milgram, eds. *Cloning: For and Against.* Chicago: Open Court, 1999.

Real, Leslie A., ed. *Ecological Genetics.* Princeton, N.J.: Princeton University Press, 1994.

Reilly, Philip R. *Abraham Lincoln's DNA and Other Adventures in Genetics.* Cold Spring Harbor, N.Y.: Cold Spring Harbor Laboratory Press, 2000.

Reiss, Michael J., and Roger Straughan, eds. *Improving Nature? The Science and Ethics of Genetic Engineering.* New York: Cambridge University Press, 2001.

Resnik, David B., Holly B. Steinkraus, and Pamela J. Langer. *Human Germline Gene Therapy: Scientific, Moral, and Political Issues.* Austin, Tex.: R. G. Landes, 1999.

Singer, Peter. *Unsanctifying Human Life: Essays onEthics.* Edited by Helga Kuhse. Malden, Mass.: Blackwell, 2002.

Singer, Peter, and Deane Wells. *Making Babies: The New Science and Ethics of Conception.* New York: Charles Scribner's Sons, 1985.

U.S. Congress. Senate. Committee on Health, Education, Labor, and Pensions. *Fulfilling the Promise of Genetics Research: Ensuring Nondiscrimination in Health Insurance and Employment.* Washington, D.C.: Government Printing Office, 2001.

_____. *Protecting Against Genetic Discrimination: The Limits of Existing Laws.* Washington, D.C.: Government Printing Office, 2002.

Veatch, Robert M. *The Basics of Bioethics.* 2d ed. Upper Saddle River, N.J.: Prentice Hall, 2003.

Vogel, Fredrich, and Reinhard Grunwald, eds. *Patenting of Human Genes and Living Organisms.* New York: Springer, 1994.

Wailoo, Keith. *Dying in the City of the Blues: Sickle Cell Anemia and the Politics of Race and Health.* Chapel Hill: University of North Carolina Press, 2001.

Walters, LeRoy, and Julie Gage Palmer. *The Ethics of Human Gene Therapy.* Illustrated by Natalie C. Johnson. New York: Oxford University Press, 1997.

Yount, Lisa, ed. *The Ethics of Genetic Engineering.* San Diego: Greenhaven Press, 2002.

BIOINFORMATICS. *See also* GENOMICS AND PROTEOMICS

Barnes, Michael R. *Bioinformatics for Geneticists.* Hoboken, N.J.: Wiley, 2003.

Baxevanis, Andreas D., and B. F. Francis Ouellette.

Bioinformatics: A Practical Guide to the Analysis of Genes and Proteins. 2d ed. Hoboken, N.J.: John Wiley & Sons, 2003.

Bergeron, Bryan P. *Bioinformatics Computing.* Upper Saddle River, N.J.: Prentice Hall, 2002.

Bird, R. Curtis, and Bruce F. Smith, eds. *Genetic Library Construction and Screening: Advanced Techniques and Applications.* New York: Springer, 2002.

Bishop, Martin J., ed. *Guide to Human Genome Computing.* 2d ed. San Diego: Academic Press, 1998.

Campbell, A. Malcolm. *Discovering Genomics, Proteomics, and Bioinformatics.* San Francisco: Benjamin Cummings, 2003.

Claverie, Jean-Michel, and Cedric Notredame. *Bioinformatics for Dummies.* Hoboken, N.J.: Wiley, 2003.

Clote, Peter. *Computational Molecular Biology: An Introduction.* New York: John Wiley, 2000.

Dwyer, Rex A. *Genomic Perl: From Bioinformatics Basics to Working Code.* Cambridge, England: Cambridge University Press, 2003.

Kohane, Isaac S. *Microarrays for an Integrative Genomics.* Cambridge, Mass.: MIT Press, 2003.

Krane, Dan E. *Fundamental Concepts of Bioinformatics.* San Francisco: Benjamin Cummings, 2003.

Krawetz, Stephen A., and David D. Womble. *Introduction to Bioinformatics: A Theoretical and Practical Approach.* Totowa, N.J.: Humana Press, 2003.

Lesk, Arthur M. *Introduction to Bioinformatics.* New York: Oxford University Press, 2002.

Lim, Hwa A. *Genetically Yours: Bioinforming, Biopharming, Biofarming.* River Edge, N.J.: World Scientific, 2002.

Meller, Jaroslaw, and Wieslaw Nowak, eds. *Applications of Statistical and Machine Learning Methods in Bioinformatics.* Frankfurt: Peter Lang, 2007.

Mount, David W. *Bioinformatics: Sequence and Genome Analysis.* Cold Spring Harbor, N.Y.: Cold Spring Harbor Laboratory Press, 2001.

Rashidi, Hooman H. *Bioinformatics Basics: Applications in Biological Science and Medicine.* Boca Raton, Fla.: CRC Press, 2000.

Westhead, David R. *Bioinformatics.* Oxford, England: BIOS, 2002.

CELLULAR BIOLOGY

Attardi, Giuseppe M., and Anne Chomyn, eds. *Methods in Enzymology: Mitochondrial Biogenesis and Genetics.* Vols. 260, 264. San Diego: Academic Press, 1995.

Becker, Peter B. *Chromatin Protocols*. Totowa, N.J.: Humana Press, 1999.

Becker, W. M., L. J. Kleinsmith, and J. Hardin. *The World of the Cell*. 5th ed. San Francisco: Benjamin Cummings, 2003.

Bell, John I., et al., eds. *T Cell Receptors*. New York: Oxford University Press, 1995.

Bickmore, Wendy A. *Chromosome Structural Analysis: A Practical Approach*. New York: Oxford University Press, 1999.

Blackburn, Elizabeth H., and Carol W. Greider, eds. *Telomeres*. Cold Spring Harbor, N.Y.: Cold Spring Harbor Laboratory Press, 1995.

Broach, J., J. Pringle, and E. Jones, eds. *The Molecular and Cellular Biology of the Yeast Saccharomyces*. 3 vols. Cold Spring Harbor, N.Y.: Cold Spring Harbor Laboratory Press, 1991-1997.

Carey, M., and S. T. Smale. *Transcriptional Regulation in Eukaryotes: Concepts, Strategies and Techniques*. Cold Spring Harbor, N.Y.: Cold Spring Harbor Laboratory Press, 2000.

Darnell, James, et al. *Molecular Cell Biology*. 4th ed. New York: W. H. Freeman, 2000.

Franklin, T. J., and G. A. Snow. *Biochemistry of Antimicrobial Action*. New York: Chapman and Hall, 2001.

Freshney, R. Ian. *Culture of Animal Cells*. New York: Wiley-Liss, 2000.

Gilchrest, Barbara A., and Vilhelm A. Bohr, eds. *The Role of DNA Damage and Repair in Cell Aging*. New York: Elsevier, 2001.

Gillham, Nicholas W. *Organelle Genes and Genomes*. London: Oxford University Press, 1997.

John, Bernard. *Meiosis*. New York: Cambridge University Press, 1990.

Kipling, David, ed. *The Telomere*. New York: Oxford University Press, 1995.

Lewis, Claire E., and James O'D. McGee. *The Macrophage: The Natural Immune System*. Oxford, England: IRL Press at Oxford University Press, 1992.

Lodish, Harvey, David Baltimore, and Arnold Berk. *Molecular Cell Biology*. 4th ed. New York: W. H. Freeman, 2000.

Marshak, Daniel R., Richard L. Gardner, and David Gottlieb, eds. *Stem Cell Biology*. Cold Spring Harbor, N.Y.: Cold Spring Harbor Laboratory Press, 2002.

Murray, A. W., and Tim Hunt. *The Cell Cycle: An Introduction*. New York: W. H. Freeman, 1993.

Pon, Liza, and Eric A. Schon, eds. *Mitochondria*. San Diego: Academic Press, 2001.

Scheffler, Immo E. *Mitochondria*. New York: John Wiley & Sons, 1999.

Sharma, Archana, and Sumitra Sen. *Chromosome Botany*. Enfield, N.H.: Science Publishers, 2002.

Vig, Baldev K., ed. *Chromosome Segregation and Aneuploidy*. New York: Springer-Verlag, 1993.

CLASSICAL TRANSMISSION GENETICS. *See also* **HISTORY OF GENETICS**

Berg, Paul, and Maxine Singer. *Dealing with Genes: The Language of Heredity*. Mill Valley, Calif.: University Science Books, 1992.

Cittadino, E. *Nature as the Laboratory*. New York: Columbia University Press, 1990.

Ford, E. B. *Understanding Genetics*. London: Faber & Faber, 1979.

Gardner, Eldon J. *Principles of Genetics*. 5th ed. New York: John Wiley & Sons, 1975.

Goodenough, Ursula. *Genetics*. 2d ed. New York: Holt, Rinehart and Winston, 1978.

Klug, William, and Michael Cummings. *Concepts of Genetics*. 4th ed. New York: Macmillan College, 1994.

Lewin, Benjamin. *Genes VII*. New York: Oxford University Press, 2001.

Mendel, Gregor. *Experiments in Plant-Hybridization*. Foreword by Paul C. Mangelsdorf. Cambridge, Mass.: Harvard University Press, 1965.

Rothwell, Norman V. *Understanding Genetics*. 4th ed. New York: Oxford University Press, 1988.

Russell, Peter. *Genetics*. 2d ed. Boston: Scott, Foresman, 1990.

Singer, Sam. *Human GGenetics: An Introduction to the Principles of Heredity*. 2d ed. New York: W. H. Freeman, 1985.

Suzuki, David T., et al., eds. *An Introduction to Genetic Analysis*. 2d ed. San Francisco: W. H. Freeman, 1981.

Weaver, Robert F., and Philip W. Hendrick. *Genetics*. 3d ed. Dubuque, Iowa: Wm. C. Brown, 1997.

Wilson, Edward O. *The Diversity of Life*. New York: W. W. Norton, 1992.

CLONING. *See also* **GENETIC ENGINEERING**

Brannigan, Michael C., ed. *Ethical Issues in Human Cloning: Cross-Disciplinary Perspectives*. New York: Seven Bridges Press, 2001.

Chen, Bing-Yuan, and Harry W. Janes, eds. *PCR Cloning Protocols*. Rev. 2d ed. Totowa, N.J.: Humana Press, 2002.

DeSalle, Robert, and David Lindley. *The Science of Jurassic Park and the Lost World.* New York: Basic-Books, 1997.

Drlica, Karl. *Understanding DNA and Gene Cloning: A Guide for the Curious.* Rev. ed. New York: Wiley, 2003.

Jones, P., and D. Ramji. *Vectors: Cloning Applications and Essential Techniques.* New York: J. Wiley, 1998.

Klotzko, Arlene Judith. *A Clone of Your Own? The Science and Ethics of Cloning.* New York: Cambridge University Press, 2006.

_____, ed. *The Cloning Sourcebook.* New York: Oxford University Press, 2001.

Lauritzen, Paul, ed. *Cloning and the Future of Human Embryo Research.* New York: Oxford University Press, 2001.

Lu, Quinn, and Michael P. Weiner, eds. *Cloning and Expression Vectors for Gene Function Analysis.* Natick, Mass.: Eaton, 2001.

MacKinnon, Barbara, ed. *Human Cloning: Science, Ethics, and Public Policy.* Urbana: University of Illinois Press, 2000.

Prentice, David A. *Stem Cells and Cloning.* New York: Benjamin Cummings, 2003.

Rantala, M. L., and Arthur J. Milgram, eds. *Cloning: For and Against.* Chicago: Open Court, 1999.

Sambrook, Joseph, and David W. Russell, eds. *Molecular Cloning: A Laboratory Manual.* 3d ed. 3 vols. Cold Spring Harbor, N.Y.: Cold Spring Harbor Laboratory Press, 2001.

Shostak, Stanley. *Becoming Immortal: Combining Cloning and Stem-Cell Therapy.* Albany: State University of New York Press, 2002.

Wilmut, Ian, Keith Campbell, and Colin Tudge. *The Second Creation: The Age of Biological Control by the Scientists That Cloned Dolly.* London: Headline, 2000.

DEVELOPMENTAL GENETICS

Beurton, Peter, Raphael Falk, and Hans-Jorg Rheinberger, eds. *The Concept of the Gene in Development and Evolution: Historical and Epistemological Perspectives.* New York: Cambridge University Press, 2000.

Bier, Ethan. *The Coiled Spring: How Life Begins.* Cold Spring Harbor, N.Y.: Cold Spring Harbor Laboratory Press, 2000.

Bowman, John L. *Arabidopsis: An Atlas of Morphology and Development.* New York: Springer-Verlag, 1993.

Carroll, Sean B., Jennifer K. Grenier, and Scott D. Weatherbee. *From DNA to Diversity: Molecular Genetics and the Evolution of Animal Design.* Malden, Mass.: Blackwell, 2001.

Cronk, Quentin C. B., Richard M. Bateman, and Julie A. Hawkins, eds. *Developmental Genetics and Plant Evolution.* New York: Taylor & Francis, 2002.

Davidson, Eric H. *Gene Activity in Early Development.* Orlando, Fla.: Academic Press, 1986.

DePamphilis, Melvin L., ed. *Gene Expression at the Beginning of Animal Development.* New York: Elsevier, 2002.

DePomerai, David. *From Gene to Animal: An Introduction to the Molecular Biology of Animal Development.* New York: Cambridge University Press, 1985.

Dyban, A. P., and V. S. Baranov. *Cytogenetics of Mammalian Embryonic Development.* Translated by V. S. Baranov. New York: Oxford University Press, 1987.

Gilbert, Scott F. *Developmental Biology.* Sunderland, Mass.: Sinauer Associates, 2003.

Gottlieb, Frederick J. *Developmental Genetics.* New York: Reinhold, 1966.

Gurdon, John B. *The Control of Gene Expression in Animal Development.* Cambridge, Mass.: Harvard University Press, 1974.

Hahn, Martin E., et al., eds. *Developmental Behavior Genetics: Neural, Biometrical, and Evolutionary Approaches.* New York: Oxford University Press, 1990.

Harvey, Richard P., and Nadia Rosenthal, eds. *Heart Development.* San Diego: Academic Press, 1999.

Hennig, W., ed. *Early Embryonic Development of Animals.* New York: Springer-Verlag, 1992.

Hsia, David Yi-Yung. *Human Developmental Genetics.* Chicago: Year Book Medical Publishers, 1968.

Hunter, R. H. F. *Sex Determination, Differentiation, and Intersexuality in Placental Mammals.* New York: Cambridge University Press, 1995.

Leighton, Terrance, and William F. Loomis, Jr. *The Molecular Genetics of Development.* New York: Academic Press, 1980.

McKinney, M. L., and K. J. McNamara. *Heterochrony: The Evolution of Ontogeny.* New York: Plenum Press, 1991.

Malacinski, George M., ed. *Developmental Genetics of Higher Organisms: A Primer in Developmental Biology.* New York: Macmillan, 1988.

Massaro, Edward J., and John M. Rogers, eds. *Folate and Human Development.* Totowa, N.J.: Humana Press, 2002.

Moore, Keith. *The Developing Human: Clinically Oriented Embryology.* 7th ed. Amsterdam: Elsevier Science, 2003.

Nusslein-Volhard, Christiane, and J. Kratzschmar, eds. *Of Fish, Fly, Worm, and Man: Lessons from Developmental Biology for Human Gene Function and Disease.* New York: Springer, 2000.

Piontelli, Alessandra. *Twins: From Fetus to Child.* New York: Routledge, 2002.

Prescott, John, and Beverly J. Tepper, eds. *Genetic Variation in Taste Sensitivity.* New York: Marcel Dekker, 2004.

Pritchard, Dorian J. *Foundations of Developmental Genetics.* Philadelphia: Taylor & Francis, 1986.

Raff, Rudolf. *The Shape of Life: Genes, Development, and the Evolution of Animal Form.* Chicago: University of Chicago Press, 1996.

Ranke, M., and G. Gilli. *Growth Standards, Bone Maturation, and Idiopathic Short Stature.* Farmington, Conn.: S. Karger, 1996.

Rao, Mahendra S., ed. *Stem Cells and CNS Development.* Totowa, N.J.: Humana Press, 2001.

Sang, James H. *Genetics and Development.* New York: Longman, 1984.

Saunders, John Warren, Jr. *Patterns and Principles of Animal Development.* New York: Macmillan, 1970.

Seidman, S., and H. Soreq. *Transgenic Xenopus: Microinjection Methods and Developmental Neurobiology.* Totowa, N.J.: Humana Press, 1997.

Stewart, Alistair D., and David M. Hunt. *The Genetic Basis of Development.* New York: John Wiley & Sons, 1982.

Tomanek, Robert J., and Raymond B. Runyan, eds. *Formation of the Heart and Its Regulation.* Foreword by Edward B. Clark. Boston: Birkhauser, 2001.

Ulijaszek, S. J., Francis E. Johnston, and Michael A. Preece. *Cambridge Encyclopedia of Human Growth and Development.* New York: Cambridge University Press, 1998.

Vijg, Jan. *Aging of the Genome: The Dual Role of the DNA in Life and Death.* New York: Oxford University Press, 2007.

Wilkins, Adam S. *Genetic Analysis of Animal Development.* New York: Wiley-Liss, 1993.

DISEASES AND SYNDROMES

GENERAL

American Psychiatric Association. *Diagnostic and Statistical Manual of Mental Disorders: DSM-IV-TR.* Rev. 4th ed. Washington, D.C.: Author, 2000.

Bennett, Robin L. *The Practical Guide to the Genetic Family History.* New York: Wiley-Liss, 1999.

Bianchi, Diana W., Timothy M. Crombleholme, and Mary E. D'Alton. *Fetology: Diagnosis and Management of the Fetal Patient.* New York: McGraw-Hill, 2000.

Brooks, G. F., J. S. Butel, and S. A. Morse. *Medical Microbiology.* 21st ed. Stamford, Conn.: Appleton and Lange, 1998.

Browne, M. J., and P. L. Thurlby, eds. *Genomes, Molecular Biology, and Drug Discovery.* San Diego: Academic Press, 1996.

Cotran, R. S., et al. *Robbins Pathologic Basis of Disease.* 6th ed. Philadelphia: Saunders, 1999.

Epstein, Richard J. *Human Molecular Biology; An Introduction to the Molecular Basis of Health and Disease.* Cambridge, England: Cambridge University Press, 2003.

Gallo, Robert C., and Flossie Wong-Staal, eds. *Retrovirus Biology and Human Disease.* New York: Marcel Dekker, 1990.

Gelehrter, Thomas D., Francis S. Collins, and David Ginsburg. *Principles of Medical Genetics.* 2d ed. Baltimore: Williams & Wilkins, 1998.

Gilbert, Patricia. *Dictionary of Syndromes and Inherited Disorders.* 3d ed. Chicago: Fitzroy Dearborn, 2000.

Hogenboom, Marga. *Living with Genetic Syndromes Associated with Intellectual Disability.* Philadelphia: Jessica Kingsley, 2001.

Jorde, L. B., J. C. Carey, M. J. Bamshad, and R. L. White. *Medical Genetics.* 2d ed. St. Louis, Mo.: Mosby, 2000.

Massimini, Kathy, ed. *Genetic Disorders Sourcebook: Basic Consumer Information About Hereditary Diseases and Disorders.* 2d ed. Detroit: Omnigraphics, 2001.

Neumann, David, et al. *Human Variability in Response to Chemical Exposures: Measures, Modeling, and Risk Assessment.* Boca Raton, Fla.: CRC Press, 1998.

New, Maria I., ed. *Diagnosis and Treatment of the Unborn Child.* Reddick, Fla.: Idelson-Gnocchi, 1999.

O'Rahilly, S., and D. B. Dunger, eds. *Genetic Insights in Paediatric Endocrinology and Metabolism.* Bristol, England: BioScientifica, 1999.

Pai, G. Shashidhar, Raymond C. Lewandowski, and Digamber S. Borgaonkar. *Handbook of Chromosomal Syndromes.* New York: John Wiley & Sons, 2002.

Pasternak, Jack J. *An Introduction to Human Molecular Genetics: Mechanisms of Inherited Diseases.* Bethesda, Md.: Fitzgerald Science Press, 1999.

Petrikovsky, Boris M., ed. *Fetal Disorders: Diagnosis and Management.* New York: Wiley-Liss, 1999.

Pilu, Gianluigi, and Kypros H. Nicolaides. *Diagnosis of Fetal Abnormalities: The 18-23-Week Scan.* New York: Parthenon Group, 1999.

Rakel, Robert E., et al., eds. *Conn's Current Therapy.* Philadelphia: W. B. Saunders, 2003.

Sasaki, Mutsuo, et al., eds. *New Directions for Cellular and Organ Transplantation.* New York: Elsevier Science, 2000.

Stephens, Trent D., and Rock Brynner. *Dark Remedy: The Impact of Thalidomide and Its Revival as a Vital Medicine.* Cambridge, Mass.: Perseus, 2001.

Twining, Peter, Josephine M. McHugo, and David W. Pilling, eds. *Textbook of Fetal Abnormalities.* New York: Churchill Livingstone, 2000.

Weaver, David D., with the assistance of Ira K. Brandt. *Catalog of Prenatally Diagnosed Conditions.* 3d ed. Baltimore: Johns Hopkins University Press, 1999.

Weiss, Kenneth M. *Genetic Variation and Human Disease: Principles and Evolutionary Approaches.* New York: Cambridge University Press, 1993.

Wynbrandt, James, and Mark D. Ludman. *The Encyclopedia of Genetic Disorders and Birth Defects.* 2d ed. New York: Facts On File, 2000.

Zallen, Doris Teichler. *Does It Run in the Family? A Consumer's Guide to DNA Testing for Genetic Disorders.* New Brunswick, NJ.: Rutgers University Press, 1997.

ALZHEIMER'S DISEASE

Gauthier, S., ed. *Clinical Diagnosis and Management of Alzheimer's Disease.* 2d ed. London: Martin Dunitz, 2001.

Hamdy, Ronald, James Turnball, and Joellyn Edwards. *Alzheimer's Disease: A Handbook for Caregivers.* New York: Mosby, 1998.

Mace, M., and P. Rabins. *The Thirty-six-Hour Day: A Family Guide to Caring for Persons with Alzheimer Disease, Related Dementing Illnesses, and Memory Loss in Later Life.* Baltimore: Johns Hopkins University Press, 1999.

Nelson, James Lindemann, and Hilde Lindemann Nelson. *Alzheimer's: Answers to Hard Questions for Families.* New York: Main Street Books, 1996.

Powell, L., and K. Courtice. *Alzheimer's Disease: A Guide for Families and Caregivers.* Cambridge, Mass.: Perseus, 2001.

Richter, Ralph W., and Brigitte Zoeller Richter, eds. *Alzheimer's Disease: A Physician's Guide to Practical Management.* Totowa, N.J.: Humana Press, 2004.

Sadowski, Marcin, and Thomas M. Wisniewski. *100 Questions and Answers About Alzheimer's Disease.* Boston: Jones and Bartlett, 2004.

Terry, R., R. Katzman, K. Bick, and S. Sisodia. *Alzheimer Disease.* 2d ed. Philadelphia: Lippincott Williams & Wilkins, 1999.

CANCER

Angier, Natalie. *Natural Obsessions: Striving to Unlock the Deepest Secrets of the Cancer Cell.* Boston: Mariner Books/Houghton Mifflin, 1999.

Bowcock, Anne M., ed. *Breast Cancer: Molecular Genetics, Pathogenesis, and Therapeutics.* Totowa, N.J.: Humana Press, 1999.

Cannon, L Bishop, et al. "Genetic Epidemiology of Prostate Cancer in the Utah Mormon Genealogy." In *Inheritance of Susceptibility to Cancer in Man,* edited by W. F. Bodmer. New York: Oxford University Press, 1983.

Coleman, William B., and Gregory J. Tsongalis, eds. *The Molecular Basis of Human Cancer.* Totowa, N.J.: Humana Press, 2002.

Cooper, Geoffrey M. *Oncogenes.* 2d ed. Boston: Jones and Bartlett, 1995.

Cowell, J. K., ed. *Molecular Genetics of Cancer.* 2d ed. San Diego: Academic Press, 2001.

Davies, Kevin, and Michael White. *Breakthrough: The Race to Find the Breast Cancer Gene.* New York: John Wiley, 1996.

DeVita, V. T., S. Hellman, and S. A. Rosenberg, eds. *Principles and Practice of Oncology.* Philadelphia: Lippincott-Raven, 1997.

Dickson, Robert B., and Marc E. Lipman, eds. *Genes, Oncogenes, and Hormones: Advances in Cellular and Molecular Biology of Breast Cancer.* Boston: Kluwer Academic, 1992.

Dunbier, Anita K., and Parry J. Guilford. "Gastric Cancer: Inherited Predisposition." In *Encyclopedia of Cancer.* 2d ed. New York: Elsevier Science, 2002.

Ehrlich, Melanie, ed. *DNA Alterations in Cancer: Genetic and Epigenetic Changes.* Natick, Mass.: Eaton, 2000.

Fisher, David E., ed. *Tumor Suppressor Genes in Human Cancer.* Totowa, N.J.: Humana Press, 2001.

Goode, Ellen L., and Gail P. Jarvik. "Genetics Predisposition to Prostate Cancer." In *Encyclopedia of Cancer.* 2d ed. New York: Elsevier Science, 2002.

Greaves, Mel F. *Cancer: The Evolutionary Legacy.* New York: Oxford University Press, 2000.

Habib, Nagy A., ed. *Cancer Gene Therapy: Past Achievements and Future Challenges.* New York: Kluwer Academic/Plenum, 2000.

Hanski, C., H. Scherubl, and B. Mann, eds. *Colorectal Cancer: New Aspects of Molecular Biology and Immunology and Their Clinical Applications.* New York: New York Academy of Sciences, 2000.

Heim, S., and Felix Mitelman. *Cancer Cytogenetics.* 2d ed. New York: J. Wiley, 1995.

Hodgson, Shirley V., and Eamonn R. Maher. *A Practical Guide to Human Cancer Genetics.* 2d ed. New York: Cambridge University Press, 1999.

Kemeny, Mary Margaret, and Paula Dranov. *Beating the Odds Against Breast and Ovarian Cancer: Reducing Your Hereditary Risk.* Reading, Mass.: Addison-Wesley, 1992.

Krupp, Guido, and Reza Parwaresch, eds. *Telomerases, Telomeres, and Cancer.* New York: Kluwer Academic/ Plenum, 2003.

La Thangue, Nicholas B., and Lasantha R. Bandara, eds. *Targets for Cancer Chemotherapy: Transcription Factors and Other Nuclear Proteins.* Totowa, N.J.: Humana Press, 2002.

Lattime, Edmund C., and Stanton L. Gerson, eds. *Gene Therapy of Cancer: Translational Approaches from Preclinical Studies to Clinical Implementation.* 2d ed. San Diego: Academic Press, 2002.

Maruta, Hiroshi, ed. *Tumor-Suppressing Viruses, Genes, and Drugs: Innovative Cancer Therapy Approaches.* San Diego: Academic Press, 2002.

Mendelsohn, John, et al. *The Molecular Basis of Cancer.* 2d ed. Philadelphia: Saunders, 2001.

Mulvihill, John J. *Catalog of Human Cancer Genes: McKusick's Mendelian Inheritance in Man for Clinical and Research Oncologists.* Foreword by Victor A. McKusick. Baltimore: Johns Hopkins University Press, 1999.

National Cancer Institute. *Genetic Testing for Breast Cancer. It's Your Choice.* Bethesda, Md.: Author, 1997.

Ruddon, Raymond. *Cancer Biology.* 3d ed. New York: Oxford University Press, 1995.

Schneider, Katherine A. *Counseling About Cancer: Strategies for Genetic Counseling.* 2d ed. New York: Wiley-Liss, 2002.

Varmus, Harold, and Robert Weinberg. *Genes and the Biology of Cancer.* New York: W. H. Freeman, 1993.

Vogelstein, Bert, and Kenneth W. Kinzler, eds. *The Genetic Basis of Human Cancer.* 2d ed. New York: McGraw-Hill, 2002.

Wilson, Samuel, et al. *Cancer and the Environment: Gene-Environment Interaction.* Washington, D.C.: National Academy Press, 2002.

CHOLERA

Coleman, William, and I. Edward Alcamo, eds. *Cholera.* Philadelphia: Chelsea House, 2003.

Keusch, Gerald, and Masanobu Kawakami, eds. *Cytokines, Cholera, and the Gut.* Amsterdam: IOS Press, 1997.

Wachsmuth, Kate, et al., eds. *Vibrio Cholerae and Cholera: Molecular to Global Perspectives.* Washington, D.C.: ASM Press, 1994.

COLOR BLINDNESS

Rosenthal, Odeda, and Robert H. Phillips. *Coping with Color Blindness.* Garden City Park, N.Y: Avery, 1997.

CONGENITAL ADRENAL HYPERPLASIA

Speiser, Phyllis W., ed. *Congenital Adrenal Hyperplasia.* Philadelphia: W. B. Saunders, 2001.

CYSTIC FIBROSIS

Hodson, Margaret E., and Duncan M. Geddes, eds. *Cystic Fibrosis.* 2d ed. New York: Oxford University Press, 2000.

Orenstein, David M., Beryl J. Rosenstein, and Robert C. Stern. *Cystic Fibrosis: Medical Care.* Philadelphia: Lippincott Williams & Wilkins, 2000.

Shale, Dennis. *Cystic Fibrosis.* London: British Medical Association, 2002.

Tsui, Lap-Chee, et al., eds. *The Identification of the CF (Cystic Fibrosis) Gene: Recent Progress and New Research Strategies.* New York: Plenum Press, 1991.

Yankaskas, James R., and Michael R. Knowles, eds. *Cystic Fibrosis in Adults.* Philadelphia: Lippincott-Raven, 1999.

DIABETES

American Diabetes Association. *American Diabetes Association Complete Guide to Diabetes: The Ultimate Home Reference from the Diabetes Experts.* New York: McGraw-Hill, 2002.

Becker, Gretchen. *The First Year: Type 2 Diabetes, an Essential Guide for the Newly Diagnosed.* New York: Marlowe, 2001.

Flyvbjerg, Allan, Hans Orskov, and George Alberti, eds. *Growth Hormone and Insulin-like Growth Factor*

I in Human and Experimental Diabetes. New York: John Wiley & Sons, 1993.

Kahn, C. R., et al. *Joslin's Diabetes Mellitus.* 14th ed. Philadelphia: Lippincott Williams and Wilkins, 2003.

Lowe, William L., Jr., ed. *Genetics of Diabetes Mellitus.* Boston: Kluwer Academic, 2001.

Milchovich, Sue K., and Barbara Dunn-Long. *Diabetes Mellitus: A Practical Handbook.* 8th ed. Boulder, Colo.: Bull, 2003.

Pinette, Gilles. *Diabetes and Diet: Ivan's Story.* Owen Sound, Ont.: Ningwakwe Learning Press, 2002.

Roith, Derek Le, and Haim Werner. *Insulin Growth Factors.* In *Encyclopedia of Cancer.* 2d ed. New York: Elsevier Science, 2002.

DOWN SYNDROME AND MENTAL RETARDATION

Broman, Sarah H., and Jordan Grafman, eds. *Atypical Cognitive Deficits in Developmental Disorders: Implications for Brain Function.* Hillsdale, N.J.: Lawrence Erlbaum, 1994.

Cohen, William I., Lynn Nadel, and Myra E. Madnick, eds. *Down Syndrome: Visions for the Twenty-first Century.* New York: Wiley-Liss, 2002.

Cunningham, Cliff. *Understanding Down Syndrome: An Introduction for Parents.* 1988. Reprint. Cambridge, Mass.: Brookline Books, 1999.

Dykens, Elisabeth M., Robert M. Hodapp, and Brenda M. Finucane. *Genetics and Mental Retardation Syndromes: A New Look at Behavior and Interventions.* Baltimore: Paul H. Brookes, 2000.

Faraone, Stephen V., Ming T. Tsuang, and Debby W. Tsuang. *Genetics of Mental Disorders: A Guide for Students, Clinicians, and Researchers.* New York: Guilford Press, 1999.

Jobling, Anne, and Naznin Virji-Babul. *Down Syndrome: Play, Move and Grow.* Burnaby, B.C.: Down Syndrome Research Foundation, 2004.

Lubec, G. *Protein Expression in Down Syndrome Brain.* New York: Springer, 2001.

Newton, Richard. *The Down's Syndrome Handbook: A Practical Guide for Parents and Caregivers.* New York: Arrow Books, 1997.

Selikowitz, Mark. *Down Syndrome: The Facts.* 2d ed. New York: Oxford University Press, 1997.

Shannon, Joyce Brennfleck, ed. *Mental Retardation Sourcebook: Basic Consumer Health Information About Mental Retardation and Its Causes, Including Down Syndrome, Fetal Alcohol Syndrome, Fragile X Syndrome,*

Genetic Conditions, Injury, and Environmental Sources. Detroit: Omnigraphics, 2000.

FRAGILE X SYNDROME

Hagerman, Paul J. *Fragile X Syndrome: Diagnosis, Treatment, and Research.* 3d ed. Baltimore: Johns Hopkins University Press, 2002.

Hagerman, Randi Jenssen, and Paul J. Hagerman, eds. *Fragile X Syndrome: Diagnosis, Treatment, and Research.* Baltimore: Johns Hopkins University Press, 2002.

Parker, James N., and Philip M. Parker, eds. *The 2002 Official Parent's Sourcebook on Fragile X Syndrome.* San Diego: Icon Health, 2002.

GENDER IDENTITY AND SEX ERRORS

Berch, Daniel B., and Bruce G. Bender, eds. *Sex Chromosome Abnormalities and Human Behavior.* Boulder, Colo.: Westview Press, 1990.

Dreger, Alice Domurat. *Hermaphrodites and the Medical Invention of Sex.* Cambridge, Mass.: Harvard University Press, 1998.

Gilbert, Ruth. *Early Modern Hermaphrodites: Sex and Other Stories.* New York: Palgrave, 2002.

Money, John. *Sex Errors of the Body and Related Syndromes: A Guide to Counseling Children, Adolescents, and Their Families.* 2d ed. Baltimore: Paul H. Brookes, 1994.

HEART DISEASES AND DEFECTS

Braunwald, Eugene, Douglas P. Zipes, Peter Libby, and Douglas D. Zipes. *Heart Disease: A Textbook of Cardiovascular Medicine.* 6th ed. Philadelphia: W. B. Saunders, 2001.

Edwards, Jesse E. *Jesse E. Edwards' Synopsis of Congenital Heart Disease.* Edited by Brooks S. Edwards. Armonk, N.Y.: Futura, 2000.

Goldbourt, Uri, Kare Berg, and Ulf de Faire, eds. *Genetic Factors in Coronary Heart Disease.* Boston: Kluwer Academic, 1994.

Kramer, Gerri Freid, and Shari Maurer. *The Parent's Guide to Children's Congenital Heart Defects: What They Are, How to Treat Them, How to Cope with Them.* Foreword by Sylvester Stallone and Jennifer FlavinStallone. New York: Three Rivers Press, 2001.

Marian, Ali J. *Genetics for Cardiologists: The Molecular Genetic Basis of Cardiovascular Disorders.* London: ReMEDICA, 2000.

HEMOPHILIA

Buzzard, Brenda, and Karen Beeton, eds. *Physiotherapy Management of Haemophilia.* Malden, Mass.: Blackwell, 2000.

Jones, Peter. *Living with Haemophilia.* 5th ed. New York: Oxford University Press, 2002.

Monroe, Dougald M., et al., eds. *Hemophilia Care in the New Millennium.* New York: Kluwer Academic/Plenum, 2001.

Resnik, Susan. *Blood Saga: Hemophilia, AIDS, and the Survival of a Community.* Berkeley: University of California Press, 1999.

Steinberg, Martin H., et al., eds. *Disorders of Hemoglobin: Genetics, Pathophysiology, and Clinical Management.* Foreword by H. Franklin Bunn. New York: Cambridge University Press, 2001.

IMMUNE DISORDERS AND ALLERGIES

Abbas, Abul K., and Richard A. Flavell, eds. *Genetic Models of Immune and Inflammatory Diseases.* New York: Springer, 1996.

Bona, Constantin A., etal., eds. *The Molecular Pathology ofAutoimmune Diseases.* 2d ed. New York: Taylor and Francis, 2002.

Clark, William R. *At War Within: The Double-Edged Sword of Immunity.* New York: Oxford University Press, 1995.

Cutler, Ellen W. *Winning the War Against Asthma and Allergies.* Albany, N.Y: Delmar, 1998.

Hadley, Andrew G., and Peter Soothill, eds. *Alloimmune Disorders ofPregnancy: Anaemia, Thrombocytopenia, and Neutropenia in the Fetus and Newborn.* New York: Cambridge University Press, 2002.

Shomon, MaryJ. *Living Well with Chronic Fatigue Syndrome and Fibromyalgia: What Your Doctor Doesn't Tell You That You Need to Know.* New York: Quill, 2004.

Walsh, William. *The Food Allergy Book.* New York: J. Wiley, 2000.

INFECTIOUS AND EMERGING DISEASES

Anderson, R. M., and R. M. May. *Infectious Diseases of Humans: Dynamics and Control.* Oxford, England: Oxford University Press, 1992.

DeSalle, Rob, ed. *Epidemic! The World ofInfectious Disease.* New York: The New Press, 1999.

Drexler, Madeline. *Secret Agents: The Menace ofEmerging Infections.* Washington, D.C.: Joseph Henry Press, 2002.

Garrett, Laurie. *The Coming Plague: Newly Emerging Diseases in a World Out of Balance.* New York: Penguin, 1995.

Hacker, J., andJ. B. Kaper, eds. *Pathogenicity Islands and the Evolution ofPathogenic Microbes.* 2 vols. New York: Springer, 2002.

Kolata, Gina. *Flu: The Story of the Great Influenza Pandemic of 1918 and the Search for the Virus That Caused It.* New York: Simon and Schuster, 2001.

Lappe, Marc. *Breakout: The Evolving Threat of DrugResistant Disease.* San Francisco: Sierra Club Books, 1996.

Levy, Stuart B. *The Antibiotic Paradox: How Miracle Drugs Are Destroying the Miracle.* New York: Plenum Press, 1992.

McNeill, William H. *Plagues and Peoples.* New York: Anchor Books, 1998.

Parker, James N., and Philip M. Parker, eds. *The Official Patient's Sourcebook on "E. coli."* San Diego: Icon Health, 2002.

World Health Organization. *Future Research on Smallpox Virus Recommended.* Geneva, Switzerland: World Health Organization Press, 1999.

KLINEFELTER SYNDROME

Bock, Robert. *Understanding Klinefelter Syndrome: A Guide for XXY Males and Their Families.* Bethesda, Md.: Department of Health and Human Services, Public Health Service, National Institutes of Health, National Institute of Child Health and Human Development, 1997.

Parker, James N., and Philip M. Parker, eds. *The Official Parent's Sourcebook on Klinefelter Syndrome: A Revised and Updated Directory for the Internet Age.* San Diego: Icon Health, 2002.

Probasco, Terri, and Gretchen A. Gibbs. *Klinefelter Syndrome: Personal and Professional Guide.* Richmond, Ind.: Prinit Press, 1999.

LACTOSE INTOLERANCE

Auricchio, Salvatore, and G. Semenza, eds. *Common Food Intolerances 2: Milk in Human Nutrition and Adult-Type Hypolactasia.* New York: Karger, 1993.

METABOLIC DISORDERS

Econs, Michael J., ed. *The Genetics of Osteoporosis and Metabolic Bone Disease.* Totowa, N.J.: Humana Press, 2000.

Evans, Mark I., ed. *Metabolic and Genetic Screening.* Philadelphia: W. B. Saunders, 2001.

Pacifici, G. M., and G. N. Fracchia, eds. *Advances in Drug Metabolism in Man*. Brussels: European Commission, 1995.

Scriver, Charles, etal., eds. *The Metabolic and Molecular Bases of Inherited Disease*. 8th ed. 4 vols. New York: McGraw-Hill, 2001.

Tew, K. D., et al., eds. *Structure and Function of Glutathione Transferases*. Boca Raton, Fla.: CRC Press, 1993.

MITOCHONDRIAL DISEASES

Lestienne, Patrick, ed. *Mitochondrial Diseases: Models and Methods*. New York: Springer, 1999.

NEURAL DEFECTS

Bock, Gregory, and Joan Marsh, eds. *Neural Tube Defects*. New York: Wiley, 1994.

Goldstein, Sam, and Cecil R. Reynolds, eds. *Handbook of Neurodevelopmental and Genetic Disorders in Children*. New York: Guilford Press, 1999.

PHENYLKETONURIA

Koch, Jean Holt. *Robert Guthrie, the PKU Story: A Crusade Against Mental Retardation*. Pasadena, Calif.: Hope, 1997.

Parker, James N., ed. *The Official Parent's Sourcebook on Phenylketonuria*. San Diego: Icon Health, 2002.

PRION DISEASES

Baker, Harry F., ed. *Molecular Pathology of the Prions*. Totowa, N.J.: Humana Press, 2001.

Groschup, Martin H., and Hans A. Kretzschmar, eds. *Prion Diseases: Diagnosis and Pathogenesis*. New York: Springer, 2000.

Klitzman, Robert. *The Trembling Mountain: A Personal Account of Kuru, Cannibals, and Mad Cow Disease*. New York: Plenum Trade, 1998.

_____, ed. *Prion Biology and Diseases*. Cold Spring Harbor, N.Y.: Cold Spring Harbor Laboratory Press, 1999.

Rabenau, Holger F., Jindrich Cinatl, and Hans Wilhelm Doerr, eds. *Prions: A Challenge for Science, Medicine, and Public Health System*. New York: Karger, 2001.

Ratzan, Scott C., ed. *The Mad Cow Crisis: Health and the Public Good*. New York: New York University Press, 1998.

PRADER-WILLI SYNDROME

Eiholzer, Urs. *Prader-Willi Syndrome: Effects of Human Growth Hormone Treatment*. New York: Karger, 2001.

SICKLE-CELL DISEASE

Anionwu, Elizabeth N., and Karl Atkin. *The Politics of Sickle Cell and Thalassaemia*. Philadelphia: Open University Press, 2001.

Gordon, Melanie Appel. *Let's Talk About Sickle Cell Anemia*. New York: PowerKids Press, 2000.

Harris, Jacqueline. *Sickle Cell Disease*. Brookfield, Conn.: Twenty-First Century Books, 2001.

Parker, James N., and Philip M. Parker, eds. *The 2002 Official Patient's Sourcebook on Sickle Cell Anemia*. San Diego: Icon Health, 2002.

Platt, Allan F., and Alan Sacerdote. *Hope and Destiny: The Patient's and Parent's Guide to Sickle Cell Disease and Sickle Cell Trait*. Roscoe, Ill.: Hilton, 2002.

Serjeant, Graham R., and Beryl E. Serjeant. *Sickle Cell Disease*. 3d ed. New York: Oxford University Press, 2001.

Simon, Dyson M. *Ethnicity and Screening for Sickle Cell/Thalassaemia: Lessons for Practice from the Voices of Experience*. Edinburgh: Elsevier Churchill Livingstone, 2005.

Tapper, Melbourne. *In the Blood: Sickle Cell Anemia and the Politics of Race*. Philadelphia: University of Pennsylvania Press, 1999.

Wailoo, Keith, and Stephen Pemberton. *The Troubled Dream of Genetic Medicine: Ethnicity and Innovation in Tay-Sachs, Cystic Fibrosis, and Sickle Cell Disease*. Baltimore: Johns Hopkins University Press, 2006.

TAY-SACHS DISEASE

Desnick, Robert J., and Michael M. Kaback, eds. *Tay-Sachs Disease*. San Diego: Academic Press, 2001.

National Tay-Sachs and Allied Diseases Association. *A Genetics Primer for Understanding Tay-Sachs and the Allied Diseases*. Brookline, Mass.: Author, 1995.

Parker, James N., and Philip M. Parker, eds. *The Official Parent's Sourcebook on Tay-Sachs Disease: A Revised and Updated Directory for the Internet Age*. San Diego: Icon Press, 2002.

TURNER SYNDROME

Albertsson-Wikland, Kerstin, and Michael B. Ranke, eds. *Turner Syndrome in a Life Span Perspective: Research and Clinical Aspects*. New York: Elsevier, 1995.

Rieser, Patricia A., and Marsha Davenport. *Turner Syndrome: A Guide for Families*. Houston: Turner Syndrome Society, 1992.

Rosenfeld, Ron G. *Turner Syndrome: A Guide forPhysicians.* 2d ed. Houston: Turner Syndrome Society, 1992.

EVOLUTION

Avital, Eytan, and Eva Jablonka. *Animal Traditions: Behavioural Inheritance in Evolution.* New York: Cambridge University Press, 2000.

Baxter, Brian. *A Darwinian Worldview: Sociobiology, Environmental Ethics and the Work of Edward O. Wilson.* Aldershot, England: Ashgate, 2007.

Beurton, Peter, Raphael Falk, and Hans-Jorg Rheinberger, eds. *The Concept of the Gene in Development and Evolution: Historical and Epistemological Perspectives.* New York: Cambridge University Press, 2000.

Calos, Michele. *Molecular Evolution of Chromosomes.* New York: Oxford University Press, 2003.

Calvin, William H. *A Brain for All Seasons: Human Evolution and Abrupt Climate Change.* Chicago: University of Chicago Press, 2002.

_____. *A Brief History of the Mind: From Apes to Intellect and Beyond.* New York: Oxford University Press, 2004.

Campbell, Bernard G., ed. *Sexual Selection and theDescent ofMan: The Darwinian Pivot.* New Brunswick, N.J.: AldineTransaction, 2006.

Cronk, Lee, Napoleon Chagnon, and William Irons, eds. *Adaptation and Human Behavior: An Anthropological Perspective.* New York: Aldine de Gruyter, 2000.

Darwin, Charles. *The Descent of Man and Selection in Relation to Sex.* London: John Murray, 1871. Reprint. Princeton, N.J.: Princeton University Press, 1981.

_____. *On the Origin of Species by Means of Natural Selection: Or, The Preservation ofFavored Races in the Struggle for Life.* London: John Murray, 1859. Reprint. New York: Random House, 1999.

Davidson, Iain. *Sex, Politics, and Religion: Archaeology for a Polite Society.* Armidale, N.S.W.: University of New England, 1999.

Dawkins, Richard. *The Blind Watchmaker: Why the Evidence ofEvolution Reveals a Universe Without Design.* New York: W. W. Norton, 1996.

_____. *ClimbingMount Improbable.* New York: W. W. Norton, 1997.

_____. *Extended Phenotype: The Long Reach of the Gene.* Rev. 2d ed. Afterword by Daniel Dennett. New York: Oxford University Press, 1999.

_____. *The Selfish Gene.* 2d ed. New York: Oxford University Press, 1990.

Depew, David, and Bruce Weber. *Darwinism Evolving: Systems Dynamics and the Genealogy of Natural Selection.* Boston: MIT Press, 1995.

Dessalles, Jean-Louis. *Why We Talk: The Evolutionary Origins of Language.* Translated by James Grieve. Oxford, England: Oxford University Press, 2007.

Dickens, Peter. *Society and Nature: Changing Our Environment, Changing Ourselves.* Cambridge, England: Polity Press, 2004.

Dobzhansky, Theodosius G. *Genetics and the Origin of Species.* New York: Columbia University Press, 1937.

Edey, Maitland A., and Donald C. Johnson. *Blueprints: Solving the Mystery of Evolution.* Reprint. New York: Viking, 1990.

Fisher, Helen. *Why We Love: The Nature and Chemistry ofRomantic Love.* New York: Henry Holt, 2004.

Fisher, Ronald Aylmer. *The Genetical Theory of Natural Selection: A Complete Variorum Edition.* 1958. Edited with a foreword and notes by J. H. Bennett. New York: Oxford University Press, 1999.

Foley, R. A. *Unknown Boundaries: Exploring Human Evolutionary Studies.* Cambridge, England: Cambridge University Press, 2006.

Freeman, Scott, and Jon C. Herron. *Evolutionary Analysis.* 2d ed. Upper Saddle River, N.J.: Prentice Hall, 2000.

Gesteland, Raymond F., Thomas R. Cech, and John F. Atkins, eds. *The RNA World: The Nature of Modern RNA Suggests a Prebiotic RNA.* 2d ed. Cold Spring Harbor, N.Y.: Cold Spring Harbor Laboratory Press, 1999.

Gould, Stephen Jay. *Eight Little Piggies.* New York: W. W. Norton, 1994.

_____. *The Panda's Thumb.* New York: W. W. Norton, 1980.

_____. *The Structure of Evolutionary Theory.* Cambridge, Mass.: Harvard University Press, 2002.

Graur, Dan, and Wen-Hsiung Li. *Fundamentals of Molecular Evolution.* 2d ed. Sunderland, Mass.: Sinauer Associates, 1999.

Heinrich, Bernd. *Why We Run: A Natural History.* New York: Ecco, 2002.

Herrmann, Bernd, and Susanne Hummel, eds. *Ancient DNA: Recovery and Analysis of Genetic Material from Paleographic, Archaeological, Museum, Medical, and Forensic Speciments.* New York: SpringerVerlag, 1994.

Jones, Martin. *The Molecule Hunt: Archaeology and the Search for Ancient DNA.* New York: Arcade, 2002.

Keller, Laurent, ed. *Levels of Selection in Evolution.* Princeton, N.J.: Princeton University Press, 1999.

Kimura, Motoo, and Naoyuki Takahata, eds. *New Aspects of the Genetics of Molecular Evolution.* New York: Springer-Verlag, 1991.

Landweber, Laura F., and Andrew P. Dobson, eds. *Genetics and the Extinction of Species: DNA and the Conservation of Biodiversity.* Princeton, N.J.: Princeton University Press, 1999.

Langridge, John. *Molecular Genetics and Comparative Evolution.* New York: John Wiley & Sons, 1991.

Levy, Charles K. *Evolutionary Wars, a Three-Billion Year Arms Race: The Battle of Species on Land, at Sea, and in the Air.* Illustrations by Trudy Nicholson. New York: W. H. Freeman, 1999.

Lewontin, R. *The Genetic Basis of Evolutionary Change.* New York: Columbia University Press, 1974.

Li, Wen-Hsiung. *Molecular Evolution.* Sunderland, Mass.: Sinauer Associates, 1997.

Lloyd, E. *The Structure of Evolutionary Theory.* Westport, Conn.: Greenwood Press, 1987.

Lynch, John M., ed. *Darwin's Theory of Natural Selection: British Responses, 1859-1871.* 4 vols. Bristol, England: Thoemmes Press, 2002.

Magurran, Anne E., and Robert M. May, eds. *Evolution of Biological Diversity: From Population Differentiation to Speciation.* New York: Oxford University Press, 1999.

Mayr, Ernst. *One Long Argument: Charles Darwin and the Genesis of Modern Evolutionary Thought.* Cambridge, Mass.: Harvard University Press, 1991.

Michod, Richard E. *Darwinian Dynamics: Evolutionary Transitions in Fitness and Individuality.* Princeton, N.J.: Princeton University Press, 1999.

Miller, Stanley L. *From the Primitive Atmosphere to the Prebiotic Soup to the Pre-RNA World.* Washington, D.C.: National Aeronautics and Space Administration, 1996.

Nei, Masatoshi, and Sudhir Kumar. *Molecular Evolution and Phylogenetics.* New York: Oxford University Press, 2000.

Persell, Stuart Michael. *Neo-Lamarckism and the Evolution Controversy in France, 1870-1920.* Lewiston, N.Y.: Edwin Mellen Press, 1999.

Pollard, Tessa M. *Western Diseases: An Evolutionary Perspective.* Cambridge, England: Cambridge University Press, 2008.

Prothero, Donald R. *Bringing Fossils to Life: An Introduction to Paleobiology.* New York: McGraw-Hill, 2003.

Quammen, David. *Song of the Dodo.* New York: Simon & Schuster, 1997.

Raff, Rudolf. *The Shape of Life: Genes, Development, and the Evolution of Animal Form.* Chicago: University of Chicago Press, 1996.

Ranzi, Carlo, with illustrations by the author. *Seventy Million Years of Man.* New York: Greenwich House, 1983.

Ryan, Frank. *Darwin's Blind Spot: Evolution Beyond Natural Selection.* Boston: Houghton Mifflin, 2002.

Selander, Robert K., et al., eds. *Evolution at the Molecular Level.* Sunderland, Mass.: Sinauer Associates, 1991.

Shlain, Leonard. *Sex, Time, and Power: How Women's Sexuality Shaped Human Evolution.* New York: Penguin, 2004.

Singh, Rama S., and Costas B. Krimbas, eds. *Evolutionary Genetics: From Molecules to Morphology.* New York: Cambridge University Press, 2000.

Somit, Albert, and Steven A. Peterson, eds. *The Dynamics of Evolution: The Punctuated Equilibrium Debate in the Natural and Social Sciences.* Ithaca, N.Y.: Cornell University Press, 1992.

Stanford, Craig. *Upright: The Evolutionary Key to Becoming Human.* Boston: Houghton Mifflin, 2003.

Steele, Edward J., Robyn A. Lindley, and Robert V. Blanden. *Lamarck's Signature: How Retrogenes Are Changing Darwin's Natural Selection Paradigm.* Reading, Mass.: Perseus Books, 1998.

Wessen, K. P. *Simulating Human Origins and Evolution.* New York: Cambridge University Press, 2005.

Williams, George C. *Adaptation and Natural Selection: A Critique of Some Current Evolutionary Thought.* 1966. Reprint. Princeton, N.J.: Princeton University Press, 1996.

Wolf, Jason B., Edmund D. Brodie III, and Michael J. Wade. *Epistasis and the Evolutionary Process.* New York: Oxford University Press, 2000.

Zimmer, Carl. *Smithsonian Intimate Guide to Human Origins.* Washington, D.C.: Smithsonian Books, 2005.

FORENSIC GENETICS

Ballantyne, Jack, George Sensabaugh, and Jan Witkowski, eds. *DNA Technology and Forensic Science.* Cold Spring Harbor, N.Y.: Cold Spring Harbor Laboratory Press, 1989.

Budowle, Bruce, et al. *DNA Typing Protocols: Molecular Biology and Forensic Analysis.* Natick, Mass.: Eaton, 2000.

Buckleton, John, Christopher M. Triggs, and Simon J. Walsh. *Forensic DNA Evidence Interpretation.* Boca Raton, Fla.: CRC Press, 2005.

Burke, Terry, R. Wolf, G. Dolf, and A. Jeffreys, eds. *DNA Fingerprinting: Approaches and Applications.* Boston: Birkhauser, 2001.

Butler, John M. *Forensic DNA Typing: Biology and Technology Behind STR Markers.* London: Academic Press, 2001.

Butzel, Henry M. *Genetics in the Courts.* Lewiston, N.Y.: Edwin Mellen Press, 1987.

Carracedo, Angel. *Forensic DNA Typing Protocols.* Totowa, N.J.: Humana Press, 2005.

Coleman, Howard, and Eric Swenson. *DNA in the Courtroom: A Trial Watcher's Guide.* Seattle: GeneLex Press, 1994.

Connors, Edward, et al. *Convicted by Juries, Exonerated by Science: Case Studies in the Use of DNA Evidence to Establish Innocence After Trial.* Washington, D.C.: U.S. Department of Justice, Office of Justice Programs, National Institute of Justice, 1996.

Fridell, Ron. *DNA Fingerprinting: The Ultimate Identity.* New York: Scholastic, 2001.

Goodman, Christi. *Paternity, Marriage, and DNA.* Denver, Colo.: National Conference of State Legislatures, 2001.

Goodwin, William, Adrian Linacre, and Sibte Hadi. *An Introduction to Forensic Genetics.* Chichester, England: John Wiley & Sons, 2007.

Hummel, Susanne. *Fingerprinting the Past: Research on Highly Degraded DNA and Its Applications.* New York: Springer-Verlag, 2002.

Jarman, Keith, and Norah Rudin. *An Introduction to Forensic DNA Analysis.* 2d ed. Boca Raton, Fla.: CRC Press, 2001.

Kirby, L. T. *DNA Fingerprinting: An Introduction.* New York: Stockton Press, 1990.

Kobilinsky, Lawrence, Louis Levine, and Henrietta Margolis-Nunno. *Forensic DNA Analysis.* New York: Chelsea House, 2006.

Lincoln, Patrick J., and Jim Thompson, eds. *Forensic DNA Profiling Protocols.* Vol. 98. Totowa, N.J.: Humana Press, 1998.

National Research Council. *DNA Technology in Forensic Science.* Washington, D.C.: National Academy Press, 1992.

Rose, David, and Lisa Goos. *DNA: A Practical Guide.* Toronto: Thomson Carswell, 2004.

Rudin, Norah, and Keith Inman. *An Introduction to Forensic DNA Analysis.* Boca Raton, Fla.: CRC Press, 2002.

Sonenstein, Freya L., Pamela A. Holcomb, and Kristin S. Seefeldt. *Promising Approaches to Improving Paternity Establishment Rates at the Local Level.* Washington, D.C.: Urban Institute, 1993.

United States National Research Council. *The Evaluation of Forensic DNA Evidence.* Rev. ed. Washington, D.C.: National Academy Press, 1996.

GENETIC ENGINEERING AND BIOTECHNOLOGY. *See also* AGRICULTURE AND GENETICALLY MODIFIED FOODS; CLONING

Aldridge, Susan. *The Thread of Life: The Story of Genes and Genetic Engineering.* New York: Cambridge University Press, 1996.

Bassett, Pamela. *Emerging Markets in Tissue Engineering: Angiogenesis, Soft and Hard Tissue Regeneration, Xenotransplant, Wound Healing, Biomaterials, and Cell Therapy.* Southborough, Mass.: D & MD Reports, 1999.

Boylan, Michael, and Kevin E. Brown. *Genetic Engineering: Science and Ethics on the New Frontier.* Upper Saddle River, N.J.: Prentice Hall, 2001.

Burley, Justine, and John Harris, eds. *A Companion to Genetics.* Malden, Mass.: Blackwell, 2002.

Chrispeels, Maarten J., and David E. Sadava. *Plants, Genes, and Crop Biotechnology.* Boston: Jones and Bartlett, 2003.

Crocomo, O. J., ed. *Biotechnology of Plants and Microorganisms.* Columbus: Ohio State University Press, 1986.

Curran, Brendan, ed. *A Terrible Beauty Is Born: Clones, Genes and the Future of Mankind.* London: Taylor & Francis, 2003.

Dale, Jeremy. *Molecular Genetics of Bacteria.* New York: John Wiley & Sons, 1994.

Davis, Bernard D., ed. *The Genetic Revolution: Scientific Prospects and Public Perceptions.* Baltimore: Johns Hopkins University Press, 1991.

Emery, Alan E., and H. Emery. *An Introduction to Recombinant DNA.* Chichester, Sussex, England: Wiley, 1984.

Ettore, Elizabeth. *Reproductive Genetics, Gender and the Body.* London: Routledge, 2002.

Evans, Gareth M. *Environmental Biotechnology: Theory and Application.* Hoboken, N.J.: Wiley, 2003.

Fincham, J. R. S. *Genetically Engineered Organisms: Benefits and Risks.* Toronto: University of Toronto Press, 1991.

Gaillardin, Claude, and Henri Heslot. *Molecular Biology and Genetic Engineering of Yeasts.* Boca Raton, Fla.: CRC Press, 1992.

Glick, Bernard R. *Molecular Biotechnology: Principles and Applications of Recombinant DNA.* Washington, D.C.: ASM Press, 2003.

Goodnough, David. *The Debate over Human Cloning.* Berkeley Heights, N.J.: Enslow, 2003.

Grange, J. M., et al., eds. *Genetic Manipulation: Techniques and Applications.* Boston: Blackwell Scientific, 1991.

Hill, Walter E. *Genetic Engineering: A Primer.* Newark, N.J.: Harwood Academic, 2000.

Jacobson, G. K., and S. O. Jolly. *Gene Technology.* New York: VCH Verlagsgesellschaft, 1989.

Joyner, Alexandra L., ed. *Gene Targeting: A Practical Approach.* New York: Oxford University Press, 1993.

Kiessling, Ann, and Scott C. Anderson. *Human Embryonic Stem Cells: An Introduction to the Science and Therapeutic Potential.* Boston: Jones and Bartlett, 2003.

Kontermann, Roland, and Stefan Dubel, eds. *Antibody Engineering.* New York: Springer, 2001.

Kowalski, Kathiann M. *The Debate over Genetically Engineered Food: Healthy or Harmful?* Berkeley Heights, N.J.: Enslow, 2002.

Kreuzer, Helen, and Adrianne Massey. *Recombinant DNA and Biotechnology: A Guide for Teachers.* Washington, D.C.: ASM Press, 2001.

Krimsky, Sheldon. *Biotechnics and Society: The Rise of Industrial Genetics.* New York: Praeger, 1991.

Lappe, Marc. *Broken Code: The Exploitation of DNA.* San Francisco: Sierra Club Books, 1984.

Le Vine, Harry, III. *Genetic Engineering: A Reference Handbook.* Santa Barbara, Calif.: ABC-CLIO, 1999.

McGee, Glenn. *The Perfect Baby: A Pragmatic Approach to Genetics.* Lanham, Md.: Rowman & Littlefield, 1997.

McKay, David, and Mark Walker. *Unravelling Genes: A Layperson's Guide to Genetic Engineering.* Frenchs Forest, N.S.W.: Pearson Prentice Hall, 2006.

McKelvey, Maureen D. *Evolutionary Innovations: The Business of Biotechnology.* New York: Oxford University Press, 1996.

Mak, Tak W., et al., eds. *The Gene Knockout Factsbook.* 2 vols. San Diego: Academic Press, 1998.

Mayforth, Ruth D. *Designing Antibodies.* San Diego: Academic Press, 1993.

Nicholl, Desmond S. T. *An Introduction to Genetic Engineering.* 3d ed. New York: Cambridge University Press, 2008.

Nossal, Gustav J. V., and Ross L. Coppel. *Reshaping Life: Key Issues in Genetic Engineering.* New York: Cambridge University Press, 1985.

Nottingham, Stephen. *Genescapes: The Ecology of Genetic Engineering.* New York: Zed Books, 2002.

Old, R. W., and S. B. Primrose. *Principles of Gene Manipulation: An Introduction to Genetic Engineering.* Boston: Blackwell Scientific, 1994.

Olson, Steve. *Biotechnology: An Industry Comes of Age.* Washington, D.C.: National Academy Press, 1986.

Oxender, Dale L., and C. Fred Fox, eds. *Protein Engineering.* New York: Liss, 1987.

Prokop, Ales, and Rakesh K. Bajpai. *Recombinant DNA Technology I.* New York: New York Academy of Sciences, 1991.

Ronald, Pamela C., and R. W. Adamchak. *Tomorrow's Table: Organic Farming, Genetics, and the Future of Food.* Oxford, England: Oxford University Press, 2008.

Rothman, Barbara Katz. *The Book of Life: A Personal and Ethical Guide to Race, Normality, and the Implications of the Human Genome Project.* Boston: Beacon Press, 2001.

Russo, V. E. A., and David Cove. *Genetic Engineering: Dreams and Nightmares.* New York: W. H. Freeman, 1995.

Shannon, Thomas A., ed. *Genetic Engineering: A Documentary History.* Westport, Conn.: Greenwood Press, 1999.

Singer, Maxine, and Paul Berg, eds. *Exploring Genetic Mechanisms.* Sausalito, Calif.: University Science Books, 1997.

Sofer, William. *Introduction to Genetic Engineering.* Boston: Butterworth-Heinemann, 1991.

Spallone, Patricia. *Generation Games: Genetic Engineering and the Future for Our Lives.* Philadelphia: Temple University Press, 1992.

Steinberg, Mark, and Sharon D. Cosloy, eds. *The Facts On File Dictionary of Biotechnology and Genetic Engineering.* New ed. New York: Checkmark Books, 2001.

Thomas, John, et al., eds. *Biotechnology and Safety Assessment.* 2d ed. Philadelphia: Taylor & Francis, 1999.

Vega, Manuel A., ed. *Gene Targeting.* Boca Raton, Fla.: CRC Press, 1995.

Wade, Nicholas. *The Ultimate Experiment: Man-Made Evolution.* New York: Walker, 1977.

Walker, Mark, and David McKay. *Unravelling Genes: A Layperson's Guide to Genetic Engineering.* St. Leonards, N.S.W.: Allen & Unwin, 2000.

Walker, Matthew R., with Ralph Rapley. *Route Maps in Gene Technology.* Oxford, England: Blackwell Scientific, 1997.

Wang, Henry Y., and Tadayuki Imanaka, eds. *Antibody Expression and Engineering.* Washington, D.C.: American Chemical Society, 1995.

Warr, J. Roger. *Genetic Engineering in Higher Organisms.* Baltimore: E. Arnold, 1984.

Watson, James D., et al. *Recombinant DNA.* 2d ed. New York: W. H. Freeman, 1992.

Williams, J. G., A. Ceccarelli, and A. Wallace. *Genetic Engineering.* 2d ed. New York: Springer, 2001.

Wu-Pong, S., and Y. Rojanasakul. *Biopharmaceutical Drug Design and Development.* Totowa, N.J.: Humana Press, 1999.

GENOMICS AND PROTEOMICS. *See also* BIOINFORMATICS

Bradbury, E. Morton, and Sandor Pongor, eds. *Structural Biology and Functional Genomics.* Boston: Kluwer Academic, 1999.

Dunn, Michael J., ed. *From Genome to Proteome: Advances in the Practice and Application of Proteomics.* New York: Wiley-VCH, 2000.

Gibson, Greg. *A Primer of Genome Science.* Sunderland, Mass.: Sinauer, 2002.

Innis, Michael A., David H. Gelfand, and John J. Sninsky, eds. *PCR Applications: Protocols for Functional Genomics.* San Diego: Academic Press, 1999.

Jolles, P., and H. Jornvall, eds. *Proteomics in Functional Genomics: Protein Structure Analysis.* Boston: Birkhauser, 2000.

Kang, Manjit S. *Quantitative Genetics, Genomics, and Plant Breeding.* Wallingford, Oxon, England: CABI, 2002.

Liebler, David G. *Introduction to Proteomics: Tools for the New Biology.* Totowa, N.J.: Humana Press, 2001.

Link, Andrew J., ed. *2-D Proteome Analysis Protocols.* Totowa, N.J.: Humana Press, 1999.

Liu, Ben-Hui. *Statistical Genomics: Linkage, Mapping, and QTL Analysis.* Boca Raton, Fla.: CRC Press, 1998.

Pennington, S. R., and M. J. Dunn, eds. *Proteomics: From Protein Sequence to Function.* New York: Springer, 2001.

Rabilloud, Thierry, ed. *Proteome Research: Two-Dimensional Gel Electrophoresis and Identification Methods.* New York: Springer, 2000.

HISTORY OF GENETICS

Alibeck, Ken, with Stephen Handelman. *Biohazard: The Chilling True Story of the Largest Covert Biological Weapons Program in the World, Told from the Inside by the Man Who Ran It.* New York: Random House, 1999.

Ayala, Francisco J., and Walter M. Fitch, eds. *Genetics and the Origin of Species: From Darwin to Molecular Biology Sixty Years After Dobzhansky.* Washington, D.C.: National Academies Press, 1997.

Beighton, Peter. *The Person Behind the Syndrome.* Rev. ed. New York: Springer-Verlag, 1997.

Bowler, Peter J. *Evolution: The History of an Idea.* Berkeley: University of California Press, 1990.

Brookes, Martin. *Fly: The Unsung Hero of Twentieth Century Science.* San Francisco: HarperCollins, 2001.

Corcos, A., and F. Monaghan. *Mendel's Experiments on Plant Hybrids: A Guided Study.* New Brunswick, N.J.: Rutgers University Press, 1993.

Darwin, Charles. *Charles Darwin's Notebooks, 18361844.* Edited by P. H. Barrett et al. Ithaca, N.Y.: Cornell University Press, 1987.

_____. *The Correspondence of Charles Darwin.* Cambridge, England: Cambridge University Press, 1994.

Dover, Gabriel A. *Dear Mr. Darwin: Letters on the Evolution of Life and Human Nature.* Berkeley: University of California Press, 2000.

Dunn, L. C. *A Short History of Genetics: The Development of Some of the Main Lines of Thought, 18641939.* New York: McGraw-Hill, 1965.

Edelson, Edward. *Gregor Mendel and the Roots of Genetics.* New York: Oxford University Press, 1999.

Fast, Julius. *Blueprint for Life: The Story of Modern Genetics.* New York: St. Martin's Press, 1965.

Fitzgerald, Patrick J. *From Demons and Evil Spirits to Cancer Genes: The Development of Concepts Concerning the Causes of Cancer and Carcinogenesis.* Washington, D.C.: American Registry of Pathology, Armed Forces Institute of Pathology, 2000.

Fredrickson, Donald S. *The Recombinant DNA Controversy, a Memoir: Science, Politics, and the Public Interest, 1974-1981.* Washington, D.C.: ASM Press, 2001.

Fujimura, Joan H. *Crafting Science: A Sociohistory of the Quest for the Genetics of Cancer.* Cambridge, Mass.: Harvard University Press, 1996.

Gillham, Nicholas Wright. *A Life of Sir Francis Galton: From African Exploration to the Birth of Eugenics.* New York: Oxford University Press, 2001.

Haldane, J. B. S. *Selected Genetic Papers of J. B. S. Haldane.* Edited with an introduction by Krishna R. Dronamraju, foreword by James F. Crow. New York: Garland, 1990.

Harper, Peter S. *A Short History of Medical Genetics.* New York: Oxford University Press, 2008.

Henig, Robin Marantz. *The Monk in the Garden: The Lost and Found Genius of Gregor Mendel, the Father of Genetics.* Boston: Houghton Mifflin, 2000.

Hubbell, Sue. *Shrinking the Cat: Genetic Engineering Before We Knew About Genes.* Illustrations by Liddy Hubbell. Boston: Houghton Mifflin, 2001.

Iltis, Hugo. *Life of Mendel.* Translated by Eden Paul and Cedar Paul. London: Allen & Unwin, 1932.

Jacob, Franyois. *The Logic of Life: A History of Heredity.* New York: Pantheon, 1973.

Johnson, George B. *How Scientists Think: Twenty-one Experiments That Have Shaped Our Understanding of Genetics and Molecular Biology.* Dubuque, Iowa: Wm. C. Brown, 1996.

Judson, Horace Freeland. *The Eighth Day of Creation: Makers of the Revolution in Biology.* Rev. ed. Cold Spring Harbor, N.Y.: Cold Spring Harbor Laboratory Press, 1997.

Kay, Lily E. *Who Wrote the Book of Life? A History of the Genetic Code.* Stanford, Calif.: Stanford University Press, 2000.

Keller, Evelyn Fox. *A Feeling for the Organism: The Life and Work of Barbara McClintock.* 10th anniversary ed. New York: W. H. Freeman, 1993.

Kornberg, Arthur. *For the Love of Enzymes: The Odyssey of a Biochemist.* Reprint. Cambridge, Mass.: Harvard University Press, 1991.

Kuhl, Stefan. *The Nazi Connection: Eugenics, American Racism, and German National Socialism.* New York: Oxford University Press, 2002.

Laffin, John. *Hitler Warned Us: The Nazis' Master Plan for a Master Race.* Totowa, N.J.: Barnes and Noble, 1998.

McCarty, Maclyn. *The Transforming Principle: Discovering That Genes Are Made of DNA.* New York: W. W. Norton, 1994.

Maddox, Brenda. *Rosalind Franklin: The Dark Lady of DNA.* New York: HarperCollins, 2002.

Mayr, Ernst. *One Long Argument: Charles Darwin and the Genesis of Modern Evolutionary Thought.* Cambridge, Mass.: Harvard University Press, 1991.

Mendel, Gregor. *Experiments in Plant-Hybridization.* Foreword by Paul C. Mangelsdorf. Cambridge, Mass.: Harvard University Press, 1965.

Olby, Robert C. *Origins of Mendelism.* New York: Schocken Books, 1966.

Orel, Vitezslav. *Gregor Mendel: The First Geneticist.* Translated by Stephen Finn. New York: Oxford University Press, 1996.

Palladino, Paolo. *Plants, Patients, and the Historians: On (RE)Membering in the Age of Genetic Engineering.* New Brunswick, N.J.: Rutgers University Press, 2003.

Persell, Stuart Michael. *Neo-Lamarckism and the Evolution Controversy in France, 1870-1920.* Lewiston, N.Y.: Edwin Mellen Press, 1999.

Potts, D. M., and W. T. W. Potts. *Queen Victoria's Gene: Haemophilia and the Royal Family.* Stroud, Gloucestershire, England: Sutton, 1999.

Rutter, Michael Sir, ed. *Genetic Effects on Environmental Vulnerability to Disease.* New York: Wiley, 2008.

Shannon, Thomas A., ed. *Genetic Engineering: A Documentary History.* Westport, Conn.: Greenwood Press, 1999.

Shermer, Michael. *In Darwin's Shadow: The Life and Science of Alfred Russel Wallace, a Biographical Study on the Psychology of History.* New York: Oxford University Press, 2002.

Stubbe, H. *A History of Genetics.* Cambridge, Mass.: MIT Press, 1968.

Sturtevant, A. H. *A History of Genetics.* 1965. Reprint. Introduction by Edward B. Lewis. Cold Spring Harbor, N.Y.: Cold Spring Harbor Laboratory Press, 2001.

Sulston, John, and Georgina Ferry. *The Common Thread: A Story of Science, Politics, Ethics, and the Human Genome.* Washington, D.C.: Joseph Henry Press, 2002.

Tudge, Colin. *In Mendel's Footnotes: An Introduction to the Science and Technologies of Genes and Genetics from the Nineteenth Century to the Twenty-Second.* London: Jonathan Cape, 2000.

Watson, James. *The Double Helix.* New York: Simon and Schuster, 2001.

Weiner, Jonathan. *The Beak of the Finch: A Story of Evolution in Our Time.* New York: Random House, 1995.

Wood, Roger J., and Vitezslav Orel. *Genetic Prehistory in Selective Breeding: A Prelude to Mendel.* New York: Oxford University Press, 2001.

HUMAN GENETICS

Adolph, Kenneth W., ed. *Human Molecular Genetics.* New York: Academic Press, 1996.

Alcock, John. *The Triumph of Sociobiology.* Reprint. New York: Oxford University Press, 2003.

Andreasen, Nancy C. *Brave New Brain: Conquering Mental Illness in the Era of the Genome.* New York: Oxford University Press, 2001.

Arking, Robert, ed. *Biology of Aging: Observations and Principles.* 2d ed. Sunderland, Mass.: Sinauer, 2001.

Austad, Steven N. *Why We Age: What Science Is Discovering About the Body's Journey Throughout Life.* New York: John Wiley & Sons, 1997.

Badcock, C. R. *Evolutionary Psychology: A Critical Introduction.* Malden, Mass.: Polity Press in association with Blackwell, 2000.

Baudrillard, Jean. *The Vital Illusion.* Edited by Julia Witwer. New York: Columbia University Press, 2000.

Blackmore, Susan J. *The Meme Machine.* Foreword by Richard Dawkins. New York: Oxford University Press, 1999.

Bock, Gregory R., and Jamie A. Goode. *Genetics of Criminal and Antisocial Behaviour.* New York: John Wiley & Sons, 1996.

Bock, Gregory R., Jamie A. Goode, and Kate Webb, eds. *The Nature of Intelligence.* New York: John Wiley & Sons, 2001.

Boyer, Samuel, ed. *Papers on Human Genetics.* Englewood Cliffs, N.J.: Prentice-Hall, 1963.

Brierley, John Keith. *The Thinking Machine: Genes, Brain, Endocrines, and Human Nature.* Rutherford, N.J.: Fairleigh Dickinson University Press, 1973.

Briley, Mike, and Fridolin Sulser, eds. *Molecular Genetics of Mental Disorders: The Place of Molecular Genetics in Basic Mechanisms and Clinical Applications in Mental Disorders.* Malden, Mass.: Blackwell, 2001.

British Medical Association. *Biotechnology, Weapons, and Humanity.* Amsterdam, Netherlands: Harwood Academic, 1999.

Burnet, Sir Frank Macfarlane. *Endurance of Life: The Implications of Genetics for Human Life.* New York: Cambridge University Press, 1978.

Burnham, Terry, and Jay Phelan. *Mean Genes: From Sex to Money to Food—Taming Our Primal Instincts.* Cambridge, Mass.: Perseus, 2000.

Carson, Ronald A., and Mark A. Rothstein. *Behavioral Genetics: The Clash of Culture and Biology.* Baltimore: Johns Hopkins University Press, 1999.

Carter, Cedric O. *Human Heredity.* Baltimore: Penguin Books, 1962.

Cartwright, John. *Evolution and Human Behavior: Darwinian Perspectives on Human Nature.* Cambridge, Mass.: MIT Press, 2000.

Cavalli-Sforza, L. L., and Francesco Cavalli-Sforza. *The Great Human Diasporas: The History of Diversity and Evolution.* Translated by Sarah Thorne. Reading, Mass.: Addison-Wesley, 1995.

Centers for Disease Control and Prevention. "Bioterrorism-Related Anthrax." *Emerging Infectious Diseases* 8 (October, 2002): 1013-1183.

Clark, William R., and Michael Grunstein. *Are We Hardwired? The Role of Genes in Human Behavior.* New York: Oxford University Press, 2000.

Clegg, Edward J. *The Study of Man: An Introduction to Human Biology.* London: English Universities Press, 1968.

Cole, Leonard A. *The Eleventh Plague: The Politics of Biological and Chemical Warfare.* New York: W. H. Freeman, 1996.

Cooper, Colin. *Intelligence and Abilities.* New York: Routledge, 1999.

Cooper, Necia Grant, ed. *The Human Genome Project: Deciphering the Blueprint of Heredity.* Foreword by Paul Berg. Mill Valley, Calif.: University Science Books, 1994.

Cronk, Lee. *That Complex Whole: Culture and the Evolution of Human Behavior.* Boulder, Colo.: Westview Press, 1999.

Crow, Tim J., ed. *The Speciation of Modern Homo Sapiens.* Oxford, England: Oxford University Press, 2002.

Cummings, Michael J. *Human Heredity: Principles and Issues.* 5th ed. Pacific Grove, Calif.: Brooks/Cole, 2000.

Curran, Charles E. *Politics, Medicine, and Christian Ethics: A Dialogue with Paul Ramsey.* Philadelphia: Fortress Press, 1973.

Cziko, Gary. *The Things We Do: Using the Lessons of Bernard and Darwin to Understand the What, How, and Why of Our Behavior.* Cambridge, Mass.: MIT Press, 2000.

DeMoss, Robert T. *Brain Waves Through Time: Twelve Principles for Understanding the Evolution of the Human Brain and Man's Behavior.* New York: Plenum Trade, 1999.

Dennis, Carina, and Richard Gallagher. *The Human Genome.* London: Palgrave Macmillan, 2002.

Diamant, L., and R. McAnuity, eds. *The Psychology of Sexual Orientation, Behavior, and Identity: A Handbook*. Westport, Conn.: Greenwood Press, 1995.

Dobzhansky, Theodosius G. *Mankind Evolving: The Evolution of the Human Species*. New Haven, Conn.: Yale University Press, 1967.

Edlin, Gordon. *Human Genetics: A Modern Synthesis*. Boston: Jones & Bartlett, 1990.

Fish, Jefferson M., ed. *Race and Intelligence: Separating Science from Myth*. Mahwah, N.J.: Lawrence Erlbaum, 2002.

Fishbein, Diana H., ed. *The Science, Treatment, and Prevention of Antisocial Behaviors: Application to the Criminal Justice System*. Kingston, N.J.: Civic Research Institute, 2000.

Fooden, Myra, et al., eds. *The Second X and Women's Health*. New York: Gordian Press, 1983.

Gallagher, Nancy L. *Breeding Better Vermonters: The Eugenics Program in the Green Mountain State*. Hanover, N.H.: University Press of New England, 2000.

Gardner, Howard. *Frames of Mind: The Theory of Multiple Intelligences*. 10th anniversary ed. New York: Basic Books, 1993.

Glassy, Mark C. *The Biology of Science Fiction Cinema*. Jefferson, N.C.: McFarland, 2001.

Goldhagen, Daniel J. *Hitler's Willing Executioners: Ordinary Germans and the Holocaust*. New York: Random House, 1996.

Gould, Stephen Jay. *The Mismeasure of Man*. Rev. ed. New York: W. W. Norton, 1996.

Graves, Joseph L., Jr. *The Emperor's New Clothes: Biological Theories of Race at the Millennium*. New Brunswick, N.J.: Rutgers University Press, 2001.

Hahn, Martin E., et al., eds. *Developmental Behavior Genetics: Neural, Biometrical, and Evolutionary Approaches*. New York: Oxford University Press, 1990.

Haldane, J. B. S. *Selected Genetic Papers of J. B. S. Haldane*. Edited with an introduction by Krishna R. Dronamraju, foreword by James F. Crow. New York: Garland, 1990.

Hamer, Dean, and Peter Copeland. *Living with Our Genes: Why They Matter More than You Think*. New York: Doubleday, 1998.

Harris, Harry. *The Principles of Human Biochemical Genetics*. New York: Elsevier/North-Holland Biomedical Press, 1980.

Herrnstein, Richard J., and Charles Murray. *The Bell Curve: Intelligence and Class Structure in America*. New York: Free Press, 1994.

Heschl, Adolf. *The Intelligent Genome: On the Origin of the Human Mind by Mutation and Selection*. Drawings by Herbert Loserl. New York: Springer, 2002.

Hsia, David Yi-Yung. *Human Developmental Genetics*. Chicago: Year Book Medical Publishers, 1968.

Jacquard, Albert. *In Praise of Difference: Genetics and Human Affairs*. Translated by Margaret M. Moriarty. New York: Columbia University Press, 1984.

Jensen, Arthur Robert. *Genetics and Education*. New York: Harper & Row, 1972.

Karlsson, Jon L. *Inheritance of Creative Intelligence*. Chicago: Nelson-Hall, 1978.

Kevles, Daniel J. *In the Name of Eugenics: Genetics and the Uses of Human Heredity*. New York: Alfred A. Knopf, 1985.

Korn, Noel, and Harry Reece Smith, eds. *Human Evolution: Readings in Physical Anthropology*. New York: Holt, 1959.

Krebs, J., and N. Davies. *An Introduction to Behavioral Ecology*. Malden, Mass.: Blackwell, 1991.

Lasker, Gabriel W., ed. *The Processes of Ongoing Human Evolution*. Detroit: Wayne State University Press, 1960.

Levitan, Max. *Textbook of Human Genetics*. New York: Oxford University Press, 1988.

Lewis, Ricki. *Human Genetics: Concepts and Applications*. 5th ed. New York: McGraw-Hill, 2003.

Lewontin, Richard C. *Human Diversity*. New York: Scientific American Library, 1995.

Ludmerer, Kenneth M. *Genetics and American Society: A Historical Appraisal*. Baltimore: Johns Hopkins University Press, 1972.

Lynn, Richard. *Dysgenics: Genetic Deterioration in Modern Populations*. Westport, Conn.: Praeger, 1996.

McConkey, Edwin H. *Human Genetics: The Molecular Revolution*. Boston: Jones & Bartlett, 1993.

Macieira-Coelho, Alvaro. *Biology of Aging*. New York: Springer, 2002.

McKusick, Victor A., comp. *Mendelian Inheritance in Man: A Catalog of Human Genes and Genetic Disorders*. 12th ed. Baltimore: Johns Hopkins University Press, 1998.

McWhirter, David P., et al. *Homosexuality/Heterosexuality: Concepts of Sexual Orientation*. New York: Oxford University Press, 1990.

Mange, Elaine Johansen, and Arthur P. Mange. *Basic Human Genetics*. 2d ed. Sunderland, Mass.: Sinauer Associates, 1999.

Manuck, Stephen B., et al., eds. *Behavior, Health, and Aging*. Mahwah, N.J.: Lawrence Erlbaum, 2000.

Marks, Jonathan M. *Human Biodiversity: Genes, Race, and History*. New York: Aldine de Gruyter, 1995.

Marteau, Theresa, and Martin Richards, eds. *The Troubled Helix: Social and Psychological Implications of the New Human Genetics*. New York: Cambridge University Press, 1999.

Medina, John J. *The Clock of Ages: Why We Age, How We Age—Winding Back the Clock*. New York: Cambridge University Press, 1996.

Mielke, James H., and Michael H. Crawford, eds. *Current Developments in Anthropological Genetics*. New York: Plenum Press, 1980.

Miller, Judith, Stephen Engelberg, and William Broad. *Germs: Biological Weapons and America's Secret War*. New York: Simon & Schuster, 2001.

Miller, Orlando J., and Eeva Therman. *Human Chromosomes*. 4th ed. New York: Springer Verlag, 2001.

Moffitt, Terrie E., Avshalom Caspi, Michael Rutter, and Phil A. Silva. *Sex Differences in Antisocial Behaviour: Conduct Disorder, Delinquency, and Violence in the Dunedin Longitudinal Study*. New York: Cambridge University Press, 2001.

Moody, Paul Amos. *Genetics of Man*. New York: W. W. Norton, 1967.

Nelkin, Dorothy, and Laurence Tancredi. *Dangerous Diagnostics: The Social Power of Biological Information*. New York: Basic Books, 1989.

Ostrer, Harry. *Non-Mendelian Genetics in Humans*. New York: Oxford University Press, 1998.

Ott, Jurg. *Analysis of Human Genetic Linkage*. Baltimore: Johns Hopkins University Press, 1991.

Pearson, Roger. *Eugenics and Race*. Los Angeles: Noontide Press, 1966.

Pierce, Benjamin A. *The Family Genetic Sourcebook*. New York: John Wiley & Sons, 1990.

Plomin, Robert, et al. *Behavioral Genetics*. 4th ed. New York: Worth, 2001.

Puterbaugh, Geoff. *Twins and Homosexuality: A Casebook*. New York: Garland, 1990.

Resta, Robert G., ed. *Psyche and Helix: Psychological Aspects of Genetic Counseling*. New York: Wiley-Liss, 2000.

Ricklefs, Robert E., and Caleb E. Finch. *Aging: A Natural History*. New York: W. H. Freeman, 1995.

Rifkin, Jeremy. *The Biotech Century: Harnessing the Gene and Remaking the World*. New York: Putnam, 1998.

Roderick, Gordon Wynne. *Man and Heredity*. New York: St. Martin's Press, 1968.

Rosenberg, Charles, ed. *The History of Hereditarian Thought: A Thirty-two Volume Reprint Series Presenting Some of the Classic Books in This Intellectual Tradition*. New York: Garland, 1984.

Ruse, M. *Sociobiology: Sense or Nonsense?* Boston: D. Riedel, 1979.

Santos, Miguel A. *Genetics and Man's Future: Legal, Social, and Moral Implications of Genetic Engineering*. Springfield, Ill.: Thomas, 1981.

Segerstrale, Ullica. *Defenders of the Truth: The Battle for Science in the Sociobiology Debate and Beyond*. New York: Oxford University Press, 2000.

Singh, Jai Rup, ed. *Current Concepts in Human Genetics*. Amritsar, India: Guru Nanak Dev University, 1996.

Steen, R. Grant. *DNA and Destiny: Nurture and Nature in Human Behavior*. New York: Plenum, 1996.

Strachan, Tom, and Andrew P. Read. *Human Molecular Genetics*. 2d ed. New York: Wiley-Liss, 1999.

Sussman, Robert, ed. *The Biological Basis of Human Behavior: A Critical Review*. 2d ed. New York: Simon and Schuster, 1998.

Suzuki, D., and P. Knudtson. *Genethics: The Clash Between the New Genetics and Human Value*. Cambridge, Mass.: Harvard University Press, 1989.

Terwilliger, Joseph Douglas, and Jurg Ott. *Handbook of Human Genetic Linkage*. Baltimore: Johns Hopkins University Press, 1994.

Thorner, M., and R. Smith. *Human Growth Hormone: Research and Clinical Practice*. Vol. 19. Totowa, N.J.: Humana Press, 1999.

Timiras, Paola S. *Physiological Basis of Aging and Geriatrics*. 3d ed. Boca Raton, Fla.: CRC Press, 2003.

Toussaint, Olivier, et al., eds. *Molecular and Cellular Gerontology*. New York: New York Academy of Sciences, 2000.

Turney, Jon. *Frankenstein's Footsteps: Science, Genetics, and Popular Culture*. New Haven, Conn.: Yale University Press, 1998.

Underwood, Jane H. *Human Variation and Human Microevolution*. Englewood Cliffs, N.J.: Prentice-Hall, 1979.

U.S. Congress. Office of Technology Assessment. *Mapping Our Genes: Genome Projects—How Big, How Fast?* Baltimore: Johns Hopkins University Press, 1988.

Vandenberg, Steven G., ed. *Methods and Goals in Human Behavior Genetics.* New York: Academic Press, 1965.

Van der Dennen, Johan M. G., David Smillie, and Daniel R. Wilson, eds. *The Darwinian Heritage and Sociobiology.* Westport, Conn.: Praeger, 1999.

Varmus, Harold, and Robert Weinberg. *Genes and the Biology of Cancer.* New York: W. H. Freeman, 1993.

Vogel, Friedrich, and A. G. Motulsky. *Human Genetics: Problems and Approaches.* New York: SpringerVerlag, 1997.

Wasserman, David, and Robert Wachbroit, eds. *Genetics and Criminal Behavior.* New York: Cambridge University Press, 2001.

Weil, Jon. *Psychosocial Genetic Counseling.* New York: Oxford University Press, 2000.

Weir, Bruce S. *Human Identification: The Use of DNA Markers.* New York: Kluwer Academic, 1995.

Weiss, Kenneth M. *Genetic Variation and Human Disease: Principles and Evolutionary Approaches.* New York: Cambridge University Press, 1993.

Wexler, Alice. *Mapping Fate: A Memoir of Family, Risk, and Genetic Research.* Berkeley: University of California Press, 1996.

Whittinghill, Maurice. *Human Genetics and Its Foundations.* New York: Reinhold, 1965.

Wright, Lawrence. *Twins: And What They Tell Us About Who We Are.* New York: John Wiley & Sons, 1997.

Wright, William. *Born That Way: Genes, Behavior, Personality.* New York: Knopf, 1998.

Young, Ian D. *Introduction to Risk Calculation in Genetic Counseling.* 2d ed. New York: Oxford University Press, 1999.

Yu, Byung Pal, ed. *Free Radicals in Aging.* Boca Raton, Fla.: CRC Press, 1993.

IMMUNOGENETICS

Bell, John I., et al., eds. *T Cell Receptors.* New York: Oxford University Press, 1995.

Bernal, J. E. *Human Immunogenetics: Principles and Clinical Applications.* Translated by Derek Roberts. London: Taylor & Francis, 1986.

Bibel, Debra Jan. *Milestones in Immunology.* New York: Springer-Verlag, 1988.

Bona, Constantin A., etal., eds. *The Molecular Pathology ofAutoimmune Diseases.* 2d ed. New York: Taylor and Francis, 2002.

Clark, William R. *At War Within: The Double-Edged Sword of Immunity.* New York: Oxford University Press, 1995.

Coleman, Robert M., et al. *Fundamental Immunology.* Dubuque, Iowa: Wm. C. Brown, 1989.

Dwyer, John M. *The Body at War: The Miracle of the Immune System.* New York: New American Library, 1988.

Falus, Andras, ed. *Immunogenomics and Human Disease.* Chichester, West Sussex, England: John Wiley, 2006.

Frank, Steven A. *Immunology and Evolution of Infectious Disease.* Princeton, N.J.: Princeton University Press, 2002.

Fudenberg, H. Hugh, et al. *Basic Immunogenetics.* New York: Oxford University Press, 1984.

Gallo, Robert C., and Flossie Wong-Staal, eds. *Retrovirus Biology and Human Disease.* New York: Marcel Dekker, 1990.

Holland, J. J., ed. *Current Topics in Microbiology and Immunology: Genetic Diversity of RNA Viruses.* New York: Springer-Verlag, 1992.

Janeway, Charles A., Paul Travers, et al. *Immunobiology: The Immune System in Health and Disease.* 5th rev. ed. Philadelphia: Taylor & Francis, 2001.

Joneja, Janice M. V., and Leonard Bielory. *Understanding Allergy, Sensitivity, and Immunity.* New Brunswick, N.J.: Rutgers University Press, 1990.

Kimball, John W. *Introduction to Immunology.* 3d ed. New York: Macmillan, 1990.

Kreier, Julius P., and Richard F. Mortensen. *Infection, Resistance, and Immunity.* New York: Harper & Row, 1990.

Kuby, Janis. *Immunology.* 4th ed. New York: W. H. Freeman, 2000.

Litwin, Stephen D., David W. Scott, et al., eds. *Human Immunogenetics: Basic Principles and Clinical Relevance.* New York: Dekker, 1989.

Mak, Tak W., and John J. L. Simard. *Handbook of Immune Response Genes.* New York: Plenum Press, 1998.

Mizel, Steven B., and Peter Jaret. *In Self-Defense.* San Diego: Harcourt Brace Jovanovich, 1985.

Panayi, Gabriel S., and Chella S. David, eds. *Human Immunogenetics.* London: Butterworths, 1984.

Pines, Maya, ed. *Arousing the Fury of the Immune System.* Chevy Chase, Md.: Howard Hughes Medical Institute, 1998.

Oksenberg, Jorge, and David Brassat, eds. *Immunogenetics of Autoimmune Disease.* Georgetown, Tex.: Landes Bioscience/Eurekah.com, 2006.

Roitt, Ivan, Jonathan Brostoff, and David Male, eds. *Immunology.* New York: Mosby, 2001.

Samter, Max. *Immunological Diseases.* 4th ed. Boston: Little, Brown, 1988.

Sasazuki, Takehiko, and Tomio Tada, eds. *Immunogenetics: Its Application to Clinical Medicine.* Orlando, Fla.: Academic Press, 1984.

Silverstein, Arthur M. *A History of Immunology.* San Diego: Academic Press, 1989.

Smith, George P. *The Variation and Adaptive Expression of Antibodies.* Cambridge, Mass.: Harvard University Press, 1973.

Stewart, John. *The Primordial VRM System and the Evolution of Vertebrate Immunity.* Austin, Tex.: R. G. Landes, 1994.

Theofilopoulos, A. N., ed. *Genes and Genetics of Autoimmunity.* New York: Karger, 1999.

Tizard, Ian R. *Immunology: An Introduction.* 2d ed. New York: W. B. Saunders, 1988.

MOLECULAR GENETICS

Adolph, Kenneth W., ed. *Gene and Chromosome Analysis.* San Diego: Academic Press, 1993.

_____. *Human Molecular Genetics.* San Diego: Academic Press, 1996.

Alberts, Bruce, Dennis Bray, Julian Lewis, Martin Raff, Keith Roberts, and James D. Watson. *Molecular Biology of the Cell.* 4th ed. New York: Garland, 2002.

Ausubel, Fredrick, Roger Brent, Robert Kingston, David Moore, J. Seidman, and K. Struhl. *Current Protocols in Molecular Biology.* Hoboken, N.J.: John Wiley & Sons, 1998.

Baltimore, David, ed. *Nobel Lectures in Molecular Biology, 1933-1975.* New York: Elsevier North-Holland, 1977.

Barry, John Michael, and E. M. Barry. *Molecular Biology: An Introduction to Chemical Genetics.* Englewood Cliffs, N.J.: Prentice-Hall, 1973.

Benjamin, Jonathan, Richard P. Ebstein, and Robert H. Belmaker, eds. *Molecular Genetics and the Human Personality.* Washington, D.C.: American Psychiatric Association, 2002.

Berul, Charles I., and Jeffrey A. Towbin, eds. *Molecular Genetics of Cardiac Electrophysiology.* Boston: Kluwer Academic, 2000.

Bishop, T., P. Sham, Pak Sham, and D. Timothy Bishop. *Analysis of Multifactorial Disease.* Oxford, England: BIOS, 2000.

Branden, Carl-Ivar, and John Tooze. *Introduction to Protein Structure.* 2d ed. New York: Garland, 1999.

Broach, J., J. Pringle, and E. Jones, eds. *The Molecular and Cellular Biology of the Yeast Saccharomyces.* 3 vols. Cold Spring Harbor, N.Y.: Cold Spring Harbor Laboratory Press, 1991-1997.

Brown, Terence A. *Genetics: A Molecular Approach.* 3d ed. New York: Chapman & Hall, 1998.

Browning, Michael, and Andrew McMichael, eds. *HLA and MHC: Genes, Molecules, and Function.* New York: Academic Press, 1999.

Capy, Pierre, et al. *Dynamics and Evolution of Transposable Elements.* New York: Chapman & Hall, 1998.

Cotterill, Sue, ed. *Eukaryotic DNA Replication: A Practical Approach.* New York: Oxford University Press, 1999.

Crick, Francis. *Life Itself: Its Origin and Nature.* New York: Simon & Schuster, 1981.

_____. *What Mad Pursuit.* New York: Basic Books, 1988.

DePamphilis, Melvin L., ed. *Concepts in Eukaryotic DNA Replication.* Cold Spring Harbor, N.Y.: Cold Spring Harbor Laboratory Press, 1999.

De Pomerai, David. *From Gene to Animal: An Introduction to the Molecular Biology of Animal Development.* New York: Cambridge University Press, 1985.

Dillon, Lawrence S. *The Gene: Its Structure, Function, and Evolution.* New York: Plenum Press, 1987.

Dizdaroglu, Miral, and Ali Esat Karakaya, eds. *Advances in DNA Damage and Repair: Oxygen Radical Effects, Cellular Protection, and Biological Consequences.* New York: Plenum Press, 1999.

Eckstein, Fritz, and David M. J. Lilley, eds. *Catalytic RNA.* New York: Springer, 1996.

Elgin, Sarah C. R., and Jerry L. Workman, eds. *Chromatin Structure and Gene Expression.* 2d ed. New York: Oxford University Press, 2000.

Erickson, Robert P., and Jonathan G. Izant, eds. *Gene Regulation: Biology of Antisense RNA and DNA.* New York: Raven Press, 1992.

Frank-Kamenetskii, Maxim D. *Unraveling DNA.* Reading, Mass.: Addison-Wesley, 1997.

Freedman, Leonard P., and M. Karin, eds. *Molecular Biology of Steroid and Nuclear Hormone Receptors.* Boston: Birkhauser, 1999.

Friedberg, Errol C., et al., eds. *DNA Repair and Mutagenesis.* Washington, D.C.: ASM Press, 1995.

Gomperts, Kramer, et al. *Signal Transduction.* San Diego, Calif.: Academic Press, 2002.

Gros, Franyois. *The Gene Civilization.* New York: McGraw-Hill, 1992.

Gwatkin, Ralph B. L., ed. *Genes in Mammalian Reproduction.* New York: Wiley-Liss, 1993.

Hancock, John T. *Molecular Genetics.* Boston: Butterworth-Heinemann, 1999.

Harris, David A., ed. *Prions: Molecular and Cellular Biology.* Portland, Oreg.: Horizon Scientific Press, 1999.

Hatch, Randolph T., ed. *Expression Systems and Processes for rDNA Products.* Washington, D.C.: American Chemical Society, 1991.

Hatfull, Graham F., and William R. Jacobs, Jr., eds. *Molecular Genetics of Mycobacteria.* Washington, D.C.: ASM Press, 2000.

Hawkins, John D. *Gene Structure and Expression.* New York: Cambridge University Press, 1996.

Hekimi, Siegfried, ed. *The Molecular Genetics of Aging.* New York: Springer, 2000.

Henderson, Daryl S., ed. *DNA Repair Protocols: Eukaryotic Systems.* Totowa, N.J.: Humana Press, 1999.

Hoch, James A., and Thomas J. Silhavy, eds. *TwoComponent Signal Transduction.* Washington, D.C.: ASM Press, 1995.

Holmes, Roger S., and Hwa A. Lim, eds. *Gene Families: Structure, Function, Genetics and Evolution.* River Edge, N.J.: World Scientific, 1996.

Joklik, Wolfgang K., ed. *Microbiology: A Centenary Perspective.* Washington, D.C.: ASM Press, 1999.

Kimura, Motoo, and Naoyuki Takahata, eds. *New Aspects of the Genetics of Molecular Evolution.* New York: Springer-Verlag, 1991.

Langridge, John. *Molecular Genetics and Comparative Evolution.* New York: John Wiley & Sons, 1991.

Lewin, Benjamin M. *Gene Expression.* New York: John Wiley & Sons, 1980.

Litvack, Simon. *Retroviral Reverse Transcriptases.* Austin, Tex.: R. G. Landes, 1996.

McDonald, John F., ed. *Transposable Elements and Genome Evolution.* London: Kluwer Academic, 2000.

McGuffin, Peter, Michael J. Owen, and Irving I. Gottesman, eds. *Psychiatric Genetics and Genomics.* Oxford, England: Oxford University Press, 2002.

MacIntyre, Ross J., ed. *Molecular Evolutionary Genetics.* New York: Plenum Press, 1985.

Maraia, Richard J., ed. *The Impact of Short Interspersed Elements (SINEs) on the Host Genome.* Austin, Tex.: R. G. Landes, 1995.

Miesfeld, Roger L. *Applied Molecular Genetics.* New York: John Wiley, 1999.

Muller-Hill, Benno. *The Lac Operon: A Short History of a Genetic Paradigm.* New York: Walter de Gruyter, 1996.

Murphy, Kenneth P. *Protein Structure, Stability, and Folding.* Totowa, N.J.: Humana Press, 2001.

Murray, James A. H., ed. *Antisense RNA and DNA.* New York: Wiley-Liss, 1992.

Nei, Masatoshi. *Molecular Evolutionary Genetics.* New York: Columbia University Press, 1987.

Pasternak, Jack J. *An Introduction to Human Molecular Genetics: Mechanisms ofInherited Diseases.* Hoboken, N.J.: Wiley, 2005.

Pfeifer, John D., ed., with Daniel A. Arber et al. *Molecular Genetic Testing in Surgical Pathology.* Philadelphia: Lippincott, Williams & Wilkins, 2006.

Pollack, Robert. *Signs of Life: The Language and Meanings of DNA.* New York: Houghton Mifflin, 1994.

Ptashne, Mark, and Alexander Gann. *Genes and Signals.* Cold Spring Harbor, N.Y.: Cold Spring Harbor Press, 2002.

Roe, Bruce A., Judy S. Crabtree, and Akbar S. Khan, eds. *DNA Isolation and Sequencing.* New York: John Wiley & Sons, 1996.

Sarma, Ramaswamy H., and M. H. Sarma. *DNA Double Helix and the Chemistry of Cancer.* Schenectady, N.Y.: Adenine Press, 1988.

Schleif, Robert F. *Genetics and Molecular Biology.* Reading, Mass.: Addison-Wesley, 1986.

Selander, Robert K., et al., eds. *Evolution at the Molecular Level.* Sunderland, Mass.: Sinauer Associates, 1991.

Simons, Robert W., and Marianne GrunbergManago, eds. *RNA Structure and Function.* Cold Spring Harbor, N.Y.: Cold Spring Harbor Laboratory Press, 1997.

Smith, Paul J., and Christopher J. Jones, eds. *DNA Recombination and Repair.* New York: Oxford University Press, 2000.

Smith, Thomas B., and Robert K. Wayne. *Molecular Genetic Approaches in Conservation.* New York: Oxford University Press, 1996.

Snyder, Larry, and Wendy Champness. *Molecular Genetics of Bacteria.* Washington, D.C.: ASM Press, 1997.

Stone, Edwin M., and Robert J. Schwartz. *Intervening Sequences in Evolution and Development.* New York: Oxford University Press, 1990.

Strachan, Tom, and Andrew P. Read. *Human Molecular Genetics.* 2d ed. New York: Garland Press, 2004.

Trainor, Lynn E. H. *The Triplet Genetic Code: The Key to Molecular Biology*. River Edge, N.J.: World Scientific, 2001.

Turner, Bryan. *Chromatin and Gene Regulation: Mechanisms in Epigenetics*. Malden, Mass.: Blackwell, 2001.

Watson, James D. *The Double Helix*. New York: Atheneum, 1968.

_____, et al. *Molecular Biology of the Gene*. 5th ed. 2 vols. Menlo Park, Calif.: Benjamin Cummings, 2003.

Weaver, Robert F. *Molecular Biology*. 2d ed. New York: McGraw-Hill, 2002.

White, Robert J. *Gene Transcription: Mechanisms and Control*. Malden, Mass.: Blackwell, 2001.

POPULATION GENETICS

Avise, John, and James Hamrick, eds. *Conservation Genetics: Case Histories from Nature*. New York: Chapman and Hall, 1996.

Ayala, Francisco J. *Population and Evolutionary Genetics: A Primer*. Menlo Park, Calif.: Benjamin/Cummings, 1982.

Boorman, Scott A., and Paul R. Levitt. *The Genetics of Altruism*. New York: Academic Press, 1980.

Bushman, Frederick. *Lateral Gene Transfer: Mechanisms and Consequences*. Cold Spring Harbor, N.Y: Cold Spring Harbor Laboratory Press, 2001.

Charlesworth, Brian. *Evolution in Age-Structured Populations*. New York: Cambridge University Press, 1980.

Christiansen, Freddy B. *Population Genetics of Multiple Loci*. New York: Wiley, 2000.

Conner, Jeffrey K., and Daniel L. Hartl. *A Primer of Ecological Genetics*. Sunderland, Mass.: Sinauer Associates, 2004.

Costantino, Robert F., and Robert A. Desharnais. *Population Dynamics and the Tribolium Model: Genetics and Demography*. New York: Springer-Verlag, 1991.

Crow, James F. *Basic Concepts in Population, Quantitative, and Evolutionary Genetics*. New York: W. H. Freeman, 1986.

Dawson, Peter S., and Charles E. King, eds. *Readings in Population Biology*. Englewood Cliffs, N.J.: Prentice-Hall, 1971.

De Waal, Franz. *Good Natured: The Origins of Right and Wrong in Humans and Other Animals*. Cambridge, Mass.: Harvard University Press, 1996.

Falconer, D. S., and Trudy F. MacKay. *Introduction to Quantitative Genetics*. 4th ed. Reading, Mass.: Addison-Wesley, 1996.

Gale, J. S. *Population Genetics*. New York: John Wiley & Sons, 1980.

Gavrilets, Sergey. *Fitness Landscapes and the Origin of Species*. Princeton, N.J.: Princeton University Press, 2004.

Gillespie, John H. *Population Genetics: A Concise Guide*. Baltimore: Johns Hopkins University Press, 2004.

Gould, Steven Jay. *Ontogeny and Phylogeny*. Cambridge, Mass.: Belknap Press, 1977.

Halliburton, Richard. *Introduction to Population Genetics*. Upper Saddle River, N.J.: Pearson/Prentice Hall, 2004.

Harper, J. L. *Population Biology of Plants*. New York: Academic Press, 1977.

Hartl, Daniel L. *A Primer of Population Genetics*. Rev. 3d ed. Sunderland, Mass.: Sinauer Associates, 2000.

Hartl, Daniel L., and Andrew G. Clark. *Principles of Population Genetics*. Sunderland, Mass.: Sinauer Associates, 2007.

Hedrick, Philip W. *Genetics of Populations*. 3d ed. Boston: Jones and Bartlett, 2005.

Hoelzel, A. R., ed. *Molecular Genetic Analysis of Populations: A Practical Approach*. New York: IRL Press at Oxford University Press, 1992.

Kang, Manjit S., and Hugh G. Gauch, Jr. *Genotype-byEnvironment Interaction*. Boca Raton, Fla.: CRC Press, 1996.

Kingsland, S. E. *Modeling Nature: Episodes in the History of Population Ecology*. Chicago: University of Chicago Press, 1985.

Lack, D. *The Natural Regulation of Animal Numbers*. Oxford, England: Clarendon Press, 1954.

Laikre, Linda. *Genetic Processes in Small Populations: Conservation and Management Considerations with Particular Focus on Inbreeding and Its Effects*. Stockholm: Division of Population Genetics, Stockholm University, 1996.

Lynch, Michael. *The Origins of Genome Architecture*. Sunderland, Mass.: Sinauer Associates, 2007.

Lynn, Richard. *Dysgenics: Genetic Deterioration in Modern Populations*. Westport, Conn.: Praeger, 1996.

McKinney, M. L., and K. J. McNamara. *Heterochrony: The Evolution of Ontogeny*. New York: Plenum Press, 1991.

Magurran, Anne E., and Robert M. May, eds. *Evolution of Biological Diversity: From Population Differentiation to Speciation*. New York: Oxford University Press, 1999.

Papiha, Surinder S., Ranjan Deka, and Ranajit Chakraborty, eds. *Genomic Diversity: Applications in*

Human Population Genetics. New York: Kluwer Academic/Plenum, 1999.

Provine, William B. *The Origins of Theoretical Population Genetics.* 2d ed. Chicago: University of Chicago Press, 2001.

Real, Leslie A., ed. *Ecological Genetics.* Princeton, N.J.: Princeton University Press, 1994.

Rousset, Franyois. *Genetic Structure and Selection in Subdivided Populations.* Princeton, N.J.: Princeton University Press, 2004.

Ruse, M. *Sociobiology: Sense or Nonsense?* Boston: D. Riedel, 1979.

Schmitt, L. H., Leonard Freedman, and Rayma Pervan. *Genes, Ethnicity, and Ageing.* Nedlands: Centre for Human Biology, University of Western Australia, 1995.

Schonewald-Cox, Christine M., et al., eds. *Genetics and Conservation: A Reference for Managing Wild Animal and Plant Populations.* Menlo Park, Calif.: Benjamin/Cummings, 1983.

Slatkin, Montgomery, and Michel Veuille, eds. *Modern Developments in Theoretical Population Genetics: The Legacy of Gustave Malecot.* New York: Oxford University Press, 2002.

Syvanen, Michael, and Clarence Kado. *Horizontal Gene Transfer.* 2d ed. Burlington, Mass.: Academic Press, 2002.

Templeton, Alan R. *Population Genetics and Microevolutionary Theory.* Hoboken, N.J.: Wiley-Liss, 2006.

Thornhill, Nancy Wilmsen, ed. *The Natural History of Inbreeding and Outbreeding: Theoretical and Empirical Perspectives.* Chicago: University of Chicago Press, 1993.

Wilson, E. O. *Sociobiology: The New Synthesis.* Cambridge, Mass.: Belknap Press, 1975.

REPRODUCTIVE TECHNOLOGY

Andrews, Lori B. *The Clone Age: Adventures in the New World of Reproductive Technology.* New York: Henry Holt, 1999.

Bentley, Gillian R., and C. G. Nicholas Mascie-Taylor. *Infertility in the Modern World: Present and Future Prospects.* New York: Cambridge University Press, 2000.

Bonnicksen, Andrea L. *In Vitro Fertilization: Building Policy from Laboratories to Legislature.* Reprint. New York: Columbia University Press, 1991.

Brinsden, Peter R., ed. *A Textbook of In Vitro Fertilization and Assisted Reproduction: The Bourn Hall Guide to Clinical and Laboratory Practice.* 2d ed. New York: Parthenon, 1999.

Campbell, Annily. *Childfree and Sterilized: Women'sDecisions and Medical Responses.* New York: Cassell, 1999.

Elder, Kay, and Brian Dale. *In Vitro Fertilization.* 2d ed. New York: Cambridge University Press, 2000.

Ettore, Elizabeth. *Reproductive Genetics, Gender, and the Body.* New York: Routledge, 2002.

Heyman, Bob, and Mette Henriksen. *Risk, Age, and Pregnancy: Case Study of Prenatal Genetic Screening and Testing.* New York: Palgrave, 2001.

Jansen, Robert, and D. Mortimer, eds. *Towards Reproductive Certainty: Fertility and Genetics Beyond 1999.* Boca Raton, Fla.: CRC Press, 1999.

McElreavey, Ken, ed. *The Genetic Basis of Male Infertility.* New York: Springer, 2000.

McGee, Glenn. *The Perfect Baby: A Pragmatic Approach to Genetics.* Lanham, Md.: Rowman & Littlefield, 1997.

Mader, Sylvia S. *Human Reproductive Biology.* 3d ed. New York: McGraw-Hill, 2000.

Marrs, Richard, et al. *Dr. Richard Marrs'Fertility Book.* New York: Dell, 1997.

Parry, Vivienne. *Antenatal Testing Handbook: The Complete Guide to Testing in Pregnancy.* Collingdale, Pa.: DIANE, 1998.

Rapp, Rayna. *Testing Women, Testing the Fetus: The Social Impact of Amniocentesis in America.* New York: Routledge, 1999.

Rosenthal, M. Sara. *The Fertility Sourcebook: Everything You Need to Know.* 2d ed. Los Angeles: Lowell House, 1998.

Rothman, Barbara Katz. *The Tentative Pregnancy: How Amniocentesis Changes the Experience ofMotherhood.* Rev. ed. New York: Norton, 1993.

Seibel, Machelle M., and Susan L. Crockin, eds. *Family Building Through Egg and Sperm Donation.* Boston: Jones and Bartlett, 1996.

Trounson, Alan O., and David K. Gardner, eds. *Handbook of In Vitro Fertilization.* 2d ed. Boca Raton, Fla.: CRC Press, 2000.

TECHNIQUES AND METHODOLOGIES. *See also* **BIOINFORMATICS**

Adolph, Kenneth W., ed. *Gene and Chromosome Analysis.* San Diego: Academic Press, 1993.

Braman, Jeff, ed. *In Vitro Mutagenesis Protocols.* 2d ed. Totowa, N.J.: Humana Press, 2002.

Budowle, Bruce, et al. *DNA Typing Protocols: Molecular Biology and Forensic Analysis.* Natick, Mass.: Eaton, 2000.

Butler, John M. *Forensic DNA Typing: Biology, Technology, and Genetics of STR Markers.* Amsterdam: Elsevier Academic Press, 2005.

Chen, Bing-Yuan, and Harry W. Janes, eds. *PCR Cloning Protocols.* Rev. 2d ed. Totowa, N.J.: Humana Press, 2002.

Crawley, Jacqueline N. *What's Wrong with My Mouse? Behavioral Phenotyping of Transgenic and Knockout Mice.* New York: Wiley-Liss, 2000.

Davis, Rowland H. *Neurospora: Contributions of a Model Organism.* New York: Oxford University Press, 2000.

Double, John A., and Michael J. Thompson, eds. *Telomeres and Telomerase: Methods and Protocols.* Totowa, N.J.: Humana Press, 2002.

Farrell, Robert. *RNA Methodologies.* 2d ed. San Diego, Calif.: Academic Press, 1998.

Gjerde, Douglas T., Christopher P. Hanna, and David Hornby. *DNA Chromatography.* Weinheim, Germany: Wiley-VCH, 2002.

Grange, J. M., et al., eds. *Genetic Manipulation: Techniques and Applications.* Boston: Blackwell Scientific, 1991.

Guilfoile, P. *A Photographic Atlas for the Molecular Biology Laboratory.* Englewood, Colo.: Morton, 2000.

Hall, Walter A., ed. *Methods in Molecular Biology: Immunotoxin Methods and Protocols.* Vol. 166. Totowa, N.J.: Humana Press, 2000.

Hames, B. D., and D. Rickwood, eds. *Gel Electrophoresis of Nucleic Acids: A Practical Approach.* 2d ed. New York: Oxford University Press, 1990.

Harlow, Ed, and David Lane, eds. *Using Antibodies: A Laboratory Manual.* Rev. ed. Cold Spring Harbor, N.Y.: Cold Spring Harbor Laboratory Press, 1999.

Jackson, J. F., H. F. Linskens, and R. B. Inman, eds. *Testing for Genetic Manipulation in Plants.* New York: Springer, 2002.

Kochanowski, Bernd, and Udo Reischl, eds. *Quantitative PCR Protocols.* Methods in Molecular Medicine 26. Totowa, N.J.: Humana Press, 1999.

Lai, Eric, and Bruce W. Birren, eds. *Electrophoresis of Large DNA Molecules: Theory and Applications.* Cold Spring Harbor, N.Y.: Cold Spring Harbor Laboratory, 1990.

Lewis, Ricki. *Human GGenetics: Concepts and Applications.* Boston: McGraw-Hill Higher Education, 2007.

Lloyd, Ricardo V., ed. *Morphology Methods: Cell and Molecular Biology Techniques.* Totowa, N.J.: Humana Press, 2001.

McPherson, M. J., and S. G. M0ller. *PCR Basics.* Oxford, England: BIOS Scientific, 2000.

McRee, Duncan Everett. *Practical Protein Crystallography.* 2d ed. San Diego: Academic Press, 1999.

O'Connell, Joe, ed. *RT-PCR Protocols.* Totowa, N.J.: Humana Press, 2002.

Pacifici, O. G. M., Julio Collado-Vides, and Ralf Hofestadt, eds. *Gene Regulation and Metabolism: Postgenomic Computational Approaches.* Cambridge, Mass.: MIT Press, 2002.

Perlmann, P., and H. Wigzell, eds. *Handbook of Experimental Pharmacology.* Heidelberg: Springer, 1999.

Pretlow, T. G., and T. P. Pretlow, eds. *Biochemical and Molecular Aspects of Selected Cancers.* Vol. 1. San Diego: Academic Press, 1991.

Sandor, Suhai, ed. *Theoretical and Computational Methods in Genome Research.* New York: Plenum Press, 1997.

Silver, Lee. *Mouse Genetics: Concepts and Applications.* New York: Oxford University Press, 1995.

Suzuki, D. T., et al. *An Introduction to Genetic Analysis.* 7th ed. New York: W. H. Freeman, 2000.

Wilson, Zoe A. *Arabidopsis: A Practical Approach.* New York: Oxford University Press, 2000.

VIRAL GENETICS

Becker, Yechiel, and Gholamreza Darai, eds. *Molecular Evolution of Viruses: Past and Present.* Boston: Kluwer Academic, 2000.

Cann, Alan J. *DNA Virus Replication.* New York: Oxford University Press, 2000.

Carlberg, David M. *Essentials of Bacterial and Viral Genetics.* Springfield, Ill.: Charles C Thomas, 1976.

Domingo, Esteban, Robert Webster, and John Holland, eds. *Origin and Evolution of Viruses.* New York: Academic Press, 1999.

Gallo, Robert C., and Flossie Wong-Staal, eds. *Retrovirus Biology and Human Disease.* New York: Marcel Dekker, 1990.

Holland, J. J., ed. *Current Topics in Microbiology and Immunology: Genetic Diversity of RNA Viruses.* New York: Springer-Verlag, 1992.

Kolata, Gina. *The Story of the Great Influenza Pandemic of 1918 and the Search for the Virus That Caused It.* New York: Simon and Schuster, 2001.

World Health Organization. *Future Research on Smallpox Virus Recommended.* Geneva, Switzerland: World Health Organization Press, 1999.

Updated by Oladayo Oyelola, Ph.D, S.C. (ASCP)

WEB SITES

Because URLs frequently change or are moved, their accuracy cannot be guaranteed; however, long-standing sites—such as those of university departments, national organizations, and government agencies—generally maintain links when sites move or otherwise may upgrade their offerings and hence remain useful.

GENERAL GENETICS

https://rarediseases.info.nih.gov/diseases/6866/
bardet-biedl-syndrome
https://ghr.nlm.nih.gov/condition/bardet-biedl-
syndrome
http://www.medscape.com/viewarticle/479108_3
https://rarediseases.org/rare-diseases/bardet-
biedl-syndrome/

Children Living with Inherited Metabolic Diseases (CLIMB)
http://www.climb.org.uk
FOD (Fatty Oxidation Disorder) Family Support Group
http://www.fodsupport.org
Genetic and Rare Diseases Information Center
https://rarediseases.info.nih.gov/diseases
Genetics Home Reference
https://ghr.nlm.nih.gov/condition
MitoAction
http://www.mitoaction.org
OMIM® - Online Mendelian Inheritance in Man
http://www.omim.org/about

https://rarediseases.info.nih.gov/diseases/5899/
congenital-contractural-arachnodactyly
https://www.ncbi.nlm.nih.gov/books/NBK1386/
https://ghr.nlm.nih.gov/condition/congenital-
contractural-arachnodactyly
https://ghr.nlm.nih.gov/gene/FBN2#
https://www.marfan.org/download/file/fid/154/
Beals%20Syndrome.pdf

https://www.ncbi.nlm.nih.gov/pubmed/26276910
http://emedicine.medscape.com/article/
426003-overview
http://www.childrenshospital.org/conditions-
and-treatments/conditions/t/tracheomalacia/
testing-and-diagnosis
http://www.ashg.org/2009meeting/abstracts/full-
text/f10691.htm

Costello Syndrome Family Network
http://www.costellosyndromeusa.org/

Genetic and Rare Diseases Information Center
https://rarediseases.info.nih.gov/diseases
Genetics Home Reference
https://ghr.nlm.nih.gov/condition
International Costello Syndrome Support Group
http://www.costellokids.com
RASopathies Network U.S.A.
https://rasopathiesnet.org/

https://ghr.nlm.nih.gov/condition/
ehlers-danlos-syndrome
https://rarediseases.info.nih.gov/diseases/2088/
ehlers-danlos-syndrome-classic-type
http://emedicine.medscape.com/
article/943567-overview

Dysautonomia Foundation, Inc.
http://www.familialdysautonomia.org
Dysautonomia Youth Network of America, Inc.
http://www.dynakids.org
Dysautonomia, Familial
http://www.fdhope.org
Genetic and Rare Diseases Information Center
https://rarediseases.info.nih.gov/diseases
Genetics Home Reference
https://ghr.nlm.nih.gov/condition

Genetic and Rare Diseases Information Center
https://rarediseases.info.nih.gov/diseases
Genetic Disease Foundation
http://www.geneticdiseasefoundation.org/
genetic-diseases/
Genetics Home Reference
https://ghr.nlm.nih.gov/condition
Inspire
https://www.inspire.com/conditions/
familial-hyperinsulinism
Jewish Genetic Diseases
http://www.mazornet.com/genetics/familial_hyper-
insulinism.htm
OMIM® - Online Mendelian Inheritance in Man
http://www.omim.org/about

Center for Jewish Genetics
https://www.jewishgenetics.org/
European Network for Rare and Congenital Anaemias (ENERCA)
http://www.enerca.org
Fanconi Anemia Research Fund, Inc (FARF)
http://www.fanconi.org
Genetics Home Reference
https://ghr.nlm.nih.gov/condition
Gene Reviews
https://www.ncbi.nlm.nih.gov/books/NBK1116/
Jewish Genetic Disease Consortium (JGDC)
http://www.JewishGeneticDiseases.org
Deanna M. Neff, M.P.H.

https://rarediseases.info.nih.gov/diseases/6506/
gigantism
http://emedicine.medscape.com/
article/925446-overview
https://medlineplus.gov/ency/article/001174.htm

http://www.orpha.net/consor/cgi-bin/OC_Exp.
php?lng=EN&Expert=36412
http://emedicine.medscape.com/
article/1085087-overview
https://ghr.nlm.nih.gov/gene/DNASE1L3

https://ghr.nlm.nih.gov/condition/
jackson-weiss-syndrome
https://rarediseases.info.nih.gov/diseases/6796/
jackson-weiss-syndrome
https://rarediseases.org/rare-diseases/
jackson-weiss-syndrome/
https://rarediseases.info.nih.gov/diseases/6796/
jackson-weiss-syndrome
https://www.omim.org/entry/123150
https://www.orpha.net/data/patho/GB/uk-Jack-
son-WeissSyndrome2005.pdf
https://www.ncbi.nlm.nih.gov/gtr/conditions/
C0795998/
http://www.wohproject.org/disorders/
jackson-weisssyndrome/

https://rarediseases.info.nih.gov/diseases/6855/
landau-kleffner-syndrome
http://emedicine.medscape.com/
article/1176568-overview
https://ghr.nlm.nih.gov/gene/GRIN2A

https://www.ninds.nih.gov/
Disorders/All-Disorders/
Landau-Kleffner-Syndrome-Information-Page

Climb (Children Living with Inherited Metabolic Diseases)
fam.svcs@climb.org.uk
Genetic Disease Foundation
http://www.knowyourgenes.org/genetic-testing.
shtml
MSUD Family Support Group
http://www.msud-support.org
OMIM® - Online Mendelian Inheritance in Man
http://www.omim.org/about
Orphanet Journal of Rare Diseases
https://ojrd.biomedcentral.com/

https://ghr.nlm.nih.gov/condition/
moyamoya-disease
https://rarediseases.info.nih.gov/diseases/7064/
moyamoya-disease
http://emedicine.medscape.com/
article/1180952-overview

Center for Jewish Genetics
www.jewishgenetics.org
Genetic and Rare Diseases Information Center
https://rarediseases.info.nih.gov/diseases
Genetics Home Reference
https://ghr.nlm.nih.gov/condition
Mucolipidosis Type IV Foundation, Inc.
http://www.ML4.org
My46 Trait Profile
www.mpssociety.org

https://rarediseases.info.nih.gov/diseases/7380/
pfeiffer-syndrome
https://ghr.nlm.nih.gov/condition/
pfeiffer-syndrome
https://www.ncbi.nlm.nih.gov/books/NBK1455/
https://www.ncbi.nlm.nih.gov/pmc/articles/
PMC1051023/

https://rarediseases.info.nih.gov/diseases/4347/
pierre-robin-syndrome
https://ghr.nlm.nih.gov/condition/
isolated-pierre-robin-sequence
https://rarediseases.org/rare-diseases/
pierre-robin-sequence/

https://ghr.nlm.nih.gov/gene/SOX9#conditions
http://emedicine.medscape.com/
    article/844143-overview
http://emedicine.medscape.com/
    article/995706-overview
http://www.orpha.net/consor/cgi-bin/OC_Exp.
    php?Lng=GB&Expert=718

Cure CMD - Congenital Muscular Dystrophy
http://curecmd.org/
Muscular Dystrophy Association (MDA)
http://www.mdausa.org/
Muscular Dystrophy Family Foundation
http://www.mdff.org
OMIM® - Online Mendelian Inheritance in Man
http://www.omim.org/about

Canadian Immunodeficiencies Patient Organization
    (CIPO)
http://cipo.ca
Genetic and Rare Diseases Information Center
https://rarediseases.info.nih.gov/diseases
Immune Deficiency Foundationhttp://www.prima-
    ryimmune.org/
Jeffrey Modell Foundation/National Primary Immu-
    nodeficiency Resource Center
http://www.info4pi.org/
National Primary Immunodeficiency Resource Center
http://www.info4pi.org
United States Immunodeficiency Network (USIDNET)
http://www.usidnet.org

https://rarediseases.info.nih.gov/diseases/7371/x-
    linked-periventricular-heterotopia
https://www.ncbi.nlm.nih.gov/books/NBK1213/
https://ghr.nlm.nih.gov/condition/
    periventricular-heterotopia#genes
https://www.omim.org/entry/300049

*Dolan DNA Learning Center, Cold Spring Harbor
    Laboratory*
Gene Almanac
http://www.dnalc.org

This is the best entry point to the Web for new-comers to genetics. An online science center devoted to public education in genetics at high school and college levels, this site provides information on DNA science, genetics and medicine, and biotechnology

through interactive features, animated tutorials, downloads, and extensive links.

*Emory University and the University of Alabama at
    Birmingham*
Ask the Geneticist
http://www.askthegen.org

This site provides answers to site visitors' questions about genetic concepts and genetic disorders. Selected questions and answers are posted within three weeks after submission and are archived in a searchable database. Genetics fact sheets and other general information are also posted.

Genetic Science Learning Center, The University of Utah
Learn.Genetics
http://learn.genetics.utah.edu

A repository of educational resources on genetics, bioscience, and health topics for students, teachers, and the public. Information about DNA, genetic disorders, cloning, stem cells, gene therapy, and genetic testing is presented through articles, animations, and interactive features. The site also describes simple experiments via a virtual lab. Comprehensive teacher resources, professional development programs, and lesson plans are available on the subsite Teach. Genetics (http://teach.genetics .utah.edu).

Genetics Society of America
Home Page
http://www.genetics-gsa.org

Although dedicated to subscribers who are professional geneticists, scientists, teachers, and engineers, this Web site supports genetics education for all ages and offers a history of the organization and short position statements on evolution and genetically modified organisms. There are also links to databases and related Web sites.

Johns Hopkins University
Genetics and Public Policy Center
http://www.dnapolicy.org

This site provides information and analysis of human genetics public policy. The site includes articles about genetics and health, genetic testing, assisted reproduction, cloning and stem cells, and genetic modification. It also provides a bibliography, reports, testimony, and statements from the Center and its staff. A video library and a searchable database of international laws are also provided.

Kimball's Biology Pages

Home Page

http://biology-pages.info

A reliable place to start for those new to genetics, this online biology textbook features clear, well-illustrated explanations of topics in biology by university professor John W. Kimball, including all aspects of genetics and biotechnology, with news updates.

MedBioWorld

Home Page

http://www.medbioworld.com

A portal providing links to several databases for medical and biotechnology professionals. Site features include Reuters Health News Explorer article database, MedBio Access full-access scholarly research collections, links to journals ranked by Thomson Scientifics' Journal Citation Reports (JCR), and the Post Genomics Blog that includes information about upcoming conferences and meetings, funding resources, and research tools. Also features job postings and links to national health observances.

National Public Radio, SoundVision Productions

The DNA Files

http://www.dnafiles.org

This Web site features radio documentaries and in-depth features that provide an informal education for nonscientists about the genomics revolution, including the science of genetics and its ethical, social, and legal implications. The third series of the Peabody Award-winning audio programs from 2007 features topics including the human genome, DNA and behavior, DNA and evolution, genetics and ecology, gene therapy, genetic medicine, biotechnology, predictive genetic testing, and more.

Nature Publishing Group

genetics@nature.com

http://www.nature.com/genetics

Part of the Web site for Nature, Britain's premier science journal. Written for educated general readers, the sections offer news and recently published articles, commentary, and an encyclopedia of life sciences. There are links to specialty journals concerning topics in genetics and biotechnology. Some articles are accessible by the public, but full use of the site requires a subscription.

Netspace

MendelWeb

http://www.mendelweb.org

An educational site for teachers and students about the origins of classical genetics, introductory data analysis, elementary plant science, and the history and literature of science. It reproduces early publications by such pioneers as Gregor Mendel and William Bateson, accompanied by commentaries and reference resources.

Rutgers University

Morgan

http://morgan.rutgers.edu/MorganWebFrames/How_to_use/HTU_intro.html

A multimedia tutorial for advanced high school students or beginning college students. Its six levels review basic principles in genetics, with particular attention to molecular interactions.

University of Massachusetts

DNA Structure

http://molvis.sdsc.edu/dna/index.htm

An interactive, animated tutorial on the molecular composition and structure of DNA for high school students and undergraduates. It can be downloaded and is available in Spanish, German, French, and Portuguese.

U.S. Department of Energy

Gene Gateway

http://genomics.energy.gov/genegateway

This Web site introduces various Internet tools that anyone can use to investigate genetic disorders, chromosomes, genome maps, genes, sequence data, genetic variants, and molecular structures. The downloadable Gene Gateway Workbook features a collection of guides and tutorials to help students and other novice users get started with some of the publicly available genetics resources.

U.S. Department of Energy Office of Science

Virtual Library on Genetics

http://www.ornl.gov/TechResources/Human_Genome/genetics.html

A comprehensive catalog of Web site links, arranged by subject, pertaining to the Human Genome Project. The links lead to gene and chromosome databases and specific information on genetics, bioinformatics, and genetic disorders.

BIOINFORMATICS

Bioinformatics Organization
Home Page
http://www.bioinformatics.org

This international organization's site is dedicated to the exchange of genetic information, serving the scientific and educational needs of bioinformatic practitioners and the public. The organization has about 25,000 members and more than three hundred projects. Membership is free to the public and is fee-based for professionals, with additional discounts and services offered. It includes free online databases and analysis tools, group hosting services, software, professional bioinformatics education, forums, and a newsletter. Fee-based data analysis and software development services are provided through the organization's Bioinformatics Core Facility.

European Bioinformatics Institute
The Path to Knowledge
http://www.ebi.ac.uk

A bioinformatics research center, this institute maintains databases concerning nucleic acids, protein sequences, and macromolecular structures. Also posts downloadable fact sheets, archived publications, news, events, training opportunities, and descriptions of ongoing scientific projects.

Technical University of Denmark DTU
Center for Biological Sequence Analysis
http://www.cbs.dtu.dk

The center conducts basic research in bioinformatics and systems biology. The site, primarily for researchers and university students, offers sequencing data sets, prediction servers, software, bioinformatics tools, information about its research groups and education programs, events, and news.

BIOTECHNOLOGY

Bio-Link
Educating the Biotechnology Workforce
http://bio-link.org

Intended for technicians, this site offers information and instruction covering recent advances in biotechnology, as well as a virtual laboratory and library, news, discussion forums, job links, and internship postings. A U.S. map also links to directories of regional biotechnology education centers, organizations, and industries.

Biotechnology Industry Organization (BIO)
Home Page
http://bio.org

BIO provides advocacy, business development, and communications services for more than 1,200 international members involved in the research and development of health care, agricultural, industrial, and environmental biotechnology technologies. The site provides free access to articles on national, state, and local biotechnology issues with links to testimonies, statements, and fact sheets. Additional site features are provided to members.

Carolina Biological Supply Company
Biotechnology and Genetics
http://www.carolina.com/biotech

This supplier of biological, science, and math supplies and teaching materials provides a rich educational resource for elementary and high school teachers and students. Resources include classroom activities, articles, a newsletter, workshops, and videos, all focusing on the use of biotechnology and laboratory techniques.

Dow AgroSciences LLC
Plant Genetics and Biotechnology
http://www.dowagro.com

This corporate Web site concerns the marketing of its agricultural biotechnology. Given that bias, it contains news releases, descriptions of products, labels and safety data sheets, articles, publication links, and a media kit of interest to general readers.

The Hastings Center
Home Page
http://www.thehastingscenter.org

The Hastings Center is an independent, nonpartisan, and nonprofit bioethics research institute that addresses ethical issues in health, medicine, and the environment. Its site contains news postings, articles on bioethics and aspects of genetics science, research project overviews, and announcements of events and publications.

National Institutes of Health

National Center for Biotechnology Information
http://www.ncbi.nlm.nih.gov

This Web site for the main health agency of the United States contains links to the various specialized institutes under its umbrella as well as public databases in genomics and sequencing, articles and handbooks on a wide range of biotechnology topics, and more than a dozen types of free software for analyzing genetic data. Primarily intended for researchers, but also includes a comprehensive science primer and other resources for educators, students, and other nonspecialists.

GENOMICS

American Institute of Biological Sciences (AIBS)

ActionBioscience.org
http://www.actionbioscience.org/genomic

Includes a growing collection of articles by distinguished scientists, educators, and other writers on a wide range of biological subjects for K-12 and undergraduate educators, as well as students and the public. The site's genomics subsection features articles on genomic mapping, ethics, genetic information, genetic manipulation, and genomes.

BioMed Central Ltd.

Genome Biology
http://genomebiology.com

A print journal that serves as an international forum for the biological research community to aid the dissemination, discussion, and critical review of information. The journal articles are accessible online to subscribers, and a sampling of full-text articles is posted for public access, including select reviews, reports, and research.

Göteborg University, Sweden

RatMap, the Rat Genome Database
http://ratmap.gen.gu.se

A professional database of information on approximately six thousand rat genes, their positions on chromosomes, pertinent nomenclature, and gene functions.

Massachusetts Institute of Technology and Harvard University

The Broad Institute
http://www.broad.mit.edu/

Intended for scientists and university students, the site provides access to genomics research news, software, and sequencing databases. It also features press releases and news archives, organized by research areas. The Outreach section features programs and events to teach high school students and the public about genomics.

National Center for Biotechnology Information

Human Genome Resources
http://www.ncbi.nlm.nih.gov/genome/guide/human

An integrated, one-stop genomic resource for biomedical researchers who can use the site's search and analysis tools to find a gene's location in the genome, find other genes in the same region, correlate diseases to genes, determine if similar genes exist in other organisms, and view genetic variations.

National Center for Biotechnology Information

A New Gene Map of the Human Genome: The International RH Mapping Consortium http://www.ncbi.nlm.nih.gov/genemap99

An electronic data supplement for the Gene Map paper, published by P. Deloukas et al. in Science 282 (1998): 744-746.

National Human Genome Research Institute

Home Page
http://www.genome.gov

In addition to information for researchers and health professionals, this site contains public information including a comprehensive introduction to the Human Genome Project, a glossary of genetic terms, fact sheets, multimedia education kits, and links to online education resources.

PHG Foundation (Foundation for Genomics and Population Health)

Home Page
http://www.phgfoundation.org

This independent not-for-profit public health organization focuses on science and biomedical innovation to improve health, especially genome-based science and technologies. The foundation's Web site, with free registration, provides access to a database of policy literature, interactive educational resources, rapid responses to genetics news stories, full-text reports, key papers, and links.

Sanger Institute, Wellcome Trust
Home Page
http://www.sanger.ac.uk

This genomics research institute's site, targeted to scientists, offers news updates, a searchable database, explanations of gene sequencing and computer software aids, and descriptions of genomics research projects. There is also a section with resources for students, teachers, and the community, including a glossary of terms, links, and information about scheduling site visits or video conferences with Sanger Institute researchers.

U.S. Department of Energy Office of Science
Genomics.Energy.gov
http://genomics.energy.gov

This gateway provides links to several subsites of the DOE including Human Genome Project Information, the Genomic Science Program, and the Microbial Genome Program. Site features include a press room with image gallery, resources for educators, a genomics primer, and articles about biofuels, medicine and genetics, as well as ethical, legal, and social issues.

U.S. Department of Energy Office of Science
Genomic Science Program
http://genomicscience.energy.gov

This research program aims to provide sufficient scientific understanding of plants and microbes to develop new strategies to produce biofuels, clean up waste, or sequester carbon. The site provides research and technology summaries, as well as links to teaching tools for educators to provide instruction on genomics, systems biology, and microbes. Includes an image library.

U.S. Department of Energy Office of Science
Joint Genome Institute (JGI)
http://www.jgi.doe.gov

The JGI unites the expertise and resources in DNA sequencing, informatics, and technology development at five national laboratories, including Lawrence Berkeley, Lawrence Livermore, Los Alamos, Oak Ridge, and Pacific Northwest, along with the HudsonAlpha Institute for Biotechnology. Primarily for researchers, the site includes a Genomic Encyclopedia of Bacteria and Archaea, sequencing information and protocols, video links, news items and meeting notices, software tools, educational opportunities, current genome project lists, research group lists, and job postings.

U.S. Department of Energy Office of Science, Office of Biological and Environmental Research, Human Genome Program
Human Genome Project Information
http://www.ornl.gov/hgmis/home.shtml

A comprehensive site about the Human Genome Project, the international thirteen-year effort to discover all of the human genes and make them accessible for further study. Although the project concluded in 2003, data analyses continue, and the site provides project information, research archives, publication links, and information and article links about ethical, legal, and social issues; gene testing; gene therapy; genetic counseling; and pharmacogenomics. A section for young students and science teachers also is provided.

World Health Organization (WHO)
The Genomic Resource Centre
http://www.who.int/genomics/en

Provides information to raise awareness on human genetics and human genomics. The site provides an A-to-Z listing of health topics and WHO initiatives, as well as a repository of articles for patients, the public, health professionals, and policy makers.

MEDICINE AND GENETICS

American College of Medical Genetics
Home Page
http://www.acmg.net

Designed for physicians, this site contains some information for patients about medical genetics, selecting a geneticist, and genetic testing, along with news articles, practice guidelines, and reference materials.

Centers for Disease Control
Office of Public Health Genomics
http://www.cdc.gov/genomics/default.htm

Intended for the public, the site provides information about human genomic discoveries and how they can be used to improve health and prevent disease. It includes a glossary, frequently asked questions, fact sheets, news articles, student and teacher resources, and state activities. It also includes information about CDC public health activities for disease prevention. Available in Spanish.

Genetic Alliance, Inc.
Home Page
http://www.geneticalliance.org
A nonprofit coalition of advocacy, research, and health care organizations that represent millions of individuals with genetic conditions. The open network connects members of parent and family groups, community organizations, disease-specific advocacy organizations, professional societies, educational institutions, corporations, and government agencies.

National Center for Biotechnology Information
Online Mendelian Inheritance in Man
http://www.ncbi.nlm.nih.gov/sites/entrez?db=omim
This catalog of human genes and genetic disorders is intended for use by physicians, genetics researchers, and advanced science and medicine students. The site's full-text, referenced overviews contain information on all known hereditary disorders and more than 12,000 genes, focusing on the relationship between phenotype and genotype. It is updated daily, and the entries contain copious links to similar sites.

The National Fragile X Foundation
Home Page
http://www.nfxf.org
Provides extensive general information about fragile X syndrome, a cause of inherited mental impairments, and advises caregivers on testing, medical treatment, education, and life planning. With links to other resources.

National Organization for Rare Disorders (NORD)
Home Page
http://www.rarediseases.org
Offers a useful and long index of genetic disorders and diseases. The rare disease database links to fact sheets on more than 1,150 indexed conditions. The organizational database, searchable by topic, provides links to more than 2,000 resources and support organizations.

National Society of Genetic Counselors
Society Home Page
http://www.nsgc.org

Although much of this site is devoted to society members, it has a search engine for locating genetic counselors in the United States, general information about genetic testing, and a newsroom with press releases and fact sheets about genetic counseling.

The University of Nottingham
INTUTE: Health and Life Sciences
http://www.intute.ac.uk/healthandlifesciences/medicine
This gateway to health and life sciences information provides education and research resources that are evaluated and selected by a network of subject specialists.

University of Washington, Seattle, and National Center for Biotechnology Information
GeneTests
http://www.ncbi.nlm.nih.gov/sites/GeneTests/?db=GeneTests
This NIH-funded site provides reliable, up-to-date genetic counseling and testing information for physicians and researchers. The site includes educational materials; expert-authored, peer-reviewed disease descriptions; a voluntary directory of U.S. and international laboratories offering genetic testing; and a voluntary directory of clinics providing genetic evaluation and genetic counseling.

TRANSGENICS

National Academy of Sciences
Transgenic Plants and World Agriculture
http://www.nap.edu/openbook.php?record_id=9889
A downloadable report published in July, 2000, by an international consortium of leading research societies. It assesses the need to modify crops genetically in order to feed the increasing world population and then discusses examples of the technology, its safety, environmental effects, funding sources, and intellectual property issues.

Syngenta Foundation for Sustainable Agriculture
Home Page
http://www.syngentafoundation.org
The Foundation provides resources to small farmers in developing countries by extending science-based knowledge, facilitating access to quality inputs, and linking them to markets in profitable ways. The

site provides resource articles, press releases, project summaries, and stories.

University of Michigan
    Transgenic Animal Model Core
    http://www.med.umich.edu/tamc

A professional Web site for researchers seeking a host animal to test transgenes. However, it contains useful general information about transgenics (especially transgenic rats), vectors, and laboratory procedures. With links and a photo gallery.

Roger Smith, Ph.D.; updated by Angela Costello

Indexes

CATEGORY INDEX

BACTERIAL GENETICS

Anthrax, 80
Bacterial genetics and cell structure, 131
Bacterial resistance and super bacteria, 136
Gene regulation: Bacteria, 557
Gene regulation: *Lac* operon, 568
MLH1 gene, 928
Model organism: *Escherichia coli*, 476
Transposable elements

BIOETHICS

Bioethics: genetics, 160
Chorionic villus sampling, 268
Cloning: Ethical issues, 313
Gene therapy: Ethical and economic issues, 481
Genetic engineering: Risks, 598
Genetic testing: Ethical and economic issues, 484
Human genetics and insurance, 735
Insurance, 810
Miscegenation and antimiscegenation laws, 910
Patents on life-forms, 1060

BIOINFORMATICS

Bioinformatics, 166
cDNA libraries, 228
Genomic libraries, 621

Icelandic Genetic Database, 773
Microarray analysis, 998

CELLULAR BIOLOGY

Archaea, 98
Bacterial genetics and cell structure, 131
Cell culture: Animal cells, 234
Cell culture: Plant cells, 237
Cell cycle, 240
Cell division, 243
Chromosome mutation, 276
Chromosome structure, 279
Cytokinesis, 374
Extrachromosomal inheritance, 504
Gene regulation: Bacteria, 557
Gene regulation: Eukaryotes, 561
Gene regulation: *Lac* operon, 568
Gene regulation: Viruses, 564
Harvey *ras* oncogene, 657
Mitosis and meiosis, 925
Nondisjunction and aneuploidy, 1011
RNA interference, 1210–1212
Stem cells, 1320
Telomeres, 1309
Totipotency, 1317

CLASSICAL TRANSMISSION GENETICS

ABO blood group system, 4
BRCA1 and *BRCA2* genes, 196

Chromosome structure, 279
Chromosome theory of heredity, 284
Classical transmission genetics, 297
Congenital adrenal hyperplasiaand genetics, 330
Complete dominance, 327
Dihybrid inheritance, 404
Epistasis, 427
Incomplete dominance, 795
Mendelian genetics, 897
Monohybrid inheritance, 942
Multiple alleles, 952
Polygenic inheritance, 1100
SRY gene, 1282

DEVELOPMENTAL GENETICS

Developmental genetics, 387
Hermaphrodites, 696
Homeotic genes, 718
Model organism: *Danio rerio*, 379
Steroid hormones, 1289
Von Gierke disease, 1356
X chromosome inactivation, 1391

DISEASES AND SYNDROMES

Aarskog syndrome, 1
Abetalipoproteinemia, 2
Achondroplasia, 6
Adrenoleukodystrophy, 9
Adrenomyelopathy, 11
Agammaglobulinemia, 13
Alagille syndrome, 26

PERSONAGES INDEX

SUBJECT INDEX

A page number or range in boldface type indicates that an entire entry devoted to that topic appears in the set.